CORONARY COLLATERALS:

Clinical &

Experimental

Observations

Michael V. Cohen, M.D.

Associate Attending Physician
Montefiore Medical Center
Professor of Medicine
Albert Einstein College of Medicine
Bronx, New York

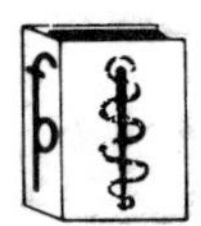

FUTURA PUBLISHING COMPANY, INC.
Mount Kisco, New York
1985

Library of Congress Cataloging-in-Publication Data

Cohen, Michael V. (Michael Victor), 1944–
    Coronary collaterals.

    Includes bibliographies and index.
      1. Coronary circulation.   2. Collateral circulation.
3. Coronary heart disease—Animal models.   I. Title.
[DNLM: 1. Collateral Circulation.   2. Coronary
Circulation.   WG 300 C6782c]
QP108.C65   1985   612'.17   85-70609
ISBN 0-87993-168-X

Published by
Futura Publishing Company, Inc.
295 Main Street, P. O. Box 330
Mount Kisco, New York 10549

L.C. no.: 85-70609
ISBN no.: 0-87993-168-x

to my mother and father,
Florence and Jules

PREFACE

Coronary collaterals have intrigued anatomists, physiologists, and clinicians for hundreds of years. Numerous treatises and investigations have sought to describe the importance of these channels. Despite the length of time available for study and analysis, the role of collaterals has been misunderstood for almost as long as their existence has been documented, and even the mere presence of these channels in normal hearts was contested until recently. One would like to believe that these accessory channels have some biologic significance, and improve function of ischemic myocardium or preserve myocardial integrity. Careful study of existing reports has uncovered some of the reasons for the confusion surrounding these collateral vessels. In large part, inappropriate analytical techniques have accounted for the impression that collaterals were merely indicators of severe underlying disease without appreciable functional value. This treatise has attempted to indicate the flaws in these latter studies. The well-designed clinical studies and numerous experimental investigations have clearly demonstrated that coronary collaterals have important salutary functional effects. It is hoped that readers will share this optimistic view after considering the data.

Acknowledgments

It is clear that a book of this size and scope could not have been written without the assistance and forbearance of numerous individuals. I would like to express my appreciation to all of those people behind the scenes who have provided me with services that made it possible to undertake and successfully complete this project. I credit Dr. Edward S. Kirk with having stimulated me to study coronary collaterals and their physiologic significance in experimental animals, and Dr. Robert Hamby for helpful discussions about collateral vessels in clinical situations. The library staff of Montefiore Medical Center and especially Mr. Vernon Bruette must be thanked for their efforts in securing hundreds of books, monographs, and journal articles. Mrs. Anna-Maria Loretto and Drs. Jules Cohen and Hiltrud Mueller helped with the translation of numerous foreign language publications. The manuscript could not have been prepared without the secretarial services of Ms. Janet E. Holwell who devoted countless hours to typing and retyping. Finally, the completion of this project necessitated unwitting sacrifices by my wife, Madelyn, and two sons, Ari and Andrew. Their continued support during the years of study and writing encouraged me to persevere and finish the preparation of this book. All of these individuals, and others, truly deserve my sincere thanks and appreciation for their roles in the realization of a dream.

Contents

CHAPTER ONE

Morphologic Considerations of the Coronary Collateral Circulation in Man

I. Definition

An organ's collateral circulation is alternative to a major vascular conduit that has become nonfunctional, e.g., obstructed. Thus, a collateral channel is an initially unused pathway that is recruited only after failure of the original vessel to permit normal flows. The collateral network may consist of either single or interconnecting systems of channels. Furthermore, they may be preformed, in which case there is immediate expansion and subsequent growth in response to the new stresses, or may be formed *de novo* where the potential for cellular transformation is preserved.

It is intuitively obvious that following occlusion of one of the coronary arteries, the jeopardized myocardium can be supplied with oxygen and other important metabolic precursors only by collateral channels. Do collateral vessels exist in human myocardium? Do they appear only in diseased hearts, or are they also present in normal cardiac tissue? If present, are they functionally important?

II. Historical Perspective

Although the present-day controversy about coronary collaterals revolves around their functional significance, this discussion only recently replaced another concerning the anatomic presence of collateral channels in the human heart. It is both interesting and instructive to recount briefly the travails of those anatomists and pathologists who studied the coronary collateral circulation, since details of the unravelling of the mystery of collaterals in normal myocardium supply an important object lesson of how assumptions and systematic methodologic errors may cause confusion and misinterpretation of scientific observations. The following description traces only investigations on coronary collaterals in man. For an accounting of the techniques used to study coronary arteries, Whitten's exhaustive review[1] should be consulted.

Richard Lower is generally credited with the first demonstration of coronary collaterals in a human heart. In his classical treatise, *Tractatus de Corde*, published in 1669, he described seeing fluid injected into one coronary artery pass into another.[2] While describing the course of the coronary arteries on the epicardial surface, he wrote, "From such an origin they are able to go off respectively to opposite regions of the heart, yet around the extremities they come together again, and here and there communicate by anastomoses. As a result, fluid injected into one of them spreads at one and the same time through both. There is everywhere an equally great need of vital heat and nourishment, so deficiency of these is very fully guarded against by such anastomosis."[2] Thus, Lower demonstrated anastomoses with an injection technique which would be modified and be used extensively 200 years later. The significance of his findings, however, was not appreciated by either him or his peers because of the poor understanding in the late seventeenth century of the clinical syndrome of ischemic heart disease.

Early in the eighteenth century, both Vieussens (1705, 1706)[3] and Thebesius (1708)[4,5] described direct communications between coronary vessels and the cardiac chambers. Vieussens injected saffron into the coronary arteries and observed the dye escape through small openings in the atrial and ventricular endocardium, while Thebesius observed bubbles emerge from openings in the heart walls after blowing air into the coronary veins of hearts immersed in water. This curious and perplexing second collateral network will be described in detail below. Thebesius also concluded that anastomoses existed between major coronary arteries.[5] These pioneering studies were followed by confirmatory reports of other famous and well-respected anatomists of the eighteenth and early nineteenth centuries. Meticulous dissections of the heart by de Sénac, von Haller and Morgagni revealed coronary anastomoses.[5] Von Haller stated that the anastomoses were quite numerous, especially around the root of the pulmonary artery, in the posterior sulcus longitudinalis, in the right ventricle, at the apex of the heart, and on the surface of the ventricles.[6] Of interest also were the connections between coronary and extracardiac arteries, e.g., to the aortic wall and diaphragm, first demonstrated by von Haller.[4] This third type of coronary collateral network will also be described below. Thus, in 1850, anyone who cared to express an opinion would naturally have asserted that coronary collaterals or anastomoses between the major coronary arteries existed.

Hyrtl[7] raised many doubts about the presence of collateral channels in human hearts. To facilitate visualization of potential anastomoses, he developed the injection-corrosion technique of preparing his specimens. He injected the left heart and thus filled the coronary arteries with a wax/resin mixture or red lead, a metallic alloy with a low melting point. After hardening or solidification of the injectate in the vasculature, the myocardium was digested in hydrochloric acid, leaving a skeleton or cast of the arterial network. Hyrtl stated emphatically that coronary anastomoses did not exist. The absence of large precapillary intercoronary connections was quickly confirmed by Henle[8] who used similar methods, although this latter anatomist conceded that there might be connections at the capillary level. It is likely that the physical characteristics of the injected mass prevented it from flowing into the smaller-caliber arterioles, thus precluding the possibility of identifying anastomoses.

In 1881 the results of an experimental study by Cohnheim and von Schulthess-Rechberg[9] became the cornerstone of the belief that coronary anastomoses were absent altogether or at least functionally insignificant. Although these authors made their observations in dogs, the results influenced the thinking of clinicians for more than fifty years. They noted that clamping of either main coronary artery in curarized animals resulted in cessation of effective ventricular contraction within two minutes. It was accordingly argued that the coronary arteries must be end-arteries without intercommunications, since it was assumed that the cardiac muscle would have continued to beat if perfusion through collaterals had been possible.

Coronary injection studies continued to produce conflicting results. Whereas Langer[10] proclaimed that there were numerous large collaterals between coronary arteries, Dragneff[11] found only minimal evidence of anastomoses in 4 of 22 injected hearts. West[12] injected a hot carmine-gelatin mixture into a coronary artery. As did Lower using a very similar protocol, West observed the mixture to flow from the aortic orifice of one of the other major arteries. In the early twentieth century, several new techniques were introduced that made the study of coronary collaterals more objective. Merkel[13] simultaneously injected both the right and left coronary arteries with a 10−15% suspension of red lead in gelatin. After injection the heart was chilled to allow the injectate to harden, and then stereoscopic x-rays were taken. Anastomoses filled with the radiopaque injectate could thus be visualized without the laborious dissections previously needed, and the special radiographs allowed the observer to appreciate depth and therefore to differentiate anastomoses from overlapping vessels, which was not possible with standard roentgenograms. In their monograph Jamin and Merkel[14] presented stereoscopic x-rays of 19 hearts. Despite the coarse quality of the early stereoscopic x-rays, the two authors were able to identify collaterals in normal hearts, although great individual differences were apparent. The collaterals were found most frequently in the auricle and interauricular and interventricular septa, and occasionally on the anterior wall of the right ventricle and over the papillary muscles and apex of the heart.

In 1907, the same year in which Jamin and Merkel published their clinical studies, Spalteholz[15] described an innovative approach to the study of the coronary circulation that permitted him to visualize small arterioles beyond the resolution capacity of the radiographic equipment then available. He cleared the heart, that is, made the superficial myocardium transparent, so that injected vessels below the surface could be visualized. After injecting both coronary arteries with chrome-yellow gelatin, the heart was fixed in formaldehyde and then dehydrated in a series of organic solvents including alcohol and benzene. The heart was then immersed in oil of wintergreen which penetrated the tissue, giving it a uniform refractive index similar to that of the fluid itself. Hence, the myocardium was rendered transparent, and the opaque, injected vessels stood out prominently from the cleared parenchyma. On the basis of these early studies as well as continuing investigations published in his classical text in 1924,[16] Spalteholz emphatically concluded that the coronary arteries were not end-arteries. Beneath the surface of the heart he saw rich networks of precapillary anastomoses connecting the vascular beds of adjacent coronary arteries, especially in the left atrium, wall of the right ventricle, the apex, and interventricular septum. In the thick muscle of the left ventricle, vessels perpendicular to the surface penetrated the outer layers to anastomose with vessels beneath the endocardium. The clearing technique obviously had its shortcomings, since only the superficial few millimeters of parenchyma were typically cleared. Nonetheless, collaterals were positively identified in even these superficial layers.

These studies triggered a number of subsequent reports that all but settled the question of coronary collaterals. Gross[6] and Kugel[17] used a combination of coronary injection with barium sulphate-gelatin mixtures, stereoarteriography, clearing, and dissection. Crainicianu[18] and Routier and his colleagues[19] injected the coronary arteries with red lead in an oily suspension and then used radiographs to identify collateral vessels. Campbell[20] employed barium suspension injectates and then stereoangiography to identify collateral channels in normal myocardial tissue. To avoid the possibility that overlapping vessels were being mistaken for intercoronary anastomoses in the standard stereoradiographs, Gross and Kugel[21] sliced the heart every 7 mm from apex to base after injecting the arteries with a barium sulphate-gelatin suspension, and then x-rayed the slices followed by clearing. Despite the multiplicity of techniques, the conclusion was similar: numerous collaterals connecting the individual coronary arteries were evident in normal human hearts. Even Cohnheim's experiments,[9] which had helped to launch the controversy, were refuted. Miller and Matthews[22] demonstrated that many of the deaths of Cohnheim's experimental animals could be attributed to his use of either curare or morphine. By using ether as an anesthetic, they found only an 8.7% mortality following ligation of the left anterior descending coronary artery. To be sure, there were still some who continued to deny the existence of precapillary coronary anastomoses. Amenomiya[23] injected coronary arteries of the normal hearts of seven young people with a lime mass, cleared the hearts, and then studied the circulation of the papillary muscles. Although he found capillary anastomoses, and therefore agreed that the coronary arteries were not true end-arteries, he was unable to find any of the precapillary collaterals described by Spalteholz.[15]

Hence, by the 1930s, the pendulum had swung once again, and the concept of coronary collaterals seemed to be established. Pathologists and clinicians accepted as fact that collateral vessels were present in normal hearts. The stage seemed to be set for the immensely important contributions of Schlesinger and Blumgart and their co-workers. In 1938, Schlesinger[24] published his critique of prior techniques used in the study of the coronary and collateral circulations, and described in detail his own methodology. The work of this Boston group dominated the anatomic investigation of collateral vessels for nearly twenty years, and many other investigators soon adopted the standardized method introduced by Schlesinger. He initially injected both the right and left coronary arteries simultaneously with a lead phosphate-agar mass at a pressure of 150 mmHg. The injection of the left coronary artery was then continued while the pressure in the right coronary artery was decreased to zero, followed by resumption of the pressure injection of the right coronary artery while the left injection was discontinued. After completion of the injection and setting of the agar, several incisions were made and the heart was "unrolled" so that all of the myocardium lay in the same plane. This unrolling facilitated the interpretation of radiographs since vessel overlapping was minimized. By using the x-rays as guides, vessels of interest could be dissected out (Figure 1-1). Identification of collater-

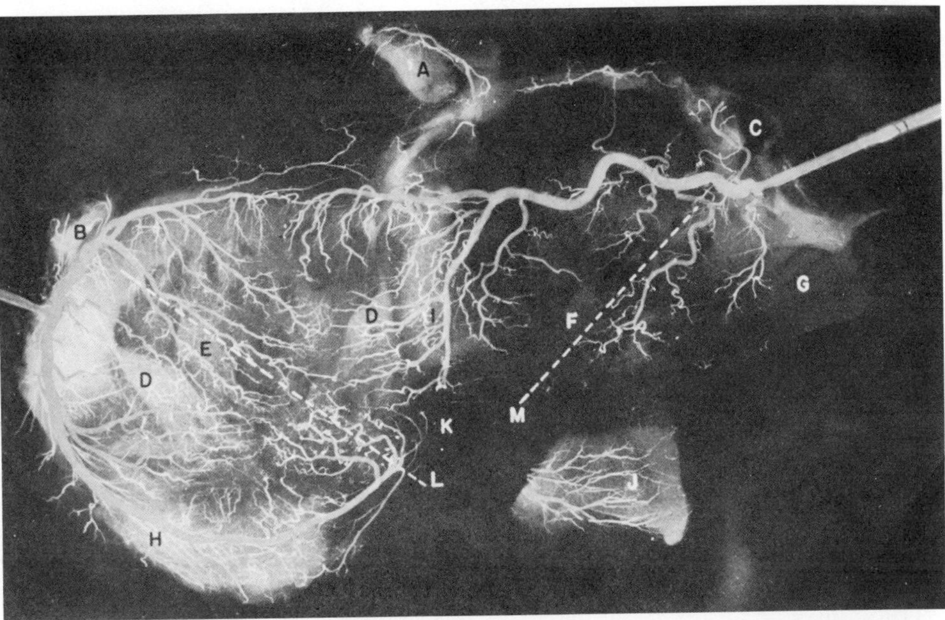

Figure 1-1   Roentgenogram of unrolled, normal heart after injection of right and left coronary arteries with lead phosphate-agar mass. The cannulae in the main coronary arteries can be seen at the two lateral borders of the photograph. The left coronary artery (left side) divides quickly into the left anterior descending artery which runs toward the anterior edge of the interventricular septum (H) and the left circumflex artery running beneath the left atrial appendage (B). The proximal portion of the right coronary artery (right side) is covered by the right atrial appendage (C), and the main vessel courses in the atrioventricular groove to meet the left circumflex artery. The letters in the photograph represent landmarks, e.g., D (2 parts) = left anterior papillary muscle; E = left posterior papillary muscle; I = posterior edge of interventricular septum; J = interventricular septum; K = apex of heart. The dashed lines L and M represent the location of the obtuse and acute borders of the heart, respectively. (Reprinted with permission of C. V. Mosby Co. from Schlesinger.[24])

als was aided by mixing the lead-agar mixtures with dyes, and injecting a different color into the right and left coronary arteries. A collateral was defined as a vessel containing a mixture of the two dyes. Further evidence of collaterals was retrograde filling of a vessel with a colored mass that had been injected into the contralateral coronary system, and appearance of injectate beyond total vascular obstructions in those individuals with coronary artery disease. Collateral vessels were routinely excised, fixed for histologic section, and examined microscopically. The lead phosphate-agar mass was three times as viscous as blood, and regularly penetrated to vessels of 40 μm diameter and irregularly to those of 20 μm caliber. Schlesinger[25] subsequently noted that vessels fixed in formalin were subject to a 50–100% correction for shrinkage from the fresh unfixed state.

Of the initial 38 hearts from subjects more than 50 years old examined by Schlesinger,[24] 7 had normal coronary arteries and 8 only minimal or moderate degrees of coronary atherosclerosis. Although he identified coronary collaterals in hearts with one or more coronary occlusions, none was apparent in the hearts with minimal or no coronary disease. Schlesinger concluded that normal hearts were devoid of significant collateral vessels, although he admitted that 10 μm precapillary anastomoses could be functionally demonstrated by observing a watery solution appear in one coronary artery after injection into the contralateral vessel. He wrote, "The coronary arteries, in *normal* human hearts, even senile hearts, are true Cohnheim end arteries, without anastomotic connections."

Over the next thirteen years, the number of hearts studied by Schlesinger and co-workers increased to over 1,200![25–29] On the basis of this extensive experience they concluded that only 9–15% of nonanemic subjects with normal coronary arteries had intercoronary anastomoses demonstrable with the Schlesinger mass. If anemic subjects were included in the tabulation, then the incidence of coronary collaterals in autopsied patients with normal coronary arteries increased to 23%. Nonetheless, these data demonstrated that a strikingly small minority of subjects with normal hearts had coronary collaterals. These reports rekindled a seemingly settled controversy. The massive number of hearts examined in these studies made it difficult for investigators with fewer preparations who believed otherwise to gain credibility.

The Schlesinger technique[24] rapidly became the standard method for detailed examinations of the coronary circulation. Others following Schlesinger's protocol[30–33] or employing slightly different injection and radiographic methods[34,35] confirmed the infrequent occurrence of coronary collaterals in normal hearts. Thus, it appeared that Cohnheim and von Schulthess-Rechberg,[9] who originally proposed that coronary arteries were end-arteries, had been vindicated. The pendulum had once again swung to the other side.

During this same period, Prinzmetal[36] employed an innovative physiologic approach to the study of the coronary vascular bed. He and his colleagues injected glass spheres ranging in diameter from 10 to 400 μm and suspended in a radiopaque mixture into the left coronary artery of normal cadaver hearts, and examined the size of the beads recovered from the ostium of the right coronary artery. Injection pressures were carefully regulated and did not exceed 160 mmHg. In 11 of 13 normal or minimally atherosclerotic hearts, beads with diameters of 70 to 180 μm were recovered from the right coronary artery, although in 8 of these 11 hearts the maximum diameter of the beads able to cross over into the right coronary vascular bed was 70−90 μm. Prinzmetal therefore assumed that collaterals in normal hearts were generally present, but did not often exceed 80 μm in diameter. Although the size of these collaterals is not different from that detected by the Schlesinger technique in normal hearts (when corrected for shrinkage), the incidence is nine times greater than that reported by Zoll et al. in 1951.[25] Wiggers,[37] however, who held that coronary anastomoses in the normal heart were inconsequential and nonfunctional, criticized Prinzmetal's experimental design. He noted that the pressure gradient between coronary arteries during the perfusion (up to 160 mmHg) was usually greater than that existing in the beating heart, and therefore believed that the glass spherules could have been forced through the elastic vessels. Furthermore, based largely on Stella's observations,[38] Wiggers claimed that blood transport between the left ventricular lumen and coronary artery in the beating heart was of little consequence. He concluded, therefore, that the recovery of 70−350 μm spherules in the ventricular cavities of a dead heart implied the passage of these and, by extension, other injected beads was an artifact perhaps caused by loss of muscle tension and subsequent maximal vascular dilatation.

Pitt[39,40] was unable to reproduce Prinzmetal's results.[35] He injected one coronary artery of excised human hearts with either 35−45 μm or 75−90 μm wax spheres at a pressure of 100 mmHg and collected the effluent from the ostium of the other coronary artery. In this manner, he demonstrated anastomoses in only 6% of normal hearts, a figure quite similar to that obtained using Schlesinger's method.[25] On the other hand, Schweizer[41] and later Gömöri,[42] whose techniques were nearly identical to Pitt's, concluded that 50% of normal hearts had intercoronary connections.

As early as 1939 Correia[43] described intercoronary connections during postmortem angiography of normal hearts with a red lead suspension. But this report was largely ignored. Then, beginning in the late 1950s, an increasing number of reports in which the investigators used radiographic techniques to evaluate the coronary collateral circulation were published that conflicted with the previously accepted data of the Boston group of Schlesinger, Blumgart, and Zoll.[24−29] Most studies[44−52] used the same lead or barium salt suspension in either agar or gelatin, as suggested by Schlesinger,[24,53] followed by radiography of the unrolled heart. Fulton[54−56] modified Schlesinger's method. He used a bismuth oxychloride-gelatin injection mass, and greatly increased the resolution of his x-rays by using industrial and crystallography films and immersing the heart in saline during the radiography. Instead of unrolling the heart, Fulton sliced the ventricles from apex to base and made x-rays of the slices. Vastesaeger[57] injected iodized oils into the coronary circulation and then took stereoscopic x-rays, while Huguet[58] performed postmortem angiography with the same radiopaque contrast medium used in vivo for diagnostic angiography. Collaterals were always present in the majority of normal hearts evaluated, and some studies detected anastomoses in 90 to 100% of the hearts.[44,49−51,54,56,58] Collateral diameters ranged up to 300 μm in most series and reached 1 mm in 7.5% of Vastesaeger's hearts.[57] The striking differences between these conclusions and those of Schlesinger and colleagues could not be overlooked.

Ethnic and geographic differences were initially considered to be possible contributing causes of the different results. In their initial report, Laurie and Woods[45] found that 75% of normal Bantu hearts from individuals older than 4 years had collateral anastomoses. Some suggested that the high incidence of megaloblastic and iron-deficiency anemias in these African natives might have contributed to the development of the multiple large collateral channels (see Chapter 3). Pepler and Meyer[46] supported this hypothesis when they noted that 57% of Bantu hearts and 26% of European hearts obtained from the same South African hospital had collaterals ($p <$ 0.01). A follow-up investigation by Laurie and Woods,[48] however, showed similar high percentages of good and excellent collaterals in Bantus (64%), Australians (60%), and Canadians (43%). Furthermore, all normal Japanese[51] and Indian[52] hearts studied more recently appeared to have abundant collaterals. It therefore seems unlikely that different ethnic origin or geographic location could account for the observed discrepancies.

Age was also not a likely explanation. Neonatal hearts had numerous coronary anastomoses.[47,57] Reiner[47] noted that there was a distinct increase in incidence and quality of collaterals with progressive gestational maturity. Laurie and Woods[45] also found collaterals in the hearts of young children. Although the observed incidence of anastomoses in hearts from children under 5 years of age was only 11%, they attributed this low percentage to technical factors related to coronary injection in very small hearts. Fifty percent of the European children who died before their tenth birthday and 80% of the Bantu children in the series of Pepler and Meyer[46] had moderate or good coronary collaterals.

Careful analysis of the methods of coronary injection used by all of these investigators suggested that minor differences in technique could account for the major discrepancies in results. Although differences in injectate viscosity or particle size, organ or injectate temperature, and perfusion pressure could very definitely affect the results of the perfusion studies, there were no consistent differences between those studies supporting and those denying the existence of collaterals. It is evident that no flow along a vessel should be expected unless a pressure gradient exists. Therefore, simultaneous injection of normal right and left coronary arteries as advocated by Schlesinger[24] precludes establishment of any pressure gradient and minimizes the chances of flow along collaterals connecting these two coronary arteries. Those injection studies where numerous collaterals were identified were almost universally characterized by injections of single coronary arteries.[43−48,50,52,57,58] By contrast, Schlesinger's reports[24−29] and those of others[30-34] injecting both coronary arteries at the same time demonstrated only sparse coronary collaterals in normal hearts. Schlesinger[24] recommended that perfusion of single arteries be continued after the simultaneous perfusion of both coronary arteries, while pressure in the contralateral vessel was allowed to fall to zero. Despite this transient unbalancing of pressures in the two coronary arteries, it is possible that already injected mass in the vessels may have impeded flow through anastomoses into a filled coronary system, thus diminishing the likelihood of visualizing right-to-left or left-to-right (intercoronary) anastomoses. Furthermore, Schlesinger's criteria for the documentation of collateral vessels virtually precluded demonstration of left-to-left or right-to-right (intracoronary) collaterals in hearts without coronary artery obstruction. In these situations, vessels conjoined by these anastomoses would be injected from the same coronary ostium and would therefore be filled with the same colored mass. The collateral would also be filled with injectate of only one color, and hence could easily be overlooked.

To substantiate this theory, Rodriguez and Robbins[49] examined 327 hearts without coronary occlusions using Schlesinger's modification of his original technique.[53] The authors found that only 12% of the injected hearts had evidence of intercoronary anastomoses. These results are similar to those reported by Schlesinger and his co-workers.[24-29] In an additional 33 normal hearts, either a primary branch of each of the three coronary arteries was ligated prior to simultaneous injection of the mass into all three arteries, or the three main coronary arteries were transected between ligatures and the proximal segments injected. Now all 33 hearts demonstrated 100−200 μm coronary collaterals, fulfilling the Schlesinger criteria. Thus, the artificial creation of a pressure gradient within the coronary bed, in spite of simultaneous injection of right and left coronary arteries, ensured retrograde filling of the vessel distal to the ligature by either intra- or intercoronary connections. Thus, anastomoses do exist in most human hearts, and the reason why Schlesinger's technique was unable to demonstrate them in hearts without naturally occurring or artificially imposed occlusions is a technical one. Rodriguez and Robbins[49] cautioned that the "current controversy in regard to the incidence of intercoronary arterial anastomoses in normal human hearts stems from the error of equating absence of anastomoses with inability to detect them." The pendulum had swung once again to the other side.

Other, newer injection media have also been used to evaluate the coronary collateral circulation. Baroldi[59-61] filled the coronary arteries either with a plastic material (Geon Latex 576) suspended in polyvinyl chloride or with latex (Neoprene 842A), and then digested the myocardium with concentrated hydrochloric acid, thus leaving a cast of the coronary tree. James[62-65] used an injectate of the plastic Vinylite dissolved in acetone, and then also placed the heart in hydrochloric acid to produce corrosion casts of the coronary vasculature (Figure 1-2 [colorplate 1*]). Almost all of their specimens showed numerous anastomoses within the ventricular wall. Baroldi[61] stated that intramyocardial arterial branches communicated at different levels with

* Colorplates for this chapter appear on pps. 53−58.

adjacent branches throughout the whole thickness of the cardiac wall with the exception of the subepicardial region. James[64] found the anastomoses to be especially numerous in the epicardium. Collaterals up to 200 μm were frequently found, while connections with diameters of 200−350 μm were less common.

Plastic casts (Geon 576) of the coronary circulation in newborns also revealed multiple large anastomoses.[66] Bloor[67] determined the maximum collateral dimension in infants by perfusing one coronary artery with suspensions of wax spheres with diameters ranging from 20 to 120 μm and collecting the effluent from the orifice of the contralateral artery. In 15 of the 20 hearts, 63−74 μm spheres were recovered in the effluent, but in no heart did larger spheres (100−120 μm) appear.

Finally, after many decades of debate and controversy, it became apparent to all but a very small minority[68] clinging to an indefensible position that coronary collaterals were present in hearts from individuals of all ages. Only technical, methodologic shortcomings prevented all from arriving at this conclusion. All investigators agree that very large coronary collaterals are present in pathologic hearts, especially those with coronary obstructive disease (see Chapter 3). However, anatomic presence cannot be equated with functional significance. Questions of the latter have generated a new debate about coronary collaterals (see Chapter 2).

III. Methods of Study

A. Postmortem Techniques

The above recounting of the history of past travails of those seeking to identify coronary collaterals has effectively summarized the major postmortem investigative techniques. Simple dissection of the coronary vasculature by the eighteenth- and nineteenth-century anatomists sometimes after intracoronary injection of metal suspensions or wax-resin mixtures to outline the coronary bed,[5,10,11] preparation of corrosion casts,[7,8,59−66] injection of radiopaque suspensions of metals, metal salts, or iodized contrast agents followed by one of several methods of slicing and x-raying the heart,[6,13,14,17−21,24−35,44−58] and clearance of superficial myocardium in organic solvents after filling the coronary vasculature with a colored gelatin[6,15−17,23] have all been used. Over the past two centuries, the successive introduction of new coronary injectates[1,24,53,59,63,69,70] has made it increasingly possible to visualize the smaller coronary branches and hence collaterals. Choice of a substance with the proper viscosity and particle size to penetrate the vascular bed and fill 40-μm arterioles but not enter the capillary venous system was an important consideration. The change from an agar to a gelatin base for the injectate made the coronary injection process much simpler.[53] And introduction of various x-ray techniques including radiography of the unrolled heart[24] and left ventricular slices[34] and stereo-radiography[13] further increased resolution and permitted clearer differentiation of collaterals from overlapping branches of adjacent coronary arteries. As detailed above, perhaps one of the most important technical factors influencing collateral identification was the precise method of introduction of the injectate into the coronary arteries. Delivery of the injectate into only one coronary artery as opposed to the simultaneous injection of both vessels was found to greatly increase the chances of demonstrating collateral channels.[49]

Perhaps the most obvious limitation of all of these techniques is their qualitative nature. Each can identify collateral vessels and possibly even measure vessel diameters, but none of the described methods can effectively estimate the quantity of blood that can flow through these channels. Nor can the collateral circulation in one heart be objectively compared to that in a second heart. Baroldi and Scomazzoni[60] addressed this issue and derived an anastomotic index to describe total collateral capacity. They determined the maximum diameter of the largest anastomotic vessel found and the average diameter and frequency of anastomoses exceeding 100 μm. The frequency was evaluated relative to the findings in the normal heart, in which the frequency was arbitrarily set as "1." Anastomotic index was defined as (maximum diameter + [average diameter × frequency]) ÷ 100. In normal hearts, the mean anastomotic index was 4.7. Fulton's anastomotic index was slightly different,[55] but was also intended to quantitate the frequency of collaterals with specified diameters. Although these anastomotic indices provided semiquantitative measures of combined collateral frequency and dimensions, the necessary laborious and time-consuming counting and sizing of collaterals in the specimens severely limited the acceptability of this technique.

Dock[71] cannulated the coronary arteries of postmortem hearts from the aorta and perfused them with kerosene at known pressures. He thus obtained coronary flows, which he felt provided information about the capacity of the coronary vascular bed and the maximum flows possible during life. Prinzmetal[72] and later Barmeyer,[73] adapted Dock's technique to measure collateral flow in the excised heart. As did Dock, Prinzmetal used kerosene as the perfusate, while Barmeyer used a mixture of paraffin oil and diesel oil. These perfusates were selected because of the similarity of their viscosities to that of blood. Each coronary artery was cannulated and perfused from separate reservoirs at similar pressures, and flows through the two vascular beds measured. Flow from one reservoir was abruptly interrupted while perfusion of the other artery was continued at the same pressure. Any increase in flow to the unobstructed vessel was felt to represent flow passing along collateral channels to the obstructed vessel. Therefore, collateral flow as a percentage of normal antegrade flow could be calculated for each vessel. In normal hearts, collateral flow averaged 4.2% of forward coronary flow.[72] These interesting measurements can obviously not be equated with actual collateral flow in the beating heart, but they did stimulate the search for more physiologic means of assessing anastomotic flow.

Prinzmetal[36] devised many ingenious ways of evaluating collateral flow in the human heart. As noted above, he perfused the coronary arteries of cadaver hearts with glass spheres of various diameters in order to size collateral diameters. He and his co-workers also perfused human radioactive red blood cells at 100 mmHg through either the left anterior descending or the left circumflex branch of the left coronary artery, and measured the distribution and concentration of these erythrocytes in multiple areas of the unrolled left ventricle with either a Geiger counter or radioautography. By calibrating the radioactivity of a known volume of the ^{32}P-tagged red blood cells, the amount of blood in each of the examined areas of the left ventricle could be determined. In the seven normal hearts studied, radioactivity was detected in all left ventricular areas despite the regional injection, and often the amount of radioactivity in the remote areas closely approximated that detected in the perfusion territory of the injected vessel.

Postmortem studies are useful for the demonstration of coronary collaterals, but cannot be relied on to approximate the in-vivo value of anastomotic connections. In the past twenty years, however, techniques have been developed both to visualize collaterals in living man and to quantitate myocardial perfusion.

B. Clinical Techniques

1. Coronary Angiography

Opacification of the coronary arteries with iodinated radiopaque contrast media has become a routine diagnostic procedure, and numerous reports[74-79] and atlases and monographs[80-84] detail the angiographic anatomy of coronary collaterals. Although angiography has traditionally been regarded as the gold standard, many aspects of the technical procedure have not been standardized. Because of the variety of techniques, the quality of results may be expected to be variable. Furthermore, angiography can provide only qualitative descriptive information about collaterals and therefore is no better than postmortem evaluation for the assessment of functional adequacy.

Multiple factors influence the quality and value of the angiographic study. Perhaps of paramount importance is the experience of the angiographer. But many other factors must also be taken into account: quality of imaging equipment; type of image intensifier; tube current and voltage; focal spot; x-ray film; processing technique; catheters; contrast media; patient size. Even the position of the catheter within the coronary ostium and the pressure with which the contrast injection is made may influence collateral visualization.[85] Vessels as small as 100 μm may be visualized with angiographic techniques.[75,77,79,82] However, this resolution is predicated on optimal function of the equipment and other ideal conditions. Suboptimal resolution and inability to visualize vessels with diameters as small as 100 μm would be expected under other circumstances.

After the angiographic procedure is complete, evaluation of the films by one or more individuals is then necessary. This evaluation is quite subjective, and the lack of precision and reproducibility must be recognized. Estimation of the degree of coronary stenosis is one of the tasks of the radiologist or cardiologist viewing the films. These data are particularly important in the evaluation of collateral vessels since patients in clinical correlative studies are frequently grouped according to the severity of their coronary lesions. The accuracy of the angiographic quantitation of luminal narrowing was first assessed by comparing postmortem angiographic determinations with direct measurements of the luminal diameter or area from arterial cross-sections.[86-88] It was apparent that the angiogram frequently underestimated stenosis severity as much as 40% of the time, but also in a smaller percentage of cases overestimated luminal narrowing. Others have contrasted the accuracy of angiograms done shortly before death to pathologic measurements of coronary stenosis. Although Kemp et al.[89] and Trask and colleagues[90] were impressed with the close correlation, most observers[91-98] have documented a disappointingly high rate of discordance. Both Schwartz[93] and Hutchins[94] noted discrepancies of at least 25% in stenosis severity in 20–30% of the

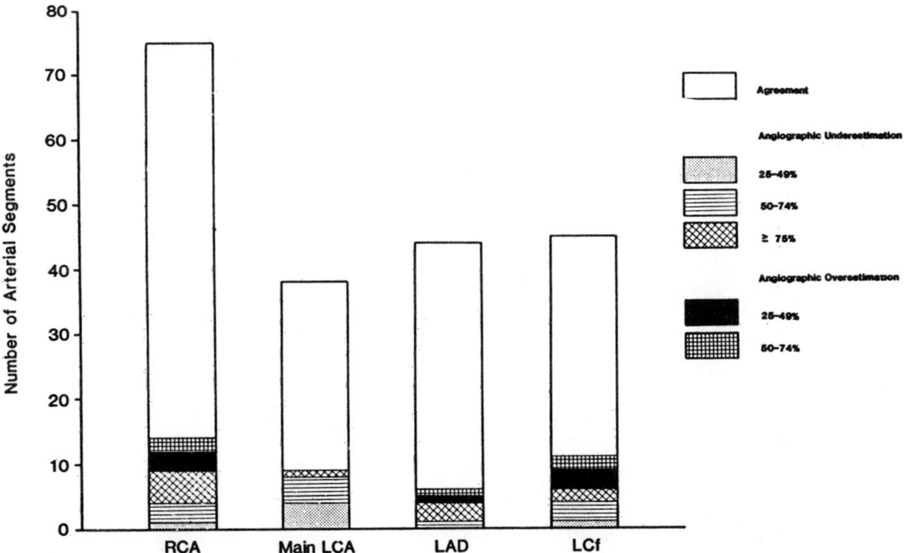

Figure 1-3 Correlation between angiographic estimates and pathologic measurements of coronary artery stenoses. In approximately 20% of arterial segments, at least a 25% angiographic under- or overestimate was made. LAD = left anterior descending artery; LCA = left coronary artery; LCf = left circumflex coronary artery; RCA = right coronary artery. (Drawn from data presented by Schwartz et al.[93])

coronary arterial segments examined (Figure 1-3). Perhaps Trask's experience[90] is better than that of others because of the exceptionally short interval between angiography and the patient's demise (median 17 days). He noted that the angiographers were able to correctly categorize the degree of coronary arterial narrowing as either less or more severe than 75% in nearly 90% of cases when compared to postmortem estimates of luminal narrowing. Nonetheless, there continued to be both under- and overestimations. As discussed by Klocke,[99] difficulties in angiographic estimation of stenosis severity should not be surprising. Stenoses are rarely concentric. Errors in evaluation of nonconcentric or nonelliptical stenosis geometry are nearly impossible to avoid. Furthermore, it is startling to realize that radiographic measurements of coronary artery narrowings created in dogs with plastic cylinders[100,101] or stenoses in plastic tubes filled with radiopaque contrast medium and placed in water baths,[102] models where abnormal geometry is not a factor, are also frequently inaccurate.

Aside from the limitations of the radiographic technique in the quantitation of severity of coronary lesions, there is appreciable inter-[95,96,103−107] and intraobserver[103,104,108] variability, which further diminishes the reliability of the interpretation of the angiogram. The same angiogram shown to several cardiologists or radiologists may elicit a disappointingly wide spectrum of stenosis estimates. In fact, the second estimate of an individual seeing the same angiogram on two occasions frequently disagrees with the first. Trask's report,[90] in which overall agreement between two angiographers was 86%, is considerably more encouraging. Computer-assisted measurement[109] of luminal narrowing at the site of a stenosis may eliminate much of the subjectivity and hence improve reliability and reproducibility.

Angiographic study of coronary collaterals has mainly been limited to documentation of either the presence or absence of these anastomotic channels. In general, most viewers are able to agree whether collaterals are present or not on the angiogram.[103,104,106] Opacification of the collateral itself, appearance of contrast medium in that portion of a coronary artery distal to a total occlusion, and opacification of branches of one coronary artery following selective injection of contrast medium into the contralateral vessel are the usual angiographic criteria of coronary collateralization. In an attempt to derive more information from the angiographic appearance of collaterals, grading systems have been used whereby the collaterals are classified as good, fair, or poor. Unfortunately, these subjective impressions depend on the degree of opacification of the collateral or recipient vessel, and therefore may be influenced by multiple exogenous factors, such as force of injection of contrast medium.[85] Despite the obvious limitations, this classification is better than merely documenting the presence of collaterals. Attempts to increase the objectivity of angiographic evaluation of collaterals have been made.[110−112] Hecht and co-workers[111] graded collaterals according to width and number, density of contrast filling of the recipient vessel, and washout time from the opacified artery. Levin[110] and Rowe[112] also measured the time necessary for opacification of or washout from arterial segments beyond occlusions. Even these classification schemes, however, are primitive and imprecise. Yet there are few alternatives. Consequently, these classifications have been used in numerous studies seeking to document the functional importance of collaterals (see Chapter 2).

Despite the obvious qualitative nature of angiographic estimation of coronary collaterals, both Webb et al.[113] and Goldstein and his colleagues[114] have demonstrated favorable correlations between the collateral indices retrograde flow and peripheral coronary pressure (see below) and the angiographic appearance of collaterals (see Chapter 3 and Figure 3-5). Thus, as the angiographic quality of collaterals improved, collateral function also improved, lending credibility to the use of the angiogram in classification of collaterals. However, others have shown discordance between angiographic estimates of collateral function and radionuclide measurements of myocardial perfusion[115,116] (see below).

2. Nuclear Medicine Methods

(a) Noble gases

Kety and Schmidt[117] devised a method to measure organ blood flow with diffusible indicators; this technique was subsequently adapted for the evaluation of regional myocardial flows. The radioactive noble gases krypton (^{85}Kr) and xenon (^{133}Xe) have been used clinically, although the latter is currently preferred. They decay by electron emission and detectable release of photons. The diffusible tracers dissolved in saline are injected selectively into a coronary artery[118] or directly into the myocardium at the time of thoracotomy.[119] During the initial pass through the capillaries, the radioisotope diffuses into the myocardial cells. Disappearance or washout of radioactivity is measured by an external radiation detection system placed over the heart. Kety[120] showed that the rate of washout from the tissue into the blood was a function of tissue blood flow. From the exponential washout curves, blood flow can be calculated (see Chapter 4). Because 95% of a bolus of noble gas entering the coronary circulation reaches the alveoli during the first circulation through the lungs and is excreted, there is little accumulation in the blood and hence no recirculating isotope to affect the washout curves.

There are certain assumptions inherent in the application of the Kety-Schmidt formula for calculation of coronary flows that are probably not violated when the myocardium is normally perfused, but which may be inaccurate when blood flow to the ventricular muscle is unevenly distributed.[121−123] Desaturation measurements require that the indicator is initially homogeneously distributed throughout the tissue under study, and there must be continuous diffusion equilibrium of indicator between the capillary blood and the tissue. In patients with coronary artery lesions and low regional flows, the radioisotope enters the poorly perfused myocardium slowly and is likewise washed out slowly. Therefore, uniformity of tissue tracer concentration cannot be achieved. If the washout is monitored for only a brief time to avoid the problems of isotope recirculation and uptake by noncardiac tissues within the field of interest (a problem mainly for indicators not excreted by the lungs), then washout from the poorly perfused area will be monitored inadequately. Therefore, when regional flow heterogeneity exists, washout and hence coronary flow calculations are principally reflections of flow to normally perfused areas. When the field of interest contains several tissue components in each of which the radioactive indicator has a different solubility (e.g., muscle, scar, adipose tissue), the lack of uniform distribution is especially evident. Maseri[124] has demonstrated a significant xenon diffusion hold-up in fat, which he felt influenced total myocardial washout to such an extent that quantitation of myocardial flow in man was impossible. Cannon,[123] on the other hand, has minimized the significance of xenon diffusion into adipose tissue.

Because of these limitations, techniques were developed to reflect regional changes in flow patterns of hearts with diseased vasculature. Using large, single crystal NaI scintillation cameras and computer image data processing, it was possible to store data in a 64×64, 128×128, or 256×256 matrix.[125] Specific areas of interest corresponding to regions of high or low myocardial flow could then be selected, and washout from the corresponding cells of the matrix could then be processed and flows calculated. Cannon and his colleagues[123,126,127] perhaps did the most for development of this technique. They performed selective precordial counting by using a multiple-crystal scintillation camera consisting of a rectangular array of 294 NaI crystals arranged in 21 columns of 14 crystals. Pulses were accumulated as digital information on a computer disc and stored on magnetic tape. Each crystal, therefore, recorded radioactive counts from a very small area. The counts recorded by individual crystals could be displayed as a matrix of varying light intensities proportional to the amount of radioactivity or as dynamic digital data. A frame from the coronary arteriogram obtained a few minutes before the isotope injection was aligned and superimposed on the radioactivity data matrix. Monoexponential rate constants of xenon clearance could be calculated for each component of the matrix following bolus intracoronary injection of ^{133}Xe using data recorded in the first 39 seconds after the peak of the local xenon curve. The regional clearance rates could then be correlated with the coronary anatomy. Obviously, any flow into myocardium beyond a complete arterial occlusion must have been delivered by collaterals. Hence this technique was able to quantitate collateral flow in patients with total occlusions.

Cannon[123] used a 1½-inch multichannel collimator in his studies of regional myocardial perfusion. The radius of myocardium viewed by each crystal was 6 mm at 3 cm distance (approximately the distance between the chest wall and the anterior wall of the heart) and 12 mm at 8−9 cm from the target (approximately the distance between the chest wall and the posterior wall of the heart). Overlap of field of view of adjacent crystals was noted to be $< 3\%$ at 5 cm from the face of the collimator and 16% at 8 cm. Regional myocardial perfusion rates will be imprecise if counts recorded by one crystal actually represent radioactivity originating from myocardium remote to the conical field of that crystal. It is assumed that this overlap is small.

(b) 201-Thallous chloride

Recently, perfusion myocardial imaging with the cation 201-thallium has become popular and has largely supplanted investigations with noble gases. As detailed in Chapter 4, initial myocardial distribution of 201-thallium is proportional to blood flow, whereas late (3−4 hours after injection) distribution of the isotope is related to mass of viable myocardium. The chloride salt of 201-thallium is dissolved in saline and injected intravenously while the subject is at rest or exercising on a treadmill or stationary bicycle. The subject is then positioned beneath a scintillation camera which is set to detect the 80 kev x-rays of the isotope's mercury daughter. Low-flow myocardial areas take up less 201-thallium than normally perfused regions and therefore appear as defects in the scintigram. The left ventricular scintigram can be divided into segments corresponding to territories perfused by specific coronary branches.[128,129] Hence, the effect of a coronary arterial narrowing on myocardial perfusion can be assessed directly. As with noble gases, any 201-thallium appearing in myocardium beyond a total occlusion must have been delivered by collaterals. In these cases the adequacy of collateral perfusion can be assessed.

201-Thallium scintigrams may be interpreted by visual inspection. However, this method of analysis, as with coronary arteriograms, tends to be very subjective. To circumvent this difficulty, various computer techniques have been developed to enable objective quantification of the scan. One such technique is that of circumferential profiles,[130] in which left ventricular activity is measured along radii constructed from the center of the chamber to each point on the circumference and then displayed as a function of the highest radial activity.

To increase the sensitivity of 201-thallium scintigraphy for detection of regional hypoperfusion, attempts have been made to create greater disparities between the low and normal flow areas. Thus, exercise[131] and the vasodilator dipyridamole[132] have been used clinically to demonstrate poorly perfused myocardium more clearly. Both exercise and arteriolar vasodilators increase flow to normal tissue severalfold, while flow to myocardium distal to critical arterial stenoses or occlusions changes little or even decreases. This exaggerated flow gradient is more easily appreciated with the 201-thallium scintigram.

(c) Radioactive macroaggregated albumin particles

Unless the native coronary artery is completely occluded, it is not possible to distinguish collateral flow to the myocardium from residual antegrade flow with 201-thallium scintigraphy. Myocardial imaging with particulate radiopharmaceuticals, however, can help to define specific sources of collateral flow.[133−137] Twenty- to thirty-micrometer macroaggregated albumin particles labeled with an isotope, usually technetium-99m or indium-113m, may be injected selectively into the coronary arteries at the time of coronary angiography. One label is injected into the right and the other into the left coronary artery. With adequate mixing, the particles travel as if they were red blood cells and their distribution is proportional to blood flow. The particles are trapped in the precapillary arterioles or capillaries. Because only approximately 50,000 particles are injected, the small number of blocked capillaries does not significantly disturb the microcirculation of the vascular bed in which the particles are lodged. Twenty to thirty minutes following injection, images are obtained with a gamma camera. Because blood to the right and left coronary arteries is differentially tagged, it is possible to determine whether blood flow to myocardium is derived only from the native vessel or whether a contribution from the contralateral artery exists. As with 201-thallium imaging, various stresses may be used to exaggerate the difference between flows to high- and low-flow areas. One radioactive label would then be injected before, and the second after, initiation of the stress. Exercise[137] and coronary hyperemia following Renografin injection[134] have been used to uncover perfusion defects.

3. Intraoperative Measurements

Exposure of the heart at the time of thoracotomy for attachment of vein grafts to coronary arteries distal to stenotic lesions[113,114,138] and cannulation of the arteries through an aortotomy[139] have provided unique opportunities to evaluate collateral function in man. As described in Chapter 4, peripheral coronary pressure and retrograde flow are collateral indices that have been used extensively in the experimental animal. The former is a measure of the residual pressure in the arterial bed after antegrade flow has been stopped, and the latter is the rate of blood flow from the distal arterial bed issuing from a proximal arteriotomy site after elimination of antegrade flow. Neither index measures collateral flow directly. Whereas several factors may influence these indices, in general, both retrograde flow and peripheral coronary pressure increase as collateral capacity and flow increase.

Reactive hyperemia is a measure of vascular reserve, and is the increased flow that appears following release of a transient coronary occlusion (see Chapter 5). Briefly, coronary occlusion results in myocardial ischemia and maximal arteriolar vasodilatation. Flow through the dilated vessels following restoration of antegrade perfusion is typically four to five times the baseline level. Several investigators have evaluated the magnitude of reactive hyperemia at the time of surgery in patients receiving saphenous vein bypass grafts.[140−144] By preventing or attenuating ischemia following elimination of antegrade flow, a well-developed collateral circulation may result in diminution of the expected arteriolar dilatation and reactive hyperemia response. Therefore, the functional adequacy of intercoronary anastomoses may be assessed. It should be noted, however, that factors other than a well-developed collateral circulation may also diminish reactive hyperemia (see Chapters 2 and 5).

It is also possible to assess collateral flow directly at the time of thoracotomy. Sullivan[119] injected [85]Kr and Horwitz[145] injected [133]Xe 3 mm below the epicardial surface, and then followed washout with a scintillation probe, as has been described above. Quantitation of collateral flow was possible if the isotope was injected into myocardium in the perfusion territory of an occluded vessel. Obviously this type of flow measurement, as well as determination of peripheral coronary pressure, retrograde flow, and reactive hyperemia, has limited application and usefulness because of the requirement for thoracotomy.

4. Measurements during Cardiac Catheterization

Since the introduction of coronary angioplasty, clinicians have had another method to evaluate collateral function.[146] During this procedure, a balloon dilatation catheter is advanced through a guiding catheter into a stenotic coronary artery and across the lesion. During balloon dilatation, antegrade flow ceases and pressure in the distal coronary artery represents the collateral index peripheral coronary pressure. A multithermistor catheter advanced into the coronary sinus can be selectively positioned to record changes in flow from the myocardial territory perfused by the artery containing the balloon. Thus, residual flow following balloon expansion and cessation of antegrade flow is a measure of collateral flow to that region. Finally, an index of collateral resistance can be calculated by dividing the difference between aortic and distal coronary pressures by the residual coronary flow during transient balloon occlusion of the coronary artery. Hence, this new technique permits extensive in-vivo evaluation of collateral function.

IV. Anatomy of the Coronary Arterial and Collateral Circulations

The coronary collateral circulation is a complex network consisting of mainly preformed but also some newly formed (transepicardial) vascular channels that can redistribute available blood supply to virtually any region of the heart and can supplement the traditional coronary blood supply from extracardiac and even intraluminal sources (Figure 1-4). The collateral circulation may be subdivided into two major anatomical groups: intracardiac and extracardiac anastomoses. Each of these two major divisions may be further subdivided on the basis of site and origin. Thus, interarterial and endomural channels are intracardiac, while retrocardiac and transepicardial connections are extracardiac. Not all four subgroups are equally important, but each will be described below. To better appreciate the course of special

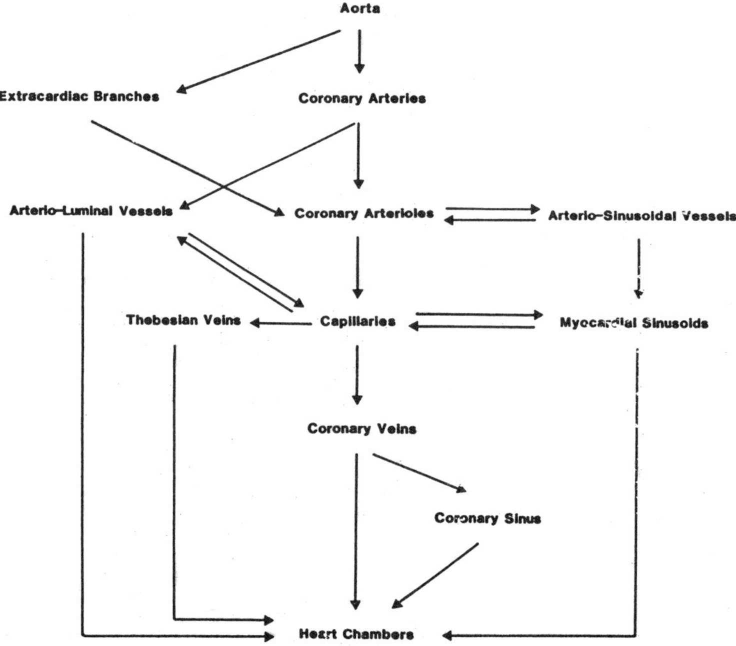

Figure 1-4   Schematic representation of the many possible sources of collateral flow to the myocardium. Whereas intercoronary collaterals redistribute blood within the cardiac tissue, endomural and extracardiac anastomotic channels supplement the traditional coronary blood supply.

intercoronary anastomoses, a brief review of the anatomy of the major epicardial coronary arteries and transmural perforating branches will precede description of the distribution of coronary collateral vessels.

A. Normal Coronary Arteries

The coronary artery network itself may easily be divided into two parts: extramural or epicardial arteries, and mural or intramyocardial vessels. The former are well known to most clinicians because of the standard use of coronary angiography as a diagnostic tool, and therefore require less description. The latter, on the other hand, are less well appreciated. It should be noted that even epicardial vessels, especially the left anterior descending artery, may plunge beneath the surface for variable distances and be covered by myocardial bridges.[147,148]

1. Epicardial Arteries

The right coronary artery arises from the right or anterior aortic sinus and courses in the right atrioventricular groove toward the apex of the heart.

It initially passes beneath the right atrial appendage, extends to the acute margin of the heart, and then loops around onto the heart's diaphragmatic surface (Figure 1-5). The length of the diaphragmatic portion of the right coronary artery is quite variable and depends largely on the length of the terminal segment of the left circumflex artery.[16,149,150] The right and left atrioventricular grooves through which the right coronary and left circumflex arteries course form a circle, and meet near the cardiac apex. The further the left circumflex vessel extends into the right atrioventricular groove, the shorter is the right coronary artery. The reciprocal relationship between terminations of the two vessels affects the pattern of coronary dominance or preponderance, a useful topographic classification of the extramural coronary circulation. The artery extending beyond the crux, a major crossroads at which the two principal sulci of the heart (the left and right atrioventricular sulci being halves of one and the interventricular and posterior interatrial sulci joining to form the other) meet, determines dominance.[151] In a right dominant system, the right coronary artery extends beyond the crux to supply the posterior aspect of the left ventricle (Figure 1-5), while the left

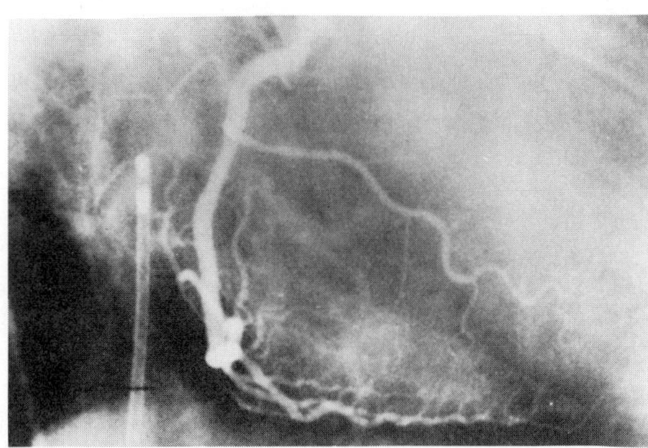

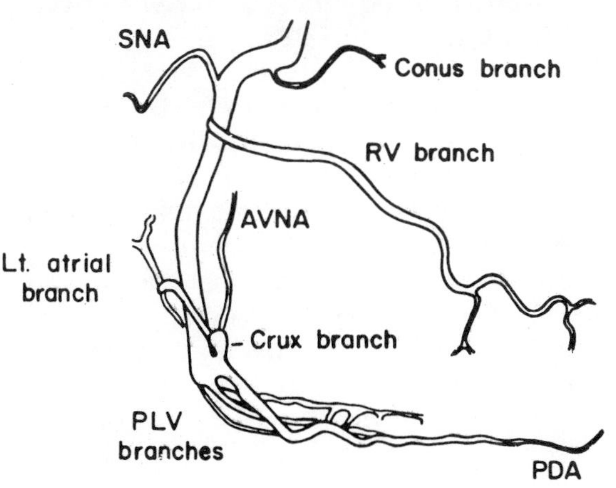

Figure 1-5A Angiographic frame and artist's drawing from right coronary angiogram in the right anterior oblique projection. This is a right dominant coronary system in which the right coronary artery gives rise to the atrioventricular node (AVNA) and the posterior descending (PDA) arteries. The crux branch is the continuation of the right coronary artery in the atrioventricular groove beyond the crux. PLV = posterior left ventricular; RV = right ventricular; SNA = sinus node artery. (Angiogram provided by Hugo Spindola-Franco, M.D., Department of Radiology, Montefiore Medical Center, Bronx, NY.)

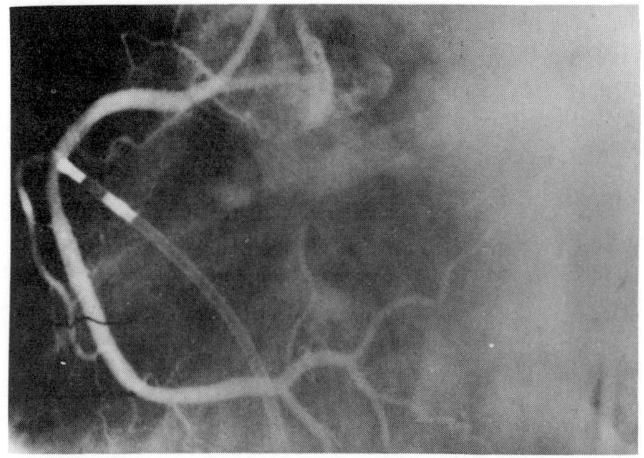

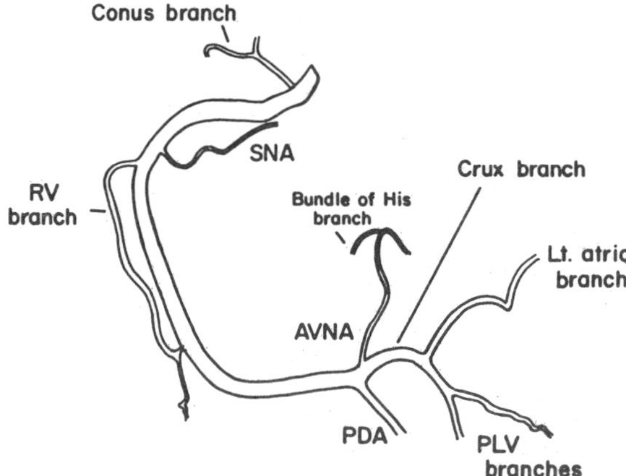

Figure 1-5B Angiographic frame and artist's drawing from right coronary angiogram in the left anterior oblique projection. See Figure 1-5A. (Angiogram provided by Hugo Spindola-Franco, M.D., Department of Radiology, Montefiore Medical Center, Bronx, NY.)

circumflex artery crosses the crux in left dominance. If neither vessel crosses the crux, the circulation is balanced. The terminal portion of the right coronary artery frequently divides into two or three branches which then descend on the posterior surface of the left ventricle.

Atrial branches of the right coronary artery are variable in size, number, and location. The sinoatrial node artery (Figures 1-5 and 1-6 [colorplate]) is usually the first major branch of this artery, and is an integral part of a special anastomotic pathway (see below). The artery to the sinoatrial node typically ramifies into ascending and descending branches that perfuse the atrial myocardium. In 8–20% of hearts,[20,152] an even more proximal branch of the right coronary artery, the descending septal artery, is evident. This vessel courses down the aortic root, sending branches to the periaortic connective tissue and parts of the crista supraventricularis before entering the superior border of the interventricular septum and ramifying. Small arterial twigs from the main coronary artery extend for short distances over the surface of the right atrium and can form intracoronary anastomoses to bypass proximal obstructions. One last atrial branch, an intermediate atrial artery, ascends to anastomose with the branch of the sinus node artery encircling the ostium of the superior vena cava.

Ventricular branches of the right coronary artery are also variable in length and importance. In 50% of hearts,[153] the first ventricular branch is the right conus branch which crosses the root of the pulmonary artery to anastomose with a similar branch from the left coronary artery. On the anterior surface of the right ventricle two main branches descend to the lower third of the heart, giving off several parallel twigs that extend horizontally to anastomose with similar branches of the left anterior descending artery. The acute marginal branch originates at the heart's acute margin and follows the margin toward the apex. At the level of the caudal third of the ventricle, this branch often turns posteriorly and extends transversely across the right ventricle's posterior surface to reach the posterior interventricular sulcus.

Greater than 77% of hearts are either right dominant or balanced.[6,16,18,31,60,63,149,151,154,155] In these hearts the right coronary artery reaches or passes the crux and gives off the posterior descending artery (Figure 1-5). This major branch descends in the posterior interventricular sulcus toward the apex, but usually ends before reaching it. The posterior descending artery gives rise to a variable number of posterior septal or penetrating branches which perfuse the posterior one-third to one-half of the interventricular septum and anastomose with the anterior septal branches from the left anterior descending artery (see below).

When the right coronary artery reaches the crux, it makes a sharp U-shaped turn, and at the apex of the U, the atrioventricular nodal artery originates (Figures 1-5 and 1-7 [colorplate]). This latter branch (see below) runs anteriorly to the base of the interatrial septum and supplies the atrioventricular node, bundle of His, and proximal bundle branches. This vessel makes numerous important anastomoses with atrial arteries in the interatrial septum and with perforating branches from the left coronary artery (Kugel's arteria anastomotica auricularis magna; see below).

The left (main) coronary artery arises from the left anterior sinus of Valsalva and courses anteriorly and to the left where, under cover of the left atrial appendage, it bifurcates into two large branches: the left anterior descending and left circumflex arteries (Figures 1-8 and 1-9). The length of the left main coronary artery is typically less than 2 cm. Occasionally (0.6–0.9%), there is no distinct left main coronary artery[60,63] and the left anterior descending and circumflex arteries originate from a common orifice or possibly separate ostia in the aortic wall.

The left anterior descending artery is almost a direct continuation of the left main coronary artery (Figures 1-8 and 1-9). It emerges from behind the left atrial appendage in the anterior interventricular sulcus. This artery descends toward the apex, and in a majority of hearts rounds the apex and ascends in the posterior interventricular sulcus for 5–30 mm (ramus recurrens).[154] In 3.8–5% of hearts the left anterior descending artery bifurcates shortly after its own origin into two vessels of equal size that descend toward the apex along either side of the anterior interventricular sulcus.[60,63]

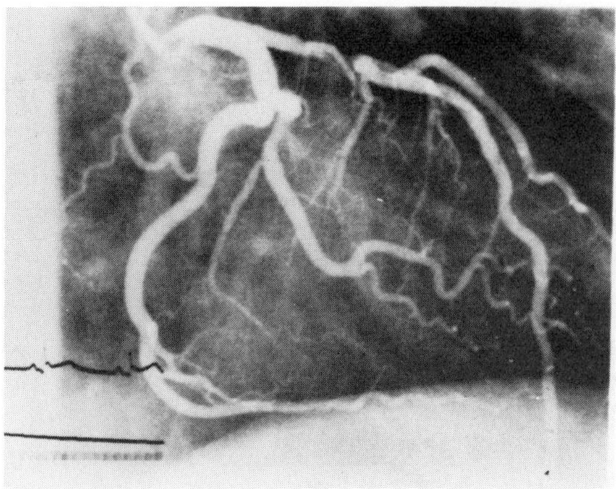

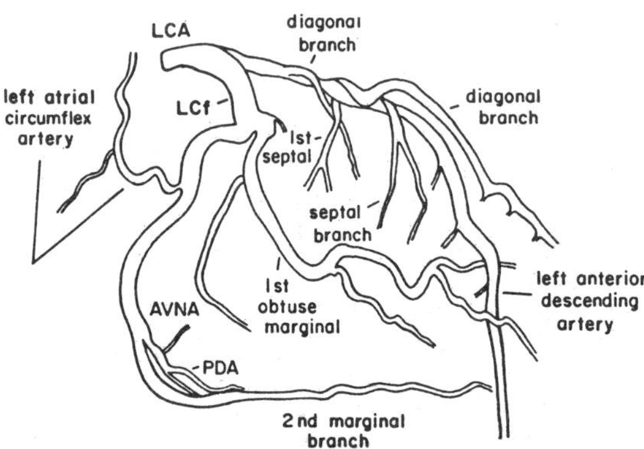

Figure 1-8A   Angiographic frame and artist's drawing from left coronary (LCA) angiogram in the right anterior oblique projection. This is a left dominant coronary system in which the left circumflex artery gives rise to the atrioventricular node (AVNA) and the posterior descending (PDA) arteries. (Angiogram provided by Hugo Spindola-Franco, M.D., Department of Radiology, Montefiore Medical Center, Bronx, NY.)

As the left anterior descending artery descends, it supplies three or four transverse twigs to the right ventricle. The first of these branches, the left conus artery, is larger than the others and ascends to the pulmonary conus where it may anastomose with a similar artery from the right coronary artery, forming the circle of Vieussens (see below).

Left ventricular branches arise from the main vessel at acute angles and course in parallel fashion over the anterior surface of the left ventricle toward the heart's obtuse margin. Of these diagonal branches, the first is the biggest. This latter artery may originate in the fork of the left main coronary artery bifurcation where the anterior interventricular and left atrioventricular sulci meet. In such cases it is called a median branch (ramus medianus). Smith[32] noted a median branch in 20% of his hearts, while Baroldi and Scomazzoni[60] found it in 33% of their autopsy material. When a median artery is present, adjacent diagonal and obtuse marginal branches tend to be smaller since their perfusion territories are in part usurped by that of the median branch. The latter usually bifurcates and the two branches extend downward toward the apex. Less commonly, diagonal branches may arise from the left circum-

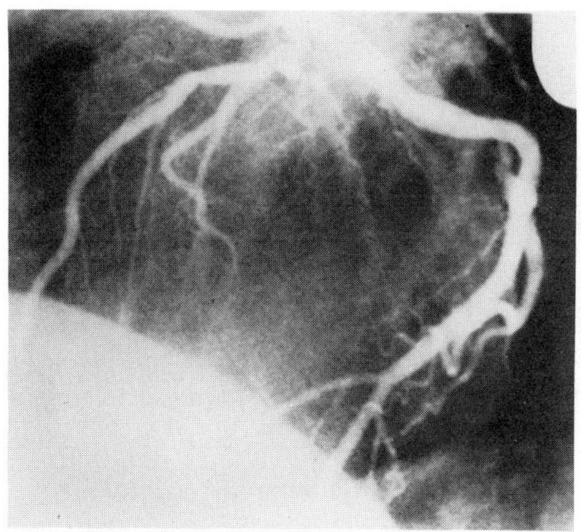

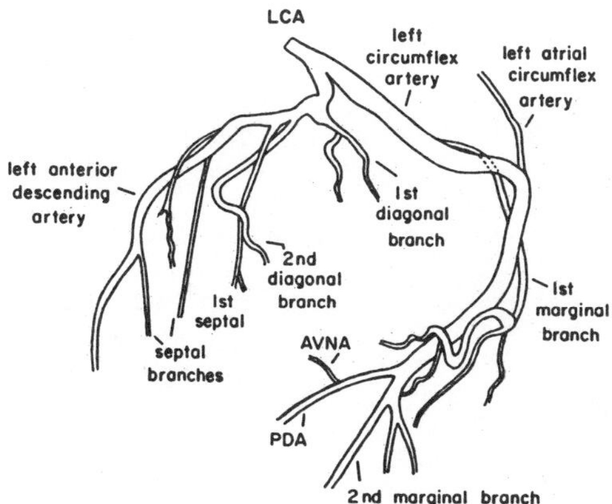

Figure 1-8B Angiographic frame and artist's drawing from left coronary angiogram in the left anterior oblique projection. See Figure 1-8A. (Angiogram provided by Hugo Spindola-Franco, M.D., Department of Radiology, Montefiore Medical Center, Bronx, NY.)

flex artery. The diagonal left ventricular branches of the left anterior descending artery generally extend beyond the obtuse margin and end in the posterior left ventricular wall. In addition to these epicardial branches, the left anterior descending artery gives rise along its length to eight to fourteen septal or perforating vessels. These septal arteries originate from the posterior aspect of the left anterior descending artery, immediately penetrate the interventricular septum, and course downward and diagonally in an anteroposterior direction (see below). The septal arteries perfuse the anterior two-thirds of the interventricular septum. Either the first or second septal artery is usually the largest perforating branch.[60,156] Because of the proximity of these anterior septal branches to the posterior septal branches arising from the posterior descending artery, numerous anastomoses may be visualized (see below).

The second major branch of the left main coronary artery is the left circumflex artery (Figures 1-8 and 1-9). This vessel runs in the left atrio-

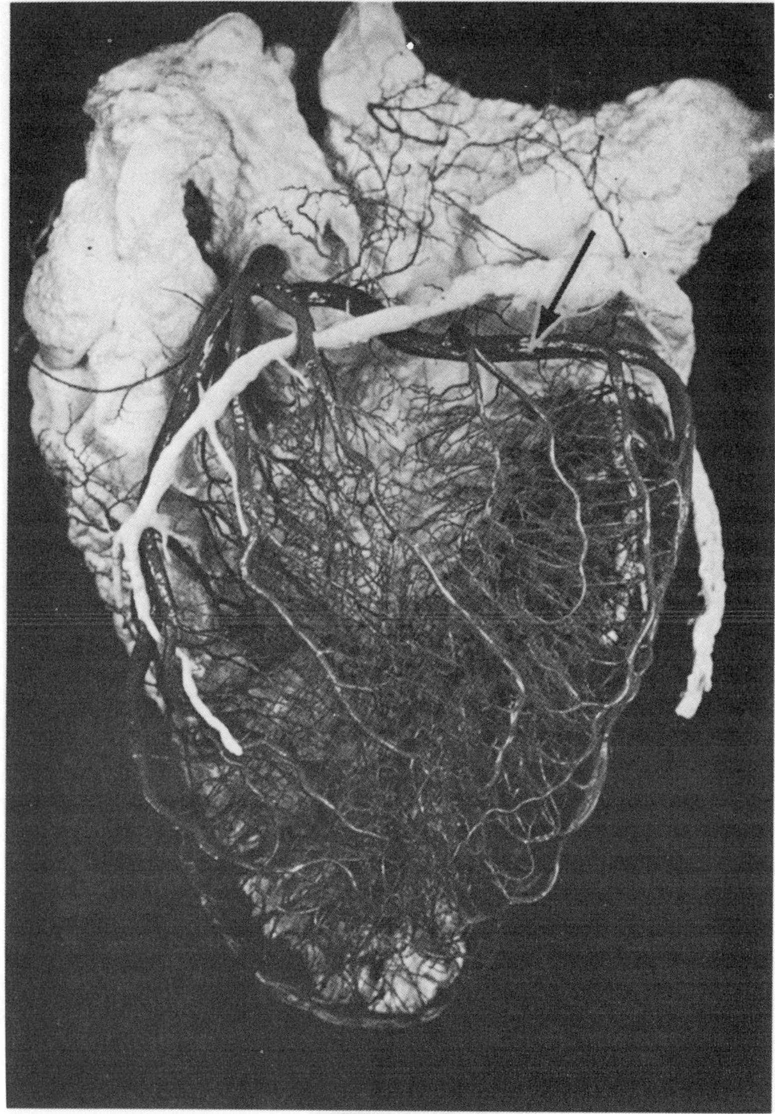

Figure 1-9   Cast viewed from the anterolateral surface of the uncast left ventricle demonstrating origin of main left coronary artery from the aorta. It quickly bifurcates into left circumflex artery (arrow) which passes laterally in the left atrioventricular groove and the left anterior descending artery, which descends along the left border of the specimen in the anterior interventricular groove to the apex. Parts of the coronary venous system are cast in white and are seen crossing superficial to the coronary arteries. (Reprinted with permission of Harper & Row, Publishers, from James.[63])

ventricular sulcus. Its proximal portion is often obscured by the left atrial appendage. This vessel initially runs roughly parallel to the base of the heart. After bending around the heart's obtuse margin onto the posterior aspect of the left ventricle, the left circumflex artery more or less abruptly curves downward toward the apex. The termination of this artery is extremely variable. It may terminate before or at the left margin, or continue onto the posterior wall and end either before, at, or beyond the posterior interventricular groove. As already described, the terminations of the left circumflex and right coronary arteries are reciprocally related. In approximately 15–20% of hearts, the posterior descending artery is a continuation of the left circumflex artery in the posterior interventricular groove[6,16,18,31,60,149,151,154,155] (Figure 1-10). In the majority of these cases the posterior descending artery is a single branch. However, in a few hearts, two equally large vessels—one a continuation of the circumflex and the other a branch of the right coronary artery—may be found running in a parallel fashion down the posterior interventricular sulcus.

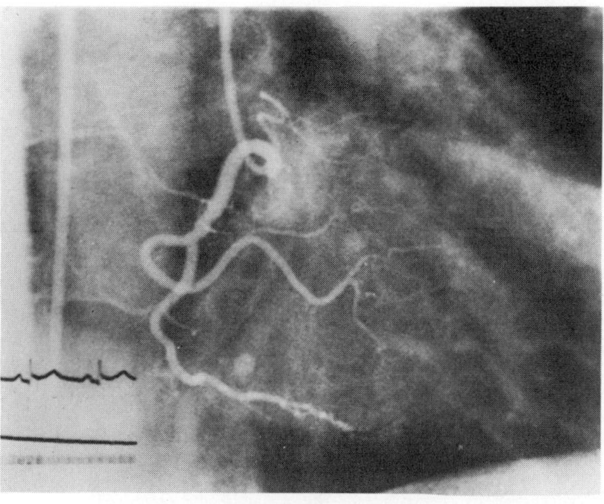

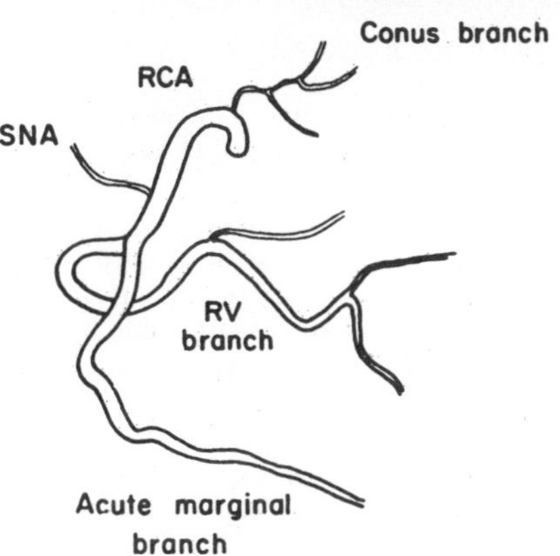

Figure 1-10A   Angiographic frame and artist's drawing from right coronary (RCA) angiogram in the right anterior oblique projection. This is a left dominant coronary system. Therefore, the right coronary artery perfuses mainly right ventricular myocardium and very little left ventricular tissue. The course of this nondominant RCA should be compared to that of the dominant RCA in Figure 1-5A. See Figure 1-5A for abbreviations. (Angiogram provided by Hugo Spindola-Franco, M.D., Department of Radiology, Montefiore Medical Center, Bronx, NY.)

Anterior, intermediate or marginal, and posterior atrial branches of the left circumflex artery course over the epicardial surface of the left atrium. The distribution and number of these branches are very variable. The sinus node artery, an anterior atrial branch, may originate from the left circumflex artery, and does so in approximately 40% of hearts[6,16,18,60,63] (see below). A second atrial branch involved in special anastomotic pathways is Kugel's artery (see below). A third large atrial branch is the left atrial circumflex artery. This proximal branch of the left circumflex artery runs along the lower margin of the left atrium parallel to the left atrioventricular sulcus and its source artery. It extends around the obtuse margin to the posterior left atrial surface. If sufficiently long, the left atrial circumflex artery may also provide arterial twigs to the posterior wall of the right atrium.

There are anterior and posterior extramural left ventricular branches. The number of these branches is dependent on the point of termination of the left circumflex artery. In some hearts right posterior ventricular branches can be found. One anterior left ventricular branch arises 0.8−1.5 cm from the origin of the left circumflex artery and perfuses the anterosuperior aspect of the left ventricle. This obtuse marginal artery is a large, fairly constant

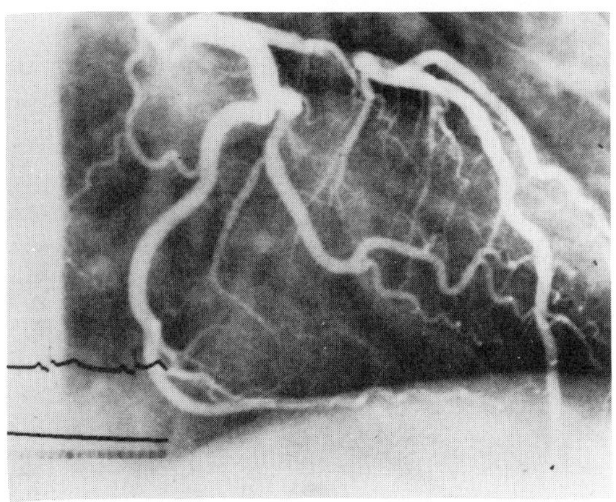

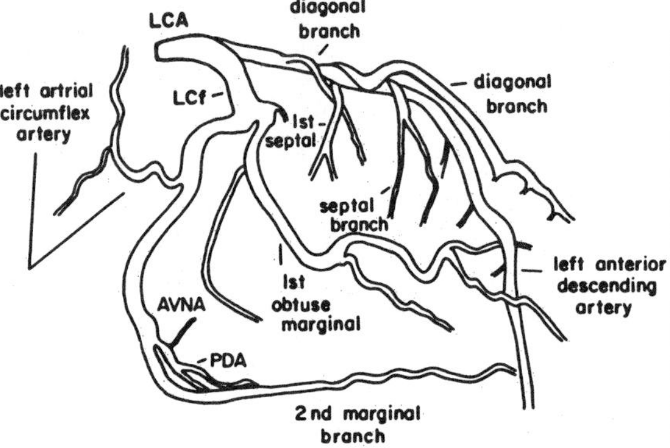

Figure 1-10B Angiographic frame and artist's drawing from left coronary (LCA) angiogram in the right anterior oblique projection. The dominant left circumflex artery gives rise to both the atrioventricular node (AVNA) and the posterior descending (PDA) arteries. (Angiogram provided by Hugo Spindola-Franco, M.D., Department of radiology, Montefiore Medical Center, Bronx, NY.)

(90%)[60] branch that arises at a right or acute angle from the circumflex artery on the anterior or lateral surface of the left ventricle, and then descends vertically or more rarely obliquely toward the apex. The obtuse marginal artery is sometimes really two parallel vessels, each with two or three secondary branches. Posterior or diaphragmatic branches may also be present. In left dominant hearts in which the posterior descending artery is a continuation of the left circumflex artery, the atrioventricular nodal artery arising at the crux is also usually a left circumflex branch (Figure 1-11 [colorplate]).

2. *Intramyocardial Vasculature*

Although the epicardial vessels described above are easily identified with either clinical angiographic or postmortem injection techniques, intramural arteries are not often visualized during routine angiographic procedures. Furthermore, because obstructive disease of the coronary arteries is mainly restricted to extramural vessels, most clinicians know little of the intramyocardial vasculature. This latter arterial network is vital, however, for formation of critical anastomotic pathways and flow redistribution following obstruction of epicardial vessels.

As the large epicardial vessels leave the atrioventricular ring, they course over the left ventricular epicardial surface. As they pass toward the apex, these vessels generally give off some superficial branches. After attaining a size of 1–3 mm, deep tributaries branch off the main vessels at right angles and penetrate the myocardium.[56,157–161] Although the radiographs of left ventricular cross-sections following intracoronary injection of barium sulphate-gelatin mixtures published by Gross[6,21] nicely demonstrated these intramural branches, a detailed description of the mural circulation was not available until Estes[157] published his observations in 1966. His reports were soon followed by the confirmatory studies of Farrer-Brown[159,160] and Kato.[161] The tributaries branching from the main epicardial vessels range in diameter from 400–1,500 μm, and can be grouped into two distinct classes. The Class A branches of Estes,[157] the branching type arteries of Farrer-Brown,[159] and the Type I vessels of Kato[161] are similar. These arteries quickly divide soon after their origin into cascading treelike structures (Figures 1-12 and 1-13). Numerous branches supply the myocardium, and the caliber of the main perforating vessel gradually diminishes as it extends toward the endocardium. Estes[157] observed these vessels to supply only the outer three-fourths to four-fifths of the myocardial wall, but technical difficulties probably prevented him from following the arterioles into the endocardial layers. Both Farrer-Brown[159] and Kato[161] noted that this type of intramural vessel extended to within several millimeters of the endocardial surface, and many terminal branches supplied the subendocardial zone. This type of myocardial perforator has few anastomoses as it passes from the surface of the left ventricle to the subendocardial myocardium.

The second type of perforating myocardial vessel—Estes's Class B

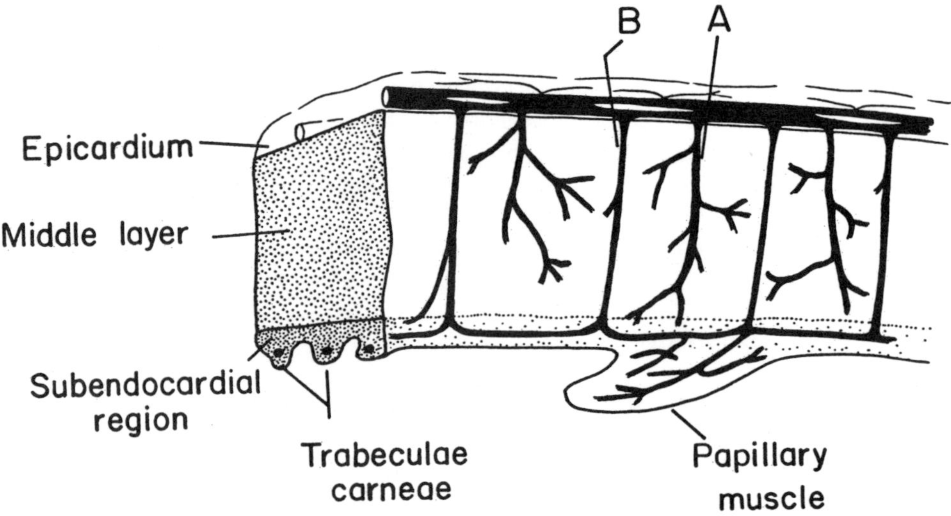

Figure 1-12   Schematic drawing of longitudinal section through left ventricular wall demonstrating branching of the two major types of perforating vessels from the epicardial artery. The one type (A) quickly divides after its origin into cascading treelike structures, and numerous branches supply the myocardium. The second type (B) passes almost directly from its point of origin to the subendocardium with minimal decrease in diameter and infrequent mid-myocardial branches. At or near the subendocardium these vessels subdivide into multiple branches that anastomose with similar branches from adjacent perforating vessels to form looping arcades. (Modified and printed with permission of Japanese Circulation Society from Kato.[161])

branch,[157] Farrer-Brown's straight-type artery,[159] and Kato's Type II vessel [161]—follows a very different course (Figures 1-12 and 1-13). At their origin these vessels generally have diameters of $50-500$ μm, and reach the subendocardium with almost no decrease in size since few mid-wall branches are given off. At or near the subendocardium these vessels subdivide into multiple branches that form looping arcades. These arcades anastomose freely in the subendocardium and form a large subendocardial plexus (see below).

This pattern of left ventricular free wall vascularity is also observed in the right ventricle.[162] However, because of the latter's thinner wall, the perforators generally arise at acute rather than right angles from the epicardial vessels on the surface.

Blood supply to the left ventricle's anterolateral papillary muscle generally comes from the left anterior descending coronary artery, although the left circumflex artery occasionally is the source. The posteromedial papillary muscle usually derives its blood supply from the posterior descending artery which in turn is most often a branch of the right coronary artery, except in left dominant hearts where the left circumflex artery may give rise to it (see above). The fingerlike papillary muscles which extend into the ventricular lumen are supplied by straight-type arteries.[158,163] Single, nonanastomosing central

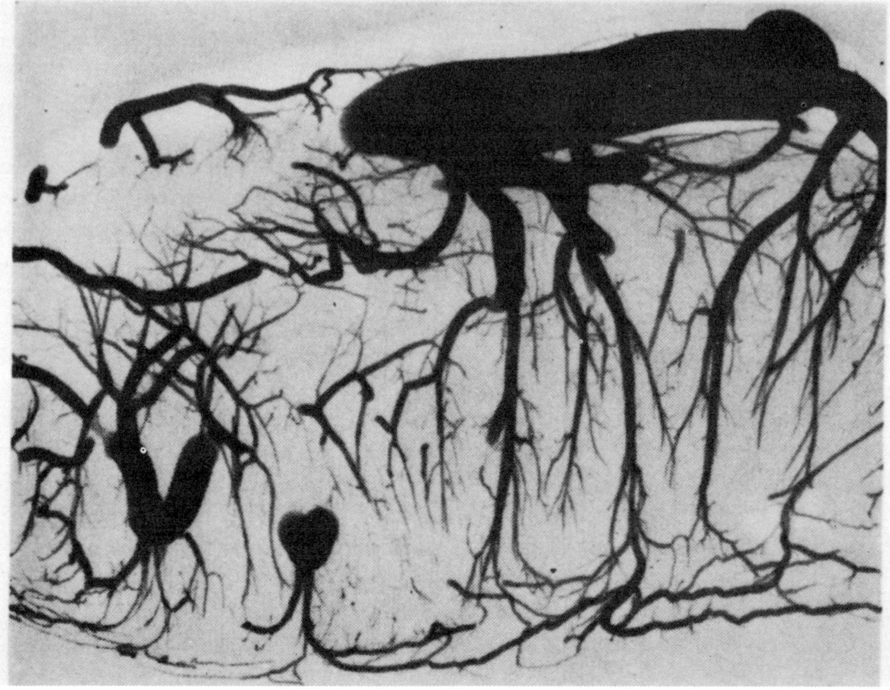

Figure 1-13   Microradiograph of perforating vessels in the left ventricular wall. A portion of an epicardial artery lying on top gives rise to type A and B mural branches. The latter terminate in the subendocardial plexus on the bottom of the photograph. (Reprinted with permission of Charles C. Thomas, Publisher, from Fulton.[56])

arteries extend to the muscle's tip. The flatter, tethered papillary muscles have a different pattern of vascular supply. There is no single central artery, but instead a segmental distribution of several long, penetrating arteries that have rich anastomoses between themselves as well as with the adjacent extra-papillary subendocardial vascular plexus.

B. Coronary Collateral Circulation

1. Intracardiac Anastomoses

(a) Histology and morphology

Although the histology of coronary collaterals has been well defined in the experimental animal (see Chapter 5), few reports of examinations in man are available.[61,161,164,165] As in the experimental animal, the histologic pattern of human collaterals is dependent on the collateral's size and stage of development. In larger collaterals, the endothelial intimal layer is separated from the muscular tunica media by an internal elastic membrane that is often incomplete. The latter observation suggests that collateral development and transformation may never be complete in man, although Schaper[164,165] has noted that well-developed collaterals have normal arterial structure. The thickness of the muscular layer is variable. Whereas muscle cells in the wall of a small collateral may be rare or even absent, resulting in a capillarylike vessel, the larger collateral may have a tunica media consisting of multiple layers of muscle cells. The tunica media acounts for the ability of the collateral to respond to pharmacologic and other vasomotor stimuli (see Chapter 3).

As extensively detailed above, coronary collaterals are present in a majority of, and probably even all, normal hearts.[36,44−52,54−67] The timing of appearance of collaterals in the developing fetus is not known. Vastesaeger[57] examined the heart from one five-month-old fetus and was unable to detect any evidence of anastomoses, although all term fetuses and newborns dying shortly after birth had collaterals with 70−200 μm diameters. These latter data confirm the earlier observations of Spalteholz.[16] Reiner's[47] extensive analysis of hearts of stillborns and premature and term infants dying several days after birth revealed that 11 of 16 hearts from stillborns and 22 of 39 hearts from infants born alive had collaterals. These frequencies are similar. However, the appearance of collaterals was affected by the degree of fetal maturity. Thus, more mature babies (24 of 30) than premature infants (9 of 25) had detectable collaterals ($p = 0.01$). Reiner[47] also felt that good collaterals progressively involuted during the first decade of life, and then reappeared during the second decade. On the other hand, Bloor et al.,[67] who injected wax sphere suspensions into coronary arteries of 20 children ranging in age from 0−14 years observed that the size and frequency of intercoronary anastomoses were the same in the first and second decades of life. Laurie and Woods[45] observed that only 11% of children under the age of five years had collaterals, although they attributed this low frequency to technical difficulties experienced during injection of the small arteries of these hearts. In a group of hearts examined after the main series had been compiled, Laurie and Woods[45] found rich anastomoses in three newborn hearts. Pepler and Meyer[46] also injected the hearts of children, and observed that 50% of European children dying before their tenth birthday and 80% of Bantu children had either moderate or good coronary collaterals.

There was no difference in the incidence of collateralization between male and female fetuses of comparable gestational age.[47] Baroldi[61,166] was also unable to detect any effect of sex. On the other hand, Omar and Rao[52] observed bigger collaterals in male hearts.

In Baroldi's series,[166] the maximum collateral diameter in newborns was 50 μm. Vastesaeger[57] noted larger collaterals ranging from 70−200 μm in hearts from term fetuses and newborn infants. In Bloor's postmortem studies,[67] in children without cardiac disease, wax spheres of 63−74 μm diameter passed from one coronary artery to the other in 15 of the 20 hearts, while in the others, smaller spheres were recovered in the effluent recovered from the nonperfused artery. In no hearts were 100–120 μm spheres recovered. In normal adult human hearts the diameters of collaterals have generally ranged from 20–350 μm.[36,44,49,51,52,54,56,57,59,61,63,166,167] Fulton[54] noted smaller collaterals in the atrial walls (20–100 μm) than in the interventricular septum (100–300 μm). Some studies have also revealed larger collaterals in these normal hearts. Omar and Rao[52] and Fulton[167] occasionally observed collaterals as large as 500 μm, and Tsuchiya[51] noted that 16% of his normal hearts had collaterals with diameters exceeding 400 μm. In Vastesaeger's series[57] of normal hearts, 6.5% had collateral diameters ranging from 300 μm to 1 mm. Baroldi[166] counted all collaterals with diameters exceeding 100–150 μm. The mean diameter ranged from 150–280 μm in the normal adult heart, while the average diameter was 200 μm.

Collaterals appear in virtually all parts of the heart,[57,61,63,167] especially the interventricular septum and free walls of the atria and left ventricle,[51,57,63] and at all depths.[44,52,61,164–166,168] Rodriguez and Robbins[49] have claimed that one-third of anastomoses are in the atrial walls. Robbins et al.[50] observed that right coronary artery perfusion with an injectate mass revealed the greatest number of collaterals, while left anterior descending coronary artery perfusion was a close second. In contrast, perfusion of the left circumflex artery was a distant third. In general, most intramyocardial arterial branches communicate at different levels with adjacent branches throughout the whole thickness of the left ventricular wall. Therefore, a diffuse anastomotic network is apparent in any intramyocardial area except the true immediate subepicardial region where only occasional anastomoses are apparent. Fulton[54,167] found that most collaterals in man were deep within the myocardial wall, while epicardial anastomoses were seen mainly at the apex. Schaper[164,165] also noted a relative paucity of subepicardial collaterals. On the other hand, James[63] observed the largest collaterals to be near the epicardium. Both Bellman and Frank[44] and Omar and Rao[52] felt that the collateral distribution was densest in the innermost and outermost layers of the myocardium.

Intramyocardial collaterals course obliquely or parallel to the muscle layers,[61] and are often finely coiled.[59,67] In the septum, bundles of parallel collateral vessels join the anterior and posterior descending branches. A fine netlike reticulum of vessels running parallel to the surface is found in the subendocardium, while a meshlike pattern is observed in the walls of the atria.[61]

In hearts with obstructed coronary arteries, a biochemical and/or biophysical stimulus results in collateral transformation (see Chapters 3, 5, and 7). Collateral diameters are greatly increased in coronary artery disease.[34,36,49,51,54,56,59–61,63,166,169] Baroldi[166] has concluded that the increase in size of the collaterals is proportional to the severity of the arterial narrowing. Thus, there is minimal change for stenoses under 60%. For lesions compromising 60–80% of the luminal diameter, the anastomotic index (see above) doubled. This index was maximally increased when the artery was obstructed. Rodriguez and Robbins[49] noted collateral diameters as large as 5 mm in hearts with severe obstructive disease. Baroldi et al.[59] observed that the average collateral diameter in pathologic hearts exceeded 500 μm, while the maximum diameter was 2 mm. This greatly increased collateral size accounts for the ease with which collaterals can be identified in hearts with coronary lesions. The apparent increase in numbers of collaterals in these latter hearts is most likely a reflection of this ease of identification and probably not the result of de-novo formation.

(b) Interarterial collaterals

(i) Intercoronary

Intercoronary or primary anastomoses are interconnections between any two coronary arteries or their respective branches (Figures 1-14A and 1-15). These collateral channels are generally present in border or watershed regions supplied by branches of two or more coronary arteries, and are found at all depths in the myocardial wall.[44] When the source and recipient arteries are patent, the numerous normal intercoronary anastomoses are slender and straight or gently curving.[65] Their diameter is most frequently less than 100 μm,[65] but may range from 20−350 μm,[59,166] and their length is 2−3 cm.[59] Because of their size and absence of a pressure gradient along their length, collaterals in normal hearts of living patients are rarely visualized with clinical angiographic techniques.[170,171] However, in individuals without

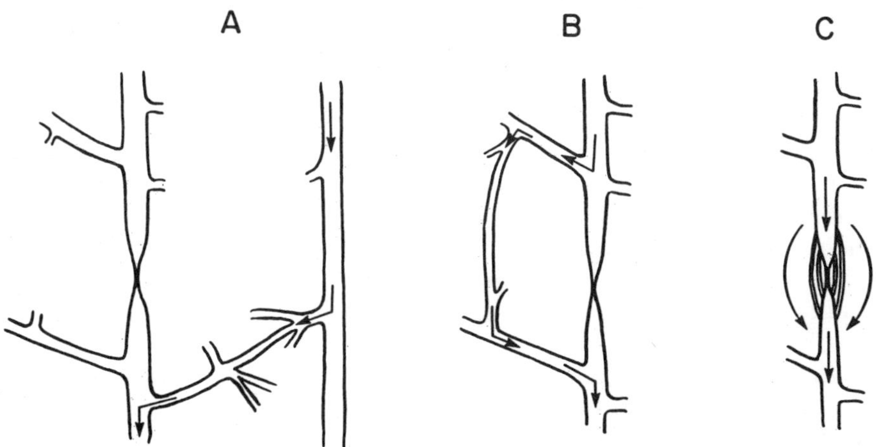

Figure 1-14   Diagrammatic representation of the three different types of inter-arterial collateral vessels. (A) Intercoronary collateral or primary anastomosis connects two different arteries. (B) Intracoronary collateral or secondary anastomosis links branches of the same artery. (C)Bridging collateral or tertiary anastomosis, a special kind of intracoronary collateral, bridges an obstruction and connects the proximal and distal segments of the artery. Arrows indicate direction of blood flow through the collateral channel.

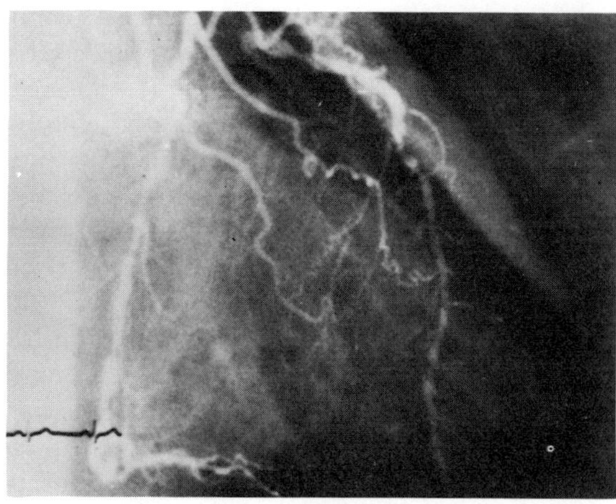

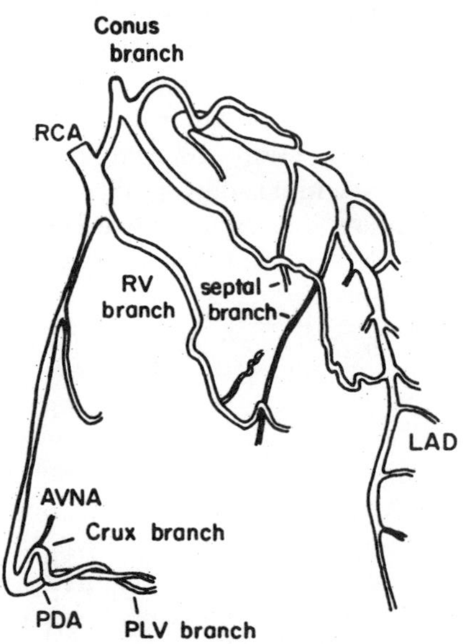

Figure 1-15 Angiographic frame and artist's drawing from right coronary (RCA) angiogram in the right anterior oblique projection. The left anterior descending (LAD) coronary artery is completely occluded at its origin. Yet the entire course of the LAD beyond this obstruction is clearly seen because of opacification by large intercoronary collaterals coursing from the proximal RCA to the LAD. The major source of collaterals is the conus branch of the RCA, which crosses the pulmonary conus and forms a semicircle as it anastomoses with analogous branches from the proximal LAD. This arterial circle or ring is called the Circle of Vieussens. The RCA is critically narrowed in its proximal third. See Figure 1-5A for abbreviations.

fixed lesions, intercoronary collaterals may be visualized angiographically if a pressure gradient is established between adjacent coronary beds. Thus, spontaneous or catheter-induced spasm of one coronary artery,[172–179] creation of a coronary arteriovenous fistula with consequent decrease of intracoronary pressure in the involved arterial bed,[180] or injection of angiographic contrast agent through a catheter wedged into a coronary artery[85,170] produce the proper hemodynamic conditions allowing collateral visualization. In individual cases, collaterals may also be identified with angiography in the absence of documented spasm, catheter wedging, or other recognized abnormality.[171,181] All of these reports again emphasize that coronary collaterals are present, even in hearts without coronary atherosclerosis. As noted above, collaterals are significantly larger when the coronary arteries are obstructed. When stenoses exceed 90%, the presssure gradient across the collateral entering the diseased vessel distal to the lesion favors angiographic opacification of the anastomotic channel.[168] Cosby and colleagues[182] have noted that intercoronary collaterals are visualized mainly in those with prior myocardial infarctions.

Rodriguez and Robbins[49] concluded that intercoronary anastomoses in the normal heart accounted for two-thirds of the heart's collaterals, and Omar and Rao[52] and Robbins et al.[50] concurred. Tsuchiya[51] detected this type of collateral in all of his specimens. Approximately 80% of normal or minimally atherosclerotic hearts injected by Robbins[50] also had primary intercoronary anastomoses. However, Baroldi[166] believes that intercoronary collaterals make up only a small part of the heart's collateral network. The greatest density of intercoronary collaterals appears to be in the interventricular septum[49–51,59] and anterior left ventricular wall.[50] Anastomoses between the left anterior descending and right coronary arteries are the most typical intercoronary collaterals in hearts free of coronary stenoses, and were present in 95% of hearts studied by Tsuchiya[51] with postmortem angiography. In contrast, only 58% of hearts had connections betwen the left anterior descending and left circumflex arteries, while as few as 19% of the cases demonstrated right coronary–left circumflex collaterals. In hearts with coronary obstructive disease the distribution of left anterior descending–left circumflex (81%) and right coronary–left circumflex (55%) collaterals increased dramatically.[51]

(ii) Intracoronary

Intracoronary, or homocoronary, anastomoses connect parts or branches of the same coronary artery. Two subtypes have been described: the secondary anastomosis links branches of the same coronary artery (Figures 1-14B and 1-16), while the tertiary collateral joins proximal and distal segments of the same branch (Figures 1-14C, 1-16, and 1-17). Secondary connections are generally smaller than intercoronary collaterals, with diameters ranging from 20–250 μm and lengths of 1–2 cm.[59,166] Baroldi and co-workers[59] estimated that there was approximately one intracoronary vessel for every arborization of branches having a lumen of approximately 500–1,000 μm. These secondary intracoronary collaterals are only occasionally subepicardial in location, and are most often found deep within the wall.[59] However, Bellman and Frank[44] observed them at all depths. These vessels form approximately one-third of the normal heart's collateral network.[49] Fifty to sixty percent of normal hearts and hearts with minimal coronary atherosclerosis have secondary intracoronary anastomoses.[50,51] The latter are more frequent in the divisions of the left than the right coronary artery.[51] Thus, right-to-right coronary artery anastomoses were visualized in 31% of normal hearts, while collaterals between left anterior descending branches were observed in 51%

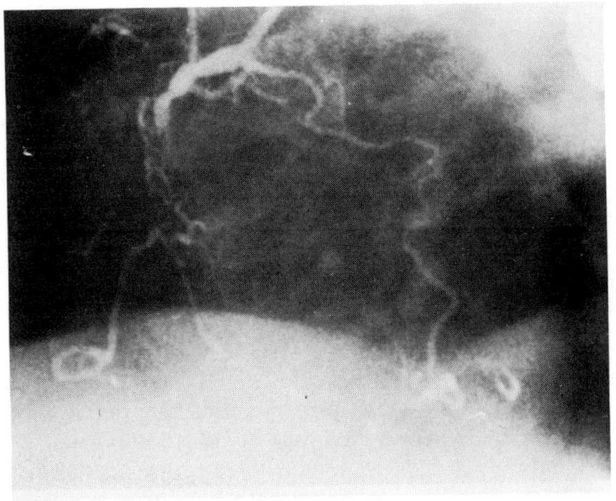

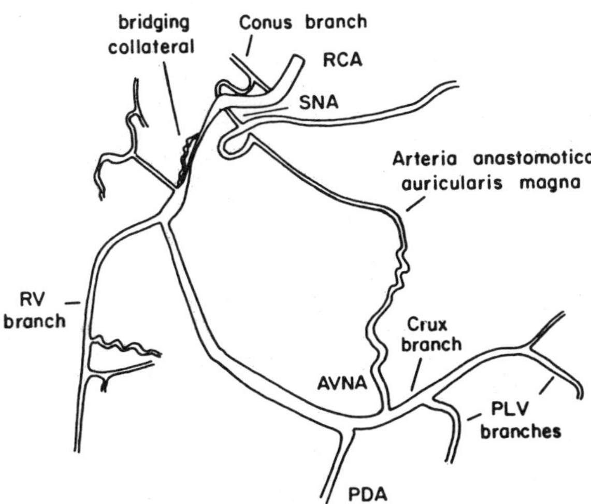

Figure 1-16 Angiographic frame and artist's drawing from right coronary (RCA) angiogram in the left anterior oblique projection. A 99% stenosis is apparent in the proximal third of the RCA. This nearly complete coronary occlusion is bypassed by a small bridging or tertiary collateral. A larger, more important collateral pathway connects the sinus node artery (SNA), a proximal branch of the RCA, to the atrioventricular node artery (AVNA), a distal branch of the same parent vessel. This intracoronary pathway is one of the forms of the arteria anastomotica auricularis magna or Kugel's artery. See Figure 1-5A for abbreviations. (Angiogram provided by Hugo Spindola-Franco, M.D., Department of Radiology, Montefiore Medical Center, Bronx, NY.)

of hearts. Left circumflex intracoronary anastomoses were present in only 23% of cases. In hearts with coronary stenoses narrowing the lumen by more than 50%, intracoronary collaterals were visualized more often in all three vascular beds (left anterior descending—78%; right coronary—45%; left circumflex—61%).[51] Clinically, secondary intracoronary anastomoses are rarely detected with angiography in the absence of coronary artery disease.

Tertiary collaterals represent a special subgroup of intracoronary anastomoses observed only in occlusive coronary disease.[51,65,79,169,183] These anastomoses are in essence local bypasses connecting arterial segments proximal and distal to a stenosis or obstruction (Figures 1-14C, 1-16, and 1-17). Tertiary collaterals are usually quite short, and are rarely more

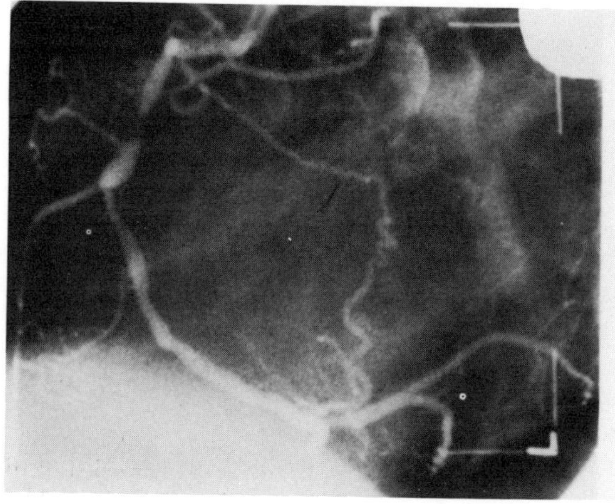

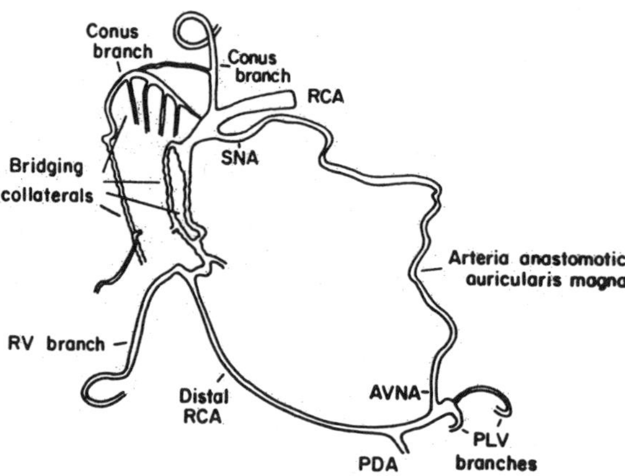

Figure 1-17 Angiographic frame and artist's drawing from right coronary (RCA) angiogram in the left anterior oblique projection. The proximal RCA is completely occluded, but flow to the distal RCA has been partially restored by numerous, unusually long, bridging collaterals which bypass the diseased arterial segment as well as one form of Kugel's artery or arteria anastomotica auricularis magna. The tertiary or bridging collateral channels are usually enlarged vasa vasorum or adventitial arteries. See Figure 1-5A for abbreviations. (Angiogram provided by Hugo Spindola-Franco, M.D., Department of Radiology, Montefiore Medical Center, Bronx, N.Y.)

than several millimeters in length.[65,79] These anastomoses are most often enlarged vasa vasorum or adventitial arteries, and form a multichannel cuff of fine, delicate vessels surrounding the arterial lesion.[65,79,169] Campbell[20] described one patient in whom numerous arteriae telae adiposae, superficial vessels in the epicardial fat pads, successfully bridged a proximal occlusion of the right coronary artery and prevented infarction in the vessel's perfusion territory. On coronary angiograms, tertiary anastomoses have a "starburst" appearance as multiple small vessels radiate outward from an abruptly terminating large artery.[65,183] In his postmortem injection studies, Tsuchiya[51] observed tertiary anastomoses in 19% of hearts with significant coronary artery disease, but never in normal hearts or hearts with minimal coronary atherosclerosis. Clinically, Cosby[182] noted tha the majority of subjects with angiographically demonstrated tertiary anastomoses had an anginal syndrome without prior myocardial infarction.

(iii) Specific pathways

Review of coronary angiograms in patients with coronary artery disease reveals numerous interarterial collateral pathways. However, there are several that recur repeatedly (Figures 1-18 through 1-20). Several of these preferred routes are described below.

SUBENDOCARDIAL PLEXUS. A subendocardial plexus is evident in all four cardiac chambers, but has been best studied in the left ventricle. These vascular channels were first recognized by Spalteholz[15,16] and confirmed by Gross,[6] but it was not until Fulton[54,56,167] published reports of his postmortem examinations of human hearts that the significance of the subendocardial plexus became evident. This plexus is a network of intercommunicating arterial channels in the deeper layers of the myocardium (Figure 1-13). Most subendocardial arteries have diameters of 100−200 μm, although larger vessels can be found in the substance of the columnae carneae. Nearly all of the vessels in the subendocardial plexus terminate in a course parallel to the subendocardial surface and interconnect with their neighbors. In the left ventricle these vessels originate at right angles from penetrating left coronary intramural branches, which themselves are branches arising at right angles from epicardial arteries.[157,159,161] Septal branches of the anterior and posterior descending arteries course close to the right ventricular surface of the interventricular septum before ramifying and contributing branches to the subendocardial plexus on both ventricular sides of the septum.[52] Because of the interconnections between adjacent branches, the plexus appears as an extensive arcade of looping vessels in the subendocardial myocardium. The subendocardial plexus is present in normal hearts but may enlarge substantially in the presence of coronary obstructive disease.[56,184] However, the subendocardial plexus cannot be visualized during clinical coronary angiographic procedures.

The subendocardial plexus is a site of potential intercommunication between branches of all coronary arteries supplying the left ventricle or other chambers.[167] Omar and Rao[52] felt that the plexus was responsible for an equitable distribution of blood throughout the entire subendocardial zone. The importance of the subendocardial plexus as a source of collaterals is further strengthened by observations that terminal branches of major coronary arteries at the apex, usually the left anterior descending artery, can be seen to turn inward to link with the plexus.[54] Similar anastomoses have been observed near the atrioventricular groove where the wall is also thin.[54]

By linking different coronary arteries, the subendocardial plexus functions as a network of intercoronary collaterals. However, because adjacent branches of the same coronary artery are also linked, the plexus may additionally complete intracoronary collateral pathways. Obstruction of an epicardial artery may result in antegrade flow down a perforating artery proximal to the lesion and then passage through the subendocardial plexus to a second perforator. Finally, retrograde flow along this latter perforator which joins the

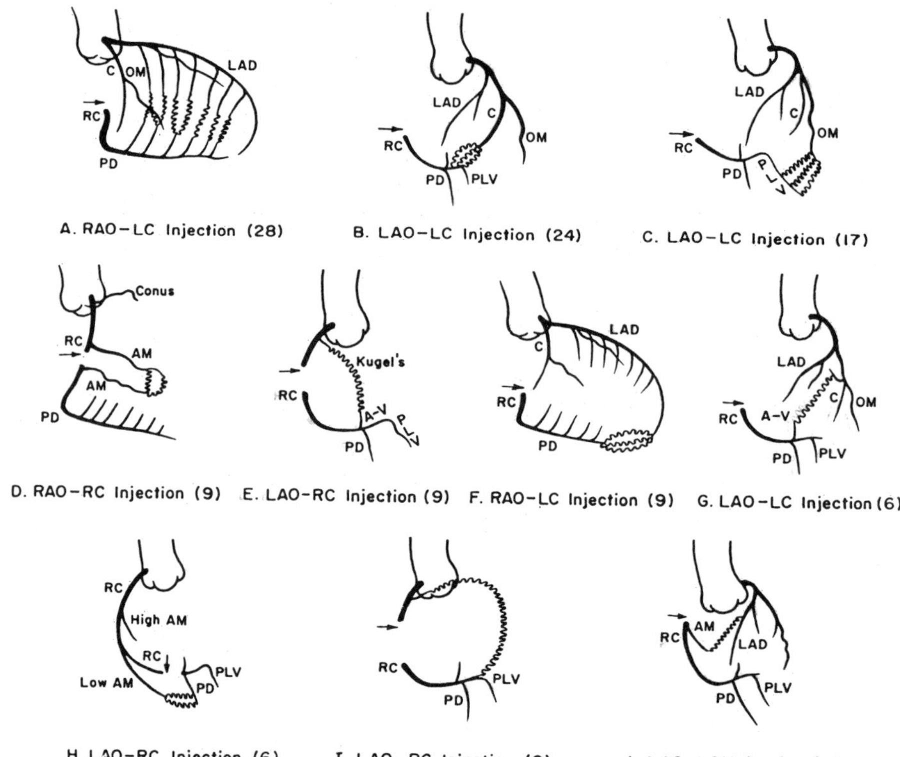

Figure 1-18 Schematic representation of collateral pathways observed with right coronary artery obstruction. Numbers in parentheses signify the frequency with which the given pathway occurred in the series. (A) LAD to PD, a branch of the RC, via ventricular septal branches. (B) Distal circumflex artery to distal RC. (C) Obtuse marginal branch of circumflex artery to posterior left ventricular branch of RC. (D) Proximal acute marginal or conus branch of RC to a more distal acute marginal branch. (E) Kugel's artery passing from either the proximal RC or LC down along the anterior margin of the atrial septum to anastomose with the A-V node branch of the distal RC. (F) Distal LAD around the cardiac apex to PD, a branch of the RC. (G) Distal circumflex artery or its left atrial circumflex branch to A-V node branch of the RC. (H) Acute marginal branch of the RC to PD branch of RC via diaphragmatic surface of right ventricle. (I) SA node branch of RC around lateral wall of the left atrium to left atrial circumflex branch, then to distal RC. (J) Right ventricular branch of LAD to acute marginal branch of RC. RAO, LAO = right, left anterior oblique projections, respectively; RC = right coronary artery; LC = left coronary artery; AM = acute marginal branch of RC; PD = posterior descending branch of RC; PLV = posterior left ventricular branch of RC; A-V = artery to atrioventricular node; LAD = left anterior descending artery; C = left circumflex artery; OM = obtuse marginal branch of C. (Reprinted with permission of the American Heart Association from Levin.[190])

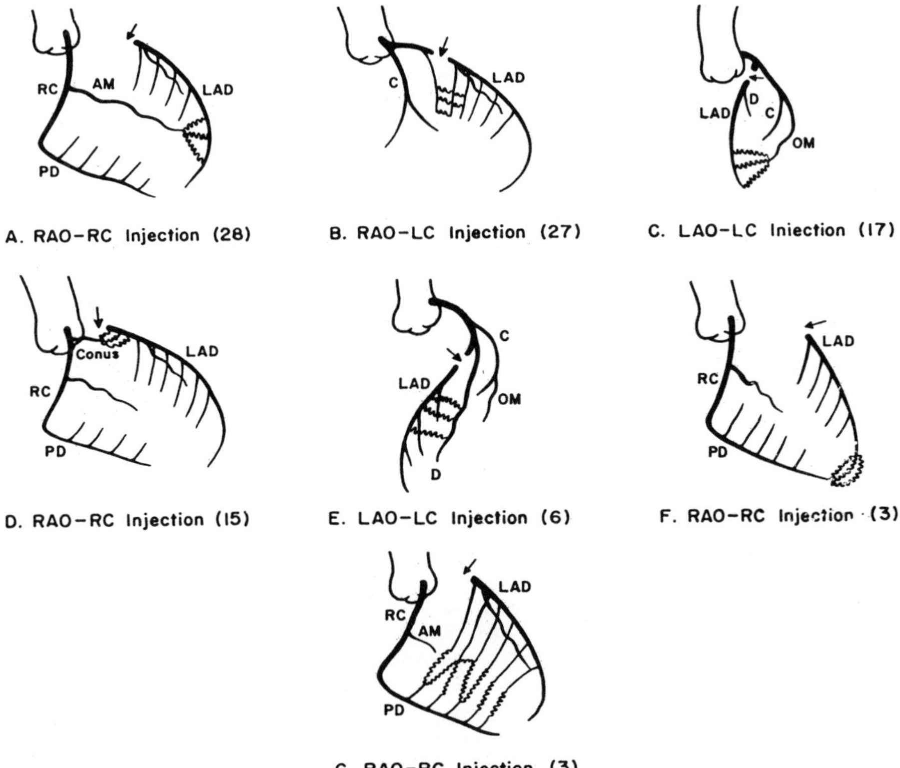

Figure 1-19   Collateral pathways in obstruction of the left anterior descending artery (LAD). Numbers in parentheses denote frequency of occurrence of each pathway in the series. (*A*) Acute marginal branch of RC to LAD. (*B*) Proximal ventricular septal branch of LAD to a more distal septal branch. (*C*) Obtuse marginal branch of the circumflex artery to LAD artery. (*D*) Conus branch of RC to LAD. (*E*) Diagonal branch of LAD to distal LAD. (*F*) PD, a branch of the RC, around the cardiac apex to LAD. (*G*) PD, a branch of the RC, to LAD via ventricular septal branches. D = diagonal branch of LAD, other abbreviations as in Figure 1-18. (Reprinted with permission of the American Heart Association from Levin.[190])

parent epicardial artery beyond the obstruction completes bypass of the lesion.

ATRIAL ANASTOMOSES.   The variability and often small size of most atrial arteries has made study of atrial anastomoses difficult. However, both intra- and transatrial anastomoses can easily be detected wih postmortem radiographic techniques and corrosion casts.[52,54,60,65,185−189] These collateral pathways greatly enlarge in the face of coronary artery disease, and therefore may at times be recognized during clinical coronary angiography.[74,77−83,190]

Fulton[54] observed that atrial connections were most frequent in the left atrial wall. For the most part, the caliber of these communications did not

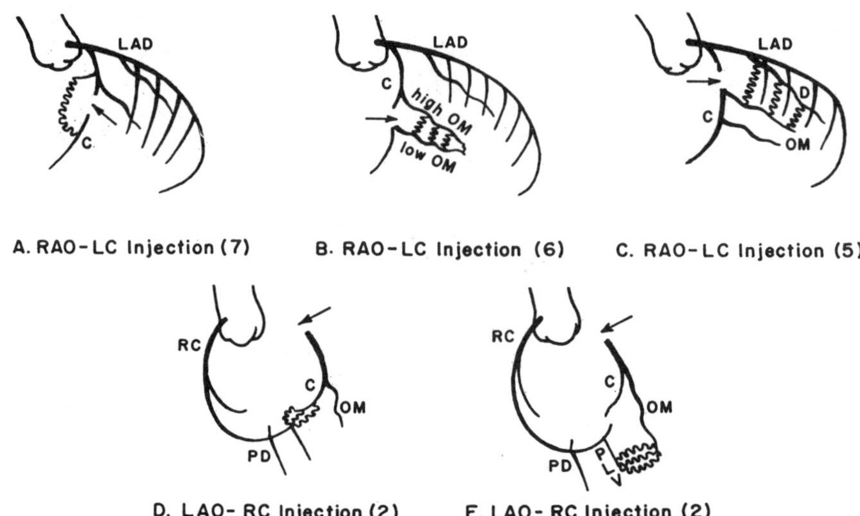

Figure 1-20   Anastomotic pathways in left circumflex artery obstruction. Numbers in parentheses reflect frequency of occurrence of pathways in the series. (*A*) Left atrial circumflex branch to distal circumflex artery. (*B*) Proximal obtuse marginal branch of circumflex artery to a more distal obtuse marginal branch. (*C*) Diagonal branch of LAD to obtuse marginal branch of circumflex artery. (*D*) Distal RC to distal circumflex artery. (*E*) Posterior left ventricular branch of the RC to obtuse marginal branch of the circumflex artery. See Figure 1-18 for abbreviations. (Reprinted with permission of the American Heart Association from Levin.[190])

exceed 100 μm, although significant enlargement did occur when major arteries were occluded. In these latter cases such communications were often intercoronary, i.e., between left circumflex and right coronary arteries. Omar and Rao[52] noted that many atrial anastomoses were superficial, and therefore grossly visible. They measured diameters of 100–300 μm. These connections were generally straight or slightly curved, and, in contrast to Fulton's results, were typically of the intracoronary type, connecting right coronary artery branches.

Anterior, intermediate, and posterior atrial branches may be derived from both the right coronary and left circumflex arteries. These branches are not constant. But when present, the branches from the right coronary artery usually supply the right atrial myocardium, while left circumflex branches generally supply left atrial tissue. Numerous intracoronary anastomoses give the appearance of multiple superficial vascular arcades.[186] Because the two atria and their arteries are located directly above the proximal portions of the right coronary and left circumflex arteries, atrial branches provide potential routes for communication between these major vessels. Indeed, numerous connections between corresponding left and right atrial branches can be identified. Thus, atrial anastomoses serve to connect several portions of the two major coronary trunks occupying the atrioventricular sulci.

The sinus node artery and Kugel's artery are two atrial vessels that are important components of specialized atrial collateral pathways (see below). The sinus node artery is an unusually large atrial vessel that may arborize extensively to form multiple intra- and intercoronary anastomoses.[185,187,189] Some of the terminal branches of the sinus node artery encircling the superior vena cava anastomose with the right atrial intermediate artery which arises from the right coronary artery near the heart's acute margin and then ascends toward the base of the heart. If the sinus node artery is a branch of the right coronary artery (see below), the resulting anastomoses are intracoronary. On the other hand, if the sinus node artery arises from the left circumflex artery, then the two atrial branches form intercoronary connections. Similarly, the left intermediate atrial artery may also ascend toward the ostium of the superior vena cava and give off branches that anastomose with the terminal twigs of the sinus node artery.

On the posterior surface of the heart, the termination of the right coronary and left circumflex arteries are reciprocally related (see above). Each gives rise to terminal atrial branches that anastomose, thus providing another source of intercoronary collaterals. In addition, small arterial branches may originate anywhere along the course of these main coronary arteries. Twigs from adjacent branches may form intracoronary networks, while small intercoronary connections are also frequent.

As noted by James,[65] atrial vessels form a particularly suitable route for collateral flow. Most atrial arteries are on the epicardial surface and are therefore subject to minimal intramyocardial compression. Furthermore, the high intraventricular pressures generated within the left and to lesser extent right ventricles have little influence on vessels located on the atrial walls. Because atrial collaterals are therefore not subjected to the same type of extravascular compression as ventricular anastomotic channels, they are potentially an important source of blood flow to ischemic myocardium, especially during exercise or other stress that raises ventricular pressure and intramyocardial compressive forces.

TRANSSEPTAL ANASTOMOSES. Whereas the atrial collaterals described above link the two major coronary trunks (right coronary and left circumflex arteries) that course in the atrioventricular sulci, anastomoses through the atrial and ventricular septa connect the two major vessels (left anterior and posterior descending arteries) occupying the anterior and posterior interventricular grooves. The planes of transatrial and transseptal anastomoses are roughly perpendicular to each other.[65] Anastomoses in the interatrial septum function much like other transatrial connections. The artery to the atrioventricular node (see below) anastomoses with perforating branches from the interatrial septum arising from any of the three major coronary arteries, as well as with the right or left posterior atrial arteries that penetrate laterally into the posterior interatrial septum.[185] One especially important channel (Kugel's artery) will be described below.

The interventricular septum is a major site of intercoronary collaterals connecting the left anterior and posterior descending arteries. In part the topographic anatomy of the heart influences the extent and importance of these collateral connections. As noted above, the posterior descending artery is a branch of the right coronary artery in approximately 85% of hearts.[6,16,18, 31,60,63,149,151,154,155] In the remainder it is a branch of the left circumflex artery. In the former situation, transseptal collaterals serve to link the right and left coronary arteries whereas in the latter case, these collaterals join only branches of the left coronary artery.

The terminations of the posterior and left anterior descending arteries in the posterior interventricular sulcus are reciprocally related. The left anterior descending artery often rounds the apex and typically (60% of cases) ascends in the sulcus for 5−30 mm as the ramus recurrens.[154] A long ramus recurrens ascending high in the interventricular groove is associated with a short posterior descending artery which itself descends toward the apex in the same groove. This interplay between the lengths of the two arteries affects the source of the posterior perfusion of the interventricular septum, and hence the extent of the potential intercoronary collaterals. Bertho and Gagnon[191] noted that in approximately one-half of the hearts studied, the interventricular septum was supplied equally by the posterior and left anterior descending arteries with each giving off four to ten septal perforators of similar caliber and dimension. In the other hearts the preponderant supply was derived from the left anterior descending artery which effectively perfused two-thirds of the septum. James and Burch[192] observed that perfusion of the interventricular septum was more dependent on the left anterior descending artery. In all hearts studied by them, the latter accounted for at least 60−70% of the septum's blood supply, while in 28% of hearts, 90−100% of septal perfusion was delivered by its branches. In the latter situation, collaterals linking the anterior and posterior septal perforators can only be of the intracoronary type. Intercoronary septal collaterals can exist only if part of the septum's blood supply is derived from the posterior descending artery when the latter is a branch of the right coronary artery. Baroldi and Scomazzoni[60] have confirmed the postmortem observations of James and Burch.[192]

The extramural vessels (left anterior and posterior descending coronary arteries) in the anterior and posterior interventricular sulci give rise to mural vessels labeled septal perforators (Figure 1-21). Anterior perforators originate in the anterior interventricular groove as perpendicular branches of the left anterior descending coronary artery. These septal arteries are usually 40−80 mm long. The anterior septal artery or the first anterior perforating vessel is usually larger than the other septal arteries. The lengths of these septal arteries decrease as the point of origin of the perforators approaches the apex. After penetrating the interventricular septum they course diagonally in an anteroposterior direction[63,192] (Figure 1-8). Closer to the apex, the inferior branches actually have an oblique ascending course, while the truly apical branches ascend in a more or less vertical direction.[60] As they pass through the septum, the anterior perforators course close to the endocardium on the septum's right ventricular side where they remain until the

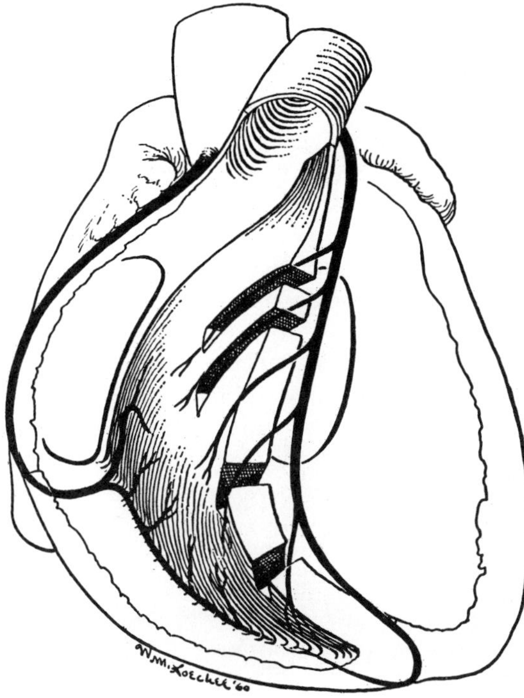

Figure 1-21   Diagram of blood supply to the interventricular septum. The anterior septal arteries arise from the left anterior descending artery and pass posteriorly along the right ventricular surface of the septum to meet the posterior septal arteries coursing anteriorly from their origin from the posterior descending artery. The anterior septal perforators are generally longer and more numerous than their posterior counterparts. (Reprinted with permission of Harper & Row, Publishers, from James.[63])

terminal arborization. This arrangement assures minimal extravascular compression during left ventricular contraction. The anterior septal branches anastomose with short penetrating branches from the posterior descending coronary artery. Posterior perforators are seldom more than 15 mm long, but are more numerous than the anterior branches, especially in the inferior portion of the septum.[60] They course diagonally parallel to the base of the heart in a posteroanterior direction. Therefore, anterior and posterior septal perforators approach each other from opposite directions (Figures 1-22 and 1-23). Anastomoses in the interventricular septum of the normal heart are numerous and have diameters ranging up to 300–350 μm.[50,54,59] In patients with obstructive disease of either the right coronary or left anterior descending artery, the diameters of these mural branches and anastomoses increase substantially (Figures 1-24 and 1-25). Hence, in such patients, septal anastomoses and collateral vessels are readily demonstrated by both postmortem examination[21,44,50–52,54,57,59–61,63,65,166,169,192] and clinical coronary angiography[74–80,190] (Figures 1-18A and 1-19G). Some investigators[51,57] have concluded that the greatest number of intercoronary collaterals may be found in the interventricular septum.

In addition to their role as intercoronary collaterals, septal perforators also may act as intracoronary anastomotic channels to bypass localized obstructive disease. Adjacent septal arteries have numerous interconnections. Thus, blood may flow antegradely along a septal perforator arising

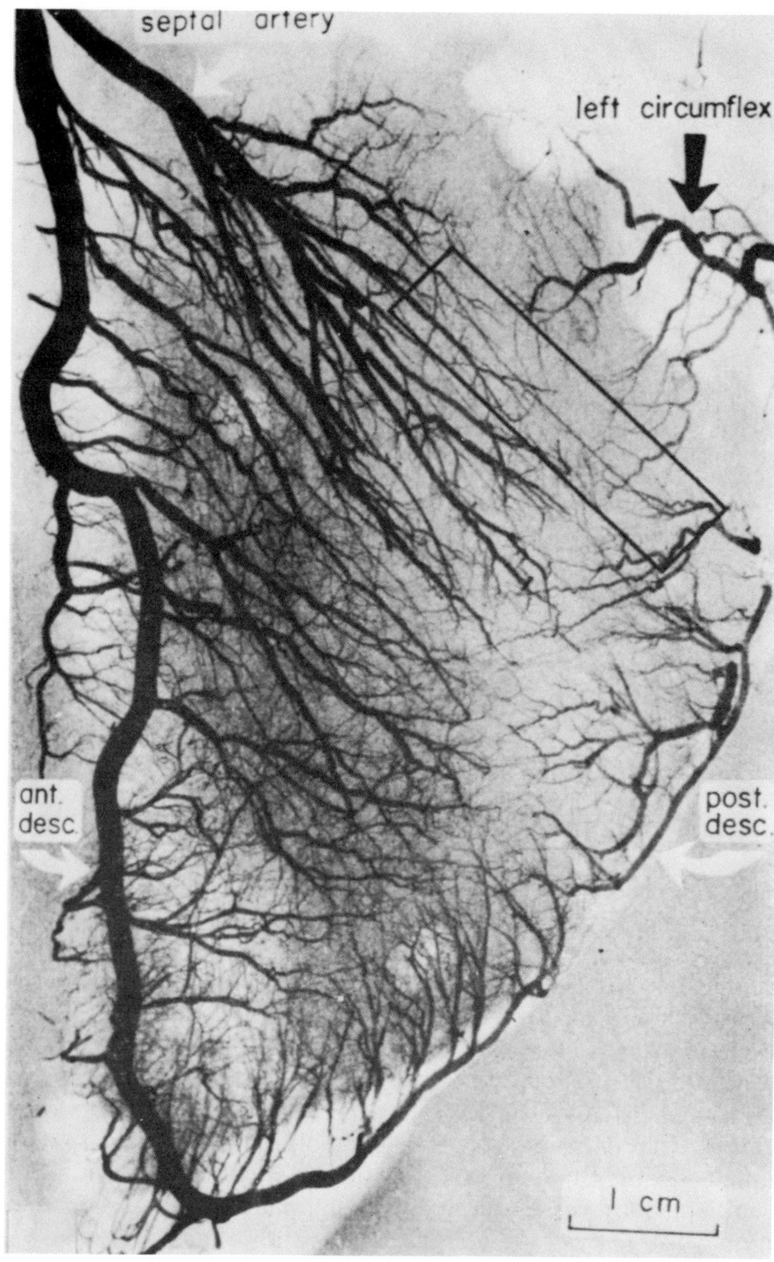

Figure 1-22   Microangiogram of interventricular septum. The long, slender septal arteries from the left anterior descending artery and smaller septal perforators from the posterior descending artery approach each other from opposite directions. Actual anastomosis between the anterior and posterior systems is observed within the rectangle in the upper right-hand corner. The first septal artery is seen to be the largest septal perforator. (Reprinted with permission of C.V. Mosby Co., from Bellman and Frank.[44])

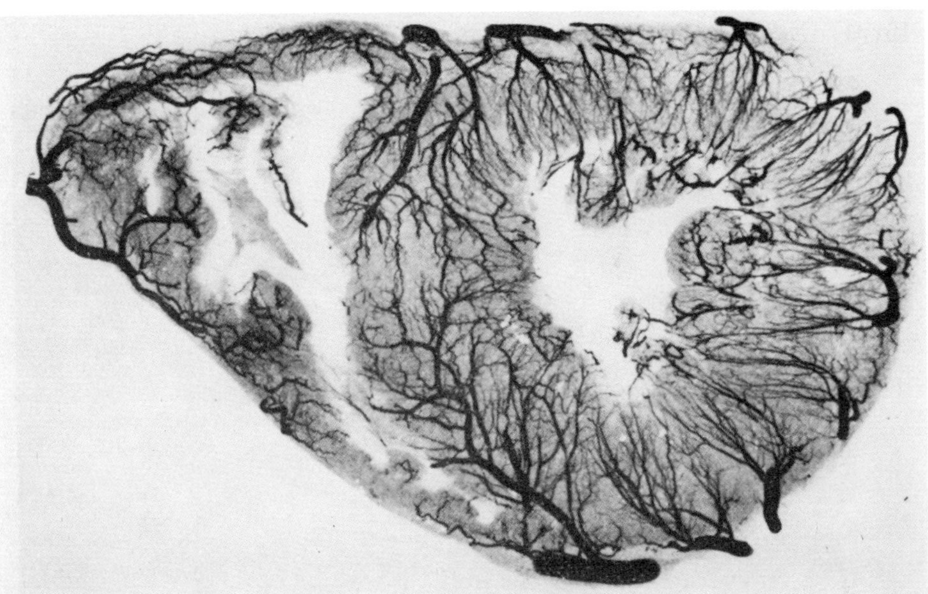

Figure 1-23 Roentgenogram of transverse section of injected heart of 29-year-old male. Right ventricle is to the left and left ventricle to the right. The two sources of septal perfusion are particularly well seen, and anastomoses between the anterior (bottom) and posterior (top) perforators are easily defined. (Reprinted with permission of C. V. Mosby Co., from Gross and Kugel.[21])

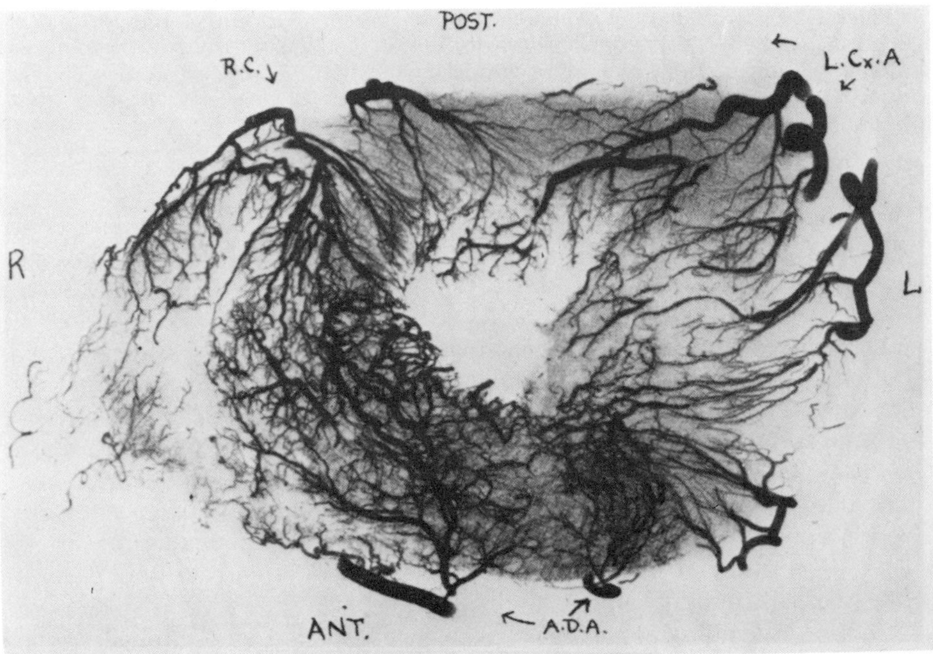

Figure 1-24 Transverse section of the ventricles after postmortem coronary injection. The left anterior descending artery (A.D.A.) had been occluded (note discontinuity in vessel). The septal perforators serving as a source of collateral blood flow to the obstructed vessel show striking enlargement. Compare this transverse section with that from a normal heart in Figure 1-23. (Reprinted with permission of the British Medical Association from Fulton.[184])

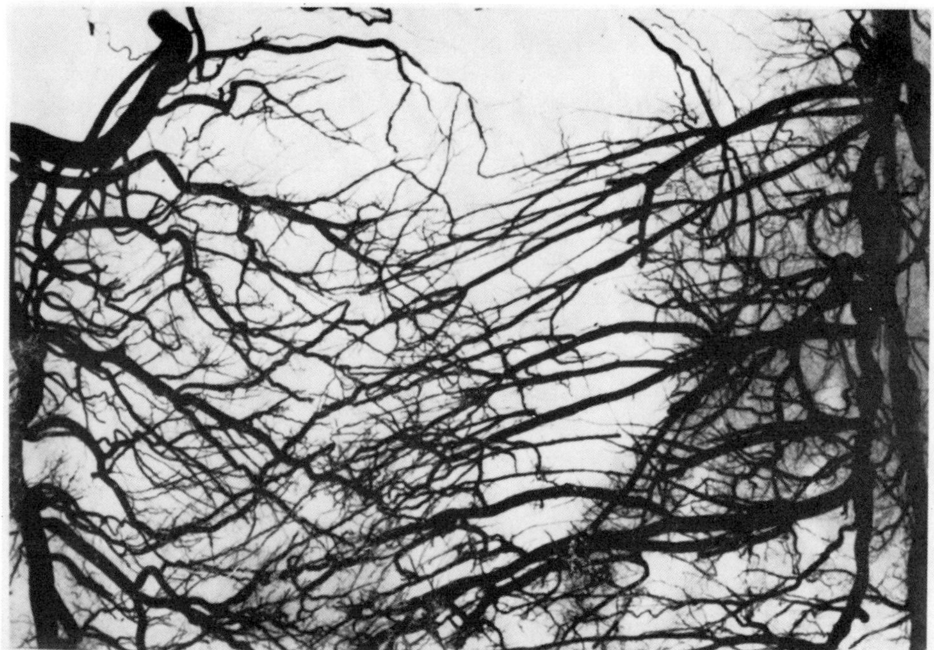

Figure 1-25   Radiograph of postmortem angiogram of portion of interventricular septum in patient with coronary artery disease. Marked enlargement of anastomoses linking the left anterior descending coronary artery (right) and posterior descending artery (left) is appreciated. (Reprinted with permission of Charles C. Thomas, Publisher, from Fulton.[56])

proximal to a lesion in the epicardial artery, and then pass to an adjacent septal artery and flow retrogradely to enter the epicardial vessel beyond the luminal obstruction (Figure 1-19B).

Vessels other than anterior and posterior septal arteries also enter the interventricular septum.[192] For example, epicardial branches from neighboring arteries in the free ventricular walls may course to the anterior and posterior interventricular sulci, where they then turn 90° and enter the septum for variable distances. On the anterior surface of the heart, these vessels originate from the left circumflex artery and its marginal branches. The right coronary ventricular branches and the left circumflex artery are sources on the heart's posterior surface. These additional penetrating arteries in the septum are neither numerous nor large, but they represent parts of potential collateral pathways.

The descending septal artery was first described by Campbell,[20] who noted it to be present in 20% of the hearts examined. Rodriguez et al.[152] found it in 12% of their postmortem human hearts. Although Campbell[20] described the descending septal artery as a proximal branch of the right coronary artery, Rodriguez observed this origin in only 63% of his material. In the remaining 37% of hearts it arose directly from the aortic sinus either from a common orifice with the right coronary or conus artery or by itself. The descending septal artery then courses down the aortic root, giving off branches to the periaortic connective tissue and parts of the crista supraventricularis. This artery enters the superior aspect of the interventricular septum and runs down the middle of the septum in contrast to the other septal arteries which run diagonally parallel to the base of the heart. But as it extends down the septum's middle, it lies between the posterior and left anterior descending arteries. This location makes it a potential source of important collaterals. The descending septal artery may also anastomose with the artery to the atrioventricular node.[74] Identification of this vessel has been easiest in postmortem specimens.[20,152,192] Because of its small size and variable origin, it has not been routinely opacified during clinical coronary angiography.[74,193]

Thus, the interventricular septum is an important location of intercoronary as well as intracoronary collaterals. These anastomoses are abundant in the normal heart, and dimensions increase strikingly in the presence of coronary obstructive disease.

VENTRICULAR EPICARDIAL ANASTOMOSES.   As already described, intercoronary and intracoronary anastomoses may be found throughout the myocardial wall in normal human hearts.[44] They are also present on the epicardial surface and in the subepicardial layers. Although Fulton[54,167] and Schaper[164,165] have described relative paucities of collaterals in these locations, James,[63] Bellman and Frank,[44] and Omar and Rao[52] have observed many subepicardial anastomoses. These superficial collateral vessels enlarge in the presence of coronary obstructive disease,[169] and it is these transformed epicardial collaterals that are so well visualized during clinical coronary angiography.[74–84,190] There is no major coronary artery that does not have numerous, potentially large epicardial connections with other arteries coursing on the ventricular surfaces.[65] These collaterals are not subject to intramyocardial compressive forces during ventricular contraction.

The most common sites for superficial ventricular intercoronary collateral channels are the right ventricular wall and left ventricular apex.[6,51,52,59,65,169] Random small vessels to the anterior surface of the right ventricle branch from the left anterior descending coronary artery all along the latter's course.[63] These right ventricular branches extend over the free wall of the right ventricle to meet similar long branches running toward the anterior interventricular groove from the right coronary artery or branches of the acute marginal artery, itself a tributary of the right coronary artery (Figures 1-18J and 1-19A). The conus artery and the circle of Vieussens is another important collateral pathway linking the left anterior descending and right coronary arteries (see below).

Collaterals on the posterior wall of the heart are also present, although they are less often visualized angiographically.[65] Ventricular branches of the obtuse marginal artery, a tributary of the left circumflex coronary artery, extend toward the heart's obtuse margin where many turn onto the posterior wall. In right dominant hearts these branches anastomose with neighboring posterolateral branches of the right coronary artery on the posterior left ventricular wall and near the apex (Figures 1-18C and 1-20E). In the small number of left dominant hearts, however, the acute marginal branch of the right coronary artery anastomoses with right posterior branches from the left circumflex artery over the posterior right ventricular wall.[169]

Epicardial collaterals extending over the anterior surface of the left ventricle are also less commonly visualized with routine coronary angiography.[65] However, small branches from the left anterior descending's diagonal arteries may anastomose with small vessels extending over the anterolateral left ventricular surface from the obtuse marginal branch of the left circumflex coronary artery (Figure 1-20C). In addition, in some hearts a median artery (ramus medianus) extends diagonally from its origin in the fork of the left main coronary artery bifurcation across the anterior surface of the left ventricle between myocardial areas perfused by diagonal arteries on one side and marginal arteries on the other. There are potential anastomoses between branches of the three arteries.

Intercoronary sulcal anastomoses link the terminal portions of the two major coronary arteries coursing in the same sulcus. Thus, the left anterior descending artery descends in the anterior interventricular groove and usually ascends for small distances in the posterior interventricular sulcus, while the posterior descending artery, most frequently a major branch of the right coronary artery, descends in the posterior interventricular sulcus. Connections near the apex between these two vessels are easily demonstrated when obstructive disease of either the left anterior descending or right coronary artery is present[51,59,190] (Figures 1-18F and 1-19F). In some hearts a single vessel may be found to link the two arteries. In other cases numerous fine arterial vessels situated in paravascular tissue form the interconnections. The latter resemble the tertiary intracoronary anastomosis appearing angiographically as a multichannel cuff bridging an obstructed arterial segment.[65,183] Terminal branches of the right coronary and left circumflex arteries which course in the atrioventricular sulcus also interconnect (Figures 1-18B and 1-20D). Most commonly, multiple small branches passing over the surface of the coronary sinus rather than a single large collateral channel link the two arterial systems.[169]

Finally, superficial intracoronary collaterals linking proximal and distal segments of an obstructed coronary artery may be visualized. Often these collaterals are in the form of tertiary anastomoses forming multichannel cuffs (Figures 1-16 and 1-17). These latter vessels are often enlarged vasa vasorum or adventitial arteries.[65,79,169]

SPECIAL ARTERIAL ANASTOMOSES.
1. *Conus artery.* The conus artery or third coronary artery[153] was first adequately described by Banchi in 1904,[149] but it was not until Schlesinger's report[153] of postmortem injection studies in 651 hearts that the functional

significance of this accessory coronary artery was truly appreciated. The conus artery is a supernumerary vessel that arises behind the right aortic valve cusp most often (64%) from a separate ostium near that of the right coronary artery (Figure 1-26), but occasionally (36%) from a common ostium with the latter artery.[60] The conus artery has been identified in 33–51% of normal or pathologic hearts.[18,60,63,149,153] When a distinct conus artery is not apparent, the homologous first ventricular branch of the right coronary artery assumes a similar course and acquires the same functional significance. After originating from the aortic root, the conus artery curves away from the right coronary artery in the right atrioventricular sulcus and courses across the anterosuperior free right ventricular wall to terminate in small arterial twigs near the anterior interventricular sulcus. The conus artery crosses the pulmonary conus at the level of the pulmonic valve and forms a semicircle where it is regularly met and joined by analogous small branches from the proximal left anterior descending coronary artery (Figure 1-27 [colorplate]). This anastomotic pathway forms an arterial circle or ring, the circle of Vieussens.

This anastomotic connection between the right coronary and left anterior descending arteries is the uppermost of a series of parallel interconnections crossing over the anterior surface of the right ventricle. But the unique qualities of the conus artery make the collateral flow to the left anterior descending artery especially valuable. The conus artery is usually small, typically with diameters of 0.4–1.0 mm, although occasionally very large vessels with diameters of 2.0 mm or more are evident.[153] Obstructive lesions of the conus artery have rarely (1.8%) been documented.[153] Therefore, the direction of collateral flow through the conus artery is virtually always antegrade toward a proximally occluded left anterior descending artery. On the other hand, when a conus artery originating directly from the aortic root is not present and when the first ventricular branch of the right coronary artery by default forms the right side of the circle of Vieussens, the direction of collateral flow is dependent on the relative location of obstructing lesions in the coronary arteries. Hence, right coronary obstruction proximal to the origin of the first ventricular branch would establish a pressure gradient from the left anterior descending artery to the right coronary artery distal to the lesion and retrograde flow through the circle of Vieussens. Conversely, antegrade flow into the left anterior descending artery would occur if this latter vessel were proximally obstructed.

The conus artery may be visualized during clinical angiography in normal hearts if the angiographic catheter is fortuitously placed in its aortic ostium. Even without catheter wedging, flow of radiographic contrast medium into the left anterior descending coronary artery may be appreciated.[171] Most angiographic studies of patients with coronary obstructive disease have documented the conus artery as an important source of collaterals to the proximally obstructed left anterior descending artery [74–84,190] (Figures 1-15 and 1-19D). When this latter artery is significantly diseased, collateral connections involving the circle of Vieussens have been observed in 12–16%

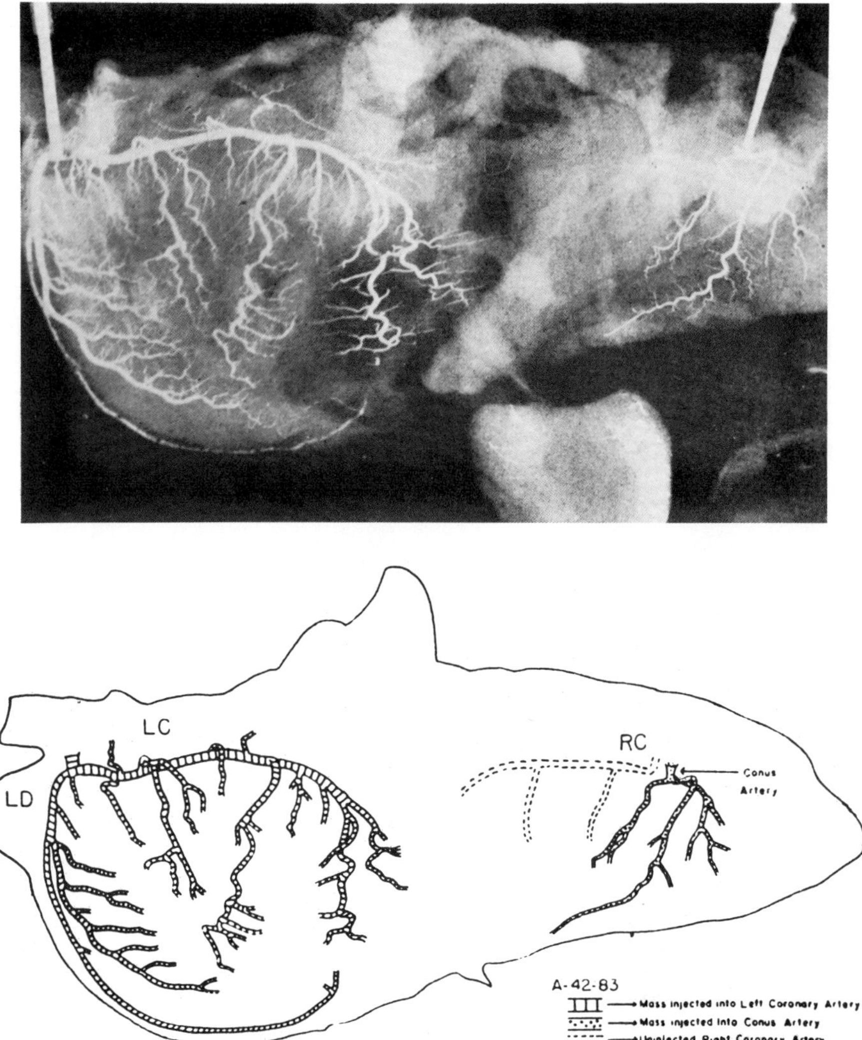

Figure 1-26   Radiograph of normal, unrolled heart after postmortem coronary injection of Schlesinger mass. The right-hand cannula was inserted into the aortic ostium of the conus artery instead of the right coronary artery (RC). The injected mass nicely demonstrates the arterial distribution of this latter vessel. In the diagram beneath the radiograph, the course of the uninjected proximal right coronary artery (dashed line) is indicated (compare with Figure 1-1). LC = left circumflex coronary artery; LD = left anterior descending coronary artery. (Reprinted with permission of C. V. Mosby Co., from Schlesinger et al.[153])

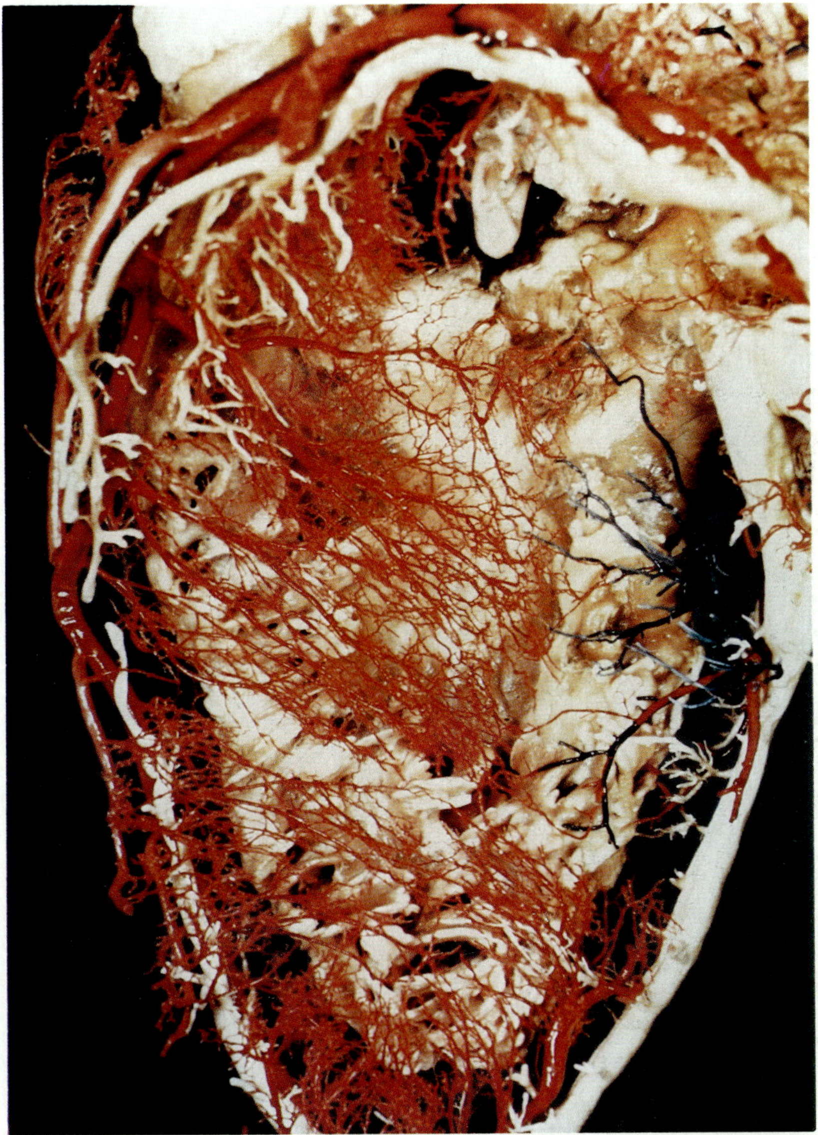

Figure 1-2   Vinylite corrosion cast of the heart of a 17-year-old male demonstrating remarkable detail of the coronary vascular bed. The left coronary arterial system is filled with red-colored vinylite, while blue vinylite fills the right coronary artery, and white vinylite the coronary venous system. In this projection, many ventricular septal arteries anastomosing anteriorly and posteriorly can easily be seen. The diameters of all of the visualized anastomoses are larger than 300 μm. (Reprinted with permission of Harper & Row, from James.[63])

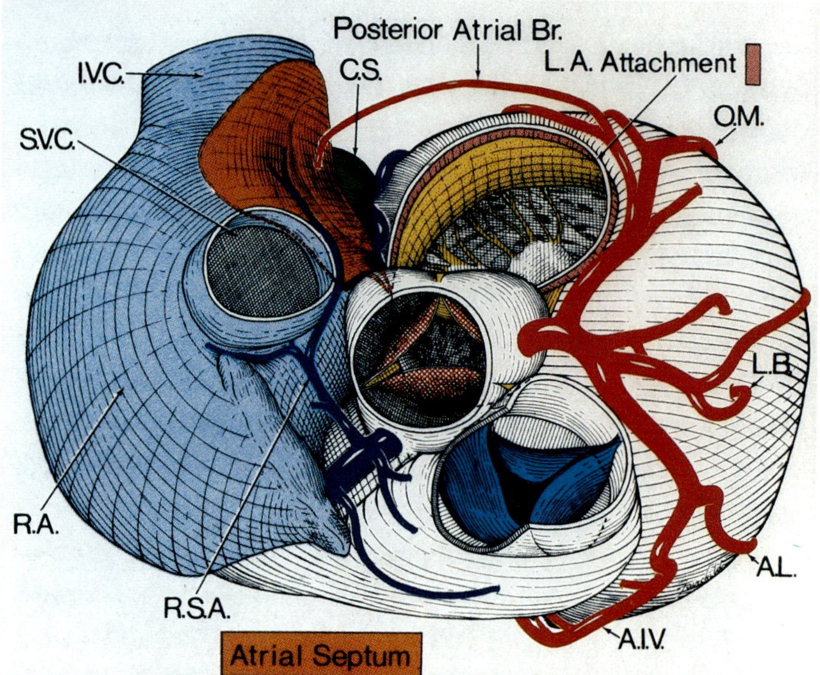

Figure 1-6   Superior view of the heart showing aortic origins of the right (blue) and left (red) coronary arteries. The right sinus node artery (RSA) usually arises within 2 cm of the origin of the right coronary artery and courses onto the anteromedial wall of the right atrium (RA). The sinus node artery gives off several branches to the atrial wall and then continues as the branch to the sinus node by passing in front of the superior vena cava (SVC). The sinus node artery terminates in the atrial septum (orange region), an important site of intra- and intercoronary collaterals. CS = coronary sinus; IVC = inferior vena cava. (Reprinted with permission of Springer-Verlag from McAlpine WA: *Heart and Coronary Arteries: An Anatomical Atlas for Clinical Diagnosis, Radiological Investigation, and Surgical Treatment.* Springer-Verlag, Berlin, 1975.)

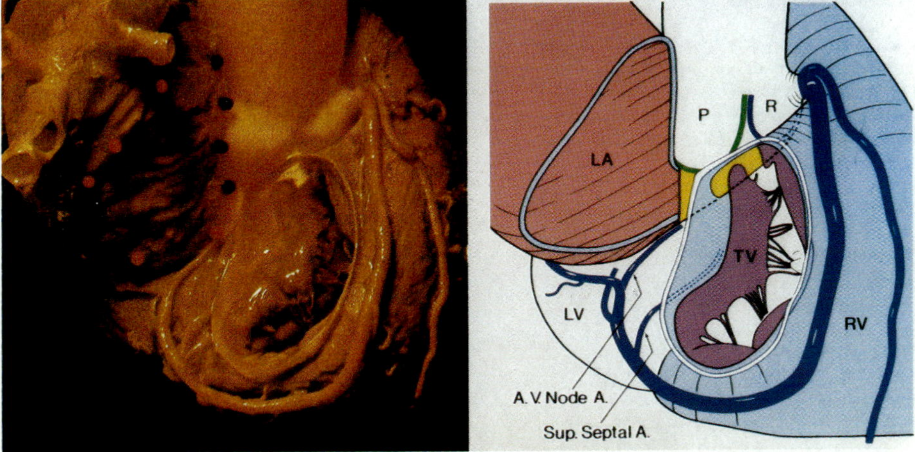

Figure 1-7   Cast (left) and schematic drawing (right) demonstrating course of right coronary artery in the right atrioventricular groove around the lateral margin of the tricuspid valve (TV). At the crux, the right coronary artery makes a sharp bend and the atrioventricular (A.V.) node artery arises from the apex of the bend. LA = left atrium; LV = left ventricle; P,R = posterior, right sinuses of Valsalva, respectively; RV = right ventricle; sup = superior. (Reprinted with permission of Springer-Verlag from McAlpine WA: *Heart and Coronary Arteries: An Anatomical Atlas for Clinical Diagnosis, Radiological Investigation, and Surgical Treatment.* Springer-Verlag, Berlin, 1975.)

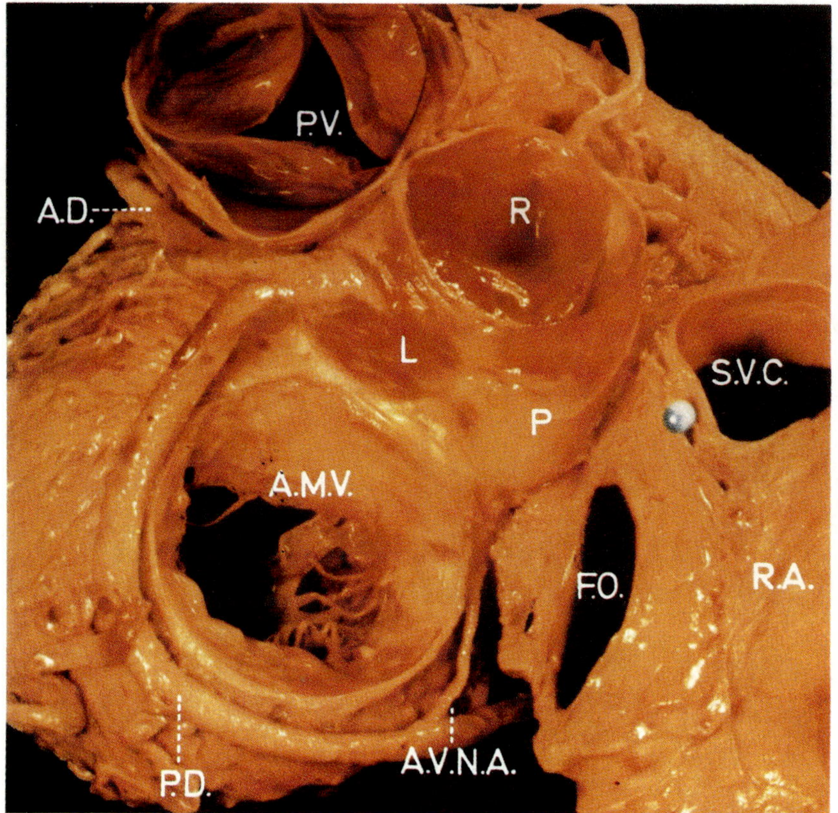

Figure 1-11   Cast viewed from the base of the heart demonstrating bifurcation of the main left coronary artery and course of the left circumflex artery in the left atrioventricular sulcus around the lateral rim of the mitral valve. In this left dominant heart, the left circumflex artery gives rise to the posterior descending (P.D.) and atrioventricular node (A.V.N.A.) arteries. A.D. = left anterior descending artery; AMV = anterior leaflet of mitral valve; F.O. = foramen ovale; R,L,P = right, left and posterior sinuses of Valsalva, respectively; RA = right atrium; SVC = superior vena cava. (Reprinted with permission of Springer-Verlag from McAlpine WA: *Heart and Coronary Arteries: An Anatomical Atlas for Clinical Diagnosis, Radiological Investigation, and Surgical Treatment.* Springer-Verlag, Berlin, 1975.)

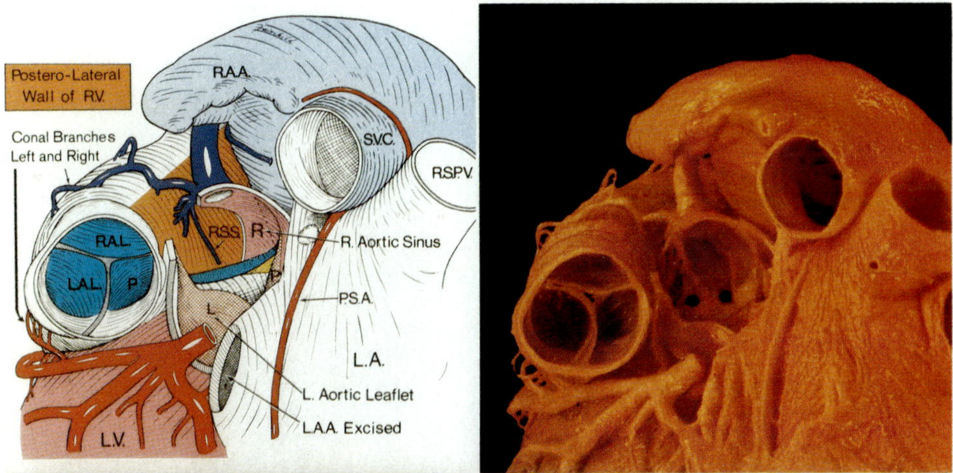

Figure 1-27   Superior view of cast (right) and diagram (left) of aortic origins of right and left coronary arteries. In this heart, the conal branch arises from the first few millimeters of the right coronary artery and then crosses the anterosuperior free right ventricular (RV) wall to reach the pulmonary conus. This artery then curves around the conus to meet similar branches from the proximal left anterior descending artery to complete the Circle of Vieussens. LA = left atrium; LAA, RAA = left, right atrial appendage,respectively; LV = left ventricle; RAL, LAL, P = right and left anterior and posterior leaflets of pulmonic valve, respectively; RSS = right superior septal artery; RSPV = right superior pulmonary vein; SVC = superior vena cava. (Reprinted with permission of Springer-Verlag from McAlpine WA: *Heart and Coronary Arteries: An Anatomical Atlas for Clinical Diagnosis, Radiological Investigation, and Surgical Treatment.* Springer-Verlag, Berlin, 1975.)

of patients.[77,78] These numbers undoubtedly underestimate the true incidence since selective catheterization of conus vessels originating from independent aortic ostia is often not accomplished.

Aside from the obvious importance of the conus artery and circle of Vieussens as an important intercoronary collateral pathway, the conus artery may also be a source of intracoronary collaterals. Either the conus vessel or first ventricular branch of the right coronary artery forms connections with adjacent right coronary marginal arterial twigs thus completing anastomotic pathways capable of bypassing proximal right coronary obstructions[52,77–79,82] (Figure 1-18D).

2. *Sinus node artery.* The sinus node artery (ramus cristae terminalis, ramus ostii cavus superioris), as its name implies, perfuses the sinus node. But it is also an important source of both intra- and intercoronary anastomotic connections. This artery arises from either the proximal right coronary or left circumflex coronary artery within 1–3 cm of the source vessel's origin. Multiple anatomic studies have defined the right coronary artery as the source of the sinus node artery in 50–68% of hearts.[6,16,18,60,63,155,185,187–189] This origin is independent of the heart's coronary artery dominance. In

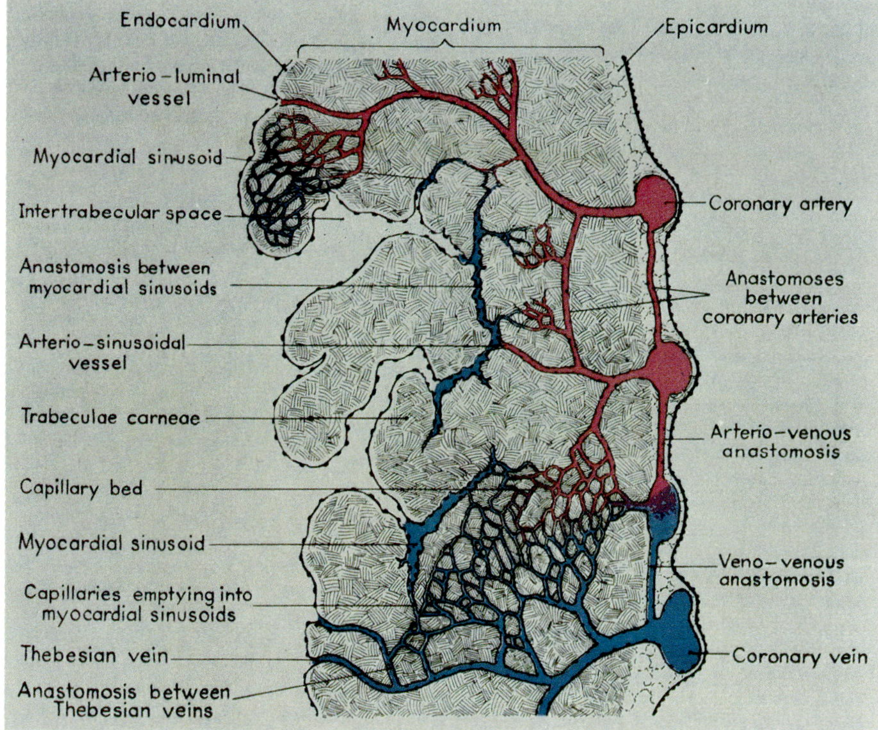

Figure 1-29   Schematic representation of the human heart's three types of endomural channels: arterioluminal and arteriosinusoidal vessels and Thebesian veins. (Reprinted with permission of Charles C. Thomas, Publisher, from Gould SE (ed): *Pathology of the Heart*, 2nd ed. Charles C. Thomas, Springfield, IL, 1960.)

the remainder of hearts the sinus node artery arises from the left circumflex artery. In rare cases the sinus node artery may be a branch of the right atrial marginal branch or even the main left coronary artery or aorta.[60,187] Despite the variable origin, the termination of the sinus node artery is quite constant: it always ends in the vicinity of the orifice of the superior vena cava and almost always does so by encircling that region.[185]

The sinus node artery is with rare exception the largest atrial branch of either the right or left coronary artery. The diameter at its origin ranges from 0.9 to 2.0 mm, and averages 1.7 mm.[187] It is easily visualized during routine clinical coronary angiography[74−84,190] (Figure 1-5). In fact, its size suggests functions other than mere arterial supply of the sinus node. Nerantzis and colleagues[189] studied 360 human hearts with either postmortem radiography following intracoronary barium sulphate-gelatin injections or corrosion casting. The vessel supplying the sinus node was not the main continuation of the sinus node artery in 37% of their hearts. The sinus node artery was also responsible for perfusion of the atrial musculature. Thus, in 19% of cases this vessel supplied the right atrium and part of the interatrial septum. In 59% of hearts, the sinus node artery additionally supplied part of the other atrium. And finally, supply of the entire atrial myocardium was dependent on the sinus node artery in 22% of cases. Hutchinson[188] has also noted that the sinus node artery is often the major arterial supply of the atria.

When arising from the proximal right coronary artery the sinus node artery passes medially and cephalad along the anterior wall of the right atrium beneath the atrial appendage.[63,187,188] It then enters the interatrial muscle band (Bachman's bundle) where it anastomoses with Kugel's artery. A stout branch continues from this junction through Bachman's bundle to the roof of the left atrium. The sinus node artery proper angles sharply rightward toward the right atrial-caval junction where it enters the sinus node. During the artery's intranodal course, at least five ascending and three or four descending collateral trunks are given off.[186] The main artery usually continues through the node to encircle most or all of the ostium of the superior vena cava (Figure 1-6). When the sinus node artery is instead a branch of the left circumflex artery, it courses along the medial aspect of the anterior part of the left atrium to Bachman's bundle.[187] The remainder of the course is similar to that for a right-sided artery.

Intercoronary collateral connections between the right coronary and left circumflex arteries established through the sinus node artery and its branches further increase the importance of this latter vessel. When arising as a proximal branch of the right coronary artery, the sinus node artery anastomoses with a proximal left circumflex branch coursing behind the aorta and pulmonary artery.[185] This grossly visible anastomosis is part of one of the variations of Kugel's arteria anastomotica auricularis magna (see below). Equally large anastomoses between the sinus node artery and Kugel's artery in the interatrial septum (a more common variety of Kugel's anastomotic pathway) also provide potential collateral connections between the right and left coronary arterial systems. A left-sided sinus node artery may anastomose with Kugel's artery originating from the right coronary artery (see below) to preserve the potential right coronary–left circumflex connection.

Intracoronary anastomoses are equally important.[185] Large connections between the intermediate right atrial artery and right-sided sinus node artery are grossly visible. A right coronary artery obstruction may be bypassed by anastomosis between branches of the sinus node artery that pass around the lateral wall of the left atrium and the left atrial circumflex branch. The circuitous path is then completed by connections between the latter vessel and the distal right coronary artery (Figure 1-18I). The left-sided sinus node artery frequently anastomoses with the left intermediate atrial artery over the body of the left atrium. Furthermore, anastomosis between a left-sided sinus node artery and Kugel's artery arising from the left circumflex artery (see below) establishes an elaborate intracoronary pathway.

3. *Atrioventricular node artery.* The atrioventricular node artery (ramus septi fibrosi) is the major source of blood to the atrioventricular node. In 10% of hearts it also is the only vessel supplying the bundle of His, while in 90% of hearts this latter specialized conduction tissue receives dual blood supply from the atrioventricular node artery and the first septal perforator from the left anterior descending coronary artery.[194] The artery to the atrioventricular node arises at the crux of the heart from the artery crossing the crux. Thus, in approximately 85% of hearts the atrioventricular node artery is a branch of the right coronary artery[63,155,156,185,188] (Figure 1-7). In the remaining 15% of hearts its origin is the left circumflex artery (Figure 1-11). In a few hearts, both the right coronary and left circumflex arteries give rise to dual atrioventricular node vessels.

The atrioventricular node artery has a predictable course, and is easily visualized during coronary angiographic procedures[74–84,190] (Figure 1-5). At the crux, the junction of the atrioventricular and interventricular septa, the vessel supplying the posterior wall of the left ventricle (either the distal right coronary or left circumflex artery) makes a U-shaped bend under the posterior descending vein. The atrioventricular node artery branches off the source artery at the apex of the bend. It then courses anteriorly, passes deep to the coronary sinus, and finally rises cephalad to the base of the interatrial septum.[185] The actual branch to the atrioventricular node leaves the main vessel at a 90° angle.

The atrioventricular node artery is also part of numerous inter- and intracoronary anastomotic pathways. Because of its proximity to both the interatrial and interventricular septa, arterial twigs branching from the atrioventricular node artery are found in both septa. Thus, anastomoses to branches of the first anterior septal perforator of the left anterior descending coronary artery have been identified in the vicinity of the His bundle.[6,194] Accordingly, the atrioventricular node, His bundle, and proximal portions of the bundle branches have an effective dual blood supply. Grossly visible anastomoses with perforating branches from the anterior interatrial septum arising from either the left anterior descending, left circumflex, or main right coronary artery are also apparent[185] (Figure 1-18E). These latter collateral connections represent parts of Kugel's arteria anastomotica auricularis magna (see below), and may represent important links between the proximal right or left coronary artery and the posterior circulation of the left ventricle. Large anastomoses between branches of the atrioventricular node artery and the right or left posterior atrial artery penetrating laterally into the posterior interatrial septum have been observed[185] (Figure 1-18G).

4. *Kugel's artery.* Contrary to its name, Kugel's artery (arteria anastomotica auricularis magna) is not a single arterial channel with a predictable origin, course, or termination. Rather, it represents an anastomotic link passing through the interatrial septum between the very proximal segment of either the right coronary or left circumflex artery and either the artery in the opposite end of the atrioventriular sulcus or the circulation of the diaphragmatic wall of the left ventricle. Four variations of this collateral connection have been described. For the purpose of simplicity, the collateral channel linking the anterior and posterior circulations of the heart through the interatrial septum has been termed simply Kugel's artery, in spite of its variable origin, course, and termination.

In 1927, Kugel[17] published descriptions of the three variations of the anastomotic connection that today bears his name. His observations were based on postmortem hearts that had first been injected with barium sulphate-gelatin and then cleared. The most common variation was observed in 66% of studied specimens. In the latter, Kugel's artery arose from either the left circumflex coronary artery 1−2 cm beyond its origin or from one of that artery's proximal branches, e.g., sinus node artery (Figure 1-28A). The vessel then plunged directly into the anterior wall of the left atrium and coursed medially ½−1 cm cephalad to the mitral annulus. Kugel's artery then entered the interatrial septum and proceeded posteriorly for its entire length. Near the crux, this anastomotic channel united directly with the distal segment of the coronary artery crossing the crux (usually the right coronary artery) or one of its major branches, e.g., the posterior descending artery or atrioventricular node artery. Thus, in right dominant hearts a right coronary−left circumflex intercoronary pathway was established. On the other hand, an intricate intracoronary left circumflex−left circumflex connection was formed in left dominant hearts. In either case, Kugel's artery linked the anterior and posterior circulations of the heart.

Kugel's second variation was observed in only 26% of cases. The origin and early course of Kugel's artery were quite similar to those observed above (Figure 1-28B). As the artery ran posteriorly in the interatrial septum, it reached a point approximately 2−3 cm anterior to the crux. The artery then turned on itself and retraced its course anteriorly through the septum. Kugel's artery exited from the interatrial septum into the anterior wall of the right atrium, and joined the proximal anterior portion of the right coronary

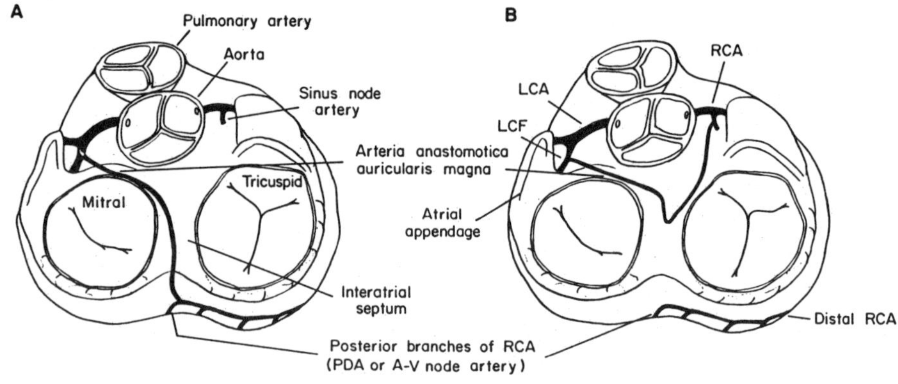

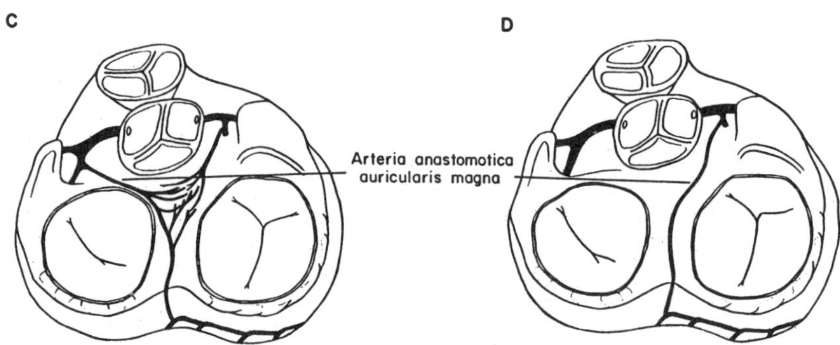

Figure 1-28   Diagrams of transverse sections of the heart at the level of the atrioventricular sulcus demonstrating four variations of Kugel's arteria anastomotica auricularis magna. A-V = atrioventricular; LCA = main left coronary artery; PDA = posterior descending artery; RCA = right coronary artery; SNA = sinus node artery. (*A* and *B* modified with permission of C. V. Mosby Co., from Kugel,[17] and *C* and *D* modified with permission of the Aerospace Medical Association, from Thompson and Froelicher.[198])

artery or one of its proximal branches. In these hearts, Kugel's artery linked the major coronary arteries coursing in opposite ends of the atrioventricular sulcus.

Finally, the third variation was observed in only 8% of hearts. Kugel's artery arose, as in the other hearts, from the anterior portion of the proximal left circumflex coronary artery (Figure 1-28C). Very early it broke up into numerous smaller branches. As the latter approached the interatrial septum, they were met by comparable anastomotic branches running through the anterior wall of the right atrium from the anterior portion of the right coronary artery. Furthermore, branches passing anteriorly through the interatrial septum from the artery crossing the crux (either the right coronary or left circumflex artery) joined the other branches. Therefore, a diffuse anastomotic network was established between branches from the anterior portions of the right coronary and left circumflex arteries and the posterior portion of the dominant vessel on the diaphragmatic wall of the heart.

James[63] described a fourth pattern that is actually similar to the first variation except for a different origin of Kugel's artery (Figure 1-28D). In this pathway Kugel's artery does not arise from the left circumflex coronary artery as described by Kugel for his three variations. Instead,the proximal right coronary artery is the source vessel. Kugel's artery then courses posterior to the tricuspid valve to the interatrial septum. As with its left-sided counterpart, the right-sided Kugel's artery plunges into the interatrial septum and surfaces near the crux to anastomose with the atrioventricular node artery and other branches of the artery crossing the crux. This anastomotic route, therefore, typically establishes an intracoronary collateral pathway from proximal to distal right coronary artery (Figures 1-16, 1-17, and 1-18E).

Kugel's artery generally anastomoses with the sinus node artery within the interatrial septum. Anastomoses with other atrial arteries penetrating the septum establish numerous intra- and transatrial connections. Thus, Kugel's artery can be an important component of many circuits bypassing obstructing right coronary or left circumflex lesions.

Although Kugel's artery may be as large as 1 mm,[195] it is not often visualized during clinical angiography. Most of the available reports documenting angiographic opacification of Kugel's artery[76−79,81−83,190,195−198] have noted origin of this vessel either directly from the right coronary artery or from the latter's sinus node artery branch (Figures 1-16 and 1-17). Left-sided Kugel's arteries have been distinctly uncommon. This is curious since all of the 50 normal hearts studied by Kugel[17] had only left-sided anastomotic pathways. Soto et al.[196] found a Kugel's artery in 6% of their patients with coronary obstructive disease. All of the latter had either right coronary and/or left circumflex arterial disease. Grollman and Heger[195] found a left-sided Kugel's artery in 3.6% of patients with right coronary or left circumflex obstructive disease. Grollman[195] also observed that a left-sided Kugel's artery was never seen unless significant coronary artery disease was present, although a right-sided Kugel's artery had been opacified in at least one subject with a normal dominant right coronary artery. The angiographic frequency probably is an underestimate. Differentiation of a Kugel's artery coursing in the interatrial septum from a superficial atrial wall or atrial circumflex collateral vessel is often not simple, and thus multiple angiographic projections may be necessary. Additionally superimposition of Kugel's artery and other vessels in various projections makes unequivocal identification of the former difficult.

(c) Endomural vessels

The coronary arterial network is obviously the prinicpal route for delivery of oxygenated blood to the myocardium. However, embryologists, anatomists, physiologists, as well as clinicians have pondered the possible significance of several accessory pathways. Vascular channels connecting the coronary vasculature directly to the heart's chambers have been identified. These endomural vessels actually represent a primitive circulatory system that is normally present only in vestigial form in man and other mammals.

The vasculature of the human heart as we know it has evolved from that of simpler vertebrate hearts which had no coronary arteries.[199-201] These latter hearts were supplied only by blood from the ventricular lumen which washed into and out of a spongework of interstices and myocardial sinusoids. Thus, muscle bundles were bathed directly by oxygenated blood. Hearts of hagfish and lampreys still demonstrate this primitive perfusion system.[202] As the evolutionary ladder was ascended, the heart became more compact, resulting in compression of the sinusoids and interference with free entry into and egress of luminal blood from the myocardium. As compensation for this dwindling luminal source, coronary arteries developed. They appeared first in elasmobranchs and bony fishes. In amphibia, the heart is partly nourished by coronary vessels and partly by luminal channels. In reptiles, birds, and mammals, coronary artery development is complete. However, as a reminder of the phylogenetic process, myocardial sinusoids persist in the innermost layers of the cardiac chambers.

Ontogenetic studies in mammals demonstrate early formation of a luminal circulation followed by its gradual disappearance as coronary vessels develop.[199-201,203,204] In the young embryo, double-layered cardiac primordia are found on either side of the developing foregut. The inner layer is the endocardium, while the outer layer is the epimyocardium. Initially, the endocardium is merely a collection of irregular clusters and cords of mesenchymal cells. These cells become organized into strands which then acquire a lumen. With time the endocardial tubes from either side migrate toward the midline and fuse. Hence, the earliest midline structure is an endocardial tube surrounded by an incompletely fused epimyocardial layer. As myocardial cells in the latter layer begin to proliferate, columns of cells extend centripetally and buckle the endocardial layer. Numerous muscular trabeculae covered by endocardium are formed which extend into the lumen. The endocardial lumen is transformed from a smooth cylinder into an irregular cavity extending into narrow channels or sinusoids between adjacent trabeculae. Thus, a sinusoidal sponge is formed, enclosing a central cavity. From the sinus venosus on the external surface of the forming heart, coronary veins develop as sprouts and ascend in the epicardium toward the bulbus arteriosus. At the same time, arterial offshoots descend from the bulbus arteriosus and form capillary anastomoses with the coronary veins. Therefore, at this point in the heart's development there are a superficial capillary network and a deep sinusoidal circulation that are wholly different in their origin. With further development there is a gradual regression of the sinusoids in the ventricles as the muscle columns continue to grow and come together, thus compressing the sinusoids and intertrabecular spaces and reducing many of them to strands of endothelium without lumens. Other sinusoids may be retained as slender channels maintaining their openings into the ventricle and frequently anastomosing within the myocardium with the more superficial coronary vascular system.

Direct connections between the coronary vessels and chambers of the heart were first recognized in adult human hearts by Vieussens in 1705 and 1706.[3] He noted that postmortem blood clots in the cavities of hearts obtained at necropsy gave off small tendrils that disappeared into small openings in the walls of the chambers. To further define the nature of these openings in the auricular and ventricular endocardium, he injected saffron dye dissolved in spirits into the left coronary artery and observed it escape through the openings into the left atrium and ventricle while little was seen to flow through veins into the right-sided chambers. Vieussens noted the openings to vary from pinpoint size to nearly 1 mm in diameter. He labeled the myocardial channels leading to the endocardial foramina "vaisseaux charnus" or "fleshy vessels."

Two years later, in 1708, Thebesius published his observations relating to communications between coronary vessels and the heart's chambers.[4,5,205,206] He placed a blow pipe in a coronary vein and noted that air blown into the vein escaped through openings in the heart wall. When the heart was immersed in water, bubbles could be seen forming at the openings. Similar experiments with glue injectate produced comparable results. Thus, Thebesius had identified vascular connections that were different from those described by Vieussens. Vieussens injected arteries while Thebesius perfused veins. Although Vieussens was the first to document luminal channels, Thebesius was memorialized and his channels were called Thebesian veins. Subsequently, all vessels passing through the myocardium to open into chamber cavities were labeled Thebesian vessels regardless of their origin. This terminology caused needless confusion among investigators, and led many to doubt the existence of direct arterial-luminal connections. Not until Wearn's meticulous studies[205,207] was it clear that there were several types of luminal channels.

Vieussens had identified direct communications between coronary arteries and the heart's chambers or arterioluminal channels. In 1798 Abernethy[208] confirmed the presence of these channels. He injected differently colored waxes directly into the coronary arteries and veins, and observed ready passage of the unmixed waxes into all cavities of the heart, especially the left ventricle. The wax injectate was too coarse to pass from one set of vessels to the other. Therefore, he actually identified direct venoluminal as well as arterioluminal channels. Oddly, most hearts with flow into the cavities had come from patients with pulmonary disease. No flow was documented in many hearts from subjects with normal lungs.

Crainicianu[18] and Kretz[209] perfused coronary arteries of postmortem hearts and noted that only 15−20% of the perfusate reached the right atrium through veins and the coronary sinus. They concluded that the rest of the injectate that was found in cardiac cavities must have escaped through Thebesian veins. Wearn[210,211] repeated these coronary artery perfusion experiments and confirmed the findings, but not the conclusions. As much as 90% of the India-ink solution escaped directly into cardiac chambers through endocardial openings in the walls of postmortem human hearts. Much less fluid was recovered from the cavities of isolated human hearts that had been permitted to resume beating following initiation of coronary perfusion.[211] Microscopic examination revealed that scarcely any capillaries contained India ink. Similar results were obtained when gum acacia was used as perfusate. After coronary arterial injection of an agar-celloidin mixture too thick to pass into the capillary bed, celloidin plugs were found protruding from endocardial foramina.[211] Mettier and his co-workers[212] made casts of the coronary arteries and ventricular chambers by injecting blue celloidin into the former and red celloidin into the latter. Coronary veins were not injected. After hydrochloric-acid digestion of the myocardium, the course of the coronary arteries was followed. There was definite fusion of the blue coronary artery mass with the red mass filling the ventricular chambers. Wearn[207] then perfused the coronary arteries with a Berlin blue-gelatin mixture that did not reach the capillaries. He cut out tissue blocks from the inner wall of the heart's chambers which contained gelatin plugs extending into the cavities. The tissue was prepared for histologic examination, and serial 8 μm sections of the gelatin plug and vessel examined. Wax reconstructions from the serial sections were also made. There were unequivocal connections between endocardial foramina and coronary arteries. Sometimes several arteries communicated with the same opening. The connecting vessels maintained their arterial structure as they branched from the parent arteriole or artery, and had diameters ranging from 0.2 to 1.0 mm. They ran more or less directly to the endocardium, and occasionally gave off branches that arborized into capillaries (Figure 1-29 [colorplate]). Sometimes the arterial structure of the arterioluminal channels was maintained until just short of the foramina, whereas in other cases the thick arterial walls were lost shortly after branching from the parent artery. The arterioluminal channels were felt to be more numerous in the ventricles than in the atria. Baroldi[61] and Watanabe[213] also found arterioluminal vessels in their plastic arterial casts of normal hearts. In Baroldi's preparations,[61] the maximum diameter of the channels was 200 μm. Arterioluminal vessels were evident in 86.4% of left ventricles and 50% of right ventricles.

Prinzmetal and his colleagues[36] perfused the cannulated main left coronary artery of postmortem human hearts with glass beads of varying diameters at pressures less than 160 mmHg. They recovered beads with diameters ranging from 70 to 350 μm from both the right and left ventricles. Obviously, these beads were too large to have passed through the capillary network.

On the basis of their histologic-morphologic studies, Wearn et al.[207] described a second endomural vessel, the arteriosinusoidal channel (Figure 1-29). They observed branches of small arteries arborizing not only into capillaries but also into vessels of irregular lumens varying from 50 to 250 μm. After branching from the parent arteriole, this vessel lost its arterial character through loss of media, thinning of intima, and gradual disappearance of the adventitia. It then broke up into thin-walled, irregular sinusoids or simple endothelial tubes sometimes supported by a small amount of subendothelial connective tissue. These sinusoids tended to meander and anastomosed with adjacent sinusoidal vessels and with capillaries before reaching an endocardial foramen, usually deep within the intertrabecular spaces. These arteriosinusoidal channels usually lay in close contact with muscle fibers, and their walls were felt to be thin enough to support exchange with the fibers.

The third type of endomural vessel is the venoluminal channel or Thebesian vein, which was originally identified by Thebesius (Figure 1-29). Other anatomists including von Haller,[205] de Sénac,[205] Bochdalek,[214] and Langer[10] acknowledged and confirmed the presence of direct connections between the coronary veins and the cavities of the heart. On the other hand, Lannelongue[215] was able to identify connections between coronary veins and endocardial foramina only in the atria. Grant and Viko[216] cannulated endocardial foramina much as Thebesius did and injected either chrome-yellow gelatin or celloidin. The myocardium was then either cleared with methyl salicylate or digested with hydrochloric acid. The Thebesian foramina ranged in size from pinpoint to 1 mm in diameter, and were usually circular but occasionally elongated like a furrow. One or more vessels emanated from them. Thebesian foramina were especially prominent on the right sides of the interatrial and interventricular septa and along the papillary muscles. Three main types of venoluminal channels were identified. The first was a vessel that quickly subdivided in the wall to form a tree ending in a capillary network continuous with that of the coronary vessels. The second was a direct vascular connection with neighboring foramina. The third was a direct link to the coronary venous system. There were never connections to coronary arteries, and no injectate was found in the latter unless the capillary bed had been traversed. Coronary venous injections of 30 μm lycopodium spores suspended in gelatin resulted in spore recovery from the ventricular lumens. However, no recovery was possible if the spores were injected into the coronary arteries. Hence, postcapillary connections between the coronary venous system and the heart's chambers had to have functional diameters of at least 30 μm, larger than that of the capillaries. Wearn's experience[211] was similar. In addition, he filled the chambers of postmortem hearts with a saline solution of 2% Berlin blue after blocking all possible egresses and ingresses. Cardiac compression resulted in flow of most of the fluid through the cardiac veins with little dye present in the capillary system. Baroldi's casts[61] of normal hearts also demonstrated Thebesian veins in the myocardium of all four chambers. The maximum diameter of these channels was 2 mm in the right atrium. In other cavities diameters ranged from 200 to 400 μm.

There is little question that anatomic channels do exist that directly link the cavities of the cardiac chambers with the coronary vasculature, both arteries and veins. However, as already noted for intercoronary collaterals, anatomy cannot be correlated with either physiologic significance or functional adequacy. Because of the nature of arterioluminal and other Thebesian vessels, investigations in intact organisms are very difficult. Numerous studies in experimental animals have addressed this issue and suggest that under certain conditions, endomural vessels may have a significant physiologic role (see Chapter 5).

Several attempts to quantitate potential coronary-luminal flow in human hearts have been made. Wearn,[210,211] and Crainicianu[18] before him, observed that 60–90% of a salt solution perfusing the coronary arteries escaped directly into the heart chambers. However, when the coronaries were perfused with dyes alone, only small amounts of perfusate were found in the ventricular lumen.[211] Furthermore, only small amounts of fluid were recovered from cardiac chambers of hearts that had been permitted to resume beating following initiation of coronary perfusion.[211] Wearn concluded that his initial observations were artifactual and were most likely the result of swelling of the distal vasculature with consequent forcing of the perfusate through the lower resistance pathway to the ventricular lumen. Hoffmann[217] cannulated the coronary arteries of human hearts through the aorta and perfused them with physiologic saline and indigo carmine. The amount of drainage into the left ventricle was quantitated. Whereas the drainage was only 4.3 ml/min/100 g in normal hearts, it increased fourfold to 18.2 ml/min/100 g in hearts with coronary obstructive disease. These results suggest that the capacity of the mural-endocardial anastomotic system may increase in individuals with coronary disease. However, even in these latter individuals the maximal flow that might be realized from this collateral system would still be only approximately one-fifth of normal antegrade myocardial perfusion, and obviously data from saline-perfused, isolated hearts cannot be directly extrapolated to the beating in-situ organ. Finally, Ravin et al.[218] estimated the volume of Thebesian venous flow into the left ventricle in beating human hearts at the time of cardiac surgery. Coronary venous flow directly entering the left ventricle accounted for 0.12–0.43% (average 0.26%) of total left ventricular flow.

Persistence of the fetal intramyocardial sinusoidal circulation linking the ventricular lumen with coronary arteries has been identified in selected patients with congenital cardiac anomalies. Most examples have been reported in hearts with pulmonic valve atresia and intact interventricular septa.[219–227] In these cases, numerous blood-filled spaces within the right ventricular wall communicating with both the right ventricular cavity and coronary arteries have been identified (Figure 1-30). Grant[219] observed anastomoses of these sinusoids with capillaries and coronary veins as well. Guidici and Becu[228] also described a patient with pulmonary atresia and a ventricular septal defect who had an aneurysmal mass of small vessels fed by the anterior and posterior descending arteries and emptying into the right ventricular cavity. Comparable left ventricular sinusoids emptying into the left ventricular cavity have been identified in a patient with aortic atresia and intact interventricular septum.[229]

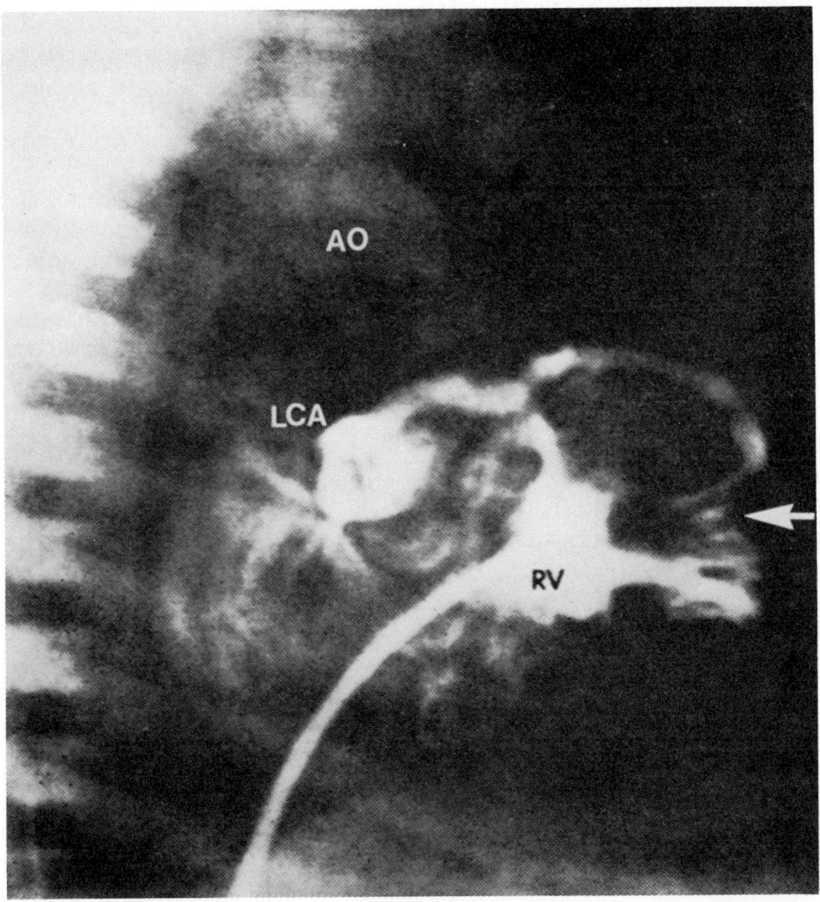

Figure 1-30   Frame from a right ventricular (RV) angiogram done in an infant with pulmonary atresia and intact interventricular septum. After injection of contrast medium into the right ventricle, opacification of myocardial sinusoids (arrow) was first apparent and then the radiopaque injectate flowed retrogradely along the left coronary artery (LCA) into the root of the aorta (AO). Thus, this patient with a congenital cardiac anomaly had obvious endomural channels anastomosing with the coronary arterial tree. (Modified and printed with permission of the British Medical Association from Freedom and Harrington.[227])

Coronary-luminal connections have also been observed in several patients with acquired heart disease and some with otherwise normal hearts. Case reports by Lovitt and Lutz[230] and Reddy et al.[231] describe individuals without anatomic anomalies who had multiple small vessels within the left ventricular wall communicating with the left ventricular lumen. The maze or plexus of vessels was supplied by coronary arterial branches. Searcy et al.[232] noted right coronary artery—right atrial communications in two patients with atherosclerotic disease involving the right coronary artery. Finally, in one patient with diffuse coronary artery disease studied by Nordenström,[233] coronary angiography produced initial opacification of the coronary arteries. As the contrast medium disappeared from the coronary arteries, it presumably filled the capillaries and opacified the left ventricular myocardium (myocardiogram). Subsequently, the contrast agent appeared in the left ventricular cavity, seemingly documenting a capillary— or coronary vein— Thebesian vessel pathway.

Ostial obstruction of both the right and left coronary artery orifices[234] or proximal occlusion of all three major coronary arteries[235] results in virtual absence of all normal antegrade flow. Continuing function of these hearts presupposes an alternate source of blood, and the endomural circulation has been proposed as a possibility. Bellet et al.[235] described the heart of a 16-year-old boy who died with myocardial tuberculosis. Tuberculous intimal involvement of the proximal portions of the main coronary arteries and external compression from surrounding caseous masses resulted in occlusion of the vessels. Even medium-sized arteries were destroyed. Only some auricular coronary branches arising from the proximal undestroyed portions of the coronary arteries were patent. Coronary veins including the coronary sinus were also obstructed. The wall of the right ventricle contained numerous vascular spaces or sinusoids, while the left ventricle had fewer. Connections between the sinusoids and coronary veins could easily be demonstrated. After long and tortuous courses, capillaries leading from smaller arterioles could also be traced to the sinusoids.

Despite these examples documenting existence and even possible salutary function of myocardial sinusoids and Thebesian vessels, their role in the average patient with atherosclerotic heart disease is difficult to define. Most likely this source of arterial blood for the myocardium is limited, and it is only the unusual case in which this primitive vascular system significantly aids the inter- and intracoronary collateral circulation.

2. Extracardiac Anastomoses

(a) Retrocardiac collaterals

Retrocardiac collaterals between coronary arteries and other systemic vessels are anastomoses located superior and posterior to the heart. The principal network of retrocardiac collaterals in man is reminiscent of the coronary arterial distribution in lower vertebrates.[236] In gill-breathing fishes the blood supply to the heart originates as hypobranchial arteries from the second collecting loops at a position comparable to the upper dorsal aorta. The hypobranchial arteries in general form branches supplying the ventral aspect of the gill region. The branches descend toward the heart and anastomose, and then on the ventral aspect of the cephalic portion of the conus fuse to form the coronary artery. This latter vessel passes caudally along the conus and bifurcates before reaching the ventricle into ventral and dorsal limbs that supply corresponding aspects of the ventricle. With replacement of gills by lungs, the origin of the coronary arteries shifts from the dorsal to the ventral aorta so that the heart is closer to its supply of oxygenated blood. Furthermore, as the heart migrates caudally from the cervical region to its final position in the thoracic cavity, the great vessels also move caudally and the origin of the coronary arteries shifts from the upper to the lower aorta. In amphibia such as the frog the coronary arteries arise as a single vessel from the right carotid subdivision of the truncus arteriosus, while in reptiles this vessel arises on the ventral aspect of the brachiocephalic trunk just above the junction of the truncus arteriosus and base of the ventricle. Finally, in man and other mammals the coronary arteries are the first aortic branches at the base of the ascending aorta immediately distal to the aortic valve.

The extracardiac coronary collateral system in mammals arises from a position homologous with the lower part of the dorsal aorta.[236] This position is reminiscent of the coronary system in gill-breathing vertebrates which arises from the upper portion of the dorsal aorta. The shift from the upper to the lower part of the dorsal aorta may be accounted for by the heart's caudal migration. Thus, in reality, the normal human heart has three vascular systems for distribution of blood and perfusion of the myocardium. In addition to the well-known system formed by the left and right coronary arteries, there are also the lesser-known luminal pathways, remnants of an intertrabecular and myocardial sinusoid network directly perfusing the myocardium in hagfish, lamprey, and some amphibia, and extracardiac accessory vessels, reminders of the coronary artery origin and pattern of gill-breathing vertebrates.

Von Haller in 1803 was the first to describe extracardiac anastomoses in man.[4,205] He observed coronary artery branches emerging from the heart and following the great vessels to anastomose with other arteries in the thoracic cavity. There were branches to the aorta, pulmonary artery, pulmonary veins, and venae cavae, as well as anastomoses with bronchial arteries. Langer,[10] in 1880, observed vascular communications between the coronary arteries and vessels in the mediastinum, parietal pericardium, diaphragm, and hila of the lungs. In 1928, Wearn[210] described anastomoses between coronary artery branches and aortic vasa vasorum. Although other nineteenth- and twentieth-century anatomists and pathologists occasionally documented anastomoses between coronary arteries and extracardiac arteries, it was not until Hudson et al.[237] reported the results of their systematic postmortem investigations that extracardiac vessels were acknowledged as potentially important collateral pathways.

Hudson and colleagues[237] cannulated the coronary arteries from the aorta either with the heart in situ or after the heart, other thoracic organs, and diaphragm had been removed *en bloc*. A lamp black suspension/acacia mixture was injected, and the extracardiac distribution of the injectate studied. The black particles were easily identified and found throughout the mediastinum, including the vasa vasorum of the aorta from the aortic valve ring to the level of the diaphragm and sometimes into the abdominal aorta, the vasa vasorum of the pulmonary artery from the latter's origin to well within the pulmonary parenchyma, the parietal pericardium, the diaphragm, the pleural surface of the lungs, the trachea and bronchi to second bifurcations or further, and the esophagus. Branches of coronary arteries usually left the heart around the ostia of pulmonary veins and arteries, the ostia of the superior and inferior venae cavae, and the root of the aorta, and in the intervascular pericardial reflection (area located posteriorly to heart between aorta, superior and inferior venae cavae, and pulmonary veins). Extensive anastomoses of atrial branches of the coronary arteries, especially the sinus node artery, and of their branches to pericardial fat were observed with the pericardiophrenic branches of the internal mammary arteries and the anterior mediastinal, pericardial, bronchial, superior and inferior phrenic, intercostal, and esophageal branches of the aorta. When the aorta was cannulated above the coronary orifices and ligated between the cannula and the heart, injectate introduced into the aorta was found in coronary arteries in the left atrial wall. Hence, Hudson[237] had clearly demonstrated a seemingly extensive extracardiac vascular network anastomosing with atrial coronary branches.

Since this extensive study of the extracardiac coronary collateral network, others have confirmed the observations in postmortem hearts and have attempted to define the incidence and characteristics of these accessory vessels in normal and pathologic hearts.[54,169,187,238–249] Hearts of newborns were studied by Halpern[238] and Moberg.[245,247] In all specimens, anastomoses between bronchial and coronary arteries were identified. Atrial branches of both the right and left coronary arteries contributed twigs that anastomosed with the mediastinal arteries and the vasa vasorum of the great vessels.[238] Moberg[245,247] also noted that injection of contrast agent into the bronchial arteries always resulted in opacification of coronary arterial branches at the ventricular level. Therefore, retrocardiac collateral vessels, as has already been demonstrated for intercoronary anastomoses, are probably present in all hearts from the time of birth.

Postmortem angiographic studies in normal adult hearts have also demonstrated the near universal presence of extracardiac collateral vessels.[54, 247,248] Moberg injected the contrast agent either nonselectively into the distal thoracic aorta after ligating the aorta more proximally,[247,248] or selectively into the bronchial arteries.[248] In either case, anastomoses between the bronchial and atrial coronary arteries were demonstrated and opacification of coronary arteries at the ventricular level was observed. Fulton[54] instead cannulated the coronary arteries and followed the passage of the injectate after it had been introduced into the vessels. He noted leakage of the injectate from the cut surface of mediastinal tissues in 8 of 13 normal or nearly normal hearts. However, because of his preparatory technique, he was unable to distinguish which mediastinal artery was responsible for the leakage.

Numerous postmortem investigations have documented anastomoses between systemic and coronary arteries in patients with pathologic hearts as well.[54,169,187,239−249] Because of the technique of thoracic aortography or selective bronchial angiography, most of these studies have been concerned with possible connections between bronchial and coronary arteries.[239−245, 247−249] In 22 of 23 hearts with coronary obstructive disease, bronchial artery injection resulted in the appearance of contrast agent in the atrial walls, and in 10 of these hearts vessels at the ventricular level were also seen.[243] Typically, the sinus node artery was involved in the anastomotic pathway.[187,239,240,243] Thus, the sinus node is often protected by this second source of arterial blood.[241] The greatest functional value of this collateral pathway would, therefore, be expected in occlusions of the right coronary artery proximal to the origin of the sinus node artery. The diameters of the anastomosing bronchial vessels were usually 200−500 μm,[247] although diameters of 1.5 mm have been observed.[239] The size of the vessels entering the atrial wall appeared to vary inversely with the number of vessels.[239] Moberg[247,248] observed that the diameters of these vessels increased with both age and severity of obstructive disease.

Whereas connection of bronchial arteries with atrial coronary branches was readily demonstrated, attempts to identify similar anastomoses with branches of the internal mammary artery were much less successful.[243,246, 248] Internal mammary artery injections of contrast agent produced no filling of coronary vessels in 30 of 49 hearts.[246,248] In 15, a few minor atrial arteries were opacified, and in only 4 hearts was there evidence of filling of ventricular vessels. Battezzati[250] injected methylene blue or India ink into the proximal internal mammary artery after ligation of the vessel in the fourth intercostal space. Following the injection, vessels of the parietal pericardium and periaortic adipose tissue were very easily identified. In two hearts the dye appeared in arterial branches of the myocardium and epicardial fat. However, Zagnoni and Ziliotto[251] never observed direct connections between the pericardial network and ventricular myocardium following injections of red lead into the internal mammary artery. In some hearts myocardial vessels could be seen to fill from mediastinal and diaphragmatic arterial branches which themselves anastomosed with the pericardium. The predilection for coronary anastomoses with the bronchial vessels is not surprising. The latter can pass directly to the region of the pericardial reflection close to the left atrium where anastomoses with the coronary vessels occur, whereas collaterals from the internal mammary artery must run along the parietal pericardium from the front to the back of the heart before reaching the pericardial reflection.

The epicardial and periaortic fat pads also participate in the extracardiac anastomotic network.[252] The fat pads surrounding the ascending aorta are vascularized by periadventitial vessels arising from both the right and left coronary arteries, as well as similar branches descending from the arch of the aorta and from pericardial and bronchial arteries. Thus, a rich anastomotic vascular bed spreading over the aortic wall is formed, resulting in multiple connections between coronary and thoracic vessels.

Fat pads cover the proximal segments of the major coronary arteries in infants and subsequently grow along the interventricular and atrioventricular sulci until the larger coronary divisions may be completely embedded.[252] Fat pads are abundant on the right and anterior left ventricles, but scanty on the posterior surface of the left ventricle. The epicardial fat is primarily vascularized by many small branches of epicardial vessels, and is the site of numerous intra- and intercoronary anastomoses. The same thoracic vessels vascularizing the periaortic fat can also extend caudally to anastomose with the vessels of the epicardial fat pads, thus establishing another extracardiac collateral pathway.

Spada[253] performed postmortem coronary angiograms in hearts of people dying of varying etiologies. He observed that the nutrient vessels of the ascending aorta, pulmonary artery and veins, and inferior vena cava originated from the proximal portions of the main coronary arteries. These same nutrient vessels received blood from the internal mammary arteries and pericardial vascular network. Thus, an anastomotic pathway from the systemic vasculature to the coronary circulation is established.

These postmortem studies can indicate only sites of potential anastomoses with the coronary vasculature. However, neither the possible direction of flow along these collaterals nor their physiologic significance can be determined. Angiographic examinations of the in-situ beating heart have at least documented that flow does occur along these extracardiac-coronary connections.[243,248,249,254–267] Because of the limitations of in-vivo radiographic procedures investigations of extracardiac collateral communications have been limited to the bronchial arterial vasculature. Aortography, selective bronchial arteriography, and coronary angiography have been employed to opacify the desired pathways. Using injections of contrast agent into the root of the aorta, Björk[255] found that 20 of 91 subjects (22%) had small collaterals connecting the atrial branches of the coronary arteries and the bronchial arteries. These observations emphasize conclusions based on postmortem material[54,247,248] that normal hearts have coronary-bronchial communications. Viamonte and colleagues[249] employed bronchial arteriography in 66 patients with bronchial carcinoma or other neoplasm and observed that extracoronary vascularization of the heart was poorly or moderately developed in 6 (9%). In two patients there was obvious flow of contrast medium into the main trunk of the coronary artery.

Flow from bronchial arteries to coronary vasculature has been documented in patients with coronary artery disease (Figure 1-31).[243,248,255,257] As already indicated, flow along a collateral pathway is dependent in part on the presence of a pressure gradient along the channel. Proximal coronary obstruction diminishes the pressure in the vascular bed beyond the lesion and promotes flow from higher pressure collaterals. In Björk's series,[255] 48% of 109 patients with coronary obstructive disease had visualized collaterals from the bronchial arteries to atrial branches of the coronary arteries. In 12%, the diameter of the anastomotic channels was at least 2 mm.

Flow from coronary to bronchial or other mediastinal arteries has also

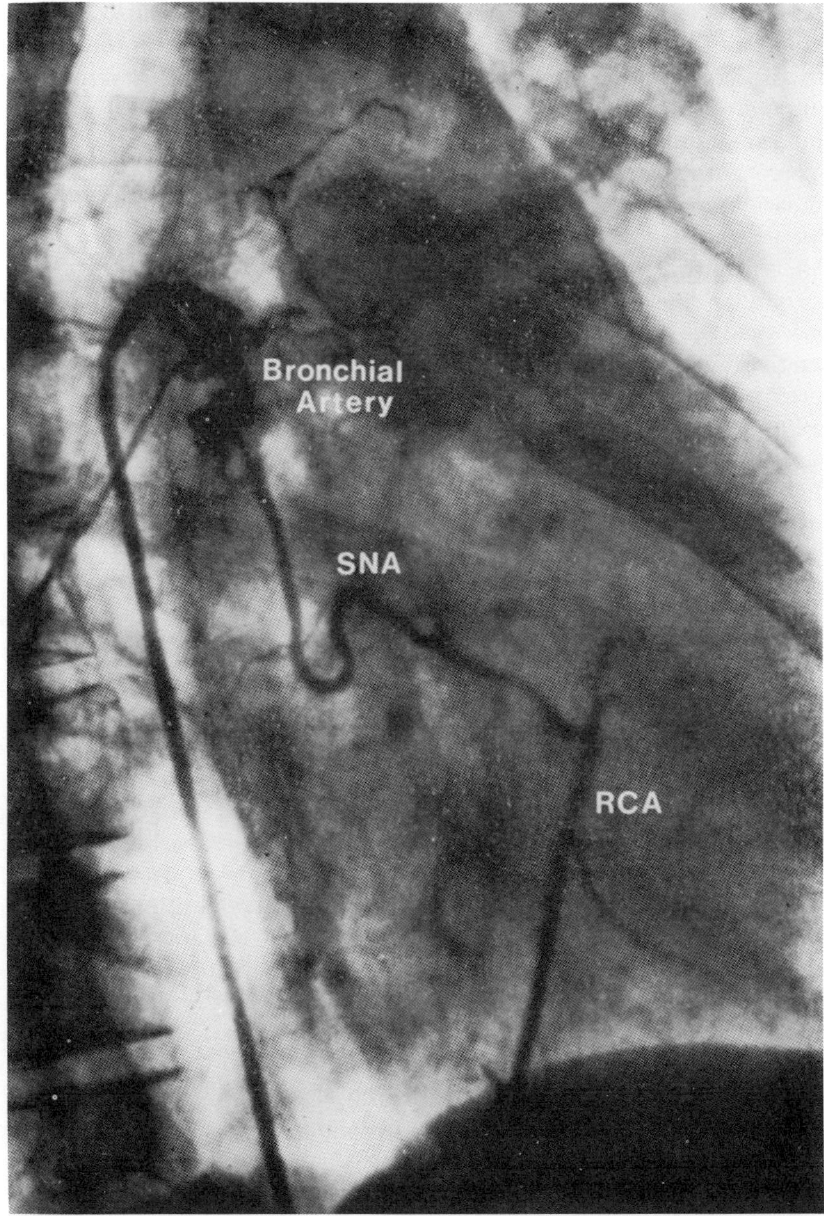

Figure 1-31   Selective bronchial artery catheterization and angiography (right anterior oblique projection). The bronchial artery filled the right coronary artery (RCA) through the sinus node artery (SNA). Coronary angiography subsequently revealed total occlusion of the RCA close to its origin. (Modified and printed with permission of the Societies of Medical Radiology in Denmark, Finland, Norway and Sweden, from Johnsson.[257])

been observed.[254,256,258–267] This diversion of coronary flow has been documented in patients with either elevated coronary pressure, as in supravalvular aortic stenosis,[254,258] or decreased bronchial and pulmonary pressures, as in cyanotic congenital heart disease with large bronchial arteries filling high-capacitance, low-pressure pulmonary vessels,[256,266] absent flow to lung segments related to chronic pulmonary emboli,[267] or congenital defect[263,265] with consequent collateral supply by bronchial arteries, or chronic lung disease with parenchymal destruction.[259–261] One 39-year-old miner with a history of bronchopneumonia and pulmonary hypertension described by Binaghi et al.[260] had coronary-bronchial anastomoses arising from both the right and left coronary arteries, specifically from the right coronary artery's sinoatrial node artery and from the left circumflex artery's atrial branch. In three other patients, fistulous communications between the coronary arterial system and peripheral pulmonary artery branches via bronchial vessels have also been described.[262,264] In each of these conditions a pressure gradient from coronary to bronchial artery was established, promoting a diversion or "steal." In fact, several patients with otherwise normal coronary arteries and shunting of blood away from the myocardium to the lung complained of angina pectoris.[260,263,265] Surgical ligation of the bronchial artery anastomosis completely relieved the ischemic symptoms.[263,265]

Finally, evidence of functioning extracardiac artery–coronary anastomoses has been obtained by cardiac surgeons during cardiopulmonary bypass.[249,268,269] In patients undergoing corrective surgery for either supravalvular aortic stenosis,[268,269] or coarctation of the aorta[249], the surgeons noted persistent and often profuse flow of oxygenated blood from the coronary ostia despite empty left ventricles and cross-clamped aortas. Obviously, oxygenated blood could have entered the coronary system only from extracardiac sources. However, it was not possible to identify the latter in these patients.

As with intra- and intercoronary collaterals, angiography cannot reliably assess the quantitative importance of extracardiac collateral vessels. Hetzer and colleagues[270] attempted to measure the flow through these accessory channels in patients on cardiopulmonary bypass. In these hearts, the aorta and pulmonary artery were cross-clamped, the inferior and superior venae cavae cannulated, and the ventricular chambers vented. Right atrial drainage was collected. It was reasoned that the only way blood could reach the right atrium was if it were delivered to the coronary arteries from extracardiac collaterals. The blood having arrived from these collaterals would then drain into the coronary venous system. Therefore, the right atrial effluent when corrected for the dilutional effect of the blood-free cardioplegic solution introduced into the coronary arteries represented extracardiac collateral flow. When perfusion pressure was in the range of 70 to 90 mmHg, the accessory collateral flow was 0–14.7 ml/min. Patients with mitral stenosis had the lowest average flow of 0.40 ml/min, whereas all patients with severe coronary artery disease had flows exceeding 8 ml/min. Therefore, in the nonworking heart, the maximum extracoronary blood flow recorded was approximately 6% of normal antegrade coronary flow.

Olinger et al.[271] also studied the effects of extracoronary collaterals in patients with coronary artery disease. After cross-clamping the aorta and venting the left ventricle, the coronary artery was opened at the site of future saphenous vein graft anastomosis. The source of any blood flowing from the cut artery must have been anastomoses between coronary and extracardiac vessels since no blood could enter the coronary arteries directly or pass from the ventricular lumen into the coronary circulation. One hundred sixty-eight coronary arteries were evaluated prior to graft attachment in 58 patients. There was evidence of noncoronary collateral flow to 22 arteries in 16 patients. The flow was considered to be moderate in 19 of these cases (frequent irrigation of surgical field) and marked in 3 (continuous irrigation of field necessary). There was no preferred distribution of these accessory collaterals to any of the three major arterial systems of the human heart. Of interest, there was a tendency for extracardiac collaterals to be more prevalent in patients with more severe obstructive disease or multivessel involvement. The functional significance of these vessels to the casual patient with coronary artery disease cannot be determined, although any collateral flow is likely to be beneficial (see Chapter 2). However, during coronary artery surgery, extracoronary collaterals may actually have detrimental effects since they may result in dilution or even removal of the cardioplegic solution injected into the coronary vessels to preserve the myocardium during cessation of antegrade coronary perfusion.

(b) Transepicardial collaterals

Transepicardial collateral vessels are formed de novo and enter the myocardium from some external source. These vessels may form naturally in granulation tissue as a consequence of disease. Moritz and colleagues[272] described four patients with normal coronary arteries who died of tuberculosis (one patient), cancer (one patient), or rheumatic pancarditis (two patients). Each had either complete or nearly complete obliteration of the pericardial space by fibrous adhesions. The coronary arteries were injected with a colloidal suspension of lamp black. In all four hearts, the vessels of the parietal pericardium were completely injected and microscopic examination of the adhesions demonstrated blackened vessels extending from the parietal pericardium to the epicardium. Blocks of myocardium and attached pericardium were cleared. The arteries of the pericardium could be seen arborizing and anastomosing with myocardial arterial branches. This neovascularization was not limited to the usual areas of epicardial fat, but was also seen in epicardial regions not ordinarily containing arterial branches.

Although the observations of Moritz et al.[272] suggested that extracardiac collaterals to the coronary circulation could form in pericardial adhesions, there was no evidence that they might have any physiologic significance. However, in 1903, Thorel[273] had presented the results of postmortem examination performed in a 68-year-old man dying of carcinoma of the penis. The pericardial space was totally obliterated, and both the right and left coronary arteries were completely occluded shortly after their origins from the aorta. This case suggested that possibly extracoronary blood delivered to the heart through the pericardial adhesions accounted for continued myocardial function despite proximal occlusion of all coronary arteries. Based on the evidence that new vessels to the heart could form in pericardial granulation tissue and suggestions that they might be able to supply enough blood to the myocardium to sustain function in the absence of normal antegrade flow, surgeons put foreign substances in the pericardial space to stimulate the formation of adhesions[274–277] (see Chapter 3). Thus, talc[274–276] or ivalon sponge[277] inserted into the pericardial space through a left thoracotomy led to the formation of vessels bridging the distance between pericardium and epicardium. Using radiopaque injectates and microscopic examination, Plachta and colleagues[276] identifed vessels with diameters up to 650 μm in the granulation tissue that formed free communication between the intracardiac channels and extracardiac vessels including vasa vasorum of the ascending aorta, pericardial branches of the internal mammary arteries, and vessels of the lung hila, mediastinum, and diaphragm.

Following these successes, other surgeons placed extracardiac tissues including skeletal muscle and omentum[278–280] within the pericardial space of patients with symptomatic coronary obstructive disease to promote formation of collaterals between the heart and the richly vascularized transplanted organs (see Chapter 3). Others[281–283] used a combination of instillation of foreign substances in the pericardial space and grafting of tissues to the myocardium. Injection of either the coronary arteries or arteries of the grafted tissue demonstrated anastomoses between the latter and vessels of the myocardium.

Further extension of these observations led Vineberg to implant the internal mammary artery directly into the myocardium to relieve angina pectoris, and he and others demonstrated numerous anastomoses between this vessel and the coronary arteries with both in-vivo angiographic techniques[283–286] and postmortem injections of the internal mammary artery[283,286] (see Chapter 3). Sewell[287–289] modified Vineberg's operation and implanted a pedicle containing the internal mammary artery as well as its accompanying vein and surrounding skeletal muscle and connective tissue, and also documented the formation of anastomoses between this systemic artery and coronary arterial branches. Thus, various techniques were developed that successfully stimulated the formation of transepicardial collateral channels.

Hence, coronary collaterals, both intracardiac and extracardiac, clearly exist. They are present in the heart of normal man from birth, and increase in diameter and length in the presence of coronary obstructive disease and other cardiac anomalies. But are these vessels functionally important? Do they help to maintain the structural integrity of the heart? Because functional adequacy cannot be addressed by the types of angiographic and postmortem injection studies presented above, different methods of interrogation had to be developed.

References

1. Whitten MB: A review of the technical methods of demonstrating the circulation of the heart: A modification of the celluloid and corrosion technic. *Arch. Intern. Med.* 42:846−864, 1928.
2. Lower R: *Tractatus de Corde item De Motu & Colore Sanguinis et Chyli in eum Transitu.* In *Early Science in Oxford,* Vol. 9, with introduction and translation by KJ Franklin (ed. RT Gunther). Oxford University Press, Oxford, 1932, p 13.
3. Vieussens R: *Nouvelles Découvertes sur le Coeur, expliquées dans une lettre écrite à Monsieur Boudin, Conseiller d'Etat, premier medecin de Monseigneur.* Laurent d'Houry, Paris, 1706.
4. Wearn JT: Morphological and functional alterations of the coronary circulation. *Harvey Lect.* 35:243−270, 1939−1940.
5. Leibowitz JO: *The History of Coronary Heart Disease.* University of California Press, Berkeley, 1970.
6. Gross L: *The Blood Supply to the Heart in Its Anatomical and Clinical Aspects.* Paul B Hoeber, Inc., New York, 1921.
7. Hyrtl J: *Die Corrosions-Anatomie und ihre Ergebnisse.* Wilhelm Braumüller, Vienna, 1873.
8. Henle J: *Handbuch der systematischen Anatomie des Menschen,* Vol. 3: *Gefässlehre,* 2nd ed. Verlag Friedrich Vieweg und Sohn, Braunschweig, 1876, p 88.
9. Cohnheim J, and von Schulthess-Rechberg A: Ueber die Folgen der Kranzarterienverschliessung für das Herz. *Virchows Arch. (Path. Anat.)* 85:503−537, 1881.
10. Langer L: Die Foramina Thebesii im Herzen des Menschen. *Sitzungsb. Akad. Wissensch. Math.-naturw. Cl.* 82:25−39, 1880.
11. Dragneff S: Recherches anatomiques sur les Artères Coronaires du Coeur chez l'Homme. (Thèse) Gérardin, Nicolle et Beugnies, Nancy, 1897.
12. West S: The anastomosis of the coronary arteries. *Lancet* 1:945−946, 1883.
13. Merkel H: Zur Kenntnis der Kranzarterien des menschlichen Herzens. *Verh. Dtsch. Path. Ges.* 10:127−131, 1906.
14. Jamin F, and Merkel H: *Die Koronararterien des menschlichen Herzens unter normalen und pathologischen Verhältnissen. Dargestellt in stereoskopischen Röntgenbildern.* Verlag von Gustav Fischer, Jena, 1907.
15. Spalteholz W: Die Coronararterien des Herzens. *Verh. Anat. Ges.* 21:141−153, 1907.
16. Spalteholz W: *Die Arterien der Herzwand. Anatomische Untersuchungen an Menschen- und Tierherzen.* Verlag von S Hirzel, Leipzig, 1924.
17. Kugel MA: Anatomical studies on the coronary arteries and their branches. I. Arteria anastomotica auricularis magna. *Am. Heart J.* 3:260−270, 1927.
18. Crainicianu A: Anatomische Studien über die Coronararterien und experimentelle Untersuchungen über ihre Durchgängigkeit. *Virchows Arch. (Path. Anat.)* 238:1−75, 1922.
19. Routier D, Heim de Balsac R, and Gerbeaux J: Étude anatomo-radiologique des artères coronaires par la radiographie après opacification. *Arch. Mal. Coeur* 31:441−446, 1938.
20. Campbell JS: Stereoscopic radiography of the coronary system. *Q. J. Med.* 22:247−267, 1929.

21. Gross L, and Kugel MA: The arterial blood vascular distribution to the left and right ventricles of the human heart. *Am. Heart J.* 9:165−177, 1933.

22. Miller JL, and Matthews SA: Effect on the heart of experimental obstruction of the left coronary artery. *Arch. Intern. Med.* 3:476−484, 1909.

23. Amenomiya R: Über die Beziehungen zwischen Koronararterien und Papillarmuskeln im Herzen. *Virchows Arch. (Path. Anat.)* 199:187−213, 1910.

24. Schlesinger MJ: An injection plus dissection study of coronary artery occlusions and anastomoses. *Am. Heart J.* 15:528−568, 1938.

25. Zoll PM, Wessler S, and Schlesinger MJ: Interarterial coronary anastomoses in the human heart, with particular reference to anemia and relative cardiac anoxia. *Circulation* 4:797−815, 1951.

26. Blumgart HL, Schlesinger MJ, and Davis D: Studies on the relation of the clinical manifestations of angina pectoris, coronary thrombosis, and myocardial infarction to the pathologic findings: With particular reference to the significance of the collateral circulation. *Am. Heart J.* 19:1−91, 1940.

27. Blumgart HL, Schlesinger MJ, and Zoll PM: Angina pectoris, coronary failure and acute myocardial infarction: The role of coronary occlusions and collateral circulation. *JAMA* 116:91−97, 1941.

28. Blumgart HL: Coronary arteries as end arteries. *Am. J. Med.* 5:321−323, 1948.

29. Blumgart HL: Coronary disease: Clinical-pathologic correlations and physiology. *Bull. NY Acad. Med.* 27:693−710, 1951.

30. Holyoke JB: Coronary arteriosclerosis and myocardial infarction as studied by an injection technic. *Arch. Pathol.* 39:268−273, 1945.

31. Ravin A, and Geever EF: Coronary arteriosclerosis, coronary anastomoses and myocardial infarction: A clinicopathologic study based on an injection method. *Arch. Intern. Med.* 78:125−138, 1946.

32. Smith GT: The anatomy of the coronary circulation. *Am. J. Cardiol.* 9:327−342, 1962.

33. Allison RB, Rodriguez FL, Higgins EA Jr, et al: Clinicopathologic correlations in coronary atherosclerosis: Four hundred thirty patients studied with postmortem coronary angiography. *Circulation* 27:170−184, 1963.

34. Miale JB, and Bledsoe A: Pathologic anatomy of coronary heart disease: Particular reference to cardiac muscle bundles. *Arch. Pathol.* 56:577−596, 1953.

35. Balduzzi G, Melis M, and Benedetti G: Introduzione allo studio arteriografico del circolo cardiaco normale ed in particolari condizioni sperimentali e patologiche con speciale riguardo alle anastomosi intercoronariche. *Arch. Ital. Chir.* 82:437−504, 1957.

36. Prinzmetal M, Simkin B, Bergman HC, and Kruger HE: Studies on the coronary circulation. II. The collateral circulation of the normal human heart by coronary perfusion with radioactive erythrocytes and glass spheres. *Am. Heart J.* 33:420−442, 1947.

37. Wiggers CJ: The problem of functional coronary collaterals. *Exp. Med. Surg.* 8:402−421, 1950.

38. Stella G: The part played by the Thebesian vessels in the blood supply to the heart. *J. Physiol.* 73:36−44, 1931.

39. Pitt B: Interarterial coronary anastomoses: Occurrence in normal hearts and in certain pathologic conditions. *Circulation* 20:816−822, 1959.

40. Pitt B, Schweizer W, and Staub H: Interarterielle koronare Anastomosen. *Experientia* 15:309−310, 1959.

41. Schweizer W: Kollateralentwicklung am Herzen. *Therapiewoche* 13:894−897, 1963.

42. Gömöri Z: Beitrag zum postmortalen Nachweis interarterieller koronarer Anastomosen im menschlichen Herzen. *Z. Kreislaufforsch.* 54:1181−1189, 1965.

43. Correia M: Les anastomoses entre les artères coronaires du coeur. *Presse Méd.* 47:1542−1544, 1939.

44. Bellman S, and Frank HA: Intercoronary collaterals in normal hearts. *J. Thorac. Surg.* 36:584−603, 1958.
45. Laurie W, and Woods JD: Anastomosis in the coronary circulation. *Lancet* 2: 812−816, 1958.
46. Pepler WJ, and Meyer BJ: Interarterial coronary anastomoses and coronary arterial pattern: A comparative study of South African Bantu and European hearts. *Circulation* 22:14−24, 1960.
47. Reiner L, Molnar J, Jimenez FA, and Freudenthal RR: Interarterial coronary anastomoses in neonates. *Arch. Pathol.* 71:103−112, 1961.
48. Laurie W, and Woods JD: Interarterial coronary anastomoses in three race groups. *Lancet* 1:13−17, 1962.
49. Rodriguez FL, and Robbins SL: Postmortem angiographic studies on the coronary arterial circulation: Intercoronary arterial anastomoses in adult human hearts. *Am. Heart J.* 70:348−364, 1965.
50. Robbins SL, Solomon M, and Bennett A: Demonstration of intercoronary anastomoses in human hearts with a low viscosity perfusion mass. *Circulation* 33: 733−743, 1966.
51. Tsuchiya G: Postmortem angiographic studies on the intercoronary arterial anastomoses. Report I. Studies on intercoronary arterial anastomoses in adult human hearts and the influence on the anastomoses of strictures of the coronary arteries. *Jpn. Circ. J.* 34:1213−1220, 1970.
52. Omar BK, and Rao NS: Functional inter-coronary anastomoses in the normal human heart: A study on the Indian material. *Indian J. Med. Res.* 60:76−88, 1972.
53. Schlesinger MJ: New radiopaque mass for vascular injection. *Lab. Invest.* 6:1−11, 1957.
54. Fulton WFM: Arterial anastomoses in the coronary circulation. I. Anatomical features in normal and diseased hearts demonstrated by stereoarteriography. *Scot. Med. J.* 8:420−434, 1963.
55. Fulton WFM: Arterial anastomoses in the coronary circulation. II. Distribution, enumeration and measurement of coronary arterial anastomoses in health and disease. *Scot. Med. J.* 8:466−474, 1963.
56. Fulton WFM: *The Coronary Arteries: Arteriography, Microanatomy, and Pathogenesis of Obliterative Coronary Artery Disease.* Charles C Thomas, Springfield, IL, 1965.
57. Vastesaeger MM, van der Straeten PP, Friart J, et al: Les anastomoses intercoronariennes telles qu'elles apparâissent à la coronarographie post mortem. *Acta Cardiol.* 12:365−401, 1957.
58. Huguet JF, Luccioni R, Navarro B, and Colonna J: Les anastomoses coronariennes: Étude radiographique post-mortem. *Ann. Radiol.* (Paris) 13:651−666, 1970.
59. Baroldi G, Mantero O, and Scomazzoni G: The collaterals of the coronary arteries in normal and pathologic hearts. *Circ. Res.* 4:223−229, 1956.
60. Baroldi G, and Scomazzoni G: *Coronary Circulation in the Normal and the Pathologic Heart.* Office of the Surgeon General, Department of the Army, Washington, DC, 1967.
61. Baroldi G: Functional morphology of the anastomotic circulation in human cardiac pathology. *Meth. Achievm. Exp. Path.* 5:438−473, 1971.
62. James TN, and Burch GE: Differences in naturally occurring arterial anastomoses of normal and pathological human hearts. (abstr) *Am. J. Med.* 27:313, 1959.
63. James TN: *Anatomy of the Coronary Arteries.* Harper & Row, Hagerstown, MD, 1961.
64. James TN: Anatomy of the coronary arteries in health and disease. *Circulation* 32:1020−1033, 1965.
65. James TN: The delivery and distribution of coronary collateral circulation. *Chest* 58:183−203, 1970.

66. Zanchi M, and Locatelli L: Le anastomosi inter-coronariche nel feto e nel neonato. *Folia Hered. Path.* 7:63−80, 1958.
67. Bloor CM, Keefe JF, and Browne MJ: Intercoronary anastomoses in congenital heart disease. *Circulation* 33:227−231, 1966.
68. Blumgart HL, and Zoll PM: Clinical pathologic correlations in coronary artery disease. *Circulation* 47:1139−1143, 1973.
69. Wagner A, and Poindexter CA: Demonstration of the coronary arteries with nylon. *Am. Heart J.* 37:258−266, 1949.
70. McClenahan JL, and Vogel FS: The use of fusible metal as a radiopaque contrast medium and in the preparation of anatomical castings. *Am. J. Roentgenol.* 68:406−412, 1952.
71. Dock W: The capacity of the coronary bed in cardiac hypertrophy. *J. Exp. Med.* 74:177−186, 1941.
72. Prinzmetal M, Kayland S, Margoles C, and Tragerman LJ: A quantitative method for determining collateral coronary circulation: Preliminary report on normal human hearts. *J. Mt. Sinai Hosp.* 8:933−945, 1942.
73. Barmeyer J: Postmortem measurement of intercoronary anastomotic flow in normal and diseased hearts: A quantitative study. *Vasc. Surg.* 5:239−248, 1971.
74. Paulin S: Interarterial coronary anastomoses in relation to arterial obstruction demonstrated in coronary arteriography. *Invest. Radiol.* 2:147−159, 1967.
75. Gensini GG, and da Costa BCB: The coronary collateral circulation in living man. *Am. J. Cardiol.* 24:393−400, 1969.
76. Baldighi G, Grugni A, Campiglio P, et al: Aspetti morfologici delle anastomosi coronariche nel vivente. *Minerva Med.* 63:4085−4098, 1972.
77. Jochem W, Soto B, Karp RB, et al: Radiographic anatomy of the coronary collateral circulation. *Am. J. Roentgenol.* 116:50−61, 1972.
78. Levin DC, Kauff M, and Baltaxe HA: Coronary collateral circulation. *Am. J. Roentgenol.* 119:463−473, 1973.
79. Paster SB: The coronary collaterals: Their development, morphology, function, and classification. *CRC Crit. Rev. Diag. Imag.* 9:51−76, 1977.
80. Paulin S: Coronary angiography: A technical, anatomic and clinical study. *Acta Radiol. Suppl.* 233:1−215, 1964.
81. Baltaxe HA, Amplatz K, and Levin DC: *Coronary Angiography.* Charles C Thomas, Springfield, IL, 1973.
82. Gensini GG: *Coronary Arteriography.* Futura Publishing Co., Inc., Mount Kisco, NY, 1975.
83. Vlodaver Z, Amplatz K, Burchell HB, and Edwards JE: *Coronary Heart Disease: Clinical, Angiographic, and Pathologic Profiles.* Springer-Verlag, New York, 1976.
84. Hamby RI: *Clinical-Anatomical Correlates in Coronary Artery Disease.* Futura Publishing Co., Inc., Mount Kisco, NY, 1979.
85. Kattus A: Relation of coronary events to spasm of coronary arteries, precariousness of obstructive lesions and availability of collateral channels. In *Current Topics in Coronary Research: Advances in Experimental Medicine and Biology,* Vol. 39 (eds CM Bloor and RA Olsson). Plenum Press, New York, 1973, pp 219−233.
86. Gray CR, Hoffman HA, Hammond WS, et al: Correlation of arteriographic and pathologic findings in the coronary arteries in man. *Circulation* 26:494−499, 1962.
87. Eusterman JH, Achor RWP, Kincaid OW, and Brown AL Jr: Atherosclerotic disease of the coronary arteries: A pathologic-radiologic correlative study. *Circulation* 26:1288−1295, 1962.
88. Staiger J, Adler CP, Dieckmann H, and Barmeyer J: Postmortem angiographic and pathologic-anatomic findings in coronary heart disease: A comparative study using planimetry. *Cardiovasc. Intervent. Radiol.* 3:139−143, 1980.
89. Kemp HG, Evans H, Elliott WC, and Gorlin R: Diagnostic accuracy of selective coronary cinearteriography. *Circulation* 36:526−533, 1967.

90. Trask N, Califf RM, Conley MJ, et al: Accuracy and interobserver variability of coronary cineangiography: A comparison with postmortem evaluation. *J. Am. Coll. Cardiol.* 3:1145−1154, 1984.
91. Vlodaver Z, Frech R, Van Tassel RA, and Edwards JE: Correlation of the antemortem coronary arteriogram and the postmortem specimen. *Circulation* 47:162−169, 1973.
92. Grondin CM, Dyrda I, Pasternac A, et al: Discrepancies between cineangiographic and postmortem findings in patients with coronary artery disease and recent myocardial revascularization. *Circulation* 49:703−708, 1974.
93. Schwartz JN, Kong Y, Hackel DB, and Bartel AG: Comparison of angiographic and postmortem findings in patients with coronary artery disease. *Am. J. Cardiol.* 36:174−178, 1975.
94. Hutchins GM, Buckley BH, Ridolfi RL, et al: Correlation of coronary arteriograms and left ventriculograms with postmortem studies. *Circulation* 56:32−37, 1977.
95. Galbraith JE, Murphy ML, and de Soyza N: Coronary angiogram interpretation: Interobserver variability. *JAMA* 240:2053−2056, 1978.
96. Arnett EN, Isner JM, Redwood DR, et al: Coronary artery narrowing in coronary heart disease: Comparison of cineangiographic and necropsy findings. *Ann. Intern. Med.* 91:350−356, 1979.
97. Waller BF, and Roberts WC: Amount of narrowing by atherosclerotic plaque in 44 nonbypassed and 52 bypassed major epicardial coronary arteries in 32 necropsy patients who died within 1 month of aortocoronary bypass grafting. *Am. J. Cardiol.* 46:956−962, 1980.
98. Isner JM, Kishel J, Kent KM, et al: Accuracy of angiographic determination of left main coronary arterial narrowing: Angiographic-histologic correlative analysis in 28 patients. *Circulation* 63:1056−1064, 1981.
99. Klocke FJ: Measurements of coronary blood flow and degree of stenosis: Current clinical implications and continuing uncertainties. *J. Am. Coll. Cardiol.* 1:31−41, 1983.
100. Conti CR, Pepine CJ, Feldman RL, and Nichols WW: The angiographic definition of critical coronary stenosis. *Acta Med. Scand. Suppl.* 615:9−17, 1978.
101. Conti CR, Pepine CJ, Feldman RL, et al: Angiographic definition of critical coronary artery stenosis. *Adv. Cardiol.* 26:100−109, 1979.
102. Björk L, and O'Keefe A: Estimation of coronary artery stenosis: Limitations of present methods. *Acta Radiol. (Diagn.)* (Stockholm) 17:777−780, 1976.
103. Björk L, Spindola-Franco H, Van Houten FX, et al: Comparison of observer performance with 16 mm cinefluorography and 70 mm camera fluorography in coronary arteriography. *Am. J. Cardiol.* 36:474−478, 1975.
104. Detre KM, Wright E, Murphy ML, and Takaro T: Observer agreement in evaluating coronary angiograms. *Circulation* 52:979−986, 1975.
105. Zir LM, Miller SW, Dinsmore RE, et al: Interobserver variability in coronary angiography. *Circulation* 53:627−632, 1976.
106. DeRouen TA, Murray JA, and Owen W: Variability in the analysis of coronary arteriograms. *Circulation* 55:324−328, 1977.
107. Fisher LD, Judkins MP, Lesperance J, et al: Reproducibility of coronary arteriographic reading in the Coronary Artery Surgery Study (CASS). *Cathet. Cardiovasc. Diagn.* 8:565−575, 1982.
108. Sanmarco ME, Brooks SH, and Blankenhorn DH: Reproducibility of a consensus panel in the interpretation of coronary angiograms. *Am. Heart J.* 96:430−437, 1978.
109. Brown BG, Bolson E, Frimer M, and Dodge HT: Quantitative coronary arteriography: Estimation of dimensions, hemodynamic resistance, and atheroma mass of coronary artery lesions using the arteriogram and digital computation. *Circulation* 55:329−337, 1977.

110. Levin DC, Sos TA, Lee JG, and Baltaxe HA: Coronary collateral circulation and distal coronary runoff: The key factors in preserving myocardial contractility in patients with coronary artery disease. *Am. J. Roentgenol.* 119:474−483, 1973.
111. Hecht HS, Aroesty JM, Morkin E, et al: Role of the coronary collateral circulation in the preservation of left ventricular function. *Radiology* 114:305−313, 1975.
112. Rowe GG: An angiographic and clinical study of coronary collateral circulation. *Basic Res. Cardiol.* 73:131−141, 1979.
113. Webb WR, Parker FB Jr, and Neville JF Jr: Retrograde pressures and flows in coronary arterial disease. *Ann. Thorac. Surg.* 15:256−262, 1973.
114. Goldstein RE, Stinson EB, Scherer JL, et al: Intraoperative coronary collateral function in patients with coronary occlusive disease: Nitroglycerin responsiveness and angiographic correlations. *Circulation* 49:298−308, 1974.
115. Kolibash AJ, Beaver BM, Fulkerson PK, et al: The relationship between abnormal echocardiographic septal motion and myocardial perfusion in patients with significant obstruction of the left anterior descending artery. *Circulation* 56:780−785, 1977.
116. Kolibash AJ, Bush CA, Wepsic RA, et al: Coronary collateral vessels: Spectrum of physiologic capabilities with respect to providing rest and stress myocardial perfusion, maintenance of left ventricular function and protection against infarction. *Am. J. Cardiol.* 50:230−238, 1982.
117. Kety SS, and Schmidt CF: The nitrous oxide method for the quantitative determination of cerebral blood flow in man: Theory, procedure and normal values. *J. Clin. Invest.* 27:476−483, 1948.
118. Ross RS, Ueda K, Lichtlen PR, and Rees JR: Measurement of myocardial blood flow in animals and man by selective injection of radioactive inert gas into the coronary arteries. *Circ. Res.* 15:28−41, 1964.
119. Sullivan JM, Taylor WJ, Elliot WC, and Gorlin R: Regional myocardial blood flow. *J. Clin. Invest.* 46:1402−1412, 1967.
120. Kety SS: The theory and applications of the exchange of inert gas at the lungs and tissues. *Pharmacol. Rev.* 3:1−41, 1951.
121. Maseri A: Pathophysiological, diagnostic and methodological problems in the study of myocardial blood flow in ischaemic heart disease. *J. Nucl. Biol. Med.* 16:259−266, 1972.
122. Klocke FJ: Coronary blood flow in man. *Prog. Cardiovasc. Dis.* 19:117−166, 1976.
123. Cannon PJ, Weiss MB, and Sciacca RR: Myocardial blood flow in coronary artery disease: Studies at rest and during stress with inert gas washout techniques. *Prog. Cardiovasc. Dis.* 20:95−120, 1977.
124. Maseri A, Pesola A, L'Abbate A, et al: Contribution of recirculation and fat diffusion to myocardial washout curves obtained by external counting in man: Stochastic versus monoexponential analysis. *Circ. Res.* 35:826−834, 1974.
125. Holman BL, Adams DF, Jewitt D, et al: Measuring regional myocardial blood flow with ^{133}Xe and the Anger camera. *Radiology* 112:99−107, 1974.
126. Cannon PJ, Dell RB, and Dwyer EM Jr: Measurement of regional myocardial perfusion in man with ^{133}Xenon and a scintillation camera. *J. Clin. Invest.* 51:964−977, 1972.
127. Cannon PJ, Sciacca RR, Fowler DL, et al: Measurement of regional myocardial blood flow in man: Description and critique of the method using Xenon-133 and a scintillation camera. *Am. J. Cardiol.* 36:783−792, 1975.
128. Bailey I, Burow R, Griffith LSC, and Pitt B: Localizing value of thallium-201 myocardial perfusion imaging in coronary artery disease. (abstr) *Am. J. Cardiol.* 39:320, 1977.
129. Lenaers A, Block P, van Thiel E, et al: Segmental analysis of Tl-201 stress myocardial scintigraphy. *J. Nucl. Med.* 18:509−516, 1977.
130. Burow RD, Pond M, Schafer AW, and Becker L: "Circumferential profiles": A new method for computer analysis of thallium-201 myocardial perfusion images. *J. Nucl. Med.* 20:771−777, 1979.

131. Verani MS, Marcus ML, Razzak MA, and Ehrhardt JC: Sensitivity and specificity of thallium-201 perfusion scintigrams under exercise in the diagnosis of coronary artery disease. *J. Nucl. Med.* 19:773–782, 1978.

132. Okada RD, Lim YL, Rothendler J, et al: Split dose thallium-201 dipyridamole imaging: A new technique for obtaining thallium images before and immediately after an intervention. *J. Am. Coll. Cardiol.* 1:1302–1310, 1983.

133. Jansen C, Judkins MP, Grames GM, et al: Myocardial perfusion color scintigraphy with MAA. *Radiology* 109:369–380, 1973.

134. Gould KL, Hamilton GW, Lipscomb K, et al: Methods for assessing stress-induced regional malperfusion during coronary arteriography: Experimental validation and clinical application. *Am. J. Cardiol.* 34:557–564, 1974.

135. Ritchie JL, Hamilton GW, Williams DL, and Kennedy JW: Myocardial imaging with radionuclide-labeled particles: Analysis of the normal image, abnormal image, and technical considerations. *Radiology* 121:131–138, 1976.

136. Kolibash AJ, Tetalman MR, Olsen JO, et al: Intracoronary radiolabeled particulate imaging. *Sem. Nucl. Med.* 10:178–186, 1980.

137. Kolibash AJ, Call TD, Tetalman MR, et al: Comparison of resting intracoronary particulate imaging and stress thallium-201 studies. *Radiology* 135:439–444, 1980.

138. Parker FB Jr, Neville JF Jr, Hanson EL, and Webb WR: Retrograde and antegrade pressures and flows in preinfarction syndrome. *Circulation* 50 (Suppl II):II-122–II-125, 1974.

139. Goldstein RE, Michaelis LL, Morrow AG, and Epstein SE: Coronary collateral function in patients without occlusive coronary artery disease. *Circulation* 51:118–125, 1975.

140. Reneman RS, and Spencer MP: The use of diastolic reactive hyperemia to evaluate the coronary vascular system. *Ann. Thorac. Surg.* 13:477–487, 1972.

141. Bittar N, Kroncke GM, Dacumos GC Jr, et al: Vein graft flow and reactive hyperemia in the human heart. *J. Thorac. Cardiovasc. Surg.* 64:855–859, 1972.

142. Flameng W, Schwarz F, Schaper W, and Hehrlein F: Functional significance of coronary collaterals. In *Coronary Heart Disease: 3rd International Symposium Frankfurt* (eds M Kaltenbach, P Lichtlen, R Balcon, and W-D Bussmann). Georg Thieme, Stuttgart, 1978, pp 67–72.

143. Oldham HN Jr, Rembert JC, Greenfield JC Jr, et al: Intraoperative relationships between aorto-coronary bypass graft blood flow, peripheral coronary artery pressure and reactive hyperemia. In *Primary and Secondary Angina Pectoris* (eds. A Masseri, GA Klassen, and M Lesch). Grune and Stratton, Inc., New York, 1978, pp 363–371.

144. McKelvie RS, Kline RL, Black LL, McKenzie FN, and Heimbecker RO: Influence of alternate sources of blood flow on the reactive hyperemia response in aorta-coronary saphenous vein bypass grafts in man. *J. Thorac. Cardiovasc. Surg.* 78:62–67, 1979.

145. Horwitz LD, Gorlin R, Taylor WJ, and Kemp HG: Effects of nitroglycerin on regional myocardial blood flow in coronary artery disease. *J. Clin. Invest.* 50:1578–1584, 1971.

146. Feldman RL, and Pepine CJ: Evaluation of coronary collateral circulation in conscious humans. *Am. J. Cardiol.* 53:1233–1238, 1984.

147. Poláček P: Relation of myocardial bridges and loops on the coronary arteries to coronary occlusions. *Am. Heart J.* 61:44–52, 1961.

148. Noble J, Bourassa MG, Petitclerc R, and Dyrda I: Myocardial bridging and milking effect of the left anterior descending coronary artery: Normal variant or obstruction? *Am. J. Cardiol.* 37:993–999, 1976.

149. Banchi A: Morfologia delle *arteriae coronariae cordis.* Arch. Ital. Anat. Embriol. 3:87–164, 1904.

150. Whitten MB: The relation of the distribution and structure of the coronary arteries to myocardial infarction. *Arch. Intern. Med.* 45:383–400, 1930.

151. Schlesinger MJ: Relation of anatomic pattern to pathologic conditions of the coronary arteries. *Arch. Pathol.* 30:403−415, 1940.
152. Rodriguez FL, Robbins SL, and Banasiewicz M: The descending septal artery in human, porcine, equine, ovine, bovine, and canine hearts: A postmortem angiographic study. *Am. Heart J.* 62:247−259, 1961.
153. Schlesinger MJ, Zoll PM, and Wessler S: The conus artery: A third coronary artery. *Am. Heart J.* 38:823−836, 1949.
154. James TN: The arteries of the free ventricular walls in man. *Anat. Rec.* 136:371−384, 1960.
155. Romhilt DW, Hackel DB, and Estes EH Jr: Origin of blood supply to sinoauricular and atrioventricular node. *Am. Heart J.* 75:279−280, 1968.
156. Lumb G, and Singletary HP: Blood supply to the atrioventricular node and bundle of His: A comparative study in pig, dog, and man. *Am. J. Pathol.* 41:65−75, 1962.
157. Estes EH Jr, Entman ML, Dixon HB II, and Hackel DB: The vascular supply of the left ventricular wall: Anatomic observations, plus a hypothesis regarding acute events in coronary artery disease. *Am. Heart J.* 71:58−67, 1966.
158. Estes EH Jr, Dalton FM, Entman ML, et al: The anatomy and blood supply of the papillary muscles of the left ventricle. *Am. Heart J.* 71:356−362, 1966.
159. Farrer-Brown G: Normal and diseased vascular pattern of myocardium of human heart. I. Normal pattern in the left ventricular free wall. *Br. Heart J.* 30:527−536, 1968.
160. Farrer-Brown G, and Tarbit MH: The vascular pattern of the left ventricle of normal hearts from East Africans in Uganda. *Afr. J. Med. Sci.* 4:419−433, 1973.
161. Kato T: A comparative study of the coronary arterial structure in the left ventricular free wall in infarcted and non-infarcted human hearts. *Jpn. Circ. J.* 40:989−1003, 1976.
162. Farrer-Brown G: Vascular pattern of myocardium of right ventricle of human heart. *Br. Heart J.* 30:679−686, 1968.
163. Ranganathan N, and Burch GE: Gross morphology and arterial supply of the papillary muscles of the left ventricle of man. *Am. Heart J.* 77:506−516, 1969.
164. Schaper W: Pathophysiology of coronary circulation. *Prog. Cardiovasc. Dis.* 14:275−296, 1971.
165. Schaper W: *The Collateral Circulation of the Heart.* North-Holland Publishing Co., Amsterdam, 1971.
166. Baroldi G: Myocardial infarct and sudden coronary heart death in relation to coronary occlusion and collateral circulation. *Am. Heart J.* 71:826−836, 1966.
167. Fulton WFM: Intercoronary anastomoses studied by postmortem stereoarteriography: Relationship to coronary occlusion and myocardial damage. In *Coronary Heart Disease: 3rd International Symposium Frankfurt* (eds M Kaltenbach, P Lichtlen, R Balcon, and W-D Bussmann). Georg Thieme, Stuttgart, 1978, pp 2−11.
168. Schaper W, Flameng W, and DeBrabander M: Comparative aspects of coronary collateral circulation. In *Comparative Pathophysiology of Circulatory Disturbances: Advances in Experimental Medicine and Biology,* Vol. 22 (ed CM Bloor). Plenum Press, New York, 1972, pp 267−276.
169. Anitschkow NN, Wolkoff KG, Kikaion EE, and Pozharisski KM: Compensatory adjustments in the structure of coronary arteries of the heart with stenotic atherosclerosis. *Circulation* 29:447−455, 1964.
170. Sheldon WC: On the significance of coronary collaterals. *Am. J. Cardiol.* 24:303−304, 1969.
171. Cheng TO: Arteriographic demonstration of intercoronary arterial anastomosis in a living man without coronary artery disease. *Angiology* 23:76−88, 1972.
172. Specchia G, Bramucci E, Angoli L, et al: Spontaneous and provoked coronary artery spasm: Are they the same? *Eur. J. Cardiol.* 8:581−588, 1978.
173. Awdeh MR: Coronary arterial spasm and collateral circulation. *Chest* 74:237, 1978.

174. Maseri A, Severi S, de Nes M, et al: "Variant" angina: One aspect of a continuous spectrum of vasospastic myocardial ischemia: Pathogenetic mechanisms, estimated incidence and clinical and coronary arteriographic findings in 138 patients. *Am. J. Cardiol.* 42:1019−1035, 1978.
175. Benacerraf A, Castillo-Fenoy A, Tonnelier M, and Wagniart P: Le test au maléate de méthyl-ergométrine au cours de la coronarographie dans les douleurs thoraciques spontanées. *Arch. Mal. Coeur* 72:39−47. 1979.
176. de Servi S, Specchia G, Angoli L, et al: Coronary arterial spasm in angina at rest associated with transient ST-segment changes. *Clin. Cardiol.* 3:54−60, 1980.
177. Metzger JP, Bor J, Rojano-Guzman A, et al: Spasme coronaire provoqué, revascularisation immédiate par suppléance hétérocoronarienne: Apport de la scintigraphie myocardique. *Arch. Mal. Coeur* 73:307−312, 1980.
178. Hattori R, Nosaka H, and Nobuyoshi M: Two cases with spontaneous spasm of left main trunk. *Br. Heart J.* 47:249−252, 1982.
179. Garfein OB, and Feit A: Dynamic intercoronary collateral flow in a patient with variant angina and coronary artery spasm. *Am. J. Med.* 72:463−466, 1982.
180. Siepser SL, Kaltman AJ, Mills N, et al: Coronary collateral flow after traumatic fistula between right coronary artery and right atrium. *N. Engl. J. Med.* 287:754−756, 1972.
181. Weiner BH, Mills RM Jr, Starobin OE, and Lingley JF: Intracoronary anastomosis in the absence of obstructive lesions of the coronary arteries. *Chest* 76:488−489, 1979.
182. Cosby RS, Giddings JA, See JR, and Mayo M: Clinicoarteriographic correlations in angina pectoris with and without myocardial infarction. *Am. J. Cardiol.* 30:472−475, 1972.
183. Cosby RS, Giddings JA, and See JR: Coronary collateral circulation. *Chest* 66:27−31, 1974.
184. Fulton WFM: Anastomotic enlargement and ischaemic myocardial damage. *Br. Heart J.* 26:1−15, 1964.
185. James TN, and Burch GE: The atrial coronary arteries in man. *Circulation* 17:90−98, 1958.
186. Lienhard G: La vascularisation du noeud de Keith et Flack chez l'homme. *Arch. Anat. Histol. Embryol.* 55:361−397, 1972.
187. Kennel AJ, and Titus JL: The vasculature of the human sinus node. *Mayo Clin. Proc.* 47:556−561, 1972.
188. Hutchinson MCE: A study of the atrial arteries in man. *J. Anat.* 125:39−54, 1978.
189. Nerantzis CE, Toutouzas P, and Avgoustakis D: The importance of the sinus node artery in the blood supply of the atrial myocardium: An anatomical study of 360 cases. *Acta Cardiol.* 38:35−47, 1983.
190. Levin DC: Pathways and functional significance of the coronary collateral circulation. *Circulation* 50:831−837, 1974.
191. Bertho E, and Gagnon G: A comparative study in three dimension of the blood supply of the normal interventricular septum in human, canine, bovine, porcine, ovine, and equine heart. *Dis. Chest* 46:251−262, 1964.
192. James TN, and Burch GE: Blood supply of the human interventricular septum. *Circulation* 17:391−396, 1958.
193. Lipchik EO, Moss AJ: Descending septal coronary artery. *N.Y. State J. Med.* 75:1755−1756, 1975.
194. Frink RJ, and James TN: Normal blood supply to the human His bundle and proximal bundle branches. *Circulation* 47:8−18, 1973.
195. Grollman JH Jr, and Heger L: Angiographic anatomy of the left Kugel's artery. *Cathet. Cardiovasc. Diagn.* 4:127−133, 1978.
196. Soto B, Jochem W, Karp RB, and Barcia A: Angiographic anatomy of the Kugel's artery: Arteria anastomotica auricularis magna. *Am. J. Roentgenol.* 119:503−507, 1973.

197. Smith C, and Amplatz K: Angiographic demonstration of Kugel's artery (arteria anastomotica auricularis magna). *Radiology* 106:113−118, 1973.
198. Thompson AJ, and Froelicher VF: Kugel's artery as a major collateral channel in severe coronary disease. *Aerospace Med.* 45:1276−1280, 1974.
199. Minot CS: On a hitherto unrecognized form of blood circulation without capillaries in the organs of Vertebrata. *Proc. Boston Soc. Natur. Hist.* 29:185−215, 1900.
200. Grant RT: Development of the cardiac coronary vessels in the rabbit. *Heart* 13:261−271, 1926.
201. Grant RT, and Regnier M: The comparative anatomy of the cardiac coronary vessels. *Heart* 13:285−317, 1926.
202. Jensen D: The hagfish. *Sci. Am.* 214(2):82−90, 1966.
203. Lewis FT: The question of sinusoids. *Anat. Anz.* 25:261−279, 1904.
204. Patten BM: The development of the heart. In *Pathology of the Heart*, 2nd ed. (ed SE Gould). Charles C Thomas, Springfield, IL, 1960, pp 24−92.
205. Wearn JT: The anatomy of the coronary vessels. In *Diseases of the Coronary Arteries and Cardiac Pain* (ed RL Levy). MacMillan Co., New York, 1936, pp 31−56.
206. Roberts JT: Arteries, veins, and lymphatic vessels of the heart. In *Cardiology: An Encyclopedia of the Cardiovascular System* (ed AA Luisada). McGraw-Hill Book Co., Inc., New York, 1959, p I-93.
207. Wearn JT, Mettier SR, Klumpp TG, and Zschiesche LJ: The nature of the vascular communications between the coronary arteries and the chambers of the heart. *Am. Heart J.* 9:143−164, 1933.
208. Abernethy J: Observations on the foramina Thebesii of the heart. *Phil. Trans. Roy. Soc. Lond.* (abridged) 18:287−290, 1809.
209. Kretz J: Über die Bedeutung der Venae minimae Thebesii für die Blutversorgung des Herzmuskels. *Virchows Arch. (Path. Anat.)* 266:647−675, 1928.
210. Wearn JT: The extent of the capillary bed of the heart. *J. Exp. Med.* 47:273−291, 1928.
211. Wearn JT: The role of the Thebesian vessels in the circulation of the heart. *J. Exp. Med.* 47:293−316, 1928.
212. Mettier SR, Zschiesche LJ, and Wearn JT: Demonstration of direct vascular communications between the coronary arteries and chambers of the heart. *Trans. Assoc. Am. Phys.* 44:345−347, 1929.
213. Watanabe Y: An experimental study on the coronary-luminal communicating channels in coronary circulation. *Jpn. Circ. J.* 24:11−26, 1960.
214. Bochdalek: Zur Anatomie des menschlichen Herzens. 1) Ueber die sogenannte pars membranacea septi ventriculorum cordis und 2) über die foramina Thebesii. *Arch. Anat. Physiol. Wissensch. Med.*:302−325, 1868.
215. Lannelongue: Recherches sur la circulation des parois du coeur. *Arch. Physiol.* 1:22−34, 1868.
216. Grant RT, and Viko LE: Observations on the anatomy of the Thebesian vessels of the heart. *Heart* 15:103−123, 1929.
217. Hoffmann E, Ringler W, and Gebhardt C: Die Bedeutung ventrikulokoronarer Verbindungen für die Ausgleichsversorgung des Herzmuskels bei Koronarsklerose. *Z. Kreislaufforsch.* 56:1218−1226, 1967.
218. Ravin MB, Epstein RM, and Malm JR: Contribution of Thebesian veins to the physiologic shunt in anesthetized man. *J. Appl. Physiol.* 20:1148−1152, 1965.
219. Grant RT: An unusual anomaly of the coronary vessels in the malformed heart of a child. *Heart* 13:273−283, 1926.
220. Currarino G, Silverman FN, and Landing BH: Abnormal congenital fistulous communications of the coronary arteries. *Am J. Roetgenol.* 82:393−402, 1959.
221. Davignon AL, Greenwold WE, DuShane JW, and Edwards JE: Congenital pulmonary atresia with intact ventricular septum: Clinicopathologic correlation of two anatomic types. *Am. Heart J.* 62:591−602, 1961.

222. Elliott LP, Adams P Jr, and Edwards JE: Pulmonary atresia with intact ventricular septum. *Br. Heart J.* 25:489−501, 1963.
223. Kauffman SL, and Andersen DH: Persistent venous valves, maldevelopment of the right heart, and coronary artery−ventricular communications. *Am. Heart J.* 66:664−669, 1963.
224. Lauer RM, Fink HP, Petry EL, et al: Angiographic demonstration of intramyocardial sinusoids in pulmonary-valve atresia with intact ventricular septum and hypoplastic right ventricle. *N. Engl. J. Med.* 271:68−72, 1964.
225. Cornell SH: Myocardial sinusoids in pulmonary valvular atresia. *Radiology* 86:421−424, 1966.
226. Lenox CC, and Briner J: Absent proximal coronary arteries associated with pulmonic atresia. *Am. J. Cardiol.* 30:666−669, 1972.
227. Freedom RM, and Harrington DP: Contributions of intramyocardial sinusoids in pulmonary atresia and intact ventricular septum to a right-sided circular shunt. *Br. Heart J.* 36:1061−1065, 1974.
228. Guidici C, and Becu L: Cardio-aortic fistula through anomalous coronary arteries. *Br. Heart J.* 22:729−733, 1960.
229. Bellet S, and Gouley BA: Congenital heart disease with multiple cardiac anomalies. Report of a case showing aortic atresia, fibrous scar in myocardium and embryonal sinusoidal remains. *Am. J. Med. Sci.* 183:458−465, 1932.
230. Lovitt WV Jr, and Lutz S Jr: Embryological aneurysm of the myocardial vessels. *Arch. Pathol.* 57:163−167, 1954.
231. Reddy K, Gupta M, and Hamby RI: Multiple coronary arteriosystemic fistulas. *Am. J. Cardiol.* 33:304−306, 1974.
232. Searcy RA, Stein PD, Ganesan G, and Bruce TA: Arterio-atrial shunting in coronary atherosclerosis. *Chest* 59:398−401, 1971.
233. Nordenström B: The Thebesian circulation in coronary angiography. *Angiology* 16:616−621, 1965.
234. Leary T, and Wearn JT: Two cases of complete occlusion of both coronary orifices. *Am. Heart J.* 5:412−423, 1930.
235. Bellet S, Gouley BA, and McMillan TM: Nourishment of the myocardium through Thebesian vessels: In a heart in which the large coronary arteries and veins were destroyed by tuberculous myocarditis. *Arch. Intern. Med.* 51:112−121, 1933.
236. Halpern MH, and May MM: Phylogenetic study of the extracardiac arteries to the heart. *Am. J. Anat.* 102:469−480, 1958.
237. Hudson CL, Moritz AR, and Wearn JT: The extracardiac anastomoses of the coronary arteries. *J. Exp. Med.* 56:919−925, 1932.
238. Halpern MH: Extracardiac anastomoses of the coronary arteries in the human newborn. (abstr) *Anat. Rec.* 118:306−307, 1954.
239. Petelenz T: Extracoronary arteries of the myocardium in man. *Folia Cardiol.* 22:223−248, 1963.
240. Petelenz T: Radiological picture of extracoronary arteries of myocardium in man. *Cardiologia* 46:65−78, 1965.
241. Petelenz T: Extracoronary blood supply of the sinu-atrial (Keith-Flack's) node. *Cardiologia* 47:57−67, 1965.
242. Petelenz T: Extracoronary shunts with coronary arteries in man. *Cardiologia* 47:323−336, 1965.
243. Arvidsson H, and Moberg A: Extracardiac anastomoses to the myocardium: Preliminary report of angiocardiographic and anatomic studies. *Acta Radiol. (Diagn.)* (Stockholm) 4:385−394, 1966.
244. Moberg A: Anatomical and functional aspects of extracardial anastomoses to the coronary arteries. *Path. Microbiol.* 30:689−694, 1967.
245. Moberg A: Anastomoses between extracardiac vessels and coronary arteries—I-Via bronchial arteries: Post-mortem angiographic study in adults and newborn infants. *Acta Radiol. (Diagn.)* (Stockholm) 6:177−192, 1967.

246. Moberg A: Anastomoses between extracardiac vessels and coronary arteries—II-Via internal mammary arteries: Post-mortem angiographic study. *Acta Radiol. (Diagn.)* (Stockholm) 6:263−272, 1967.

247. Moberg A: Anastomoses between extracardiac vessels and coronary arteries—III-Microangiographic appearance. *Acta Radiol. (Diagn.)* (Stockholm) 7:33−47, 1968.

248. Moberg A: Anastomoses between extracardiac vessels and coronary arteries. *Acta Med. Scand. Suppl.* 485:4−26, 1968.

249. Viamonte M Jr, Petelenz T, and Viamonte M: Radiologic study of extracoronary arteries in living humans with special attention to coarctation of the aorta. *South. Med. J.* 66:1403−1406, 1973.

250. Battezzati M, Tagliaferro A, and De Marchi G: La legatura delle due arterie mammarie interne nei disturbi di vascolarizzazione del miocardio: Nota preventiva relativa ai primi dati sperimentali e clinici. *Minerva Med.* 46:1178−1188, 1955.

251. Zagnoni C, and Ziliotto P: Considerazioni e raffronti sopra l'intervento di legatura delle arterie mammarie interne (Operazione di Davide Fieschi) (Studio critico sperimentale). *Acta Chir. Ital.* 14:511−538, 1958.

252. Robertson HF: The vascularization of the epicardial and periaortic fat pads. *Am. J. Pathol.* 6:209−215, 1930.

253. Spada D: Le a.a. cardioaortali, cardiopolmonari ed i vasi nutritizi della vena cava discendente e delle vene polmonari di origine coronarica. *Arch. Ital. Anat. Istol. Pat.* 33:22−33, 1959.

254. Beuren AJ, Schulze C, Eberle P, et al: The syndrome of supravalvular aortic stenosis, peripheral pulmonary stenosis, mental retardation and similar facial appearance. *Am. J. Cardiol.* 13:471−483, 1964.

255. Björk L: Angiographic demonstration of extracardial anastomoses to the coronary arteries. *Radiology* 87:274−277, 1966.

256. Björk L: Anastomoses between the coronary and bronchial arteries. *Acta Radiol. (Diagn.)* (Stockholm) 4:93−96, 1966.

257. Johnsson K-A: Collateral circulation between bronchial and coronary arteries: Report on two cases verified by selective catheterization of the bronchial arteries. *Acta Radiol. (Diagn.)* (Stockholm) 8:393−400, 1969.

258. DoValle PV, Barcia A, Bargeron LM Jr, et al: Angiographic study of supravalvular aortic stenosis and associated lesions: Report of five cases and review of literature. *Ann. Radiol.* (Paris) 12:779−796, 1969.

259. Smith SC, Adams DF, Herman MV, and Paulin S: Coronary-to-bronchial anastomoses: An *in vivo* demonstration by selective coronary arteriography. *Radiology* 104:289−290, 1972.

260. Binaghi G, Rossi GB, Caresano A, et al: Anastomosi coronarico-bronchiali: Osservazione clinico-radiologica in un caso. *G. Ital. Cardiol.* 4:739−744, 1974.

261. Morettin LB: Coronary arteriography: Uncommon observations. *Radiol. Clin. North Am.* 14:189−208, 1976.

262. Macchi RJ, Fabregas RA, Chianelli HO, et al: Anomalous communication of the left coronary artery with a peripheral branch of the right pulmonary artery. *Chest* 69:565−568, 1976.

263. Spindola-Franco H, Weisel A, and Delman AJ: Pulmonary steal syndrome: An unusual case of coronary-bronchial pulmonary artery communication. *Radiology* 126:25−27, 1978.

264. Senac JP, Adda M, Molina L, et al: Communications anormales entre artères coronaires et branches périphériques des vaisseaux pulmonaires: A propos de deux cas. *Ann. Radiol.* (Paris) 22:280−284, 1979.

265. Sutton MG St John, Miller GAH, Kerr IH, and Traill TA: Coronary artery steal via large coronary artery to bronchial artery anastomosis successfully treated by operation. *Br. Heart J.* 44:460−463, 1980.

266. Zureikat HY: Collateral vessels between the coronary and bronchial arteries in patients with cyanotic congenital heart disease. *Am. J. Cardiol.* 45:599−603, 1980.

267. Green CE, Kelley MJ, Higgins CB, and Bookstein JJ: Acquired coronary-to-bronchial artery communication: A possible cause of coronary steal. *Cathet. Cardiovasc. Diagn.* 7:191−196, 1981.

268. Rastelli GC, McGoon DC, Ongley PA, et al: Surgical treatment of supravalvular aortic stenosis: Report of 16 cases and review of literature. *J. Thorac. Cardiovasc. Surg.* 51:873−882, 1966.

269. Massimo C, Scultetus R, and Modiano C: Supravalvular aortic stenosis associated with aplasia of the left carotid artery: A case report. *J. Cardiovasc. Surg.* 15:380−382, 1974.

270. Hetzer R, Warnecke H, Wittrock H, et al: Extracoronary collateral myocardial blood flow during cardioplegic arrest. *Thorac. Cardiovasc. Surgeon* 28:191−196, 1980.

271. Olinger GN, Bonchek LI, and Geiss DM: Noncoronary collateral distribution in coronary artery disease. *Ann. Thorac. Surg.* 32:554−557, 1981.

272. Moritz AR, Hudson CL, and Orgain ES: Augmentation of the extracardiac anastomoses of the coronary arteries through pericardial adhesions. *J. Exp. Med.* 56:927−931, 1932.

273. Thorel CH: Pathologie der Kreislauforgane. *Ergebn. Allg. Path.* 9:559−1116, 1903.

274. Thompson SA, and Raisbeck MJ: Cardio-pericardiopexy; The surgical treatment of coronary arterial disease by the establishment of adhesive pericarditis. *Ann. Intern. Med.* 16:495−520, 1942.

275. Thompson SA, and Plachta A: Fourteen years' experience with cardiopexy in the treatment of coronary artery disease. *J. Thorac. Surg.* 27:64−71, 1954.

276. Plachta A, Thompson SA, and Speer FD: Pericardial and myocardial vascularization following cardiopericardiopexy: Magnesium silicate technique. *Arch. Pathol.* 59:151−161, 1955.

277. Vineberg A: Experimental background of myocardial revascularization by internal mammary artery implantation and supplementary technics, with its clinical application in 125 patients: A review and critical appraisal. *Ann. Surg.* 159:185−207, 1964.

278. O'Shaughnessy L: Surgical treatment of cardiac ischaemia. *Lancet* 1:185−194, 1937.

279. Strieder JW: Discussion of coronary sclerosis and angina pectoris. *J. Thorac. Surg.* 10:540, 1941.

280. Beck CS, and Leighninger DS: Operations for coronary artery disease. *JAMA* 156:1226−1233, 1954.

281. Beck CS: The coronary operation. *Am. Heart J.* 22:539−544, 1941.

282. Feil H, and Beck CS: Coronary sclerosis and angina pectoris: Report of thirty patients treated by the Beck operation. *J. Thorac. Surg.* 10:529−540, 1941.

283. Vineberg A: Revascularization of the right and left coronary arterial systems: Internal mammary artery implantation, epicardiectomy and free omental graft operation. *Am. J. Cardiol.* 19:344−353, 1967.

284. Favaloro RG, Effler DB, Groves LK, et al: Myocardial revascularization by internal mammary artery implant procedures: Clinical experience. *J. Thorac. Cardiovasc. Surg.* 54:359−368, 1967.

285. Langston MF Jr, Kerth WJ, Selzer A, and Cohn KE: Evaluation of internal mammary artery implantation. *Am. J. Cardiol.* 29:788−792, 1972.

286. Vineberg A: Evidence that revascularization by ventricular-internal mammary artery implants increases longevity: Twenty-four year, nine month follow-up. *J. Thorac. Cardiovasc. Surg.* 70:381−394, 1975.

287. Sewell WH: Physiological background, coronary arteriography, and the pedicle operation for coronary arterial insufficiency. *J. Natl. Med. Assoc.* 55:299−305, 1963.

288. Sewell WH, and Sealy WC: Coronary cinearteriography and pedicle operation in diagnosis and treatment of coronary insufficiency. *Surgery* 55:99−104, 1964.

289. Sewell WH: Evaluation of vascular implants for coronary insufficiency. *Ann. Thorac. Surg.* 3:439−445, 1967.

CHAPTER TWO

Functional Significance of Coronary Collaterals in Man

I. Introduction

The possibility that coronary collaterals might have a functional role has been debated for many years. Although there is agreement that coronary collaterals enlarge because of coronary obstructive disease and resultant myocardial ischemia, the significance of this histologic transformation has been doubted. On the basis of analysis of clinical presentation and myocardial function in patients with coronary artery disease, several investigators have concluded that coronary collaterals are merely markers of the underlying disease.[1-6] In a recent monograph, Gorlin[4] wrote: "In the last analysis, coronary collaterals in man are more an indication of severe regional ischemia (present or potential) than a sign of biological 'compensation' for a perfusion deficit." It would appear that careful review of the available studies does not support Gorlin's pessimistic conclusion. Most clinical and pathologic investigations support the salutary functional role of the coronary collateral. Investigations describing the functional significance of the collateral circulation as well as those denying any importance of the anastomotic network are presented in this chapter. It is hoped that the reader will recognize the difficulty encountered in performing many of these clinical studies, and will understand the reasons for the contradictory conclusions. However, it is also hoped that the reader will agree, after analyzing all of the evidence, that coronary collaterals help to preserve the functional integrity of the myocardium in hearts with coronary obstructive disease.

II. Coronary Collaterals in Angina Pectoris and Myocardial Infarction

A. Pathologic Studies

The anastomotic circulation has been extensively studied in postmortem hearts from patients who died of coronary artery disease.[7-34] Outstanding contributions have been made by Blumgart and Schlesinger and their colleagues,[7-11] Baroldi and associates,[12-16] and Fulton.[17-22] Because the earliest evaluations of the collateral circulation were necessarily limited to postmortem examinations, multiple attempts to correlate the extent of development of the anastomotic network with clinical presentations prior to the terminal events were made. These retrospective studies attempting to relate symptoms to pathologic findings in necropsy material are obviously unable to prove unequivocally that coronary collaterals play an important role during life in patients with ischemic heart disease. However, the observation that the collateral circulation was better developed in those individuals with longer durations of ischemic symptoms and the suggestive evidence that collaterals attenuated or even prevented ischemic events in patients with coronary obstructive disease helped to promote the concept of functional significance of coronary collaterals and stimulated many other clinical studies.

Pathologic investigations have identified a relationship between the symptoms of coronary obstructive disease and the frequency of enlarged collateral vessels. From a large series of 355 injected hearts, Blumgart and his co-workers[9] uncovered 38 cases in which angina pectoris had been the primary cardiac symptom. All had at least one obstructed artery, and hearts that revealed old coronary occlusions invariably had intercoronary collateral channels.[11] Zoll[10] later observed that collaterals were more common in coronary patients with angina pectoris (88%) than in asymptomatic individuals (58%). Furthermore, Allison et al.[28] observed occlusion of at least one coronary artery in 32 of 41 hearts (78%) from patients with complaints of angina pectoris, and extensive intercoronary anastomoses were noted in 36 (88%). Thus, collaterals appeared to be associated with symptomatic coronary artery disease. Fulton[19,22] documented a temporal association between duration of antecedent angina pectoris and the size and caliber of the collateral circulation (anastomotic score). Thus, in patients with angina for less than three months, the anastomotic score was not different from that found in normal hearts, whereas in patients with angina for six months to two years and seven to fourteen years prior to death, the anastomotic score progressively increased. The increased duration of symptomatic disease in these groups of patients was presumably a reflection of the more prolonged presence of critical coronary lesions,thus accounting for the more intense stimulation of coronary collateral growth (see Chapter 3). These studies do indeed imply that collaterals are markers of obstructive coronary artery disease, but functional significance can be neither confirmed nor denied. It is instructive to note that Blumgart and his colleagues[8-10] identified individual hearts with significant occlusive disease but without associated premortem histories of clinical symptoms. In such cases it is tempting to attribute some functional importance to the rich collateral supply observed in these hearts.

As early as 1941, Blumgart et al.[9] believed that the collateral circulation in hearts of patients with angina pectoris was sufficient to supply enough blood flow to satisfy basal metabolic requirements, but that myocardial needs could no longer be adequately met during stress. The investigators reasoned that it was during these episodes of stress when metabolic demand exceeded supply that the patients developed myocardial ischemia manifested as angina pectoris. Despite this early suggestion that coronary collaterals played an important functional role in maintaining at least adequate resting myocardial nutrition and oxygenation, many continued to view the mere presence of angina pectoris and other ischemic manifestations of coronary artery disease as irrefutable evidence that collateral channels were inadequate and were to be regarded solely as markers of disease without any functional role.[1-6] But one must wonder whether patients with collaterals initially might have had more intense ischemia than otherwise comparable patients without collateral vessels, and whether the collateral development initiated by the ischemia actually might have minimized that ischemia to make the clinical course of patients with and without collaterals seem similar.

Because angina pectoris is a subjective complaint which is difficult to quantitate, many investigators have attempted to relate coronary collateral development to the occurrence of myocardial infarction, a more readily defined end-point. Acute myocardial infarction is generally preceded by progressive atherosclerotic narrowing of the coronary arteries. Superimposed thrombosis in a region of critical arterial narrowing is probably the most frequent cause of progression of a subtotal coronary stenosis to a complete occlusion,[35] although coronary vasospasm and platelet aggregation have also been implicated.[36] Critical narrowing of the coronary artery prior to the events leading to complete occlusion diminishes normal antegrade flow with the consequent potential production of myocardial ischemia. The latter stimulates collateral development (see Chapter 3). The relative rates of progression of the coronary lesion and development of the compensatory collateral channels in part determine the clinical outcome subsequent to the appearance of total coronary obstruction.

Virtually all examinations of the collateral vasculature in patients with longstanding atherosclerotic disease and coronary occlusions have revealed numerous, large anastomotic vessels.[7-33] Collaterals with diameters exceeding 1 mm are not uncommon. Allison et al.[28] injected coronary arteries with a barium sulphate-gelatin mixture and then unrolled the hearts to take radiographs. Of specimens demonstrating pathologic evidence of myocardial infarction, 79.3% had intercoronary anastomoses, and all but one heart with infarction associated with occlusion of at least one coronary artery had collaterals. The one exception occurred in a heart with a recent coronary occlusion and infarct. Baroldi[16] injected the coronary arteries of the hearts in his study with latex, and then studied casts of the arterial vasculature. He graded the collateral circulation by calculating an anastomotic index based on the maximal collateral diameter observed and the frequency and average diameter of anastomotic channels with calibers exceeding 100 μm. The magnitude of this index progressively increased as the number of coronary occlusions rose. Thus, in normal hearts the index averaged 4.7, whereas it was 16.3, 18.3, and 24.3 in hearts with one, two, and three or more coronary occlusions, respectively. The index was little affected by the condition of the myocardium in the distribution of the occluded vessel.

The observed collateral enlargement in hearts with coronary occlusions is not restricted to epicardial or intramural channels. Changes in the subendocardial plexus are particularly evident.[20-22,37,38] Fulton observed diffuse enlargement of this plexus even in hearts in which only one coronary artery had been occluded.[21] Because this plexus is connected to the epicardial mural vessels by straight perforating arteries, it is obvious that diffuse enlargement of the plexus can help to redistribute the limited blood supply in hearts with obstructive disease of the epicardial arteries.

After myocardial infarction, enlargement of anastomotic channels can be considerable. Using postmortem arteriography, Hutchins et al.[33] examined the hearts of patients who died 2 days to 16 years after a myocardial infarction. As the interval between the infarction and the patient's death increased,the diameter and tortuosity of collateral vessels supplying the distal segment of the occluded vessel also increased. The authors postulated that the same process of vascular remodeling in the collateral which is known to result in dramatic increases in vessel diameter (see Chapter 5) also caused increases in collateral length. Increasing vessel length in the face of fixation of the ends of the collateral channel at the donor and recipient artery sites woud result in the observed tortuosity. Jones[29] observed that after only nine to ten days infarcted myocardium was almost avascular, whereas healed infarcts older than four weeks had a nearly normal vascular pattern attributable to the development of coronary collaterals. Thus, major collateral vessels appeared two to four weeks after acute infarction. Jones speculated that myocardial infarction following coronary occlusion in man was inevitable because of the initial paucity of collaterals, but that subsequent collateral development might influence the ultimate extent of the infarcted area. Analysis of the time course of extension of infarction following the initial episode was felt to justify this conclusion. Jones observed that extension of infarction into remaining surviving but ischemic muscle occurred in 70% of cases within three weeks of the acute infarction (before full collateral development), while extension without a new coronary occlusion never occurred more than eight weeks after the original infarction.[29] Thus, the development of major collateral channels by the end of the fourth week appeared to limit the tendency for extension of an infarcted zone.

The studies described above document that patients with coronary occlusion and myocardial infarction have extensive collateral networks, and that collaterals continue to enlarge following coronary occlusion. This morphologic evidence of collateral development, however, is not proof of functional significance. Determination of the extent and location of infarction and ischemia in hearts with coronary occlusion, however, does support the functional importance of collaterals.

Numerous reports have described cases of total coronary occlusion without evidence of myocardial damage.[7-12,14,16,20,23,28,37,39-46] In the absence of antegrade perfusion, only collateral vessels could have accounted for continuing supply of oxygen and nutrients to the jeopardized myocardium, and lack of infarction supports the functional adequacy of this alternate vascular pathway. Allison and co-workers[28] injected the coronary arteries of 430 hearts with a gelatin-barium sulphate mass and identified 227 complete arterial occlusions in 103 hearts. In 11 hearts there were 14 occlusions (6.2%) without associated myocardial infarction. All of these occluded vessels had extensive intercoronary anastomoses. Similarly, Lesbre and associates[45] noted that 6 to 8% of their cases with coronary occlusion had no evidence of infarction. Baroldi's postmortem injection studies of 217 hearts with coronary atherosclerosis suggest that the percentage of occlusions without associated infarction may be substantially higher.[16,46] Of 112 hearts with at least one coronary occlusion, 23 (20.5%) had no evidence of myocardial damage, while in 27 other hearts (24.1%) only focal areas of fibrosis were found.

One report[39] of two patients with total proximal occlusions of both the right and left main coronary arteries again supports the importance of alternate sources of myocardial blood supply. Despite absence of any antegrade blood flow, there was no evidence of either myocardial infarction and/or antecedent clinical cardiac insufficiency. Presumably, Thebesian vessels, arterioluminal channels, and/or extracoronary collaterals accounted for sparing of the myocardium.

Thus, coronary occlusion can occur without myocardial necrosis. The only logical explanation for this unexpected observation must be the availability of an alternate source of myocardial perfusion, thus supporting the functional importance of the collateral circulation. However, Baroldi[16] has noted that the collateral circulation is apparently not more extensive in those patients with coronary occlusion and no myocardial damage than it is in those with comparable coronary lesions and evidence of myocardial necrosis (focal fibrosis, old and/or recent infarction). This seemingly paradoxical observation suggests either an inherent difference of the functional capacity of the collateral circulation in some individuals, or the contribution of other factors that might affect the functional role of the collateral circulation. For example, the presence of critical stenosis of the donor artery (jeopardized collaterals)[20,22,38] may adversely influence the potential functional benefits of even a well-developed collateral circulation by limiting perfusion of the collateralized myocardium. Temporal factors must also be taken into consideration when evaluating the collateral circulation. Longer duration of disease increases the likelihood of collateral development.[19,22] Gradual progression of a coronary lesion to total occlusion provides adequate opportunity for formation of an extensive collateral circulation which can function following cessation of antegrade perfusion. However, more rapid progression may result in vessel occlusion before development of a functional collateral network with consequent myocardial infarction. Continued collateral development following infarction will then result in an extensive anastomotic system that can have no effect on the already necrotic tissue. Yet this individual and the one protected from infarction by his collateral vasculature may have comparable anastomotic networks at the time of evaluation.

When infarction does occur following coronary artery occlusion, many investigators have observed that the infarct is frequently smaller than the perfusion territory of the occluded vessel.[8,11,16,20,22,24,29,46-52] Although all of the myocardium in the vascular distribution of the obstructed vessel is theoretically in jeopardy following cessation of antegrade flow, realistically only a fraction of the tissue actually infarcts. This natural salvage of tissue is once again related to the collateral circulation and supply of an alternative source of arterial blood. Depending on the specific circumstance of the individual heart, the collateral circulation may not be able to prevent infarction, but instead might limit its size. Jones[29] analyzed hearts from patients with prior myocardial infarcts, and observed that development of a vascular network in the infarcted zone was delayed by three to four weeks following onset of the infarction. He also noted that extension of the original central infarct to the more peripheral areas of the occluded vessel's perfusion territory was rare after four weeks. Hence, the area of final necrosis rarely encompassed the entire vascular bed of the occluded artery. Jones concluded that the fate of these marginal regions was actually determined during the first few weeks after the initial myocardial damage, during which time coronary collaterals were enlarging and developing. Thus, collaterals to the jeopardized peripheral myocardial region originally supplied by the occluded coronary artery were felt to be responsible for myocardial salvage and limitation of infarct size.

Fulton[20,22,50] also evaluated the influence of collaterals on the extent of infarction. He believed that the coronary collateral circulation available at the time of coronary occlusion was the most important factor determining the extent of myocardial damage. Fulton noted that an occluded coronary artery could be associated with myocardial damage varying from massive regional infarction to patchy or confluent fibrosis, and was able to correlate infarct pattern with collateral distribution. In the normal heart, diameters of the anastomotic vessels were generally less than 200 μm, and infrequently reached 300 μm. When there was little deviation from this normal distribution and collateral diameters ranged from 200 to 500 μm (AA in Figure 2-1), sudden complete occlusion of a major coronary artery resulted in massive regional myocardial infarction involving almost the full thickness of the wall of the left ventricle and the greater part of the perfusion territory of the occluded artery (A in Figure 2-1). In such instances, death was the usual outcome. When communicating vessels with diameters as large as 500 to 800 μm were frequent (BB in Figure 2-1), considerable protection was apparent. Now acute occlusion of a major coronary artery caused only subtotal regional infarction with salvage of a considerable portion of myocardium at risk, especially in the midwall and epicardial layers (B in Figure 2-1). The margins of the final infarct were not clearly delineated, and at times the lesion was patchy with islands of surviving myocardium surrounded by fibrosis. Such infarcts were generally not fatal. In the remaining hearts collaterals with

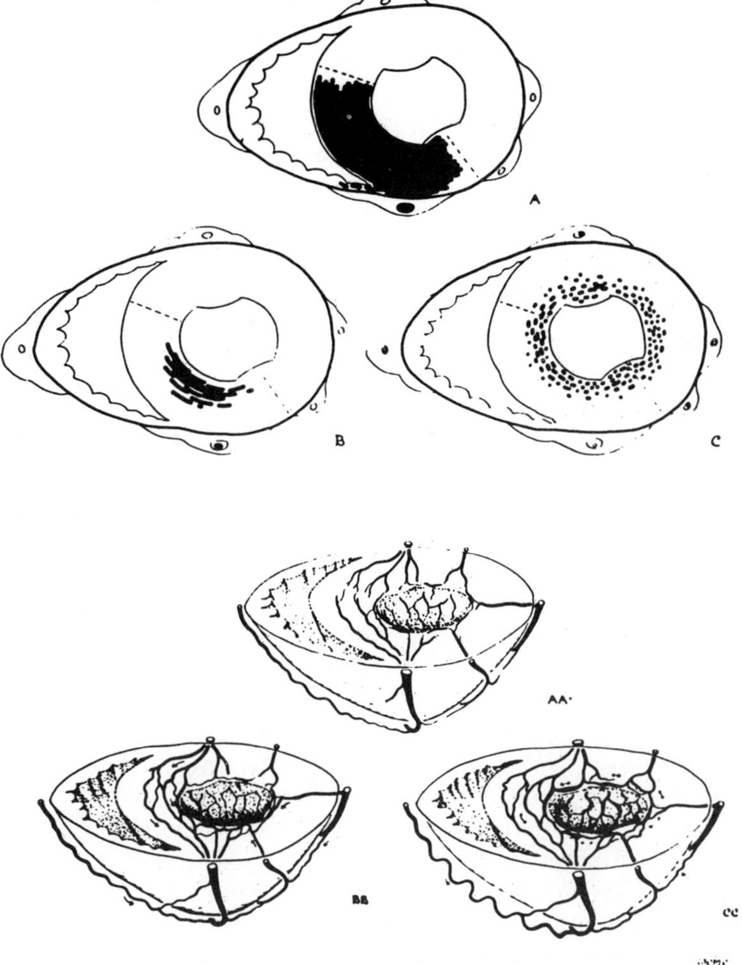

Figure 2-1   Correlation between extent of myocardial infarction (blackened areas in A, B, and C) and corresponding coronary collateral supply (AA, BB, and CC). As the collateral supply to the jeopardized myocardium becomes richer, the size of the infarct diminishes. (Reprinted with permission of the British Medical Association from Fulton.[20])

diameters of 500 to 800 μm were numerous, and smaller numbers of still larger caliber were also evident (CC in Figure 2-1). In this setting, coronary occlusion did not produce regional myocardial damage. Instead, focal necrotic and fibrotic lesions were found distributed widely throughout the endocardial layer of the left ventricle (C in Figure 2-1). In these hearts the extensive anastomotic network prevented infarction until the terminal event when multiple major coronary arteries were occluded, producing generalized myocardial ischemia. At this time many focal areas remotely placed from their usual source of blood supply became necrotic, thus forming a ring of infarcted tissue in the inner zone of the left ventricle. These studies indicate that the association between collateral size and extent and ultimate infarct size cannot be ignored.

In a recent study by Lee et al.[51] of patients dying 3 to 16 days after myocardial infarction, the vascular territory of the critically stenotic or occluded vessel was identified radiographically after perfusion of the vessel's bed with a barium sulphate-gelatin mixture. The area of the vascular bed was measured and compared to that of the infarct. The size of the infarct was always smaller than that of the jeopardized bed. From 50 to 88% (average 69 ± 3%) of the ischemic bed was infarcted. Most of the myocardial salvage was related to variation in the transmural extent of necrosis. Thus, the epicardial layers were often spared, while the subendocardial region was often totally necrotic. In only 4 of 18 hearts were the lateral zones of spared myocardium greater than 8% of the width of the vascular bed at risk. A preliminary report by Jugdutt et al.[52] also confirmed that the size of an infarct is always less than the size of the occluded vessel's vascular bed. In patients who died two to seven days after acute infarction related to total occlusion of a single major left coronary artery branch, infarct mass averaged 36% of that of the vascular bed. In these hearts significant sparing was noted at both the lateral and subepicardial margins. Thus, quantitative measurements, in addition to qualitative analyses, have clearly established that the extent of infarction is always less than the size of the perfusion bed of the occluded coronary artery.

Various investigators[9,20,22,23,40,53] have observed that the location of freshly infarcted myocardium may not correspond anatomically to the vascular bed perfused by the recently thrombosed artery, but instead may be located in the territory served by a second chronically stenotic or occluded coronary artery. This phenomenon has been termed "infarction at a distance" or "pararegional infarction." Blumgart et al.[9] described one case of an individual with a brief three-month history of angina pectoris who succumbed after an acute myocardial infarction. Examination of the heart revealed multiple coronary artery narrowings and a fresh occluding thrombus near the mouth of the right coronary artery. However, the major site of infarction was the anterior wall of the left ventricle in the distribution of a chronically narrowed left anterior descending coronary artery.

Infarction in a neighboring territory is not an uncommon event following coronary occlusion. Fulton[20] observed this type of infarction at a distance in 5 of 21 cases with coronary artery occlusion and recent myocardial damage. Of particular note was the observation that distant infarction never occurred in a territory that had not previously been the seat of ischemic damage. Earlier occlusion or critical subtotal stenosis of the artery anatomically supplying the distant region and a prominent anastomotic network linking the recently and chronically occluded arteries are necessary prerequisites for production of infarction at a distance. The sequence of events in one of Fulton's cases[20] is illustrative and begins with collateral dependency of the left coronary artery on the donor right coronary artery (Figure 2-2). Complete thrombotic occlusion of the left anterior descending artery at site 1 in the

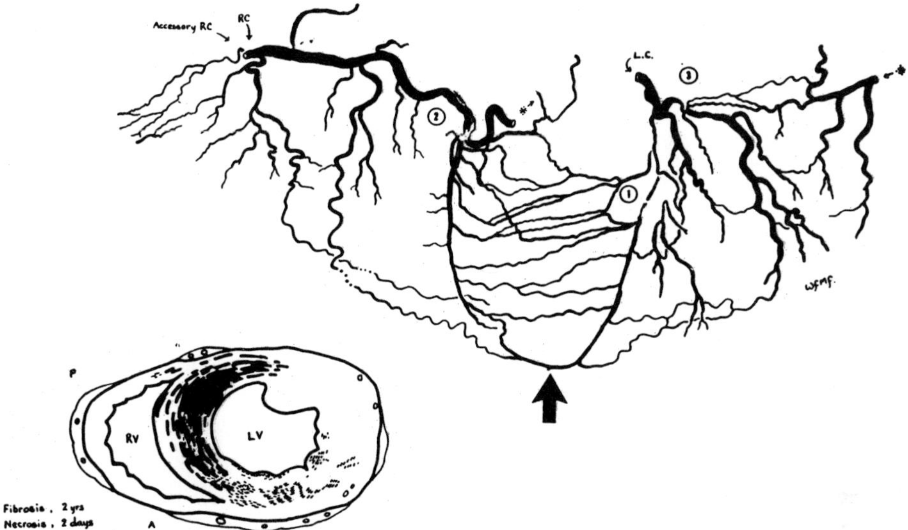

Figure 2-2   Coronary artery anatomy demonstrating the sites of obstructive disease and cross-section of the right and left ventricles showing the location of infarcted tissue (blackened areas) in a patient who died following a myocardial infarction. Left anterior descending coronary artery occlusion occurred at site 1 two years prior to the patient's demise and resulted in infarction of approximately one-third of the arterial territory at risk. The remaining jeopardized myocardium was spared by a particularly rich collateral supply passing from the right coronary artery across the interventricular septum (arrow). Two years later thrombotic occlusion of the right coronary artery at site 2 resulted in abolition of this collateral supply and resultant massive infarction of the remaining anterior wall and septum in the perfusion territory of the previously occluded left anterior descending artery. By comparison, necrosis in the inferior wall was minimal. This is an example of "infarction at a distance" where occlusion of one coronary artery results in infarction of myocardium in the distribution of a second artery. (Reprinted with permission of the British Medical Association from Fulton.[20])

diagram two years prior to the individual's death resulted in infarction of approximately one-third of the arterial territory at risk. The remaining two-thirds were spared by a rich collateral circulation (see arrow) bringing blood across the interventricular septum from the right coronary artery. Finally, two years after the left anterior descending occlusion dissection and thrombosis of the right coronary artery at site 2 in the diagram resulted in abolition of the relief blood supply to the collateral-dependent territory and resultant massive infarction of the anterior wall and septum. Parts of the inferior wall were also noted to be necrotic. In such situations infarction may actually not occur in the vascular region supplied by the acutely occluded artery, which itself may be the recipient of collaterals from other vessels. In other cases where the recently occluded vessel is not adequately collateralized, a single arterial occlusion may cause infarction, often massive, in two separate vascular beds. The phenomenon of "infarction at a distance" certainly is consistent with the important functional role that the collateral circulation plays. After the first coronary occlusion, collaterals successfully maintain perfusion of the myocardium originally served by the diseased vessel. After the second coronary occlusion, which affects the collateral source, collateral perfusion is no longer adequate to maintain myocardial integrity, and infarction ensues.

Thus, infarction is at least in part affected by the collateral circulation. The latter not only influences the occurrence of ischemia, but also its location. These pathologic observations help to establish the functional significance of the collateral circulation.

Rupture of either the left ventricular free wall or interventricular septum following acute myocardial infarction is usually a fatal complication that may also be influenced by the coronary collateral circulation. Of the 1,200 hearts evaluated by Blumgart and his co-workers[54] with postmortem angiography and radiography, 29 had isolated recent occlusions. Cardiac rupture occurred in nine of these hearts, and in each there were absent or poorly developed anastomoses distal to the acute occlusion. In a larger series of 20 cases of free wall rupture following myocardial infarction reported by Wessler et al.,[55] coronary collaterals were significantly less common than in a control series. Anastomotic filling of vessels was incomplete or entirely absent within the area of fresh infarction in all 20 hearts, a condition found in only one-third of the control group. Schuster and Bulkley[56] also analyzed the factors contributing to expansion or thinning of the myocardium after transmural myocardial infarction and subsequent rupture. Their patients typically were having their first infarct and collateralization of the occluded vessel was poor. Thus, individuals without longstanding symptoms of coronary artery disease and, therefore, without the ischemic stimulus for collateral transformation and growth, are most likely to develop free wall rupture following coronary occlusion. Inadequate collateral development cannot prevent total transmural necrosis, disruption of the wall's structure with intramural stretching and tearing of dead fibers, softening of the area, and subsequent rupture.

James[57] has observed that the dual blood supply of the interventricular septum from the left anterior descending and right coronary arteries must be compromised to produce septal perforation. Because of the many collaterals traversing the septum between the anterior and posterior descending arteries, compensation for occlusion of one of these vessels by the collateral circulation and maintenance of tissue viability are typically observed. However, when both the anterior and posterior sources of septal blood supply are occluded or compromised,the septum is deprived of both normal antegrade and collateral perfusion, and perforation is a very possible consequence. Fulton[20] described perforation of the interventricular septum in a 73-year-old woman who died eight days following thrombotic occlusion of the left anterior descending coronary artery. Although the other major coronary arteries, including the right coronary artery, were normal, collateral communications across the septum from branches of the right coronary artery were poorly developed, and the vessels of the subendocardial plexus showed little change from the normal pattern. In this patient inadequate collateral development accounted for the septal rupture. Therefore, perforation of the interventricular septum following acute coronary occlusion is related to either failure of development or compromise of functional anastomotic channels.

The evidence from these pathologic studies strongly suggests that the collateral circulation has a protective role in hearts with coronary obstructive disease. The degree of protection will depend on the inherent capabilities of preexisting collaterals to develop adequate functional capacity to deliver sufficient blood supply to a jeopardized region. Genetic factors influencing the collateral circulation are unknown, but collateral development is affected by the duration of the ischemic stimulus. Therefore, as the interval between subtotal and total coronary occlusion lengthens, the likelihood of formation of a functional collateral network increases. The latter factor may determine the final clinical and pathologic events resulting from coronary occlusion.

B. Clinical, Angiographic, and Intraoperative Studies

Clinical arteriography and intraoperative studies have permitted the correlation of symptomatic presentation and subsequent course of the various coronary artery disease syndromes with anatomic and physiologic evaluations of the coronary collateral circulation. As will be described in Chapter 3, the angiographic appearance of coronary collateral vessels is related to the severity of the underlying coronary artery disease. Assessment of clinical material must not overlook this tie between severity of disease and the collateral circulation, and conclusions about the importance of collaterals can be made only after disease severity has been taken into account.

The onset of angina pectoris is probably related to development of critical stenosis of a coronary artery. In this setting, increased workload of the heart results in increased myocardial demand in the face of impaired delivery of blood. Myocardial ischemia results. But equivalent compromise of luminal cross-sectional area of two arteries does not necessarily have the same functional consequences. Rafflenbeul and associates[58] studied patients with recent onset of anginal symptoms who had isolated stenoses of either the left anterior descending or the right coronary artery. In the 13 patients with new symptoms and right coronary artery stenosis, an average 63% decrease in cross-sectional area of the vessel was observed. In contrast, a 77% decrease in left anterior descending artery luminal area was evident in the 17 individuals with symptoms and isolated disease of that vessel ($p < 0.05$). At identical degrees of obstruction (78%) of both vessels, collaterals to the right coronary artery were seen in 53% of cases, compared to only 29% for the left anterior descending artery. Therefore, functional severity of disease may not always be accurately assessed by simple estimation of the degree of coronary stenosis. Furthermore, the startling realization that the right and left coronary systems may be functionally distinct perhaps accounts for some of the existing contradictory conclusions about collaterals.

Duration of anginal symptoms appears to influence the frequency with which coronary collaterals are visualized during coronary angiography,[2,5,59-61] although other studies[62,63] have not demonstrated the same correlation. The conclusion that the collateral circulation is likely to be better developed in those with more prolonged symptomatic courses parallels that already derived from analysis of postmortem angiographic studies. The combined angiographic-intraoperative investigation of Goldstein and co-workers[60] is particularly noteworthy. They evaluated the dilatory capacity of the collateral vasculature after nitroglycerin administration in patients undergoing elective saphenous vein bypass grafting for relief of intractable angina pectoris. After making the distal anastomosis between the saphenous vein graft and coronary artery, retrograde flow was collected from the graft while the grafted native vessel was occluded proximally. Hence, the only source of blood to the distal coronary artery was the collateral circulation. Measurements were made before and after injection of nitroglycerin into the aortic root. Because of vasodilator-induced falls in perfusion pressure, the measured changes in retrograde collateral flow were transformed into calculated resistance values (resistance = aortic pressure/retrograde flow). As shown in Figure 2-3, the duration of angina prior to surgery could be related to the change in calculated collateral resistance after nitroglycerin infusion. No patient with angina for less than six months had more than a 30% fall in collateral resistance after nitroglycerin, whereas 9 of 21 patients with angina for more than six months had greater than a 30% fall in resistance ($p < 0.05$). The results indicate increased responsiveness of the collateral circulation in patients with greater duration of angina, and also suggest that these latter patients have a better-developed functional collateral circulation.

Ramirez[64] reviewed the clinical histories of individuals who died of ischemic heart disease. Those patients with adequate collaterals had had a much longer clinical course than those without collaterals (52.7 versus 26.7 months), and were significantly more likely to have had angina before their first myocardial infarction ($p < 0.005$). Furthermore, those with collaterals had fewer complications during those infarcts, and tended to have fewer left ventricular wall motion abnormalities.

The severity of anginal symptoms and/or functional patient class has been contrasted with the degree of collateral development by several investigators.[65-69] The observations of Fuster and his colleagues[67] are typical. They compared patients with typical angina provoked by exertion or emotional excitement to those who have pain at rest. Neither the number of vessels involved, the distribution of disease, the severity of the lesions, nor the presence or absence of collaterals was related to functional disability. Schwarz and co-workers[68,69] reported that in patients with coronary artery occlusion, those with good collaterals actually had more severe angina than those with poor collaterals (New York Heart Association functional class 3.4 ± 0.2 and 1.3 ± 0.3, respectively). Dyspnea, on the other hand, was less severe in

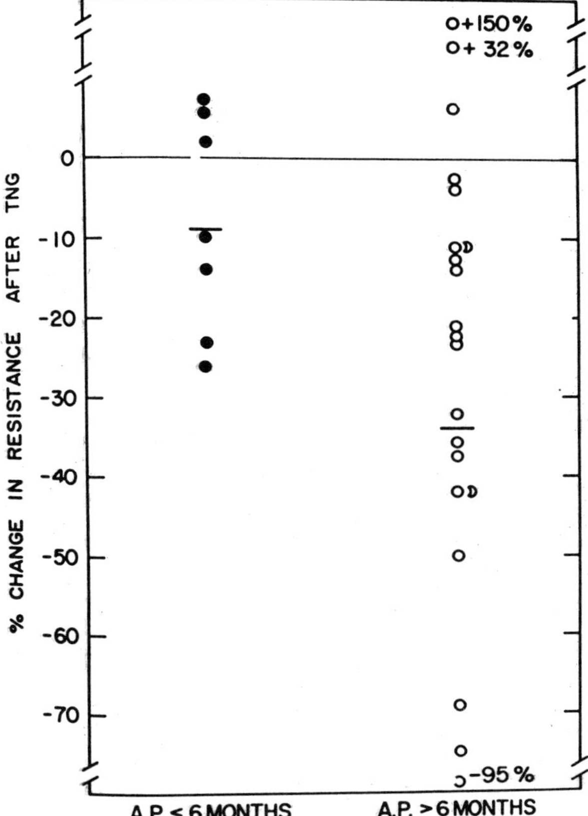

Figure 2-3   Relationship between change in coronary collateral resistance following nitroglycerin infusion and duration of anginal symptoms in patients undergoing saphenous vein bypass graft surgery. No patient with angina pectoris (A.P.) for less than 6 months had more than a 30% fall in collateral resistance, whereas nitroglycerin elicited greater than a 30% decrease in 9 of 21 patients with longer symptomatic courses ($p < 0.05$). (Reprinted with permission of the American Heart Association from Goldstein et al.[60]).

those with good collaterals. Thus, in patients with stable angina pectoris the presence of collaterals does not appear to have any easily defined salutary symptomatic effect.

Although a clinical distinction has been made between typical angina pectoris associated with ST-segment depression and Prinzmetal's variant accompanied by ST-segment elevation, few have attempted to determine possible effects of coronary collaterals on the two patterns. Yasue and co-workers[70] performed coronary angiography during both spontaneous and induced (pharmacologic agents, exercise, hyperventilation) episodes of angina pectoris, and concluded that the adequacy of the residual myocardial perfusion determined the direction of the ST-segment shift. Ninety-seven percent of patients with ST-segment elevation had total or subtotal spastic occlusion of a major coronary artery. In contrast, 77% of the anginal attacks associated with ST-segment depression were accompanied by either subtotal spastic occlusion or less severe diffuse narrowing of a major coronary artery. Six patients with ST depression had total vessel occlusion, but in three the artery was richly collateralized, and in two only small distal branches were affected by the occlusions. Two patients had both ST depression and elevation. When the latter was observed, the affected artery was totally occluded, while subtotal occlusion or diffuse narrowing of the same artery resulted in ST-segment depression. In the 31 patients with ST-segment elevation, only 2 had collateral vessels compared with 8 of 16 with angina associated with ST-segment depression ($p < 0.001$). Therefore, angina with ST-segment elevation is a reflection of more severe, noncollateralized lesions causing marked transmural myocardial ischemia, whereas angina with ST-segment depression reflects only subendocardial ischemia related to either less severe spasm and therefore partial preservation of antegrade perfusion or limitation of myocardial ischemia by a rich collateral network.

Patients with angina pectoris may present with either a chronic, stable pain syndrome or an acute, unstable preinfarction pattern representing either new or exacerbation of old symptoms. It has been suggested that the presence of an adequate collateral circulation diminishes the likelihood of unstable preinfarction angina,[61,67,71,72] although this view is not supported by others.[73-76] Fuster and associates[67] examined the collateral circulation in patients with either stable or unstable angina and symptoms for less than one year. Significantly fewer patients with unstable angina had collateral vessels ($p < 0.05$). Biffani et al.[61] reported similar differences in rates of angiographically demonstrable collateral vessels in subjects with unstable and stable angina. Parker et al.[72] observed that all patients with stable angina pectoris and more than 95% obstruction of a coronary artery had demonstrable collateral opacification, whereas only 4 of 18 subjects with unstable angina and critical coronary lesions ($> 90\%$) had collateral vessels. Furthermore, during intraoperative studies in these same patients with high-grade coronary stenoses, retrograde coronary blood flow averaged 2.5 and 7.0 ml/min in those with unstable and stable angina, respectively. Of note was the observation that patients with unstable angina and no collaterals had retrograde flows averaging 1.2 ml/min (range 0−4 ml/min), while those few with collaterals had higher flows approaching those seen in patients with stable angina.[71,72]

Although the above studies suggest that collaterals do influence clinical presentation, Neill et al.[74,76] did not find that coronary collateralization was different in patients with either preinfarction or stable angina. Thus, of 48 totally occluded arteries in patients with unstable angina, all but two had good collateral filling of the distal segment,[76] a rate comparable to that observed in a parallel clinical group with stable symptoms. Less severe coronary lesions were associated with fewer good collaterals in both groups. A four-month follow-up revealed that the patterns of coronary collateralization in the patients with initially unstable symptoms were unchanged except in those subjects who had developed new occlusions. In these latter instances new collaterals were apparent. Therefore, in light of the appearance and then subsidence of symptoms in most patients, the constancy of the collateral patterns tends to exclude the coronary collateral as an important etiologic factor in the pathophysiology of the symptoms. Iskandrian and associates[75] have made similar conclusions. They observed that 93% of patients with main left coronary artery disease without angiographically demonstrable collaterals had unstable angina, compared to 69% of those with rich collaterals. This difference was not statistically significant ($0.1 > p > 0.05$). Thus, the net effect of collaterals on clinical symptoms is unclear. Although some studies support the concept of a functional role for coronary collaterals, equal numbers conclude that collaterals make little difference.

A recent report by Feldman and Pepine[77] on the clinical effects of transient inflation of a balloon inserted into a coronary artery prior to coronary angioplasty is quite provocative. During this brief coronary occlusion, only one of six subjects with angiographically visualized collaterals to the artery being occluded developed angina or ST-segment elevation, whereas five of thirteen without collaterals complained of pain and showed electrocardiographic changes. These differences were not significant. However, the groups are small. The trend is interesting, and further data are awaited.

This review of the effect of the collateral circulation on the clinical syndrome of angina pectoris leaves many questions unanswered. The relationship between collaterals and the clinical functional status of the patient is uncertain. This may be related in part to the design of the various investigations as well as the heterogeneity of the patient populations studied. Finally, angina is a subjective complaint. Therefore, comparisons between patient groups based on this end-point may be difficult to duplicate. Perhaps more objective end-points (e.g., myocardial infarction) would result in less ambiguous and less confusing data.

The development of coronary collaterals is a dynamic process which extends over months and perhaps years. The timing of myocardial infarction can be dated more precisely. It is intuitively obvious that the infarcting myocardium will be benefited by the presence of collaterals only if they are already in evidence. Continued development of collaterals after infarction may have other biologic significance, but will not have an effect on the already necrotic tissue. It is crucial, when evaluating the collateral circulation following myocardial infarction, to realize that the timing of collateral development with reference to the index cardiac event is frequently unknown. This consideration may prevent one from either inappropriately attributing functional significance to collaterals or denying it.

The frequency of collateral circulation after a myocardial infarction is in part related to the history of angina pectoris prior to the infarction.[61,78–80] Williams et al.[78] reported on 20 individuals requiring cardiac catheterization for refractory pump failure or chest pain during the first days to weeks following myocardial infarction. They observed that 5 of 6 (83%) patients with adequate collaterals had had angina prior to the infarction, whereas only 4 of 14 (29%) without adequate collaterals gave a similar history ($p < 0.05$). Furthermore, the duration of the anginal symptoms tended to be longer in those with collaterals. Aygen[79] evaluated 100 patients with total occlusion of the left anterior descending coronary artery. He observed that 14 of 25 (56%) patients without adequate collaterals had had sudden myocardial infarction without prior angina. On the other hand, 93% of the 75 patients with adequate collaterals had had angina for long periods, averaging 56 months. Cortina et al.[80] performed coronary angiography in a group of patients four weeks after their first transmural infarction. The collateral circulation was more extensive in those having a history of angina for at least one month prior to the infarct, and the subsequent infarct was smaller than in those with no or only a brief period of symptoms. Biffani[61] also noted that individuals with infarcts and prior angina were twice as likely to have collaterals as patients with infarcts but no history of preceding angina.

As the duration between myocardial infarction and angiographic study increases, the likelihood of collateral demonstration becomes greater. Ohgitani[81] performed coronary angiography in patients from 3.5 weeks to 7 years (average 7.6 months) after an acute myocardial infarction. Fifteen of 26 (58%) studied within three months of the infarction had evidence of collateral circulation. However, in only 7 of the 15 (47%) were the collaterals judged to be effective (good opacification of the distal segment of the diseased artery and good run-off). In contrast, 18 of 23 (78%) patients had collaterals when studied three or more months after the infarct. In 14 of the latter 18 (78%) patients with collaterals, these anastomoses were considered to be adequate. Virtually all patients (12 of 13) with a totally obstructed artery studied within the initial three-month period had collaterals, but anastomoses were evident in only 25% of individuals with subtotal (90–99%) obstruction. When patients with subtotal obstruction were studied more than three months after infarction, as many as 80% had angiographic evidence of collaterals. This study indicates that documentation of an anastomotic network is at least in part related to the timing of the angiographic study. Hence, attempts to examine the influence of coronary collaterals shortly after myocardial infarction may arrive at different conclusions from those investigations that are delayed until the collaterals are fully developed.

Bertrand and associates[82] routinely did angiography in patients one to three weeks following acute myocardial infarction, and observed differences in the frequency of collaterals to an obstructed artery in the anterior and posterior vascular territories of the heart. Twenty patients sustained an anterior infarction following occlusion of the left anterior descending artery, and collaterals were either absent or judged inadequate in 12 (60%). By contrast, only 12 of 36 (33%) patients with total occlusion of the right coronary artery and posterior infarction had no or poor collaterals. This study again emphasizes that coronary artery disease and its consequences are not uniform, and significant regional differences do exist.

As previously noted in examinations of postmortem hearts, coronary occlusion may occur without evidence of myocardial infarction.[7–12,14,16,20,23,28,37,39–46] Similar observations have also been made in living patients. Pagenstecher[83] reported that the distal end of the left anterior descending coronary artery had to be ligated in an individual following a penetrating injury of the heart. During the first five postoperative days there were no apparent complications related to the ligation. The patient died of purulent pericarditis, but there is no comment about the condition of the myocardium in the account of the autopsy. Carleton and Boyd[84] described the case of a 22-year-old male with an anterior chest stab wound. At the time of exploratory thoracotomy, the proximal left anterior descending artery was noted to be lacerated, and both the proximal and distal ends of the vessel were vigorously bleeding. Despite ligation of both ends of the vessel, there was no clinical or electrocardiographic evidence of myocardial necrosis following surgery. Both Fuster[85] and Schwarz[69] have also documented angina pectoris in patients with total coronary occlusion but without evidence of myocardial infarction. These observations suggest that the collateral circulation was able to provide enough perfusion of the ischemic myocardium to avoid infarction.

Other case reports of patients with total proximal occlusion of all three major coronary arteries further emphasize the importance of the collateral circulation.[39,69,86-88] Some had minimal symptoms, while others had no evidence of infarction. In one particularly graphic example,[86] there was a total occlusion of the main left coronary artery and a complete occlusion of the proximal right coronary artery immediately beyond a large conus artery. This latter vessel collateralized the left anterior descending coronary artery, which then filled the left circumflex. The left ventricular ejection fraction in this patient was normal. In another patient[88] with no electrocardiographic or ventriculographic evidence of infarction, and total occlusion of the main left and proximal right coronary arteries, perfusion of the entire heart was provided by a sequential venous graft to the posterior descending and obtuse marginal arteries, which had been anastomosed seven years earlier for angina, and prominent collaterals from the grafted vessel to the left anterior descending artery.

Numerous examples of patients with complete occlusion of the main left coronary artery with collateralization from a normal or diseased right coronary artery are also available (Figure 2-4).[63,86,88-96] Despite loss of normal antegrade perfusion of most of the left ventricular myocardium, normal left ventricular ejection fractions and function of the anterior wall and absence of infarction again attest to the collateral circulation's important functional role in coronary artery disease.

During the course of acute myocardial infarction, some patients develop cardiogenic shock. Both Williams and associates[5,78] and Herman and Gorlin[73] have noted that those patients developing shock appear to have meager collateral circulations. Of 20 patients evaluated for either persistent pain or congestive heart failure following acute infarction, 6 had good collaterals and 14 had either no collaterals or only threadlike vessels.[5,78] Despite similar coronary vessel involvement and site of the infarct in the two groups, the patients with collaterals had better cardiac function. None of the latter group developed shock or died, whereas the postinfarct course of 10 of the 14 with inadequate collaterals was complicated by shock, and 8 died.

In Fuster's large study[85] of patients with coronary artery disease undergoing cardiac catheterization within one year of onset of symptoms, a group

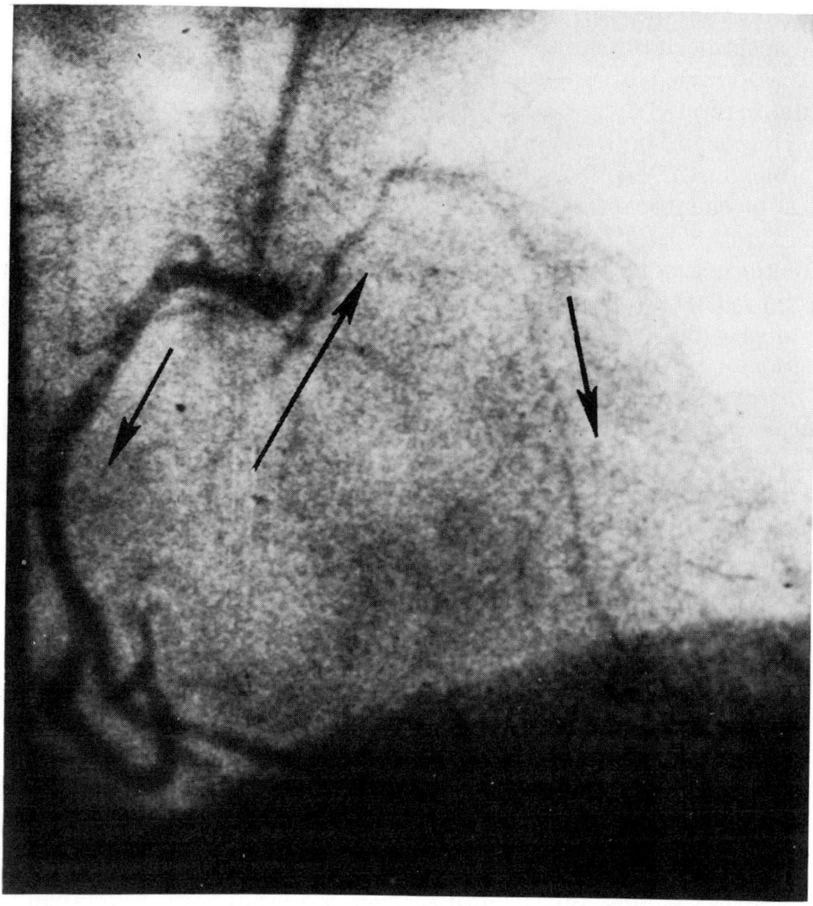

Figure 2-4   Frame from a right coronary artery angiogram in a patient with occlusion of the main left coronary artery. The normal right coronary artery is opacified. The entire left coronary artery system was also opacified by virtue of right-to-left collaterals. The contrast medium flowed from the distal right coronary artery retrogradely along the atrioventricular groove branch of the left circumflex artery and then subsequently down the left anterior descending coronary artery. (Reprinted with permission of the American Heart Association from MV Cohen et al: *Circulation* 45 [Suppl I]:I-57—I-65, 1972.)

with subendocardial infarction was identified. Ninety-three percent of these latter patients with complete coronary occlusion had coronary collaterals. The authors suggested that the collaterals were probably responsible for limiting the infarction to the inner wall of the left ventricle. Of course, this speculation cannot be proved, but it is supported by the pathologic studies which have demonstrated that infarction is almost always smaller than the occluded vessel's perfusion territory, most likely a result of collateral perfusion.[8,11,16,20,22,24,29,46—52]

Lage et al.[97] measured CPK isoenzymes in 19 patients with acute myocardial infarction and correlated calculated infarct size with angiography done on the 15th day after onset of symptoms. Five patients without collaterals and 8 with meager evidence of coronary collaterals had similar infarct sizes (38.8 ± 17.1 and 38.6 ± 15.0 CKMB-g-eq, respectively). However, the six individuals with prominent collateral channels had significantly smaller infarcts (20.5 ± 8.2 CKMB-g-eq). All patients had comparable degrees of coronary artery disease. Nohara[98] also noted that patients with their first infarct and nonjeopardized collaterals had lower peak CPK levels following thrombolysis with urokinase than individuals with jeopardized collaterals. Those with no collaterals had even higher peak enzyme levels. Although the data from the second study are confounded by the CPK washout following reperfusion, it appears that collaterals may truly help to minimize infarct size.

At the time of elective saphenous vein bypass grafting, Schwarz and co-workers[69,99−101] biopsied the anterior left ventricular wall of patients with stenoses or occlusions of the proximal left anterior descending coronary artery. There were no other significant coronary lesions in the left coronary artery system that could have affected circulation to the anterior walls. If collaterals were evident, they always originated from vessels with stenoses of less than 50%, i.e., the collaterals were not jeopardized. The amount of fibrous tissue in each biopsy was determined. Myocardial tissue from those patients with less than 75% diminution of the vessel's cross-sectional area contained only 17% fibrosis (Figure 2-5). Patients with more than 95% decrease in luminal area and no collaterals had 68% fibrosis, whereas in patients with similar obstructive disease and collaterals, the samples contained only 29% fibrosis ($p < 0.001$). There was no difference in the fibrous tissue content of samples from patients with severe disease and collaterals and those with mild disease. Therefore, collaterals appeared to account for salvage of ischemic myocardium.

In contrast to Schwarz's results and conclusions,[69,99−101] Bodenheimer's study[102] demonstrated no effect of collaterals on muscle preservation. He and his colleagues studied punch myocardial biopsies from the perfusion territories of vessels with stenosis of at least 90% in patients undergoing revascularization surgery. Muscle loss was independent of the presence of coronary collaterals (5 of 7 with and 11 of 21 without collaterals had significant muscle loss). However, the patients in this study had multivessel disease, raising the possibility that in some patients the collateral circulation may have been jeopardized. Such limitation of collateral flow might help explain the surprising lack of effect of collaterals on myocardial integrity.

Postinfarction angina is typically noted in patients with well-collateralized hearts. In a group of 58 patients with transmural myocardial infarction and coronary occlusion described by Fuster et al.,[85] 32 had postinfarction angina, while the remaining 26 were free of symptoms. Only 35% of the latter group had collateral filling of the occluded artery, while as many as 78% of the subgroup with angina had collaterals. Fuster also identified 30 patients with subendocardial infarction and coronary occlusion. All had postinfarct an-

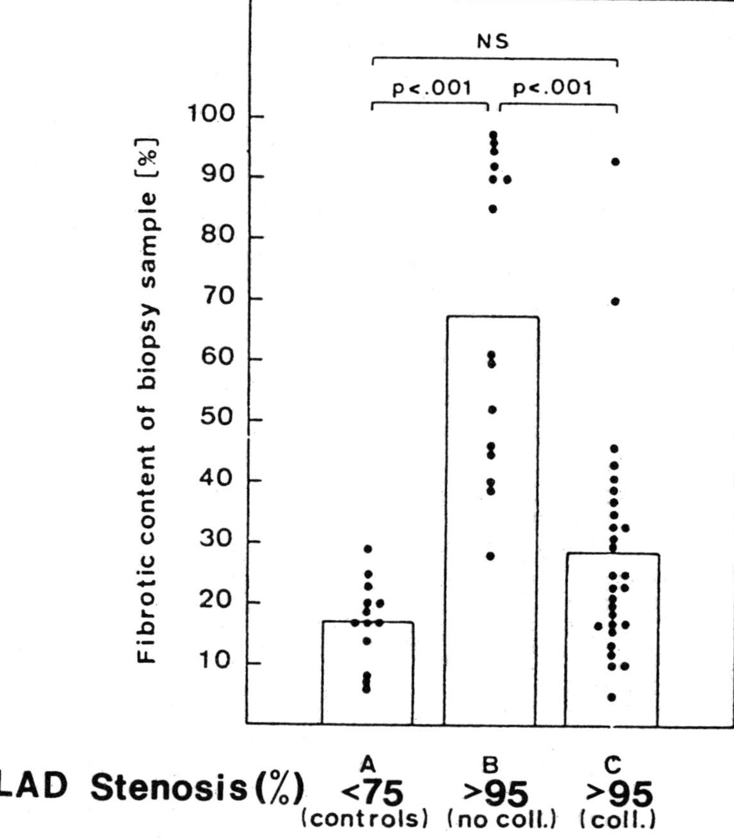

Figure 2-5   Quantitation of fibrosis in left ventricular anterior wall biopsies obtained at the time of elective saphenous vein bypass grafting in patients with stenosis of the left anterior descending artery. The fibrotic contents were similar in patients with noncritical (< 75%) lesions as well as in those with collateralized subtotal stenoses (> 95%). In contrast, fibrotic contents of the biopsy specimens of individuals with subtotal lesions but no collaterals accounted for nearly 70% of the sampled tissue's volume, significantly greater than in either of the other two groups ($p < 0.001$). (Modified and printed with permission of Dun-Donnelly Publishing Corp. from Schwarz et al.[101])

gina and in 93% of this group, the occluded vessel was well collateralized. In these patients, the collateral circulation was probably responsible for sparing of myocardium that could then become ischemic again in the postinfarction period. Cosby et al.[103] performed coronary angiography in patients with progressive symptoms of angina pectoris and identified two collateral patterns. Intercoronary anastomoses were identified in 17 subjects, 12 of whom had histories of prior infarcts. In 10 patients there were only local homocoronary collaterals bridging the obstructing arterial lesion, and 8 had not had infarcts. Therefore, the occurrence of previous infarction appeared to be an important factor predisposing to the development of a collateral network.

Although the collaterals were unable to prevent recurrent symptoms, it is unwarranted to conclude that the coronary collaterals were merely markers of severe disease without any functional significance. Recurrent symptoms and more extensive collateral circulations may both be manifestations of more intense ischemia.

Recently, Schuster and Bulkley[34] described the clinical syndrome of "ischemia at a distance." From a large series of patients who died within 30 days of an acute myocardial infarction, they identified 20 who had had postinfarction angina without enzymatic or pathologic evidence of new infarction. Electrocardiographic abnormalities (ST-T-wave changes) during anginal episodes in eight patients appeared in leads corresponding to a vascular distribution different from that of the original infarction. The myocardium involved in this ischemia at a distance was perfused by nonoccluded but critically narrowed vessels. All patients had rich anastomotic networks. The functional significance of the collateral circulation in these individuals is similar to that previously described for hearts with infarction at a distance. Acute coronary occlusion in these patients produced infarction in that vessel's distribution territory and at the same time compromise of previously existing functional collateral channels by which the newly occluded artery had provided myocardial perfusion in the distribution of the second critically stenosed artery. Thus, ischemia at a distance implies that at least two coronary arteries linked by a functional collateral network are critically narrowed or occluded.

The development of a postinfarction aneurysm may be related to failure of development of an adequate collateral circulation.[79,104–107] Rowe[107] noted that obstructed coronary arteries supplying the region of a left ventricular aneurysm had few or even no collaterals. Manvi and Ellestad[105] also found poor collateral filling in the vicinity of a ventricular aneurysm in 14 of 29 (48%) patients studied, while Cheng[104] found that in as many as 25 of 35 (71%) patients with a ventricular aneurysm, collateral filling was poor. Aygen[79] noted that of 100 patients with total occlusion of the left anterior descending coronary artery, 1 of 75 (1%) with good collaterals and 14 of 25 (56%) with inadequate collateral vessels had anterior left ventricular wall aneurysms. Mullen and co-workers[106] reviewed the coronary arteriograms from 60 patients undergoing resection of left ventricular aneurysms. All patients had at least 90% stenoses of the left anterior descending artery, while 72% had complete occlusion. Only 22 (37%) patients had collateral filling of the distal segment of this artery. In contrast, 71% of a randomly selected group of patients with total occlusion of the left anterior descending artery without left ventricular aneurysm formation had good collaterals. It is not possible to decide unequivocally whether the paucity of collateral vessels is the cause or the effect of aneurysm formation. However, observations in other patients that collaterals can perfuse infarcted myocardium suggest that poor collateralization in patients with aneurysms is more likely to be the cause of aneurysm formation. Schwarz's results[69,99–101] of increased myocardial replacement with fibrous tissue in patients with fewer collaterals support this conclusion.

This section has described the possible effects of the coronary collateral circulation on the clinical presentation of patients with coronary artery disease. The pathologic studies documenting either no infarction following coronary occlusion, infarcts smaller than the perfusion territory of the obstructed vessel, or infarction at a distance support the conclusion that collaterals have an unequivocal salutary functional role. Even clinical studies analyzing the factors contributing to postinfarction shock, rupture of the ventricular septum, or formation of ventricular aneurysms have confirmed the importance of the collateral circulation in the determination of these potential complications. Collaterals are also responsible for survival and frequently normal cardiac function of patients with main left coronary artery occlusion and even a few patients with total proximal obstruction of all major coronary arteries. These end-points of infarction, rupture, and aneurysm formation are all easily identified and quantified, and these qualities undoubtedly contribute to one's ability to identify a relationship to the collateral circulation. On the other hand, anginal symptoms are much less easily graded. The coronary collateral circulation is clearly affected by the severity of the underlying coronary obstructive disease and the duration of the clinical symptoms. But it has not been possible to prove an ameliorating effect of collaterals on anginal pains, possibly because of the complex interaction of factors that result in the anginal syndrome. Thus, in patients with angina, claims have been made that collaterals are only markers of the underlying coronary disease. It is likely, however, that without collaterals these patients with only angina would have experienced infarction. Nonetheless, it is apparent that the beneficial value of coronary collaterals is best demonstrated in those situations where ischemia or a functional defect can be quantitated.

III. Electrocardiography

Perhaps the earliest, and still the easiest, technique for recording the clinical effects of myocardial ischemia is resting electrocardiography. The significance of Q waves and recognition of infarct patterns are appreciated by even beginning medical students. The location of a myocardial infarct on the electrocardiogram generally correlates with both the coronary artery involved and the angiographic location of left ventricular dysfunction.[108] The finding of a normal electrocardiogram in the presence of severe coronary artery disease is well appreciated.[63,85,87,108–119] From a larger group of 480 patients with coronary artery disease, Martinez-Rios et al.[109] identified 21 patients who had a normal electrocardiogram. Seventeen of this group of 21 had complete obstruction of at least one major coronary artery. In a study of 106 patients with triple vessel coronary disease, Benchimol and co-workers[111] observed that 16% had a normal electrocardiogram and an additional 13% had only ST-T-wave abnormalities. Three patients with complete obstruction of at least one coronary artery had normal resting electrocardiograms. Such observations, especially in the presence of a totally obstructed coronary artery, suggest a protective role of the collateral circulation.

To determine whether coronary collaterals had any influence on the electrocardiographic pattern, investigators attempted to correlate alterations of the electrocardiogram with the angiographic appearance of the collateral circulation. In the series of Martinez-Rios,[109] 19 of the 21 patients with marked coronary obstructive disease and normal electrocardiograms had good collaterals, including 15 of the 17 with total coronary occlusions. Fuster[85] segregated patients with coronary artery disease into groups according to their clinical syndrome. Thus, 164 patients with angina pectoris were identified. Forty-two percent had coronary occlusions without clinical or electrocardiographic evidence of myocardial infarction, and 91% of this latter subgroup had coronary collaterals. To demonstrate the functional capability of these collaterals, Wolf et al.[117] quantitated collateral flow with ^{133}Xe washout curves. Patients studied had proximal left anterior descending or left circumflex occlusions. All without electrocardiographic abnormalities had collateral flows exceeding 50 ml/min/100g, while patients with evidence of myocardial infarction had considerably lower flows.

Perhaps the evidence for the beneficial effect of coronary collaterals on the electrocardiogram would be more convincing if patients with and without collateral channels but no other distinguishing clinical characteristics were compared. Ensslen et al.[87,115] studied 87 patients with complete occlusion of the left anterior descending and/or right coronary artery. If the distal segment of the obstructed vessel was opacified during coronary angiography, then the coronary collaterals were described as "good." Twenty-six, or 30% of the study population had good collaterals, while 40 (46%) had "defective" collaterals, and 21 (24%) had no evidence of collateralization. There was evidence of transmural infarction on the electrocardiogram in only 19% of the group with good collaterals, whereas 90 and 95% of the patients with defective and no collaterals, respectively, had electrocardiographic Q waves. Schwarz[114] presented similar data. Eighty-nine patients had 95−100% stenoses of the left anterior descending and/or right coronary arteries. None of the 20 with good, unjeopardized collaterals had Q waves on the electrocardiogram (Figure 2-6). In contrast, 61 of 69 patients without good collaterals had Q waves indicating transmural infarction.

In another careful study of 288 patients with total occlusion of the right coronary artery and 177 individuals with left anterior descending coronary artery occlusions, Hamby et al.[63] also demonstrated an association between coronary collaterals and electrocardiographic signs of transmural infarction. Seventy-one percent of the patients with left anterior descending occlusions had collaterals. There were no clinical or angiographic differences in the subgroups with and without collateral vessels. Yet 44 of 52 (85%) without collaterals but only 42 of 125 (34%) with collaterals had electrocardiographic evidence of anterior wall infarction, a highly significant difference ($p < 0.005$) (Figure 2-7). The striking difference continued to be evident when patients

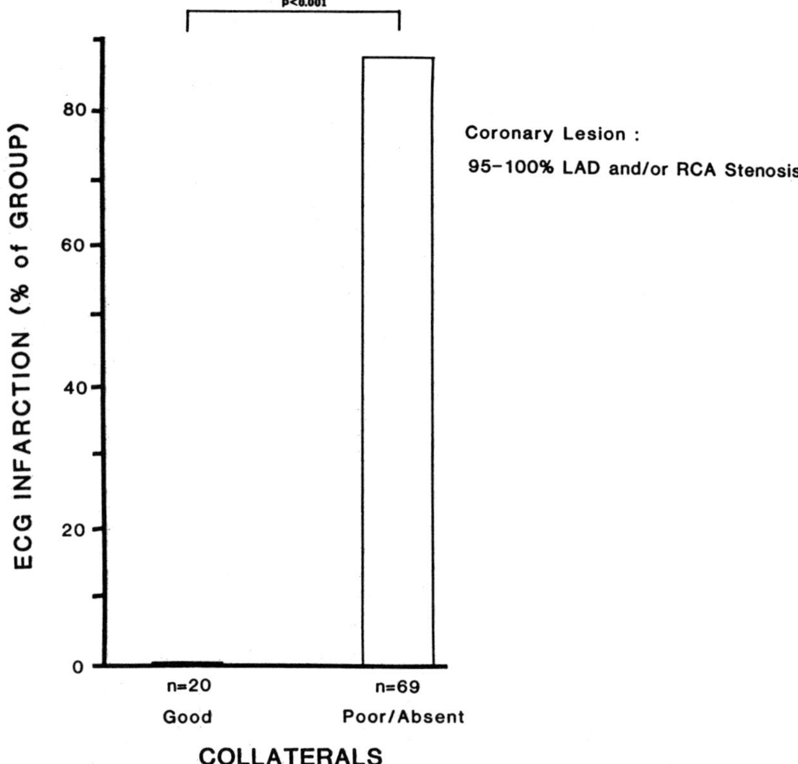

Figure 2-6   Effect of coronary collaterals on electrocardiographic pattern of infarction in patients with critical (95–100%) lesions of either the right (RCA) or left anterior descending (LAD) coronary artery. No patient with good collaterals had evidence of an infarct, whereas 81% of those with poor or no collaterals to the diseased coronary artery had Q waves indicating transmural infarction. (Drawn from data presented by Schwarz et al.[114])

with only isolated disease of the left anterior descending artery were examined (11 of 12 or 92% of those without and 11 of 39 or 28% with collaterals had Q waves). Collaterals appeared to be less important in patients with right coronary lesions, perhaps because of the frequent dual blood supply (right coronary and left circumflex arteries) to the posterior wall of the left ventricle. Of 44 patients with right coronary occlusions and no collaterals, 66% had inferior wall infarction diagnosed by electrocardiography. This proportion was not different from 53% of the 244 patients with collaterals who also had abnormal electrocardiograms. On the other hand, when only isolated right coronary disease was considered, collaterals again became important. Eight of 8 occlusions (100%) without and 17 of 29 (59%) with collaterals were associated with inferior infarction ($p < 0.05$).

This possible difference between right coronary and left anterior de-

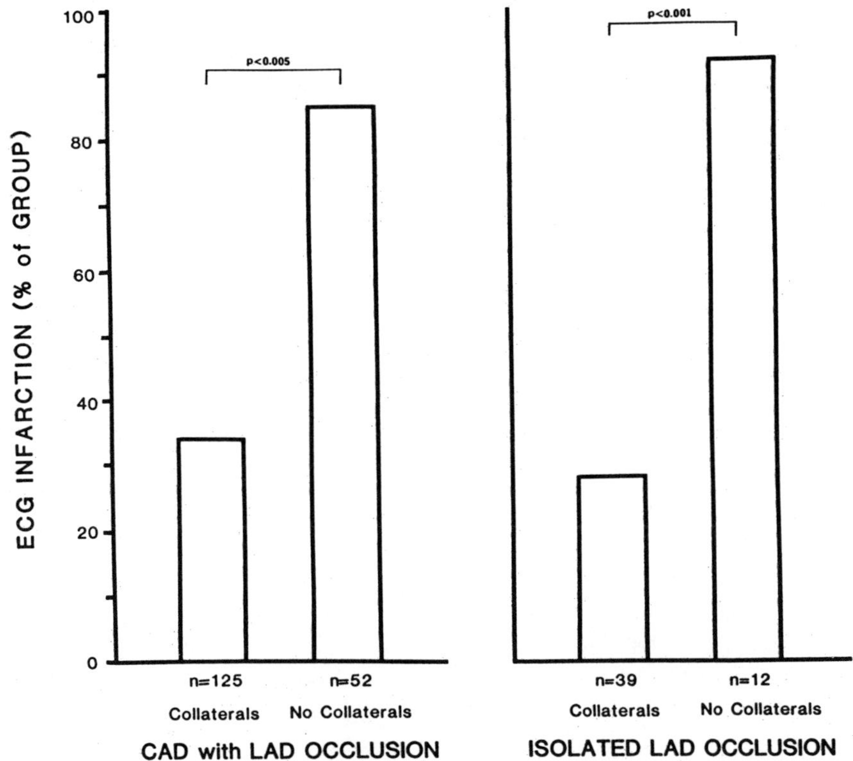

Figure 2-7   Relationship between electrocardiographic changes of anterior wall infarction in patients with occlusion of the left anterior descending coronary artery and angiographically evident coronary collaterals. Whether all patients with coronary obstructive disease (left) or only those with isolated LAD occlusion (right) were considered, abnormal electrocardiograms were observed in significantly fewer individuals with collaterals. (Drawn from data presented by Hamby et al.[63])

scending artery lesions is echoed by Bourassa's report.[112] He and his colleagues noted that collaterals influenced the occurrence of electrocardiographic Q waves in patients with total occlusions of the left anterior descending artery but had no effect on the occurrence of inferior wall infarction in right coronary occlusion. Dwyer[113] also found no difference in incidence of collateralization of right coronary artery occlusions in patients with and without Q waves in the inferior leads of the electrocardiogram. However, significantly fewer patients with infarction (3 of 22, or 13.6%) than without (13 of 28, or 46%) had evidence of dual collateral circulation to the right coronary artery from both the left anterior descending and left circumflex arteries ($p < 0.01$).

   In a study of patients with total or severe occlusive disease ($\geq$80%) of the left anterior descending coronary artery, Berndt and associates[116] found a significantly higher incidence of collateral filling of the distal segment of the diseased artery in patients without electrocardiographic evidence of anterior myocardial infarction. The groups with and without collaterals had similar coronary lesions. In 38 patients with anterior wall infarction, 25 (66%) had angiographically demonstrable collaterals, whereas 26 of 28 subjects (93%) with normal electrocardiograms had anastomotic networks ($p = 0.02$).

Curiously, Vigorito[119] was unable to document any effect of collaterals on the occurrence of abnormal electrocardiograms in 82 patients with proximal occlusion of the left anterior descending coronary artery. However, he did demonstrate a collateral effect in disease of the right coronary artery. Proximal occlusion of this vessel was noted in 105 patients. In the presence of good, nonjeopardized collaterals (23 patients), only 60% had electrocardiographic evidence of diaphragmatic infarction, whereas 100% of those without collaterals (12 patients) had abnormal electrocardiograms ($p < 0.01$). Eighty-one percent of those with poor collaterals also had diaphragmatic infarcts. This collateral effect was evident whether the patients had single- or multi-vessel disease.

Other investigators have not been able to confirm that the collateral circulation may prevent the appearance of electrocardiographic signs of infarction.[2,5,62,65,100,120−124] In patients with significant single vessel disease (stenosis > 90%), Helfant et al.[62] observed a normal resting electrocardiogram in 22 of 61 (36%) with and 16 of 58 (28%) without collaterals, respectively. Miller and co-workers[65] selected patients with significant disease (> 75% stenosis) of the left anterior descending coronary artery, and matched patients for location and severity of disease in other vessels. They then segregated study individuals into subgroups with and without collaterals. Collaterals did not affect the appearance of Q waves in the electrocardiogram. Twenty-seven percent of patients without collaterals and 36% with collaterals to the left anterior descending artery had anterior infarction. Similar observations have been made in patients with three-vessel disease.[2,5,65,123] Hecht and associates[124] also observed pathologic Q waves in 4 of 11 (36%) patients with good collaterals and 10 of 24 (42%) without collaterals. McConahay[121] noted an even higher incidence of abnormal electrocardiograms in patients with collaterals.

Bodenheimer et al.[102] recorded epicardial electrograms from the surface of the left ventricle in patients undergoing elective coronary revascularization surgery or aneurysm resection. Patients with and without angiographically visualized collaterals and at least a 90% decrease in the diameter of a major coronary artery were compared. When collaterals were present, epicardial tracings recorded R waves in 11 of 16 and Q waves in the remaining 5. Similarly, 31 of 39 patients without collaterals had R waves while only 8 had Q waves. Thus, collaterals appeared to have little effect.

As previously noted, Feldman and Pepine[77] observed that inflation of a dilating balloon causing transient occlusion of the left anterior descending coronary artery resulted in more frequent clinical symptoms and electrocardiographic abnormalities in subjects without angiographically visible collateral channels. Thus, 1 of 6 individuals with, and 5 of 13 without collaterals had anginal symptoms and ST-segment elevation. Although this difference was not significant, the trend is certainly provocative. Further reports providing results in larger groups are eagerly awaited.

The discrepancies observed between the various studies may be due in part to differences in coronary topography, the variable time needed for patients to develop occlusive disease of the coronary artery under study, the small number of patients evaluated in some studies, and insensitivity of the electrocardiogram as a tool in evaluation of the left ventricle. It is particularly noteworthy that many of the studies described above also have demonstrated numerous examples of normal electrocardiograms in the face of regional ventriculographic wall motion abnormalities.[108,116] Furthermore, it is striking that almost all of the studies demonstrating a beneficial effect of collaterals on electrocardiographic patterns were done in patients with total coronary occlusions, whereas the investigations that concluded collaterals were not helpful used patients with subtotal coronary lesions. The use of patients with subtotal stenoses introduces significant bias since coronary collaterals are generally not visualized until the stenosis exceeds 90%. Therefore, essentially all patients with collaterals will have stenoses greater than 90%, whereas some of the patients without collaterals used in the comparison will have less severe disease, with perhaps only 75% stenoses. Hence, in some of the studies, the patients with coronary collaterals may have more severe disease.

Although not unanimous, the conclusion of the preponderance of studies supports a functionally beneficial role of coronary collaterals. However, because of the electrocardiogram's insensitivity, a more specific technique for investigation of the value of the collateral vessel would be desirable.

IV. Intraoperative Studies: Reactive Hyperemia

Evidence of preservation of left ventricular function or attenuation of myocardial ischemia by coronary collaterals would justify the conclusion that these accessory channels have clinically important functional effects. Intraoperative investigations at the time of saphenous vein bypass graft surgery have attempted to document the ability of collaterals to modify ischemia by analyzing the reactive hyperemic response following transient occlusion of the venous graft.

Reactive hyperemia is the increment in flow above baseline levels that is seen after release of a transient coronary occlusion (stippled area in Figure 2-8). After coronary occlusion, the distal arteriolar resistance vessels become maximally dilated, an autoregulatory response mediated by endogenous vasodilators (e.g., adenosine), in an attempt to restore normal perfusion of the myocardium (see Chapter 5). Following release of the occlusion, antegrade flow resumes. Because the arteriolar vessels are initially maximally dilated,

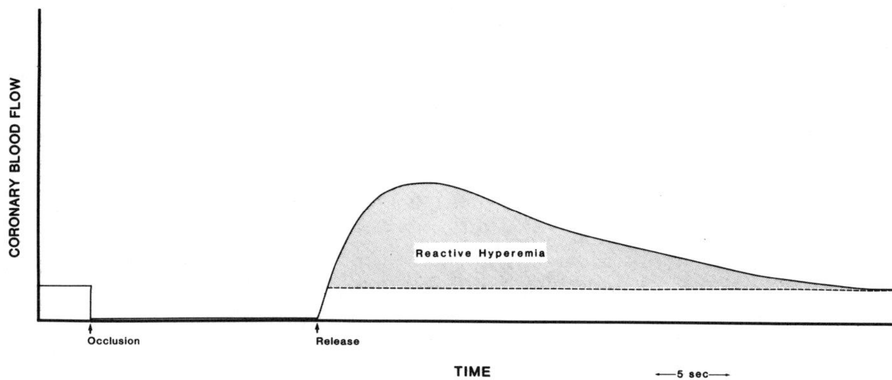

Figure 2-8   Following occlusion of a coronary artery, blood flow drops to zero. After release of the occlusion, flow increases and surpasses the level noted prior to the occlusion. The excess flow above baseline is "reactive hyperemia" and is related to restored flow through coronary arterioles which are maximally dilated because of the preceding period of myocardial ischemia.

flow quickly rises and exceeds that observed before the occlusion. Flow remains elevated until arteriolar tone increases to normal levels. The excess flow, or reactive hyperemia, frequently exceeds the flow debt incurred during the cessation of antegrade flow by 300 to 400%. If the myocardium has an alternate source of oxygenated blood, then ischemia will not be as intense and arteriolar vasodilatation will not be as marked during coronary occlusion. The reactive hyperemic response will be correspondingly weaker.

Flameng and his co-workers[125-127] measured reactive hyperemia with an electromagnetic flow probe encircling the saphenous vein graft in patients with and without angiographically visualized coronary collaterals. Those without collaterals were divided into groups according to the degree of stenosis of the grafted coronary artery: 71–80%; 81–90%; and 91–99%. In a fourth group, temporary (20-second) acute occlusion of the stenotic vessel was created with a rubber tourniquet proximal to the site of graft anastomosis. All individuals with collaterals had chronic complete arterial occlusions. Graft hyperemic flow was evaluated after release of a 20-second occlusion of the anastomosed saphenous vein. The hyperemic/basal coronary flow ratio was 1.02 in those with the least severe stenoses (Figure 2-9). The lack of graft hyperemia implies that residual antegrade flow through the stenotic native vessel was sufficient to prevent ischemia during graft occlusion. In those with 81–90% stenoses, the flow ratio averaged 1.21. There was a significant increase in the flow ratio to 1.88 in patients with 91–99% stenoses. In these latter patients the amount of residual antegrade coronary flow was not sufficient to compensate for the loss of graft flow during occlusion of the venous graft, and ischemia resulted. Ischemia was maximized when the native coronary artery was occluded at the same time as the graft resulting in a hyperemic/basal flow ratio of 2.92. In contrast to patients with acute coro-

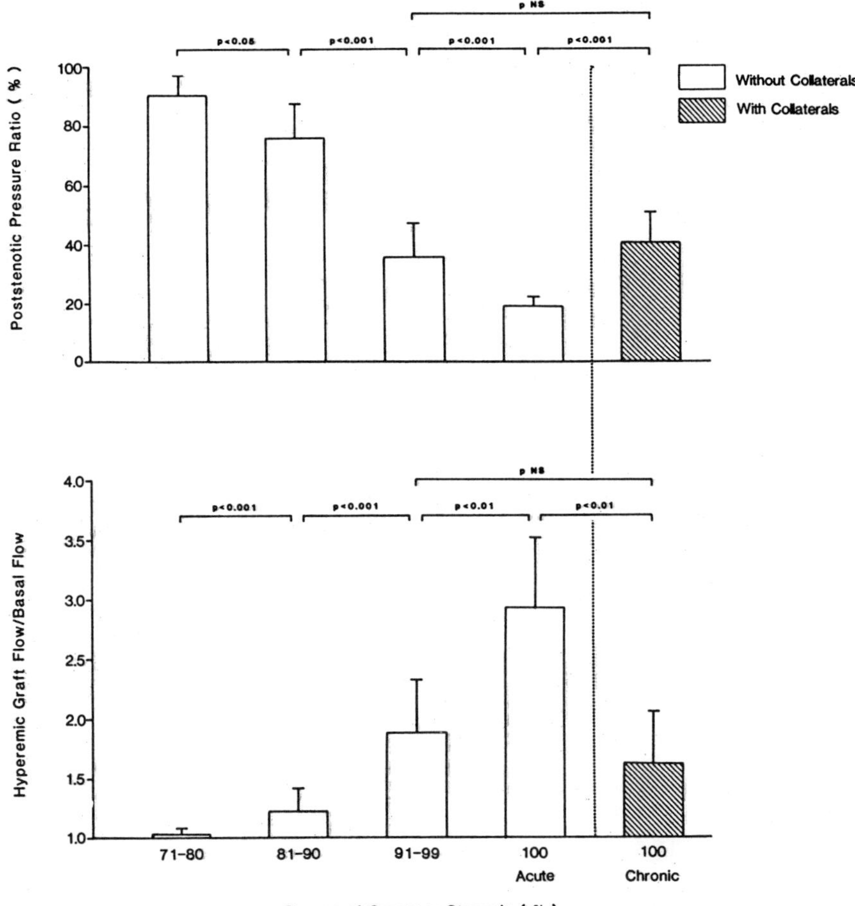

Figure 2-9   Relation between poststenotic pressure ratio (top) and hyperemic graft flow response (bottom) and the degree of coronary stenosis. Mean values ± standard deviation are depicted. In this series only individuals with chronic total coronary occlusions had angiographic evidence of coronary collaterals. Following attachment of saphenous vein grafts distal to the major coronary lesions, intragraft pressure following proximal occlusion represented poststenotic coronary pressure. This variable was normalized for diastolic aortic pressure and expressed as a ratio. Following release of the graft occlusion, increased graft flow represented the hyperemic response. In those individuals without collaterals there was a significant progressive diminution in the poststenotic pressure ratio and rise in the hyperemic graft flow response as stenosis severity increased. These trends were reversed in patients with collaterals despite presence of total occlusions. The increased poststenotic pressure ratio and lower hyperemic flow are consistent with the presence of an alternate source of blood to the ischemic myocardium, e.g., via collaterals (see text). The measurements in patients with total occlusions and collaterals were not different from those in individuals with patent vessels and noncollateralized 91−99% lesions. (Modified and printed with permission of Dun-Donnelly Publishing Corp. from Flameng et al.[125])

nary occlusion and no collaterals, patients with chronic arterial occlusion and adequate collaterals had significantly lower flow ratios averaging 1.62. This lower ratio signifies less ischemia during graft occlusion and implies partial compensation by the collateral circulation for loss of antegrade flow. Thus, the collaterals functionally transformed a chronic total occlusion into a 90% stenosis (similar reactive hyperemic flows in these two groups of patients).

Further evidence of attenuation of myocardial ischemia by coronary collaterals was apparent when the durations of the hyperemic responses of Flameng's patient groups were compared.[125-127] The response lasted only 1.5 sec in those with the least severe stenoses because of the negligible ischemia created by graft occlusion. Duration increased to 9.2 and 28.7 sec in the other two groups with subtotal obstructions, and averaged 28.3 sec after acute occlusion. In contrast, hyperemia lasted only 18.1 sec in those with chronic occlusion and coronary collaterals. The shorter duration in the latter group again signifies less ischemia than in those patients with 90−99% lesions or those with acute occlusions and no collaterals.

Flameng et al.[125-127] also measured pressure in the saphenous vein graft distal to the site of the transient occlusion, and expressed the pressure as a ratio of diastolic poststenotic coronary pressure/diastolic aortic pressure. The pressure ratio averaged 90.2% in patients with 71−80% stenoses (Figure 2-9). Thus, there was only a small pressure drop across the stenosis in the native vessel. With increasing stenosis severity, the pressure ratio progressively fell to 76.2%, 35.8%, and finally 18.9% in those with acute occlusion. Those patients with collaterals had pressure ratios of 40.2%. Hence, large collaterals effectively increased the distal coronary pressure by delivering an alternate source of blood. Again, the collateralized occlusion was approximately equivalent to a 90% stenosis.

Oldham et al.[128] measured distal coronary pressure and reactive hyperemia following release of graft occlusion in a group of patients with total proximal obstruction of the bypassed artery. In contrast to Flameng's data,[125-127] the pressure gradient across the coronary lesion averaged 63 ± 4 mmHg and the average peripheral coronary pressure was 22 ± 4 mmHg. Furthermore, there was marked graft reactive hyperemia. These observations suggest that the collateral circulation was poorly developed in Oldham's patients. Perhaps this is not so surprising. These intraoperative measurements can only be made in patients who are sufficiently symptomatic to warrant surgery. If the collateral circulation of these patients had been better developed, it is possible that surgery would not have been necessary. Obviously, comparable data cannot be obtained in the asymptomatic patient with coronary artery disease. These considerations make Flameng's results even more striking and further emphasize the physiologic significance of well-developed collateral channels.

Others have also measured graft hyperemic flows.[129-133] But these studies have been unable to separate the effects of collateral circulation from those of residual antegrade flow through subtotal coronary stenoses. Furthermore, failure to segregate the patients according to the degree of collateralization and severity of stenosis and omission of study patients with total occlusions make the results difficult to interpret. Thus, these reports supply little additional useful information.

The clinical studies described above clearly demonstrate that collaterals can effectively attenuate myocardial ischemia. It is obvious that these collateral channels are unable to abolish ischemia, but even the modest effect documented by Flameng[125–127] would be expected to have a beneficial effect on left ventricular function.

V. Left Ventricular Function

Studies designed to evaluate the relationship between the coronary collateral circulation and left ventricular function present many difficulties. Frequent uncertainties and frank errors in the angiographic determination (often underestimation) of the severity of a stenosis[134–144] and inter- and intraobserver variability in quantitation of stenosis severity[137,145–149] make segregation of patients according to the degree of coronary narrowing less reliable. It is hoped that computer calculation of lesions in several views will minimize these errors.[150] Furthermore, there is no certainty that angiographic appearance of collaterals can provide any indication of functional adequacy. Paulin's thoughtful review of this problem[151] details other angiographic clues that may be helpful in estimating functional capacity.

Previous attempts by multiple investigators to stratify patients with similar coronary lesions on the basis of the presence or absence of collaterals have probably been inadequate. The location of the obstructive lesion in the recipient vessel and the possible effects of variations in coronary topography have rarely been considered. For example, occlusion of a left anterior descending artery before the origin of the first septal perforator and diagonal artery would be expected to have greater consequences than a more distal obstruction. Thus, despite identical collateral supplies demonstrated angiographically in patients with proximal and distal lesions, one might expect different functional effects.

Although the left anterior descending artery typically supplies almost two-thirds of the interventricular septum and most of the anterior wall and apex of the left ventricle, a significant portion of the anterior wall in some cases is supplied by a median (or intermediate) artery. Furthermore, in some hearts the ramus recurrens branch of the left anterior descending artery may supply the inferoapical portion of the left ventricle. Lack of consideration of these anatomic variations might result in incorrect assessment of the functional importance of the collateral circulation.

Similarly, the extent of right coronary artery perfusion may be important. Determination of coronary preponderance (or dominance) is useful, but variability is still present among patients categorized as having right dominant circulations. A variable amount of the posterior wall of the left ventricle may be supplied by a dominant right coronary artery.[118] Thus, all occlusions of this vessel are not equivalent. Groups of patients segregated only according to the extent of disease in the three major coronary arteries may, therefore, not be as homogeneous as originally considered.

For nearly 15 years investigators have been trying to correlate cardiac function with the presence of coronary collateral channels. Hemodynamic variables including end-diastolic volume and pressure, cardiac output, and stroke work as well as ejection fraction have been used as measures of global left ventricular function, while shortening of minor and major axes of the ventricle has been used to evaluate regional function. The current controversy concerning the effect of collaterals on left ventricular function has replaced the now resolved debate that raged in the first half of this century over the assertion that all normal hearts contained collaterals. Many studies have convincingly demonstrated the salutary effect of collaterals. The majority of investigations that purport to prove the ineffectiveness of anastomotic channels are flawed because of bias against collaterals introduced during group selection.

Collaterals have been observed to affect hemodynamics in patients with chronic coronary artery disease[152–155] as well as in those with acute infarction.[78,82,98,156] Bowyer and Asato[153] studied patients with complete occlusion of the left anterior descending coronary artery. The adequacy of the collateral circulation was based on the angiographic diameter of the visualized anastomoses as well as the degree of opacification of the occluded vessel beyond the obstruction when the contrast agent was introduced into another coronary artery. The left ventricle was smallest (end-diastolic volume 203 ± 21 ml) in those individuals with the best collaterals, while the end-diastolic volume was increased (295 ± 39 ml) in those with sparse collateral circulation. Left ventricular dilatation was most marked in those individuals without any evidence of collaterals (399 ± 62 ml). Arie and colleagues[155] compared two groups of patients with complete obstruction of the left anterior descending artery, one with good and the other with poor collaterals to the diseased vessel, and made similar observations. Both end-diastolic and end-systolic volumes were normal or nearly so in the former, whereas those with inadequate collaterals had dilated hearts. Kober et al.[154] measured end-diastolic volume and pressure in groups of patients with one-, two-, and three-vessel disease. When patients were stratified for the mere presence of collaterals, no effect on hemodynamics was detected. However, when collaterals were classified as either good or poor according to their ability to opacify the distal segment of a diseased coronary artery during angiography, then an effect was observed. For similar degrees of obstructive disease, end-diastolic volume and pressure were lower in individuals with good collaterals. The effect of collaterals was most marked in patients with two-vessel disease and three-vessel disease with two occluded arteries.

Williams et al.[78] performed cardiac catheterization in 20 patients during the course of an acute myocardial infarction. Nineteen patients had obstructive lesions exceeding 90%, while nine had total occlusions. In 17 the left anterior descending artery was diseased, while in the other 3 the right coronary artery was involved. In the 6 patients with good collaterals, left ventricular end-diastolic pressure, cardiac index, and stroke work index averaged 13 mmHg, 3.0 l/min/m^2, and 45 g · m/m^2, respectively. These values were significantly different in the 14 patients with poor or no collaterals in whom average end-diastolic pressure was markedly increased to 30 mmHg ($p < 0.01$), and cardiac index and stroke work index depressed to 2.0 l/min/m^2 ($p < 0.05$) and 13 g · m/m^2 ($p < 0.01$), respectively. None of the six patients with good collaterals developed cardiogenic shock, and all survived the hospitalization. In contrast, ten of the patients with inadequate collateralization had clinical courses complicated by shock, and eight died. Nohara's data[98] are similar: in 14 patients with their first infarcts and nonjeopardized collaterals (12 with total coronary occlusion), stroke volume and left ventricular end-diastolic pressure averaged 44.3 ± 8.4 ml/beat/m^2 and 15.7 ± 5.5 mmHg, respectively. In contrast, five patients with total coronary occlusion and jeopardized collaterals had significantly lower stroke volumes (31.0 ± 6.3 ml/beat/m^2, $p < 0.01$) and higher left ventricular filling pressures (21.4 ± 1.3 mmHg, $p < 0.01$). Hemodynamic data in patients with coronary occlusions but no collaterals were similar to those in the group with jeopardized collaterals.

Bertrand's study of patients 7 to 21 days following myocardial infarction identified 20 individuals with anterior wall necrosis and complete left anterior descending artery occlusion.[82] Although collaterals did not appear to affect either left ventricular end-diastolic pressure or cardiac index, the heart was significantly smaller in those individuals with good collaterals. Left ventricular end-diastolic volume averaged 76 ml/m^2 in those with good and 109 ml/m^2 in those with poor or absent collaterals ($p < 0.01$). Curiously, collaterals did not confer the same advantage to those with posterior wall infarcts and right coronary artery occlusions. Perhaps the high incidence of associated disease of the left anterior descending artery may account for this lack of effect. In a more recent study from the same group, 52 patients with left anterior descending artery obstruction and acute infarction were identified.[156] Although there continued to be a trend for those with collaterals to have smaller hearts, the difference was not significant.

One of the useful parameters for evaluating left ventricular function is the ejection fraction which quantitates the emptying of the left ventricular chamber during the ejection phase of the cardiac cycle. Calculated as the ratio of stroke volume to end-diastolic volume, the ejection fraction normally exceeds 50%. This parameter is useful in the analysis of global function of the left ventricle. Many investigators have found an impressive correlation between presence of an adequate coronary collateral circulation and preservation of a normal or near-normal ejection fraction despite total coronary occlusions.[68,69,78,82,87,114,115,153–159]

The studies demonstrating functional significance of the coronary collateral circulation are surprisingly uniform in their approach, selection of patient groups, and methods employed. Virtually all investigators evaluating patients with chronic symptoms have selected only those with severe obstructive disease. To eliminate potential bias and the uncertainties of grading coronary stenoses, most have chosen patients with total occlusions,[68,69,87,115,153,155,158] while the remaining studies have examined patients with stenoses greater than 90%,[154,157] or in excess of 95%.[114] Perhaps equally central to the success of the studies has been the attempt to grade the quality of the collateral pathways. After identification of anastomotic channels, the investigators analyzed the degree of opacification of the distal segment of the diseased vessel during angiography and the rate of distal runoff. Because of little or no antegrade flow through the obstructed vessel, both distal opacification and runoff depended virtually entirely on the adequacy of the collateral circulation. Thus, a distinction could be made between good or adequate and bad or defective collateral channels.

Ensslen and colleagues[87,115] evaluated the collateral circulation in 87 patients with total occlusion of the left anterior descending and/or right coronary artery. The collaterals were labeled "good" in 26 (30%) and "defective" in 40 (46%) patients (Figure 2-10). Collaterals were not visualized in 21 (24%) patients. The ejection fraction in patients with good collaterals averaged 67.9%, not significantly different from 71.3% in those with normal coronary arteries. However, the ejection fraction was significantly depressed to 41.9% and 41.6% in patients with defective and no collaterals, respectively. Schwarz's data are similar.[68,69] The ejection fraction averaged 59.6% in patients with complete left anterior descending coronary artery obstruction and good collaterals and 67.8% in left ventricles with well-collateralized right coronary occlusions (Figure 2-11). Neither value was significantly different from the ejection fraction of 65.2% measured in normal hearts. In hearts with defective collaterals, left anterior descending and right coronary occlusions caused significant falls to 41.4% and 51.0%, respectively. The absence of collaterals had a much more marked effect in Bowyer's[153] patients with total occlusion of the left anterior descending artery. Good collaterals were associated with preservation of a normal ejection fraction of $51 \pm 2\%$. In contrast, the ejection fraction was only $31 \pm 4\%$ in those with defective collaterals, and fell even further to $20 \pm 2\%$ when collaterals were absent.

Sesto and Schwarz[158] stratified patients with obstructive disease of the left anterior descending coronary artery according to severity of the lesion and presence of collaterals. Group A (105 patients) had no collaterals. In patients with stenoses of less than 75%, the average ejection fraction of 68.9% was normal (Figure 2-12). As the severity of the lesion increased to 75–99% and then to complete occlusion, there were progressive falls in ejection fraction to 53.5% and 40.3%. Group B (72 patients) had adequate collaterals. No patients in this group had stenoses less than 75%. In the 75–99% subgroup the ejection fraction was 60.5%, comparable to that in group A patients with similar lesions. With total arterial occlusion the ejection fraction averaged 53.0%, significantly higher than in group A patients without collaterals ($p < 0.05$). An additional group (C, 41 patients) had a saphenous vein bypass graft anastomosed to the diseased artery. With total revascularization the

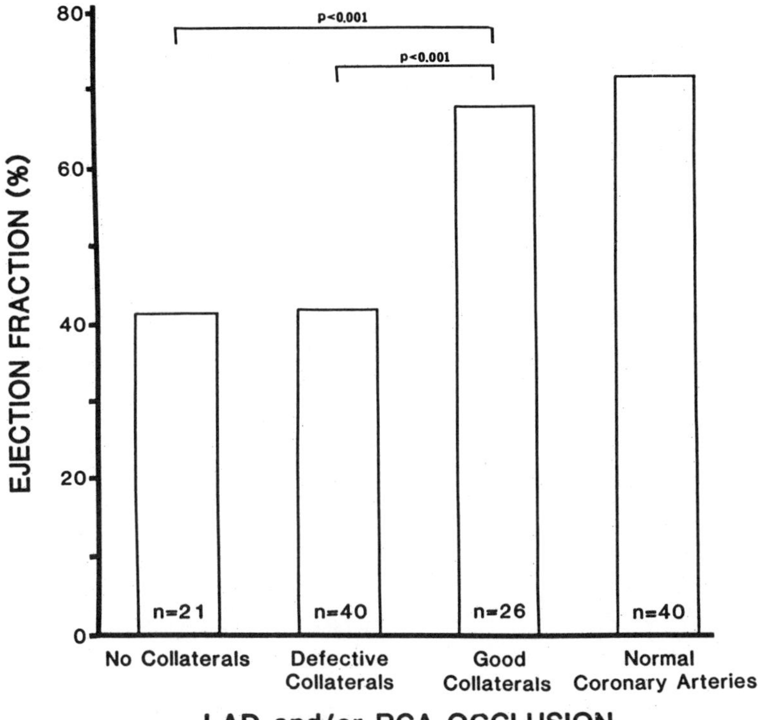

Figure 2-10   Relationship between presence and quality of angiographically visualized coronary collaterals and left ventricular ejection fraction in individuals with total left anterior descending (LAD) and/or right (RCA) coronary artery occlusion. Ejection fractions were equally depressed in patients with no or poor/defective collaterals, and were preserved (normal) when good collaterals were evident. (Drawn from data presented by Ensslen et al.[115])

ejection fraction was unaffected by the severity of disease in the native vessel (69.2% with 75–99% stenoses and 70.0% with total occlusions). Thus, collateral vessels had the effect of partial revascularization of the left ventricle and prevented some of the expected deterioration of myocardial function following coronary occlusion.

Studies by Aloan[157] and Kober[154] demonstrate the spurious conclusions that are inevitable if care is not taken to compare patients with equivalent extent of disease or judge the quality of the collateral circulation. Thirty-three patients with obstructive disease of the left anterior descending artery, 15 with and 18 without collaterals, were evaluated by Aloan.[157] All patients with collaterals had stenoses exceeding 90%, whereas some patients without collaterals had milder lesions. When all patients were considered, those with collaterals had an average ejection fraction of 56%, not different from 54% in those without collaterals (Figure 2-13). However, when only patients with and

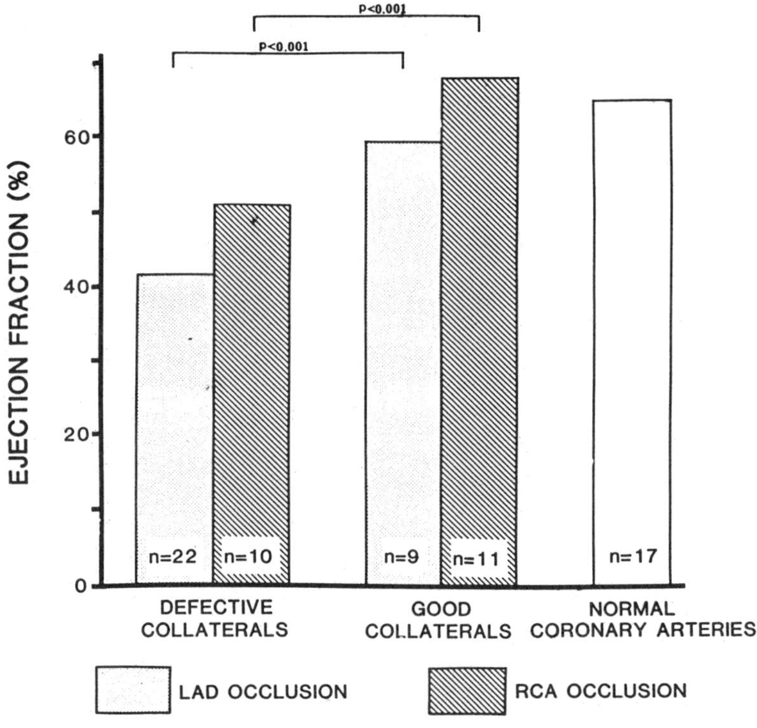

Figure 2-11   Effect of the quality of angiographically visualized coronary collaterals on left ventricular ejection fraction in patients with complete obstruction of either the left anterior descending (LAD) or right (RCA) coronary artery. Subjects with good collaterals had normal ejection fractions. However, left ventricular function was significantly depressed if the occluded vessels were poorly collateralized. (Drawn from data presented by Schwarz et al.[68])

without collaterals with equally severe disease (> 90%) were studied, there was an obvious difference in ejection fraction. Those without collaterals now had an ejection fraction of 24%, much less than that in patients with collaterals ($p < 0.05$).

Kober[154] studied patients with one-, two-, and three-vessel disease. When ejection fractions were compared in patients with and without collaterals but with similar coronary disease, there were no differences. However, if the quality of the collaterals, rather than their mere presence, was judged, then the collaterals had a definite effect on left ventricular function. Ejection fraction was higher in those with good than in those with poor collateral vessels.

Walker and colleagues[160] studied 212 patients with coronary artery disease to determine what variables might affect left ventricular dysfunction. They graded multiple factors including left ventricular function, site and

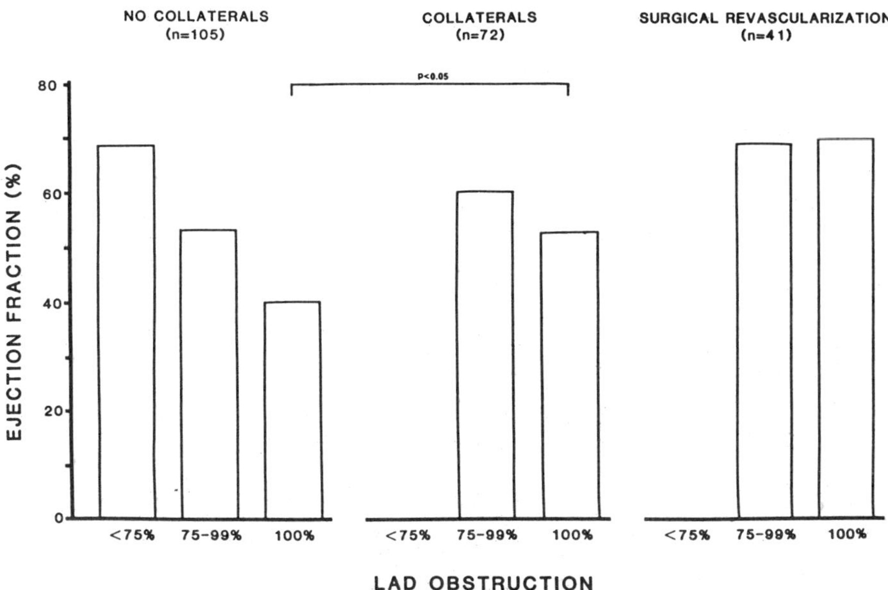

Figure 2-12   Effects of varying severity of left anterior descending coronary artery (LAD) lesions and angiographically demonstrable coronary collaterals on left ventricular ejection fraction. In patients without collaterals, progressive deterioration of ejection fraction was observed as the coronary lesion progressed to complete obstruction. However, in individuals with collaterals the fall in ejection fraction was attenuated, presumably because of the alternate source of oxygenated blood to the jeopardized myocardium. Surgical revascularization with saphenous vein grafts prevented any change in ejection fraction as the coronary lesion became more severe. Thus, adequate collateralization had the effect of a partial revascularization (Drawn from data presented by Sesto and Schwarz.[158])

severity of coronary artery disease, and coronary collaterals, and then did a multiple regression analysis. The grade of collaterals was inversely correlated with the amount of left ventricular dysfunction ($p < 0.05$).

Limited studies performed during acute myocardial infarction indicate that collaterals in this clinical setting also influence global left ventricular function.[78,82,98,156,159] Bertrand et al.[82] studied patients with acute anterior infarction associated with complete occlusion of the left anterior descending artery. These patients underwent routine cardiac catheterization within three weeks of their infarction and were not hemodynamically unstable. The authors observed that in 8 patients with an adequate collateral circulation to the left anterior descending artery, the ejection fraction averaged 54.5% compared to 34.5% in 12 patients with inadequate or no collaterals ($p < 0.01$). However, the presence ($N = 24$) or absence ($N = 12$) of adequate collaterals in patients with acute inferior wall infarction associated with complete right coronary obstruction did not significantly alter global left ventricular function (ejection fraction 50% versus 49%). Their later report[156]

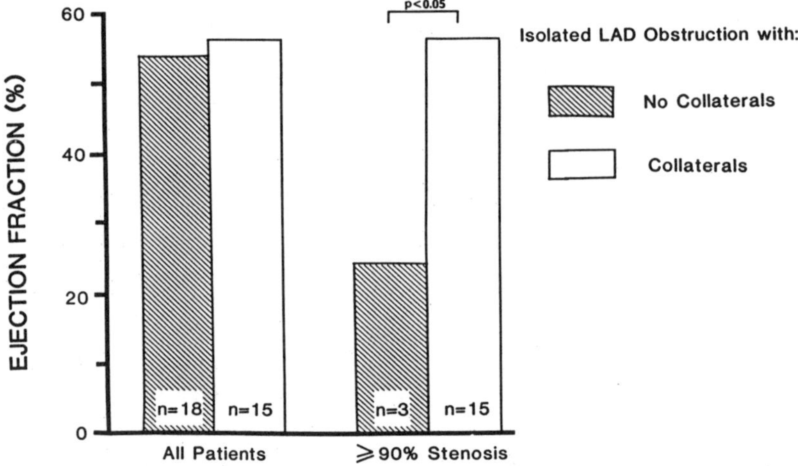

Figure 2-13   Effect of collaterals on left ventricular ejection fraction in patients with isolated disease of the left anterior descending coronary artery (LAD). When all patients were considered, collaterals had no effect. However, because the LAD lesions in patients with collaterals always exceeded 90%, the coronary disease was significantly more severe in this group than in the group without collaterals. Only three individuals without collaterals had stenoses exceeding 90%. Despite comparisons between small groups with comparable coronary artery lesions, collaterals had a significant effect in preserving ejection fractions in patients with collaterals. These data demonstrate the importance of insisting that patients with and without collaterals also have similar coronary artery lesions before meaningful comparisons can be made. (Drawn from data presented by Aloan et al.[157])

on 52 patients with left anterior descending coronary artery occlusion revealed that patients with collaterals ($N = 14$) had ejection fractions averaging 50%, while those without collaterals had average ejection fractions of 42%. This difference, however, was not significant. Betriu and colleagues[159] also routinely studied patients four weeks following infarction. There were 194 patients with lesions exceeding 90%, and 60% had total occlusions. Collaterals were observed in 115 subjects. The ejection fraction was significantly higher ($p < 0.001$) in those with well-developed collaterals than in those with none. Williams et al.[78] studied 20 patients during acute myocardial infarction, 9 with total coronary occlusion, and 10 of the remaining 11 with stenoses of at least 90%. The ejection fractions averaged 42% and 20% in 6 patients with and 14 without collaterals, respectively ($p < 0.02$). Nohara's data[98] obtained at 15 days following onset of the first infarction in a group of patients with complete coronary occlusion also confirm that ejection fraction is higher in individuals with nonjeopardized collaterals than in either those with jeopardized collaterals or those with no angiographic evidence of collateral vessels.

Complete obstruction of the left main coronary artery occurs in approximately 0.06−0.4% of the population having coronary angiography.[89,92,95,161,162] In the presence of such a totally obstructive lesion, the vascular supply to the left ventricle depends entirely on the right coronary artery and associated collateral pathways. In one case of left main coronary artery obstruction, the entire blood supply of the heart was maintained by collaterals from the conus artery and to a lesser extent the sinus node artery arising immediately proximal to an associated occlusion of the right coronary artery.[86] In another report the total coronary blood supply in a patient with proximal occlusion of both the main left and right coronary arteries was delivered by a sequential aortocoronary saphenous vein graft to the obtuse marginal and posterior descending arteries inserted seven years earlier.[88] Blood distribution to the entire left ventricle was then dependent on collaterals. Thus, an opportunity is provided to evaluate, in an extreme situation, the role of the collateral circulation in preservation of left ventricular function. Several reports[63,86,88−96,161−167] have described the effects of total occlusion of the left main coronary artery on global function of the left ventricle. Of 33 cases in which left ventricular function was quantified, 20 maintained a normal ejection fraction ($> 50\%$), while three additional patients had ejection fractions between 40 and 50%.[86,88−94,96,162,166,167] The majority of these patients had minimal or no disease of the right coronary artery. Significant obstructive lesions of the latter vessel, which thus jeopardized the collateral supply, were virtually always associated with depressed systolic function of the left ventricle. Therefore, in these patients surviving total occlusion of the left main coronary artery, the majority had well-preserved global left ventricular function, which was obviously attributable to adequate collateral flow. It is likely that the low incidence of occluded left main coronary arteries and the high proportion of patients with this lesion who have normal left ventricular function are attributable to the high attrition rate in those individuals with poor collaterals, extensive ischemia, and severely depressed ejection fractions.

The contractile pattern of the left ventricle in patients with coronary artery disease has been demonstrated by numerous investigators to be beneficially influenced by the collateral circulation.[63,68,69,78,79,82,87,99,100,107,114−117,119,124,152,155,157−159,168−179] Unlike global hemodynamic parameters, the angiographic evaluation of regional contractile pattern permits one to relate the specific local vascular supply to function of the myocardium perfused by that vessel. The left ventricular angiogram in the right anterior oblique projection reveals the anterior, apical, and inferior surfaces of the heart. The first two are supplied by the left anterior descending artery, while the last is perfused by the right coronary artery. The left anterior oblique projection defines the posterior-lateral wall supplied by the left circumflex artery and the interventricular septum perfused by the left anterior descending vessel. Abnormal regional contractile patterns may be described qualitatively as either hypokinetic, akinetic, or dyskinetic, referring to diminished, absent, or paradoxical localized movement. Regional disorders of contraction may also be quantitated. The right anterior oblique projection of the ventriculogram may be bisected by drawing a line from the middle of the aortic orifice to the apex (Figure 2-14). This is the ventricle's long axis. The

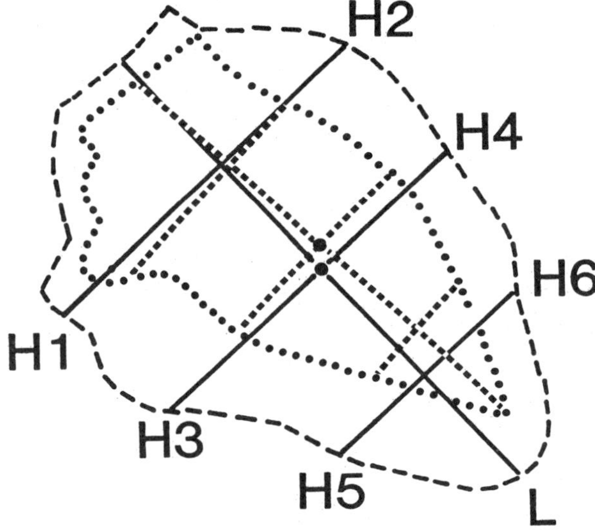

Figure 2-14   End-diastolic (dashed line) and end-systolic (dotted line) left ventricular silhouettes traced from frames of a left ventricular angiogram in the right anterior oblique projection. The long axis (L) is drawn from the aortic orifice to the apex. This line is then quadrisected by three lines drawn parallel to the plane of the aortic valve. The six halves of these three parallel lines are called hemiaxes. Shortening of hemiaxes H_1, H_3, and H_5 during systole is a reflection of contraction of myocardium supplied by the right coronary artery. On the other hand, systolic shortening of L and the hemiaxes H_2, H_4, and H_6 represents contraction of myocardium perfused by the left anterior descending coronary artery.

latter is then quadrisected into four segments of equal length by drawing three lines parallel to the plane of the aortic valve. The six halves of these three parallel lines, or hemiaxes, are labeled as indicated in Figure 2-14. The lengths of the hemiaxes and long axis are then measured in end-systolic and end-diastolic frames, and shortening is expressed as a ratio of the difference divided by the end-diastolic measurement. In general, changes of the long axis and hemiaxes H_2, H_4, and H_6 are assumed to represent contraction of myocardium perfused by the left anterior descending coronary artery, while hemiaxes H_1, H_3, and H_5 are considered to represent right coronary artery perfusion territory. A second quantitative method measures the length of the perimeter of the left ventricular silhouette in the right anterior oblique projection that contracts abnormally. The abnormal portion is expressed as a percentage of the total perimeter. Regardless of the method used to define an abnormal region, the findings can be easily related to the presence or absence of collateral vessels supplying the region.

The success of these studies in attributing a functional role to the coronary collateral circulation for the maintenance of regional myocardial function is dependent on many of the same factors evaluated previously during the discussion of the relationship between coronary collaterals and left ventricular ejection fraction. Most of the investigations concluding that there was a positive correlation between collaterals and regional function in patients with chronic anginal symptoms have studied exclusively or principally subjects with total coronary occlusions,[63,68,69,79,87,99,100,107,115–117, 119,124,152,155,158,168,169,172,175,178,179] while several additional studies have restricted evaluation to those with severe disease, either stenoses exceeding 95%[114,176] or stenoses exceeding 90%.[157,173] Furthermore, the patients selected for study often had single-vessel disease, thus eliminating concerns about jeopardized collaterals and effects of regional dysfunction in neighboring segments. Finally, the simple presence of collaterals was not considered sufficient evidence of their functional capacity. Instead, the quality of collaterals was felt to be important, and the degree of opacification of the distal segment of the occluded or critically stenosed vessel during angiography and the distal run-off were gauged.

Aygen[79] studied 100 patients with complete obstruction of the left anterior descending artery. He defined collateral flow as adequate when the left anterior descending artery was clearly visualized and its diameter approximately normal. Aygen found that regional contraction of the anterior wall of the left ventricle could be related to adequate collateral filling of the obstructed left anterior descending artery. Thus, 56% of those with adequate collaterals had normal contractions of the anterior wall despite absence of antegrade perfusion, compared to only 4% of those lacking adequate collaterals (Figure 2-15). An aneurysmal anterior wall was observed in 56% of subjects without collaterals, but was unusual (1%) in the presence of adequate collaterals. Patients with collaterals had a higher incidence of anterior wall hypokinesis, but more patients without collaterals had akinetic segments. Thus, myocardial motion abnormalities following occlusion of the left anterior descending coronary artery were more frequent and more severe in those without collaterals supplying the anterior wall.

Hamby and co-workers[63] also identified 177 patients with total occlusion of the left anterior descending coronary artery, 125 with and 52 without adequate collaterals. Most patients had multiple-vessel disease. As demonstrated in Figure 2-16, anterior wall asynergy was seen in fewer patients with than without collaterals to the obstructed vessel. When all patients with obstructive coronary disease were considered, 66% with and 92% without collaterals had regional anterior wall motion abnormalities ($p < 0.005$). This striking difference was preserved when patients with isolated obstruction of the left anterior descending coronary artery were studied (Figure 2-16). Thus, 22 of 39, or 56% of those with collaterals had anterior wall asynergy, in contrast to 11 of 12, or 92% of those without collaterals ($p < 0.05$).

Vigorito et al.[119] also studied patients with either total left anterior descending or right coronary artery occlusion. Collaterals had no effect on the frequency of anterior wall infarction in those with left anterior descending disease, and did not influence contraction of anterior left ventricular wall segments in those with infarcts. The reasons for the differing results of this

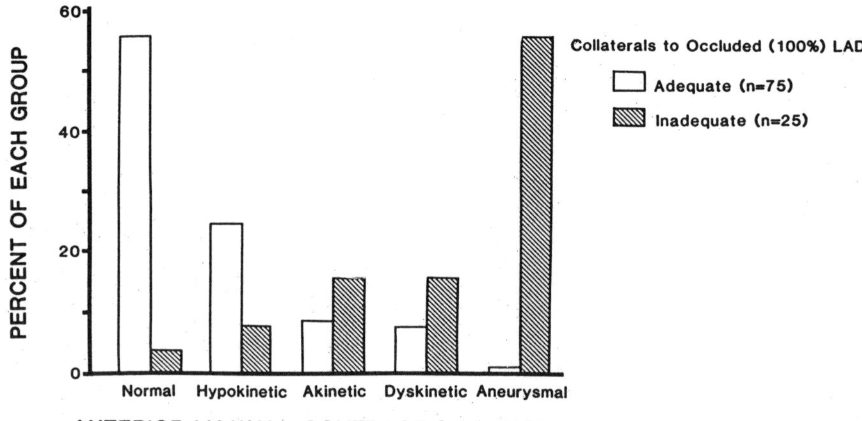

Figure 2-15   Relationship of anterior left ventricular (LV) wall contraction pattern to adequacy of collateralization of a completely occluded left anterior descending coronary artery (LAD). Whereas more than 80% of individuals with adequate collaterals had either normal or only mildly hypokinetic anterior walls, at least 70% of subjects with inadequate collaterals had either aneurysmal or dyskinetic anterior walls. Therefore, myocardial motion abnormalities following LAD occlusion were more frequent and more severe in those without collaterals supplying the anterior wall. (Drawn from data presented by Aygen.[79])

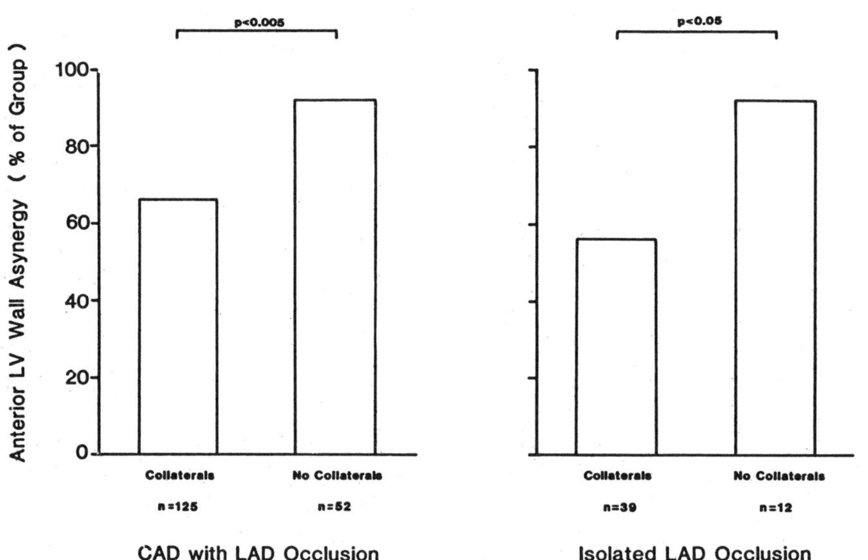

Figure 2-16   Effect of collaterals on contraction of the anterior left ventricular (LV) wall in patients with occlusion of the left anterior descending coronary artery either in combination with other coronary disease (left) or as an isolated lesion (right). In both cases fewer patients had left ventricular asynergy if coronary collaterals were present (Drawn from data presented by Hamby et al.[63])

and Hamby's[63] studies are unclear. In contrast, as noted above, the presence of good, nonjeopardized collaterals decreased the likelihood of a diaphragmatic infarct in those with right coronary occlusion.[119] In addition, only 14% of those with good collaterals and prior diaphragmatic infarcts had severe asynergy of the diaphragmatic wall, significantly better than in either those with poor (54%, $p < 0.01$) or no (92%, $p < 0.001$) collaterals.

Hecht et al.[124] evaluated two groups of patients with coronary lesions, those with stenoses of 75–99% and those with total coronary occlusions. The patients with subtotal obstructions were subdivided into groups with normal and impaired angiographic opacification of the distal segment of the diseased vessel. Collaterals were observed only in those with subtotal obstruction of the coronary artery and impaired distal filling, implying inadequate antegrade flow through the lesion (9 of 20 vessels in this group) and those with total occlusion (34 of 38 completely obstructed vessels). After consideration of the collateral width and density of opacification of the distal segment of the stenotic or occluded vessel, only one of the 20 vessels with subtotal lesions and impaired antegrade flow and 10 of the 38 occluded arteries were considered to have good collaterals. Coronary lesions compromising the lumen by less than 75%, as well as more severe lesions coupled with normal filling and angiographic opacification of the distal diseased artery and, therefore, not accompanied by coronary collaterals, were associated with normal left ventricular wall motion. Of the 11 patients with good collaterals, 7 had normal regional contraction (Figure 2-17). On the other hand, only 3 of 42 patients with inadequate or absent antegrade coronary flow and poor collaterals had normal wall motion ($p < 0.001$). Furthermore, akinesis was never observed if good collaterals were evident, whereas akinesis was noted in areas perfused by 18 of the 42 vessels with poor collateral filling. Thus, collateral perfusion clearly affected regional myocardial function. Hecht's study emphasizes the critical importance of collateral quality. As demonstrated in Figure 2-17, the effect of collaterals on wall motion is obscured if only groups with and without collaterals are examined. Arie's results[155] in patients with total occlusion of the left anterior descending coronary artery, some of whom had good and others poor collaterals, echo Hecht's observations. Rowe[107] also confirmed Hecht's data, and concluded that myocardial contraction distal to a coronary occlusion was proportional to the extent of collateral filling of the distal segment of the diseased vessel.

Levin has also been concerned with the effect of collaterals on myocardial contraction.[168,169] Like Hecht,[124] Levin and his colleagues have attributed great significance to the adequacy of distal runoff in the stenotic or occluded vessel. In vessels with lesions less severe than 90%, runoff is generally the result of antegrade flow, while collaterals are solely responsible for runoff when the vessel is totally occluded. Runoff depends on a combination of antegrade flow and collaterals when the lesion compromises the arterial lumen by 90 to 99%. Levin examined regional wall motion in three groups of patients: those with 75–89% stenoses, those with subtotal obstructions of 90–99%, and those with complete vessel occlusions. As expected, the fre-

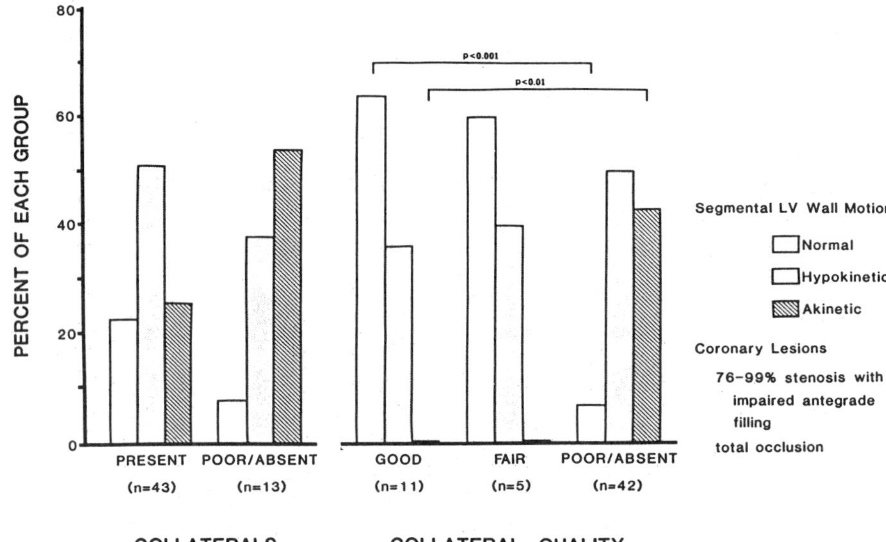

Figure 2-17   Effects of presence and qualitative grading of collateral adequacy on left ventricular (LV) wall motion. Collaterals were observed only in subjects with subtotal obstructions of 76–99% where antegrade opacification of the distal coronary artery was impaired and in those with total coronary occlusion. When patients were segregated by the mere presence or absence of collaterals, no obvious effect of these accessory vessels on LV wall motion was detected. However, when collateral grading was taken into account, it became apparent that collateral perfusion clearly affected regional myocardial function. Thus, 7 of 11 individuals with good collaterals had normal contraction patterns, and akinesis was never observed. In contrast, only 3 of 42 cases with no or only poor collaterals had normal wall motion, and 18 demonstrated akinesis. (Drawn from data presented by Hecht et al.[124])

quency of motion abnormalities increased as the severity of disease increased. But within each group subsets with either adequate or inadequate runoff had strikingly different contraction patterns. In patients with 75–89% stenoses and adequate runoff, 79% of myocardial segments perfused by the diseased vessels contracted normally, while 15% were hypokinetic and 6% were either akinetic or dyskinetic (Figure 2-18). In contrast, in patients with similar coronary lesions but with inadequate runoff, 33% of the myocardial segments were hypokinetic and 67% were akinetic or dyskinetic. Adequate runoff in patients with 90–99% lesions resulted in normal contraction in 69% of segments, hypokinesis in 27%, and akinesis or dyskinesis in 4%. Inadequate runoff was associated with marked deterioration. Only 15% of segments were normal, while 23% were hypokinetic and 62% akinetic or dyskinetic. In patients with total occlusions where runoff was dependent only on collateral flow, the results were surprisingly similar. With adequate runoff, 43% of myocardial segments were normal, 52% were hypokinetic, and 5% were akinetic or dyskinetic. When distal runoff was felt to be inadequate, only 11%

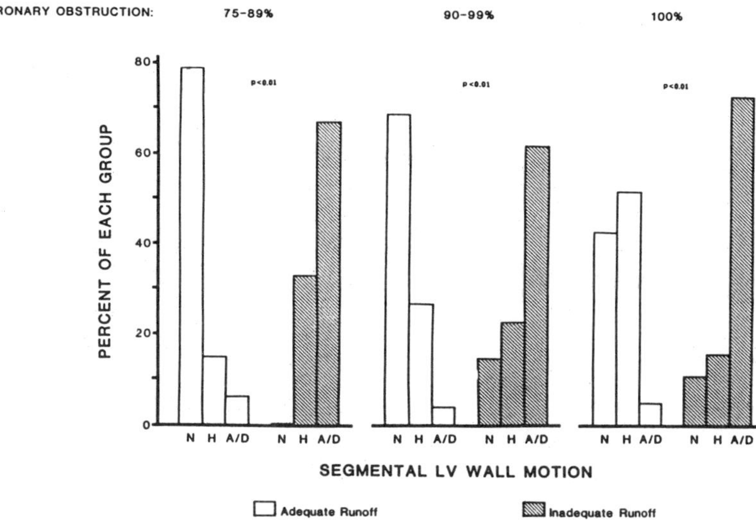

Figure 2-18   Relationship between distal coronary artery runoff, severity of coronary artery obstruction, and segmental left ventricular (LV) wall motion. Lesions less severe than 90% are generally not associated with angiographically visible coronary collaterals, and thus distal runoff is the result of residual antegrade flow. When the artery is completely obstructed, runoff is solely dependent on collaterals. For lesions between 90 and 99%, a combination of residual antegrade and collateral flows is responsible for the runoff. Normal or minimally impaired contraction is dependent on adequate runoff, whether the result of residual antegrade or collateral flow. Conversely, poor runoff is associated with imparied regional myocardial function independent of the severity of the coronary lesion. Thus, adequate collateral flow was functionally equivalent to good residual antegrade perfusion and was associated with preservation of myocardial function. (Drawn from data presented by Levin et al.[168])

of myocardial segments contracted normally. Sixteen percent of segments were hypokinetic and 73% were either akinetic or dyskinetic. The differences between subgroups with and without adequate runoff are statistically significant ($p < 0.01$). Therefore, within each grade of coronary lesions, myocardial function was much better when distal runoff was adequate. It made little difference whether distal runoff was the result of residual antegrade flow or collateral perfusion. Thus, adequate collateral flow was functionally equivalent to good residual antegrade perfusion, and was again seen to be associated with preservation of myocardial function.

Ensslen and associates[87,115] studied patients with total occlusion of the left anterior descending or right coronary artery and quantitated the effect of collaterals on regional myocardial contraction. Twenty-six of 87 individuals had good collaterals, while the remaining subjects had no or only defective collaterals. Contraction of the hemiaxes and long axis of the left ventricle was used to evaluate local function. With occlusion of the left anterior descending artery, there was an average of only 0.38 abnormal hemiaxis/patient (maximum 4-H2, 4−6 in Figure 2-14) when collaterals were good, but 3.6 hemiaxes/patient were abnormal when collaterals were defective or absent. Furthermore, average shortening of the corresponding hemiaxes and long axis was 34.7% in those with good collaterals, significantly less than 40% in normal hearts, but greater than 10.7% in those with inadequate collaterals. With right coronary artery occlusion, 0.37 hemiaxis/patient (maximum 2-H1 and 3 in Figure 2−14) was abnormal when collaterals were good and 1.5 hemiaxes/patient when they were defective or absent. Average inferior wall hemiaxis shortening was 30.2% in normal hearts and 28.6% in patients with well-collateralized arterial lesions. These values were not different. On the other hand, average shortening of 11.7% in those with inadequate collaterals was significantly worse.

Schwarz and his co-workers[68,69,99,100,114,158] have been particularly interested in the effect of collaterals on myocardial function. In one study, Sesto and Schwarz[158] examined the relationship between severity of left anterior descending coronary artery stenosis, presence of adequate collaterals, and average shortening of anterior wall hemiaxes and the long axis. There were 127 patients without and 72 with collaterals. In those without collaterals and with stenoses of less than 75%, average shortening was normal (39.4%). With progression of disease to 75−99% stenosis, shortening declined to 25.4% ($p < 0.001$). Shortening nearly ceased (5.4%) when the artery was totally occluded ($p < 0.001$). This precipitous decline in shortening with increasing severity of the coronary stenosis is graphically depicted in Figure 2-19. No patient with collaterals had a coronary stenosis less than 75%. Shortening was 23.6% in those with collaterals and 75−99% stenoses, a significant decline from that in normal hearts ($p < 0.001$), but no different from that in the group with comparable coronary lesions and no collaterals. However, with progression of the stenosis to complete occlusion, there was no further deterioration of regional contraction (18.8%) (Figure 2-19). The difference between hemiaxis shortening in those with and without collaterals and total arterial occlusions was significant ($p < 0.001$). Shortening was restored to normal in patients with surgical revascularization despite the severity of the arterial lesions. Therefore, collaterals effectively produced partial revascularization and functionally converted a total occlusion to approximately a 90% stenosis.[69]

Berndt et al.[116] altered the approach to the question of the effect of collaterals on systolic shortening. They selected 76 patients with stenoses of the left anterior descending coronary artery in excess of 80%, 62 of whom had total occlusion, and divided them into groups with (59 patients) and without (17 patients) anterior wall asynergy. Collateral vessels were visualized in 71% of the former group and 100% of the latter group. If the groups were restricted to patients with total coronary occlusion, then 80.4% of those with anterior wall asynergy and 100% of those with normal ventricles had collaterals.

When the left main coronary artery is occluded, perfusion of much of the left ventricular myocardium is dependent on collateral flow from the right coronary artery. Numerous reports[63,86,88−96,166,167] have documented absence of left ventricular contraction abnormalities in selected individuals

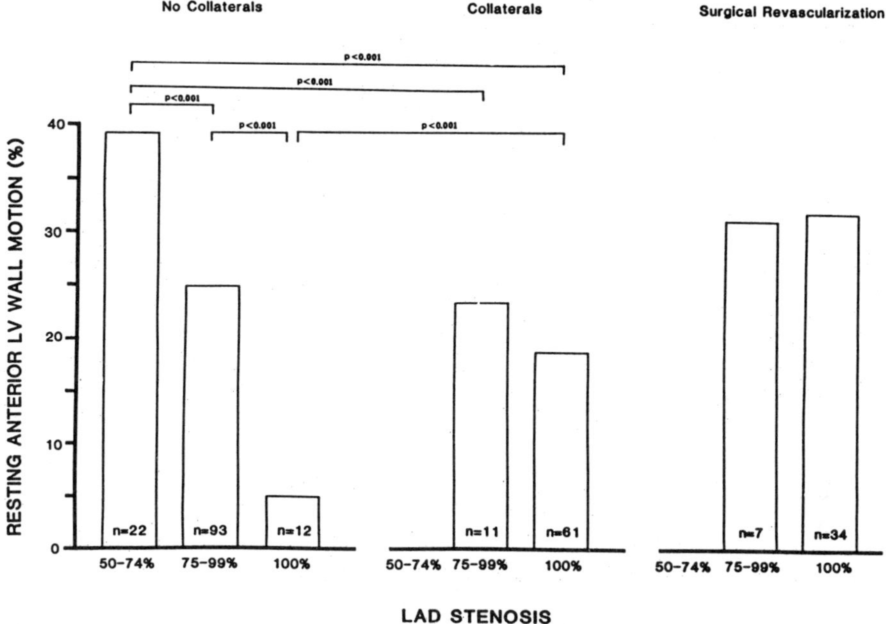

Figure 2-19   Effects of differing severity of left anterior descending coronary artery (LAD) obstruction and the presence of collaterals on averaged resting shortening of the long axis and anterior left ventricular (LV) wall hemiaxes. In individuals without collaterals, increasing coronary artery stenosis produced progressive diminution of contraction of the myocardium supplied by the diseased LAD. However, collaterals prevented any further deterioration in function when the severity of the lesions progressed from 75–99% to total occlusion. Of course, surgical revascularization produced full function of the anterior wall regardless of the severity of the LAD lesions. Thus, collaterals effectively produced partial revascularization and functionally converted a total occlusion to approximately a 90% stenosis. (Drawn from data presented by Sesto and Schwarz.[158])

with left main coronary artery occlusion. Normal resting systolic wall motion in these subjects attests to the importance and adequacy of the collateral circulation.

In the studies described above, collateral adequacy has been judged principally by the degree of opacification of the distal segment of the diseased coronary artery during angiography. Because of the unclear association between angiographic appearance and flow, other techniques have also been used to evaluate collateral function. Wolf[117] quantitated collateral flow with the ^{133}Xe clearance method in patients with total occlusion of the left anterior descending artery, and correlated directly measured flows with regional function. When anterior wall hemiaxial shortening was normal, flows averaged 69.3 ± 11.3 ml/min/100g. Hypokinetic areas had significantly lower flows of 60.6 ± 11.0 ml/min/100g, while collateral flows fell to 53.1 ± 9.9 ml/min/100g when the anterior wall was akinetic. More subjects with half-axial shortening of less than 15% had flows below 50 ml/min/100g than patients with shortening exceeding 15%. Thus, again, there is a definite relationship between coronary collaterals and myocardial function.

Kolibash et al.[179] measured resting myocardial perfusion at the time of cardiac catheterization with dual intracoronary injections of radiolabeled macroaggregated albumin particles in patients with total occlusion of the left anterior descending and/or right coronary artery. Sixty-three right coronary and 47 left anterior descending artery obstructions were evaluated in 91 patients. Collaterals to 101 of the myocardial perfusion territories beyond the occlusions were identified. In the nine areas without collaterals, all had resting perfusion defects and eight had abnormal left ventricular hemiaxis shortening (Figure 2-20). Forty-three of the 101 collateralized areas had normal resting perfusion and therefore adequate collaterals, and 28 (65%) were associated with normal segmental shortening. In contrast, the remaining 58 collateralized regions demonstrated abnormal resting perfusion

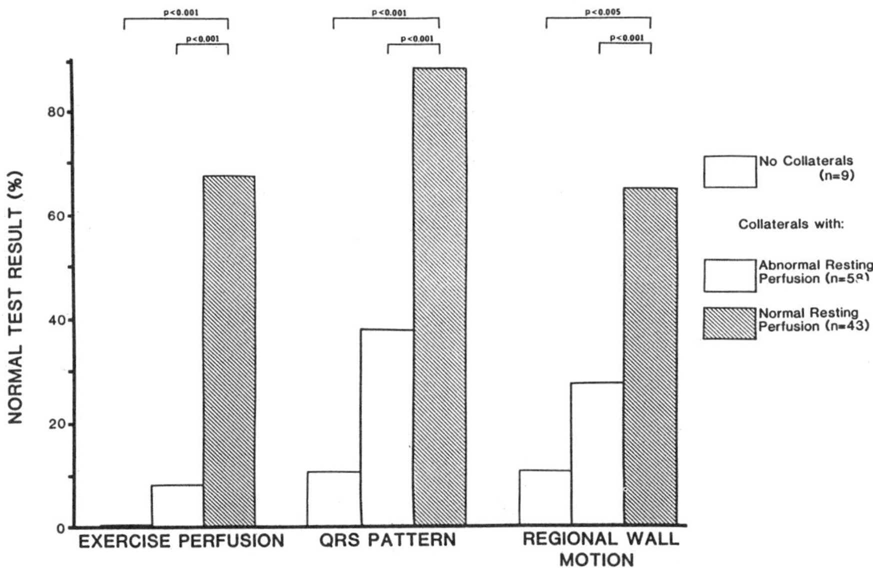

Figure 2-20   Effect of collaterals on exercise perfusion(^{201}Tl scintigraphy), the electrocardiogram, and regional left ventricular wall motion in patients with total occlusion of the left anterior descending and/or right coronary artery. The presence of collaterals was assessed by intracoronary injections of radiolabeled macroaggregated albumin particles. Virtually all tests were abnormal in patients without evidence of collaterals. Most patients with poor collaterals (abnormal resting perfusion) also had abnormal exercise perfusion, electrocardiographic Q waves, and regional wall motion abnormalities, but their responses were better than those of patients without collaterals. In contrast, when collaterals were adequate (normal resting perfusion), at least two of the other three tests were normal in 86% and all were normal in 40%. Thus, the presence of adequate collaterals attenuated and even eliminated objective evidence of myocardial ischemia in many subjects with total coronary occlusions. (Drawn from data presented by Kolibash et al.[179])

implying incomplete revascularization by collateral vessels, and only 16 (28%) had normal segmental wall motion. Thus, the ability of collaterals to furnish adequate flow to myocardium without antegrade perfusion was positively correlated with preservation of regional function. To underscore the importance of collaterals in these patients, Kolibash also evaluated the frequency of electrocardiographic Q waves and stress perfusion defects measured with ^{201}Tl-exercise scintigraphy. In the nine areas without angiographically visualized collaterals, all four variables (including resting perfusion and regional myocardial contraction) were abnormal except for the electrocardiogram in one and segmental function in another (Figure 2-20). Of the 58 regions with inadequate collaterals and resting perfusion defects, at least two of the three additional variables (regional left ventricular contraction, resting electrocardiogram, exercise scintigraphic defects) were abnormal in 47 (81%) cases, and all variables were abnormal in 32 (55%) areas. However, when resting perfusion was normal, 37 (86%) regions had at least two other variables that were also normal, and all variables were normal in 17 (40%). Only two areas with normal resting perfusion had abnormalities of all of the other three variables.

In several studies, echocardiographic assessment of septal, anterior, and posterior wall contractions has been used in lieu of angiographic analysis.[172,177] Kolibash[172] studied 12 patients with total left anterior descending artery occlusion and angiographically visualized collaterals from the right coronary artery. Septal perfusion was also assessed scintigraphically by intracoronary injection of radioactively labeled albumin macroaggregates. Seven patients had normal septal motion, whereas in five septal motion was either hypokinetic or paradoxical. Five of the seven with normal motion had normal scintigraphic perfusion of the septum. But four of the five with abnormal motion had abnormal perfusion scans despite angiographically visualized collateral channels. This study again emphasizes the importance of grading the quality of the collaterals.

Neiminen et al.[177] used echocardiographic wall excursion indices to separately evaluate walls perfused by each of the three major coronary arteries. For each diseased vessel, indices were equivalent for those with and without collaterals. However, those with collaterals had more extensive obstructive disease than those without (higher coronary obstructive index). The maintenance of similar function despite more widespread and severe coronary occlusive disease again supports the functional value of the coronary collateral.

Nitroglycerin diminishes left ventricular preload as well as afterload and, therefore, can decrease wall tension and myocardial oxygen consumption. There may also be a beneficial effect on collateral perfusion. The decreased oxygen demand and possibly increased supply attenuate myocardial ischemia with resultant improved function. Banka and associates[170,173] correlated reversibility of segmental myocardial contraction abnormalities during nitroglycerin left ventriculograms with the presence of collaterals. Thirty-six patients with stenoses of at least 75% had 61 asynergic segments in the baseline ventriculogram (36 hypokinetic, 24 akinetic, and 1 dyskinetic).

Twenty-six asynergic segments were supplied by collaterals, and 22 (84.6%) were responsive to nitroglycerin. Shortening of seven segments completely normalized. Two of the four nonresponders had jeopardized collaterals. Thirty-five segments had no collaterals. Only 19 (54.3%) improved with nitroglycerin. This difference between those with and those without collaterals is significant ($p < 0.02$). Hypokinetic segments improved equally as often in the two groups, but initially akinetic segments were more likely to respond in those with collaterals (7/9 versus 5/15, $p < 0.05$).

Kupper and Bleifeld[178] also employed nitroglycerin ventriculography to study myocardial responsiveness. Of 17 patients with proximal occlusion of the left anterior descending artery and collaterals from the right coronary artery, only seven had normalization of segmental motion after nitroglycerin. Collaterals in these seven and the remaining ten patients with irreversible left ventricular abnormalities appeared to be grossly similar during angiographic visualization. But further attempts to measure collateral flow before and after vasodilatation with the angiographic contrast agent revealed 103% increases in flow in those with reversible myocardial motion abnormalities but only negligible 19% increases in the others. Thus, those patients with collateral reserve had viable myocardium with potentially reversible contraction abnormalities. Again, the importance of grading collaterals is apparent. This report suggests that even angiographic grading may be inadequate.

Collaterals are also effective in patients with acute myocardial infarction. Williams et al.[78] performed coronary angiography and left ventriculography in 20 patients form 2 to 23 days following the onset of infarction. Nineteen of the twenty had coronary stenoses of at least 90%, and nine had total occlusions. Seventeen had disease of the left anterior descending artery, while three had right coronary artery lesions. Six of the total group had good collaterals, and 14 had no or defective anastomoses. In those patients with good collaterals, only 14 ± 7% of the total endocardial silhouette demonstrated akinetic or dyskinetic segments. In contrast, as much as 47 ± 2% of the perimeter was abnormal in those with inadequate collaterals ($p < 0.01$). These results were generally confirmed by Bertrand and associates[82] who studied patients 7 to 21 days after acute infarction. In those with anterior infarction, 20 had total occlusion of the left anterior descending coronary artery, 12 with no or inadequate collaterals and 8 with good collaterals. In those with good collaterals, 31.5% of the end-diastolic perimeter was abnormal, significantly less ($p < 0.01$) than the 47% that was abnormal in patients with poor coronary collaterals. Of interest was the lack of effect of collaterals on left ventricular function following posterior myocardial function.[82] Twenty-four of 37 patients with infarction had total occlusion of either the left circumflex or right coronary artery. The size of the akinetic area was the same in both the collateralized and noncollateralized infarcts. In the more recent report from the same group,[156] 52 patients with left anterior descending coronary artery occlusion and acute infarction were studied, of whom 14 had collaterals. Although there was a tendency for those with collaterals to have less extensive abnormal perimeter segments, the difference was not significant. In contrast, the subgroup of patients with adequate collaterals from the larger population of 194 individuals with 90–100% coronary lesions studied by Betriu and colleagues[159] four weeks following acute infarction had significantly smaller akinetic segments ($p < 0.001$) than those without collaterals.

Most of the clinical studies described above have exclusively or principally evaluated patients with left anterior descending coronary disease. This choice is probably not accidental. The right anterior oblique projection of the left ventriculogram which has almost exclusively been used for quantitation of regional function probably can more accurately predict perfusion deficits of the left anterior descending than of the right coronary artery. The former artery perfuses the anterior wall, which is well visualized in the right anterior oblique angiogram, whereas the right coronary artery is apt to perfuse the posterior as well as inferior and diaphragmatic walls of the heart. Motion of the posterior wall can be evaluated completely only if the left anterior oblique projection is also analyzed. Therefore, asynergy related to right coronary lesions might be overlooked if only one projection were employed. Perhaps this technical drawback makes some of the studies of collaterals to the right coronary artery less reliable, and accounts for the distinction made by some authors between collaterals to occluded right coronary and left anterior descending arteries. Although Hamby[63] demonstrated a significant correlation between coronary collaterals and regional function in patients with occlusions of the left anterior descending coronary artery, he and his co-workers were unable to show the same relationship for right coronary artery disease. Complete occlusion of the right coronary artery was identified in 288 patients, and 240 (87%) had collaterals. There were no clinical differences between subgroups with and without collaterals. There was also no difference in the frequency of abnormal left ventricular contractile patterns. Sixty-seven percent of the group with collaterals to the right coronary artery and 82% of those without collaterals had inferior wall asynergy. The results were not different if only patients with isolated right coronary disease were studied. However, as indicated above, Ensslen[87,115] and Vigorito[119] were able to demonstrate a beneficial effect of coronary collaterals on regional function in patients with occluded right coronary arteries. Schwarz[68] made similar observations. Inferior wall hemiaxis shortening was examined in patients with and without collaterals and right coronary artery occlusion. Shortening in those with good collaterals ranged from 22 to 36%, not very different from hearts with normal coronary arteries. In contrast, shortening in those with inadequate or no collaterals was significantly depressed ($6–13\%, p < 0.001$). Jang[175] has also concluded that the angiographic size of inferior wall myocardial infarction in patients with isolated total occlusion of the right coronary artery was inversely proportional to the angiographically graded collateral circulation. Therefore, collaterals to the right coronary artery do not appear to be very different from those to the left anterior descending coronary artery. Other studies with possible false-negative results may be related to failure to evaluate the left anterior oblique projection of the left ventriculogram.

As already indicated, the ability of these clinical studies to conclude that coronary collaterals are associated with preservation of regional myocardial function is dependent on appropriate case selection and choice of clinical features used in group comparisons. The central importance of a well-designed clinical study is nicely illustrated by the reports of Aloan,[157] Hecht,[124] and Kolibash.[172,179] These considerations perhaps account for the negative results reported by some investigators (see below).

Aloan and his colleagues[157] evaluated left ventriculograms in 33 patients with isolated obstructive disease of the left anterior descending coronary artery. Fifteen patients had collaterals, while 18 had none. When regional contractility of the base of the left ventricular anterior wall was studied, no differences were detected in the two groups. However, because all patients with collaterals had stenoses exceeding 90%, the group with collaterals had more severe obstructive disease than the patients without collateral vessels. To make the groups more comparable, Aloan selected a subset of patients without collaterals who had equally severe disease (stenoses greater than 90%). Now regional contractility was significantly better in patients with collaterals ($p < 0.01$). Hence, comparisons must be made in patients with equivalent disease. It is not reasonable to compare patients without collaterals who may have stenoses of only 75% to patients with angiographically visible anastomotic pathways who, therefore, must have lesions exceeding 90%.

The importance of the quality of the angiographically visualized collaterals cannot be stressed enough. Hecht's study[124] clearly demonstrates the pitfalls of making conclusions about the functional adequacy of coronary collaterals from data where only the presence or absence of the collaterals has been noted. As graphically depicted in Figure 2-17, the significance of the collateral circulation was obscured when the quality of the collaterals was ignored. Thus, the frequency of normal, hypokinetic, and akinetic regional contractions was similar in those with and without anastomotic vessels. But when patients were segregated according to collateral quality, those with good collaterals had significantly better function than those individuals with poor collaterals ($p < 0.001$).

The reports by Kolibash et al[172,179] suggest that not even angiographic grading of collaterals may be sufficient. These investigators correlated echocardiographically measured septal motion with septal perfusion determined by intracoronary injections of macroaggregated albumin particles and the presence of angiographically visualized coronary collaterals in patients with total occlusion of the left anterior descending coronary artery.[172] Seventy-one percent of patients with collaterals and normal septal motion also had normal septal perfusion. But 80% of those with abnormal septal motion had abnormal septal perfusion despite visualized collaterals. Therefore, there was an excellent correlation between septal motion and septal perfusion (necessarily via collaterals), but a poorer correlation between motion and the angiographic appearance of collaterals. In his more recent study,[179] Kolibash again noted the discrepancy between angiographic appearance of collaterals and resting myocardial perfusion beyond a total coronary occlusion. Collaterals to regions with normal perfusion were graded from angiograms as poor in 16 cases, good in 12, and excellent in 15. Similarly, collaterals to areas with resting perfusion defects were poor in 19 instances, good in 22, and excellent in 17. There was no difference between the two groups. Angiography is clearly not a substitute for measurement of collateral flow or functional indices. Angiographic grading of collaterals must be accepted only as a simplistic, and often inaccurate, approximation, and not as a definitive measurement, of flow.

Claims have been made that coronary collaterals have no effect on either hemodynamics,[1,2,5,59,62,65,122,123,156,158,180−183] left ventricular ejection fraction,[156,182−187] or regional myocardial contraction.[1,2,5,59,62,65,66,112,121−123,156,180−183,185−191] However, most of these studies suffer from the drawbacks previously discussed. Furthermore, the investigators have uncommonly evaluated patients with total coronary occlusion. In patients with subtotal obstruction, perfusion of myocardium is likely to be dependent on a combination of residual antegrade and collateral flows, making the specific effects of collaterals difficult to define. And as Hecht et al.[124] have indicated, consideration of distal runoff from stenotic vessels should not be overlooked. Finally, not all clinical studies evaluating regional contractility have attempted to correlate segmental abnormalities with the presence of collaterals to the diseased coronary artery subserving that portion of the ventricular wall being studied. Treating the left ventricle as a whole and simply noting the presence of asynergy without specifically relating it to the source of perfusion might result in the erroneous conclusion that asynergy occurred in the presence of demonstrated collateral vessels even though the latter supplied normally contracting myocardium in a different coronary distribution.

Miller and his colleagues[1,2,5,59,65,123,181] and Helfant et al.[62,122,180] have been principal proponents of the lack of functional value of coronary collaterals. All of Miller's reports describe patients with subtotal occlusions, multivessel disease, and either no or angiographically evident coronary collaterals. No attempts were made to grade collateral quality, exclude consideration of jeopardized collaterals, or correlate myocardial contraction and perfusion of the same segment of the left ventricle. Some efforts were made to compare patients with collaterals to patients without anastomotic vessels but with equal severity of obstructive disease, but most comparisons were between patients with stenoses exceeding 50% or 75% grouped according to the presence or absence of angiographically visualized collaterals. The latter analysis generally preselects a group with collaterals that has more severe disease than the group without collaterals since it is acknowledged that collaterals usually do not appear until the coronary stenosis reaches 90%. Because Miller and his associates have found that asynergy is more common in those with collaterals, they concluded that these channels are merely markers of the severity of the underlying coronary artery disease. However, the numerous flaws in study design make it difficult to accept these conclusions.

Helfant's initial study[180] suffered from many of the same criticisms made of Miller's reports. His second study[62] evaluated only patients with single-vessel disease and stenoses of at least 90%. Of 61 patients with collaterals, 28 had disease of the left anterior descending artery, 30 had right coronary artery involvement, and 3 had left circumflex obstruction. Fifty-eight patients had no collaterals, and disease of the left anterior descending, right coronary, and left circumflex arteries was present in 35, 20, and 3, respectively. Fifty-nine percent of those with collaterals and 53% of those without had left ventricular asynergy. Although this insignificant difference would support the conclusion that collaterals did not have a functionally apparent effect, the lack of collateral grading diminishes the study's value (see Figure 2-17).

Carroll[190] evaluated the significance of collaterals in patients with at least 75% stenoses of the right coronary and/or left anterior descending artery. Coronary collaterals were identified in 69% of the 119 patients evaluated. In contrast to Miller's and Helfant's reports, Carroll et al. graded the quality of collaterals. There was no effect of collaterals either on the number of abnormally contracting left ventricular segments or on the magnitude of hemiaxis shortening. In this study, however, patients without collaterals had lesions ranging from 75% to 100%, whereas those with collaterals most likely had more severe disease (not specified in the description of the study). Lavine's report[66] is very similar to Carroll's. He and his colleagues also evaluated patients with lesions exceeding 75%. Forty-eight of the 78 study subjects (62%) had collaterals. Forty-three of the patients with collaterals (90%) had abnormal left ventricular contraction, whereas only 16 of those without collaterals (53%) had regional functional abnormalities. This difference was significant ($p < 0.025$). There was no difference in the number of patients with two- and three-vessel disease in the two groups. But because of the study design, one would expect the group with collaterals to have had more severe disease. Lavine's data confirm this expectation. The average coronary score was 6.3 in the group without collaterals and 8.0 in the subjects with collaterals ($p = 0.05$). Therefore, because of this fundamental difference between the two groups, it is not possible to make any reasonable conclusion about the functional significance of the collateral channels.

Markis et al.[185] repeated coronary and left ventricular angiography after an average of 26 months in a group of 36 patients with angina pectoris. They attempted to correlate progression of obstructive disease with changes in the left ventricular ejection fraction. If a coronary stenosis was at least 20% greater at the time of the second study, then by definition, progression had occurred. When arteriographic progression and new collateral vessels were evident, a significant reduction in ejection fraction was also observed. When progression occurred without the appearance of new collaterals, no significant reduction in ejection fraction was documented. From these observations it is not possible to make any conclusions about the functional significance of collaterals. In the group with progression and no deterioration of left ventricular function, the increasing severity of the coronary lesion may have been minimal, e.g., from 60 to 80% stenosis, and there would therefore have been a negligible stimulus for collateral development and no significant decline in myocardial perfusion and hence function. On the other hand, progression in the other group presumably created more severe lesions that affected myocardial function. The development of coronary collaterals occurred because the stenosis had exceeded 90%. Although the collaterals may not have been able to prevent deterioration of left ventricular function, they may have minimized the decline in ejection fraction. Because of the presence of multivessel disease in many of these patients, it is also possible that the collaterals that developed were jeopardized. Therefore, because of the absence of comparable groups, this study cannot be used to deny the possible value of collaterals.

Cohn et al.[183] evaluated 24 patients with coronary stenoses greater than 75%. Eleven patients had no evidence of collaterals, seven had good collaterals, and six had either jeopardized collaterals or anastomoses that were poorly visualized during coronary angiography. There was a tendency for ejection fraction to be lower in patients with collaterals, but they also had more severe disease. The subjects in this study with collaterals were grouped with similar patients from previous studies in order to make valid statistical comparisons of larger groups. Thus, 18 patients with good collaterals were compared to 19 subjects with poor collaterals. Resting flows to the myocardium perfused by the collaterals were nearly equal in the two groups, and regional asynergy was equally frequent in those with good and poor collaterals. However, after intracoronary injection of radiographic contrast agent, a potent vasodilatory substance, flow to well-collateralized myocardium increased by 80%, significantly greater than the 31% increase to poorly collateralized myocardium ($p < 0.05$). It is not surprising that there was no apparent difference in resting ventricular function between those with good and those with poor collaterals since baseline flows were equivalent. However, the greater flow reserve of the angiographically adequate collaterals suggests they would have been better able to preserve ventricular function during stress.

Most studies have convincingly demonstrated that the presence of adequate coronary collaterals is associated with better resting global and regional left ventricular function. However, this conclusion is possible only when clinical evaluations are designed to eliminate bias in patient selection, compare otherwise comparable groups with and without collaterals, and grade collateral quality. Many studies which have determined that coronary collaterals have no functional value are misleading because of inherent systematic and/or analytic flaws. Although one may conclude that collaterals help to preserve myocardial function at rest, there is no assurance that they will be able to continue to have the same beneficial impact during stress when myocardial demand increases. However, this latter issue is important since the heart is stressed numerous times during daily activities even in the sedentary individual.

VI. Cardiac Function Following Myocardial Reperfusion

Coronary artery recanalization or thrombolysis with either streptokinase or urokinase, percutaneous transluminal coronary angioplasty, and saphenous vein bypass graft surgery are currently being used in selected patients in the first few hours after the clinical onset of myocardial infarction to restore myocardial perfusion quickly. It has been theorized that rapid restoration of blood flow would have the greatest opportunity of maximizing myocardial salvage. Several investigators have evaluated the role that coronary collaterals play in this process. All patients entered in these protocols undergo cardiac catheterization generally in the first six hours after onset of symptoms in preparation for the reperfusion procedure; left ventricular function is then assessed a second time approximately two weeks later with either contrast or radionuclide ventriculography. Recent clinical studies[192–194] have demonstrated a greater improvement in ejection fraction and more striking reduction in ^{201}Tl perfusion defect in the follow-up evaluation in those subjects with an adequate collateral supply to the infarct area before thrombolysis therapy. Furthermore, Rentrop[195,196] has suggested that the critical interval for streptokinase recanalization that would assure improvement of left ventricular function following infarction is longer in patients with good collaterals to the region of the acute infarct. These data suggest, but do not prove, that collaterals are able to forestall massive transmural necrosis in the jeopardized region until a reperfusion procedure can be successfully applied to insure long-term viability of non-necrotic, ischemic myocardium.

Rogers and co-workers[197] studied the effects of early reperfusion on infarcting myocardium, and concluded that coronary collaterals were central to the ultimate fate of jeopardized myocardium in most patients. There were 35 subjects in the "no-flow" group who had total coronary occlusion and no angiographic evidence of coronary collaterals, and 26 patients in the "limited-flow" group who had either subtotal coronary stenosis and therefore some residual antegrade flow (8 patients) or total occlusion of the infarct-related vessel with intact collaterals (18 patients). The initial cardiac catheterization was performed a mean of seven hours after onset of symptoms, and the follow-up study 12 ± 7 days after the infarct. In the "no-flow" group there was no change in global or regional ejection fraction if early reperfusion was successful, and global ejection fraction actually declined in those with unsuccessful reperfusion because of disappearance of the immediate postinfarct compensatory hyperkinesis seen in normal myocardium adjacent to the infarcted area. In contrast, successful reperfusion in the "limited-flow" group improved regional ejection fraction in the infarct zone, and thereby also increased the global ejection fraction. Unsuccessful reperfusion resulted in no change. Thus, preserved flow to the infarcted area was a necessary prerequisite for improvement in myocardial function following reperfusion, and a good collateral network was equivalent to residual antegrade flow in maintaining adequate perfusion of the jeopardized tissue in the hours before the reperfusion attempt.

Perioperative infarction following saphenous vein bypass grafting is most often not related to early graft occlusion, but usually to difficulties encountered with intraoperative myocardial preservation techniques.[198] Brindis has defined the conditions most often encountered in patients with perioperative infarcts: severe coronary stenosis in the grafted vessel and absence of collateral vessels to the region of perioperative infarction. In these circumstances the myocardium is poorly perfused, and the flow of cardioplegic solution into the area is impaired.

Hence, collateral channels play an important role in the preservation of myocardial viability before reperfusion can be initiated. The collaterals prevent necrosis and increase the likelihood that reperfusion procedures will have beneficial functional effects.

VII. Coronary Collateral Reserve

Global and regional left ventricular function is dependent on adequate perfusion of the myocardium. During stress, such as exercise, myocardial demand increases, and coronary flow also increases to keep pace with the augmented demand. During intraoperative studies, Marcus et al.[199] have measured the maximal coronary flow velocity following release of a transient occlusion of a normal coronary artery. The ratio of peak to resting velocity averaged 4.6 ± 0.4. This reactive hyperemic response implies that normal coronary arteries have the capacity to increase flow nearly fivefold. Thus, demand can virtually never outstrip supply. However, it is not reasonable to assume the same is true for coronary collaterals. Although collaterals may be able to support normal resting myocardial function, their capacity to increase flow during stress can not be inferred. Nonetheless, this information is important. Knowledge of the coronary collateral flow reserve would enable one to predict the amount of stress required to exhaust the capacity of the collaterals to increase flow. Prior to this point left ventricular function would be preserved, while beyond this point function would deteriorate.

Knoebel et al.[110] measured myocardial flow with a coincidence counting system and single bolus injections of $^{84}RbCl$ at rest and during isoproterenol stress in normal control patients and subjects with coronary artery disease. In those with normal coronary arteries the catecholamine increased flow by 87%, while in patients with mild coronary obstructive disease flow rose by 73%. There was no difference between these two peak flows. Patients with severe coronary artery disease were divided into three subgroups: those with no, those with intercoronary, and those with bridging collaterals. The former two had negligible (~5%) increases in myocardial flow following isoproterenol infusion, while in those with bridging collaterals, flow was augmented by 42%.

Horwitz and his colleagues[200] also evaluated the responses of collaterals to isoproterenol infusion. Myocardial flow beyond total coronary occlusions was measured with ^{133}Xe. Resting perfusion rates in normal subjects and in collateralized regions were identical, 63 ml/min/100g. Isoproterenol increased double product (heart rate × systolic blood pressure) by 54% in normal individuals, while average myocardial flow rose by 90%. To account for individual variability in the double product response and, therefore, in myocardial demand, myocardial flow was normalized (flow × 50/[heart rate × systolic blood pressure]). In normal subjects normalized flow increased by 91 ± 28%, whereas the increase was only 16 ± 27% in collateralized myocardium ($p < 0.01$). Therefore, despite normalization of resting myocardial flow by collaterals, collateral reserve in these patients was limited.

Cohn and colleagues[183] evaluated myocardial blood flow with ^{133}Xe washout curves before and after administration of a vasodilator. The radiographic contrast agent Renografin was injected directly into the coronary arteries to elicit regional vasodilatation. In 11 patients without coronary collaterals, only two of whom had coronary stenosis exceeding 94% of the luminal diameter, Renografin increased myocardial flow by 71 ± 8%. Of 13 patients with collateral vessels, 11 had coronary lesions in excess of 94%. In six subjects with poorly visualized or compromised collaterals, flow increased by only 31 ± 9%, whereas flow rose by 80 ± 16% in the seven patients with high-grade, unjeopardized collateral channels ($p < 0.05$). Thus, flow reserve, which was severely compromised in the patients with marked coronary artery narrowing, was restored when collaterals were well developed and unjeopardized.

Wolf et al.[117] studied 13 patients with proximal total occlusion of the left anterior descending coronary artery and two additional patients with proximal left circumflex occlusion before and during infusion of dipyridamole, 0.5 mg/kg. Myocardial flow was measured in the distribution of the occluded vessel with ^{133}Xe. All patients had nonjeopardized collaterals. Flow increased in all patients with collateral vessels. In ten patients with akinetic zones flow increased from average resting values of 58.1 to 84.2 ml/min/100g during vasodilator infusion. Flow rose from 65.5 to 99.0 ml/min/100g in two patients with hypokinetic regions, and from 71.7 to 125.0 ml/min/100g in the remaining three patients with normal regional contraction. These maximum flows were not different in the three groups, and approximated maximal antegrade flow in coronary arteries with obstructions exceeding 50%. Hence, the authors estimated the conductance of well-developed collateral vessels to be one-third to one-half that of normal coronary arteries.

At least in some individuals, collateral flow may be equivalent to normal antegrade coronary flow or nearly so at rest, and collaterals have the capacity to increase flow when needed. However, this capacity appears to be limited. Thus, one would expect left ventricular function to remain normal during low level stress only. Coronary collaterals are not perfect substitutes for the obstructed native artery.

VIII. Pacing Studies

To determine the functional reserve of coronary collaterals, some stress intended to increase myocardial oxygen consumption must be imposed. The three major determinants of oxygen utilization by cardiac tissue are wall tension, inotropic state, and heart rate.[201] Thus, an increase in any of these variables will necessitate an increased oxygen demand and consequently an increased coronary flow as the autoregulatory mechanism adjusts the supply to meet the demand. Perhaps the simplest technique for stressing the heart is augmentation of the frequency of contraction. With a catheter in either the right atrium or ventricle, heart rate can easily be increased with little change in cardiac output or blood pressure. Cardiac pacing is a safe, well-established method of stressing the heart even in patients with significant coronary obstructive disease.

Many investigators have determined that resting myocardial blood flow may be normal even with severe coronary artery obstructive disease, including total occlusion.[200,202–210] However, many of these same studies have revealed that flow to myocardium beyond coronary stenoses does not increase normally during pacing.[204–208] But the response may be modified when adequate collaterals are present. Cannon and his co-workers have extensively studied coronary blood flow responses to atrial pacing in patients with normal coronary arteries and others with obstructive disease.[204–206, 208,209] In their investigations, myocardial blood flow was measured with ^{133}Xe injected directly into the coronary arteries. Multiple regional washout curves were recorded with a multiple crystal scintillation detector. In this fashion flow to multiple myocardial areas of interest could be correlated with the presence of stenoses in the arteries perfusing those areas and the appearance of angiographically visualized collaterals. Patients with normal coronary arteries had myocardial flows averaging 61 ± 6 ml/min/100g, and the blood flow was homogeneously distributed throughout the left ventricle. On the other hand, obstructive disease of the coronary arteries resulted in variable decrements in flow to the perfused tissue causing noticeable heterogeneity. Atrial pacing usually caused flow increments of nearly 25 ml/min/100g when the coronary stenosis was less than 50%, but only 12 ml/min/100g increases when the coronary lesion was more severe ($p < 0.05$).[209] In some patients with rich collaterals, flow was normal under resting conditions and increased normally during pacing.[206]

To better examine the flow response during pacing, Cannon compared the increase in flow to the increase in demand.[205,206,208,209] The latter was estimated by calculating the double product (heart rate $\times$ blood pressure). A regional response index (regional flow $\times$ 10^3/double product) was then determined. For normal myocardial tissue in hearts with normal coronary arteries, the index during atrial pacing was approximately 3.0.[206] The index was significantly lower in patients with coronary artery disease. As shown in Figure 2-21, however, the presence of adequate collaterals was an important determinant of the regional response index during pacing. Thus, in the four patients with adequate collaterals the index was equal in both the myocardial region perfused by normal vessels and the tissue beyond the collateralized coronary lesion. In contrast, in nine subjects with poor collaterals, the increase in flow in the myocardium in the distribution of the obstructed vessel was inadequate for the rise in double product. Thus, the regional response index was only approximately 1.0, half as much as that in normally perfused tissue in hearts with obstructive disease in other areas. Therefore, collaterals do have reserve, and help to meet the increased myocardial demands of atrial

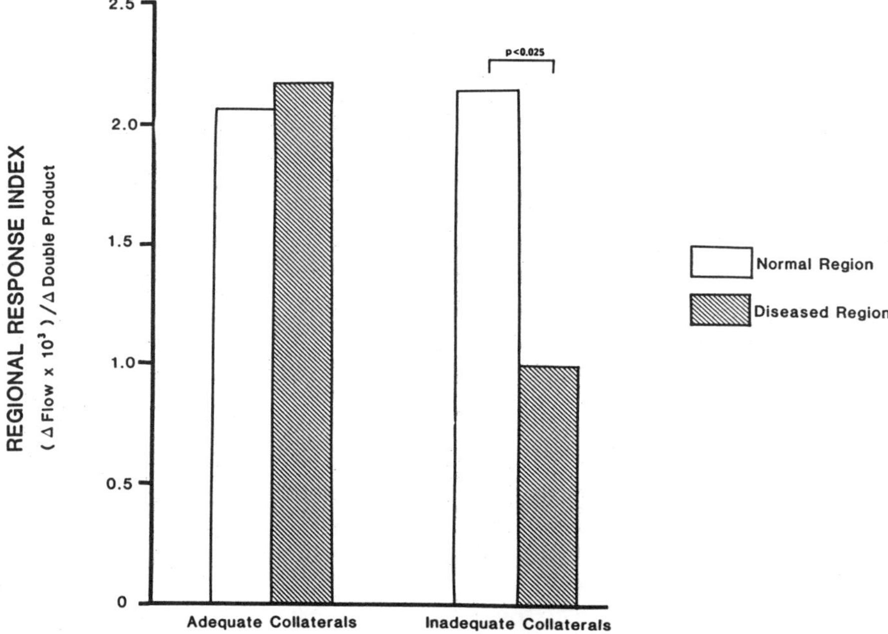

Figure 2-21   Regional response index (regional supply/demand ratio) during atrial pacing to rates of 150 bpm in patients with coronary artery disease. In patients with adequate collaterals, the increase in regional blood flow matched the rise in double product in both normally perfused tissue and collateral-dependent myocardium, and the regional response index was comparable in both areas. In contrast, the rise in blood flow during pacing in regions with inadequate collaterals was insufficient for the increase in double product. Consequently, the regional response index was significantly higher in normally perfused areas than collateralized myocardium. Hence, well-developed collaterals are capable of supplying normal flows during the stress of atrial pacing. (Modified and printed with permission of Unversity Park Press from Cannon et al.[205])

pacing. It must be pointed out, however, that the pacing rate in these studies was incrementally increased to a maximal heart rate of 150 beats/min or the onset of angina pectoris. Faster rates might have revealed a differential response between normally perfused myocardium and tissue beyond diseased coronary arteries in those with good collaterals.

Frick[207,211,212] has also studied the effects of atrial pacing on coronary artery morphology and myocardial blood flow. He and his co-workers performed selective coronary arteriography in multiple projections followed by atrial pacing at increasing rates until angina and/or dyspnea occurred with ischemic ST-segment changes. The pacing rate was then kept at this level, and a repeat selective arteriogram obtained of the coronary artery previously shown to be the source of collaterals. Basal and pacing myocardial blood flows were also measured using ^{133}Xe washout. Eighty-one percent of patients with collaterals had total occlusion of the vessel that was collateralized, while the others had stenoses in excess of 85%.[211] In 11 patients (34%) designated as positive responders, atrial pacing was associated with enhanced angiographic visualization of collateral channels. In 16 patients (50%) designated as nonresponders, there was no angiographic evidence of morphologic change in the collateral vessels. Finally, in five patients (16%) designated as negative responders, atrial pacing was accompanied by decreased angiographic visualization of collaterals. In patients without collateral vessels at rest, ischemia induced by atrial pacing was not accompanied by appearance of new collaterals.

In a second group of 24 patients with complete coronary occlusion and collaterals, 10 were responders, 10 were nonresponders, and 4 were negative responders.[207] Blood flows to the entire left ventricular myocardium prior to and during atrial pacing in the responder group averaged 50 and 66 ml/min/100g, respectively. This average increase of 34.6% was greater than the 11.1% increase in flow from 56 to 62 ml/min/100g in the others ($p < 0.01$). An attempt was made to determine the magnitude of the contribution of collateral vessels to this difference. During basal conditions blood flow to areas supplied by collaterals was only slightly less than that to regions not supplied by collaterals in responders (45 and 50 ml/min/100g, respectively) and in the combined groups of non- and negative responders (56 and 59 ml/min/100g, respectively). Myocardium not perfused by collaterals was generally supplied by vessels with no or subtotal obstructions. Thus, collaterals were able to maintain near-normal basal flows. As predicted from the coronary angiographic data, flow to collateralized myocardium increased more during atrial pacing in the responder group. Flow rose by 54.7% in the latter, and by only 13.1% in those without evidence of increased collateralization during pacing ($p < 0.05$) (Figure 2-22). This trend was also observed in noncollateralized myocardium in the same hearts where the flow increment was 33.3% in responders and 7.6% in others ($p < 0.01$). Although the flow increments to myocardium perfused by angiographically visualized collaterals tended to be higher than the increases to noncollateralized tissue, the differences were not significant. It is unclear why flow did not increase further in the normal and noncollateralized myocardium, especially in the nonresponders. Per-

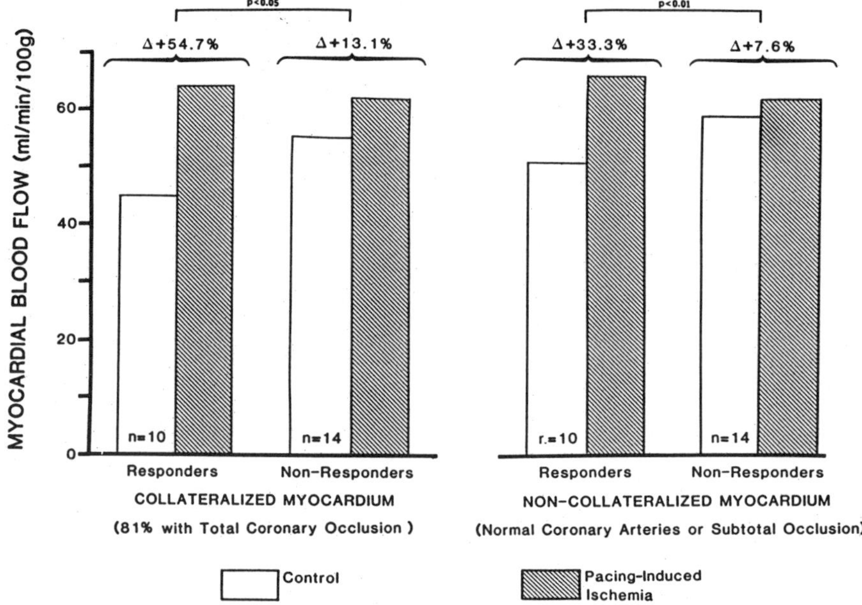

Figure 2-22   In some patients ("responders"), angiographic visualization of coronary collaterals is enhanced during atrial pacing, while in others ("non-responders") it is not. Resting regional myocardial blood flow is generally normal in the collateralized areas of the heart in these two groups, but atrial pacing results in a significantly greater flow augmentation in the responders. Hence, coronary collaterals do have reserve and help to increase flow during stress. (Drawn from data presented by Frick et al.[207])

haps flow increases were limited by subtotal coronary lesions in noncollateralized vessels, and scar tissue in their perfusion territory. It is clear, however, that collaterals do have some reserve and that they help increase flow during stress.

Schwarz and colleagues[68,69,158] examined the ability of coronary collaterals to maintain left ventricular function during right ventricular pacing. Patients with left anterior descending coronary obstructive disease had left ventriculography before and immediately after cessation of pacing at rates of 170 beats/min. For patients with stenoses less than 75% average anterior wall hemiaxial and long axis shortening did not change with pacing (39.4% before and 39.3% after pacing) (Figure 2-23). None of these individuals had coronary collaterals. In subjects with 75−99% lesions and no collaterals average shortening diminished from 25.4% to 13.7% ($p < 0.001$) with pacing. With total coronary occlusion resting regional function was further depressed (5.4%) in those without collaterals, but because of this marked depression little additional deterioration was possible with pacing (5.8%). Patients with collaterals only had coronary lesions exceeding 75%. In those with 75−99% stenoses, regional function which was nearly normal (23.6%) at baseline heart rates declined steeply (8.7%) with pacing. Although function at rest was partially preserved by collaterals when the left anterior descending became totally

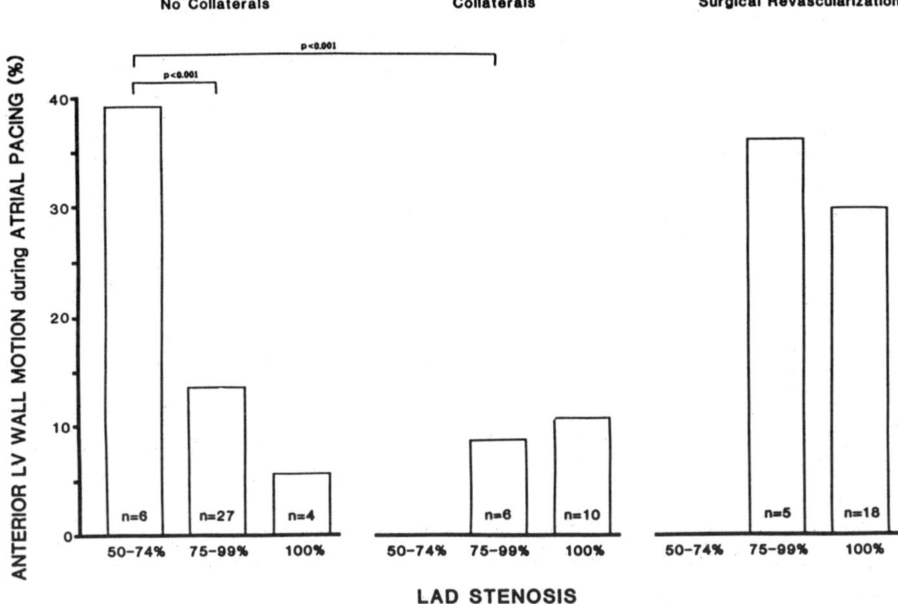

Figure 2-23   Right ventricular pacing to 170 bpm produced increasingly marked deterioration in anterior left ventricular (LV) contraction pattern in patients without collaterals as the severity of the left anterior descending coronary artery (LAD) disease progressed. Anterior wall contraction abnormalities were similar in patients with collaterals. Therefore, at a ventricular pacing rate of 170 bpm, collateral vascular reserve had been exhausted. Of course, no deterioration of anterior wall function was observed in individuals with successful surgical revascularization. (Drawn from data presented by Sesto and Schwarz.[158])

occluded (18.8%), the decline in function was marked during pacing (10.8%). The effects of pacing on global left ventricular function in these same patient groups paralleled the changes in regional myocardial function. The decrease in ejection fraction was similar in the 75–99% stenosis and total occlusion groups whether collaterals were present or not. Thus, there was only a tendency for regional function during pacing to be better if collaterals were present. However, it is noteworthy that these patients were paced at rates of 170 beats/min. With this intense stress it is likely that collateral reserve would have been exhausted, and any protective effect afforded by collaterals obscured. It is anticipated that similar studies at lower heart rates would have demonstrated the functional value of the collaterals.

Lavine et al.[66] measured left ventricular end-diastolic pressure and stroke work during right atrial pacing and then constructed ventricular function curves in 48 patients with and 30 without coronary collaterals. All had coronary stenoses greater than 75%. Those with collaterals had a greater number of abnormal pacing ventricular function curves ($p < 0.01$). However, patients with collaterals also had significantly worse coronary obstructive disease than those without these anastomotic channels. Therefore, the increased likelihood of abnormal ventricular function during pacing in individuals with collaterals was very probably a result of the more significant arterial disease, rendering it impossible to draw conclusions about the independent effect of collaterals.

Atrial or ventricular pacing is a stress which increases heart rate and, therefore, myocardial oxygen consumption. Coronary collaterals do have reserve, and hence can respond to the stress by dilating and increasing perfusion of the dependent myocardium. However, the reserve can be exhausted with subsequent regional and global myocardial failure. Coronary collaterals can only partially preserve myocardial function. They are not perfect substitutes for an occluded major coronary artery.

IX. Exercise Stress Testing

Exercise is clearly a more physiologic stress than either atrial or ventricular pacing. Furthermore, myocardial oxygen demand is likely to be much higher during exercise. Whereas heart rate is necessarily increased during pacing, cardiac output is unchanged, blood pressure is little affected, and contractility only mildly increased. During exercise, however, cardiac output as well as heart rate increase dramatically, systolic blood pressure may normally exceed 200 mmHg, and circulating cathecholamines greatly augment myocardial contractility. Hence, cardiac work and oxygen demand are substantially increased. There must also be an obligatory increase in coronary flow to satisfy the nutritional requirements of the heart if the balance between supply and demand is to be preserved. In normal man coronary flow can increase at least four- to fivefold during exercise.[213–215] It is apparent that even subtle degrees of coronary obstructive disease might interfere with this normal increase in flow during exercise, thus causing a potential imbalance between supply and demand with resultant myocardial ischemia. One would anticipate that the diminished reserve capacity of coronary collaterals would also be taxed during the exercise state. Whereas resting function might have been preserved by collateral development, myocardial function during maximal exercise would be expected to be diminished.

Attempts to demonstrate the functional value of coronary collaterals during exercise have utilized either the electrocardiographic response, thallium scintigraphic image, or radionuclide cineangiogram during standardized stress tests. There are numerous studies that have documented ST-segment shifts during exercise and correlated the abnormalities with the state of the coronary collateral vasculature.[2,3,5,62,65,66,68,85,110,120,123,188,216–226] Of these, only a handful have demonstrated a positive effect of coronary collaterals on the intensity of myocardial ischemia as indicated by the depth of ST-segment depression during or immediately after exercise.[85,110,217,218] McConahay noted a strong tendency for patients with single-vessel obstructive disease and collaterals to have a lower incidence of positive stress tests[217] as well as less ST-segment depression[218] than individuals with similar coronary artery disease but no angiographically visualized collateral vessels. This tendency was not observed in patients with two- and three-vessel disease. Fuster and his colleagues[85] identified 164 patients with angina pectoris and no evidence of prior myocardial infarction. Forty-two percent of this group had at least one coronary occlusion, and 91% of the occluded vessels were collateralized. Fuster divided patients into two groups with obstructive coronary lesions of vessels supplying either the inferior and posterior walls of the left ventricle or the anterior wall. Ninety-one percent of patients with disease of the inferior or posterior wall circulation and ST-segment shifts in the inferior leads (III, aVf) during exercise had neither total occlusion nor evidence of coronary collateralization. In contrast, 57% of those with disease in a similar distribution but with normal stress tests had coronary occlusions and collaterals. This effect of collaterals on the results of the stress test was highly significant ($p < 0.01$). Of the remaining 43% with right coronary or left circumflex obstructive disease and normal stress tests, most (36%) had stenoses of only 50−75%. Thus, in patients with right or left circumflex coronary disease, successful collateralization may revascularize the myocardium and prevent ischemic electrocardiographic changes during exercise. On the other hand, collaterals were unable to prevent ST-segment shifts in patients with obstructive disease of the left anterior descending coronary artery. Fifty-three percent of patients with occlusion of the vasculature supplying the anterior wall had collaterals, and all had precordial lead ST-segment shifts during exercise. Perhaps the different results reflect the greater amount of myocardium usually perfused by the left anterior descending artery than by either of the other two vessels.

This small number of favorable reports is dwarfed, however, by the many studies concluding that coronary collaterals are ineffective.[2,3,5,62,65,66,68,120,123,188,216,219−226] But with few exceptions the referenced investigations are subject to the same criticisms directed at studies analyzing the relationship between collaterals and left ventricular function. Most studies did not limit the patient population to those with one-vessel disease, and therefore did not account for the probable frequent occurrence of jeopardized collaterals. Furthermore, patients with collaterals were frequently acknowledged to have more severe disease than those without collateral vessels, thus biasing the comparisons in favor of the group without accessory channels. In addition, unlike Fuster's study,[85] other reports did not attempt to correlate the electrocardiographic leads where myocardial ischemia was detected with either the specific diseased vessel or the anatomic area of collateral revascularization. Thus, a patient with a collateralized left anterior descending occlusion and a noncollateralized right coronary lesion having exercise-induced ST-segment depression in the inferior electrocardiographic leads should not be considered an example of functional inadequacy of the collateral circulation. Finally, in few studies was the angiographic adequacy of the collateral circulation assessed to segregate patients into subgroups with differing probabilities of demonstrating benefits of a collateral circulation.

Bartel and co-workers[3] studied patients with coronary artery disease who had had exercise stress tests. There were 158 patients with and 118 without collateral vessels. Whereas 75% of subjects with collateral vessels had positive stress tests, only 47% of those without collaterals had tests demonstrating exercise-induced myocardial ischemia ($p < 0.001$). Although the authors assumed that these results proved that collaterals had no protective effect, their conclusion must be tempered because of the data that the patients with collaterals had more extensive coronary disease. Sixty-eight percent of the latter group had triple-vessel disease, while only 24% of those without collaterals had obstructive disease of all major coronary arteries. Bartel also divided patients into subgroups based on the number of major vessels obstructed. No difference in the frequency of positive tests was observed in patients with two-vessel disease with and without collaterals, although patients without collaterals and either one or three diseased vessels had significantly fewer positive exercise tests than their counterparts with collaterals ($p < 0.05$). There is little assurance, however, that the severity of the coronary lesions in the groups with and without collaterals was comparable even after subgrouping for the number of involved coronary arteries.

Lavine et al.[66] noted that patients with collaterals had the same incidence of positive stress tests as those without these vessels. However, their own data demonstrated that the two groups were not similar. Patients with collateral channels had a significantly higher coronary score, i.e., more obstructive disease, than those without anastomotic vessels ($p = 0.05$). Helfant and co-workers[221] exercised patients with coronary artery disease on a bicycle and correlated the magnitude of the resulting ST-segment depression with the presence of coronary collaterals and the severity of the coronary obstructive disease. Of 14 patients with either no or 1-mm ST-segment depression, only three had angiographically visualized coronary collaterals. However, of 19 patients with at least 2-mm ST-segment depression, 14 had collateral vessels. This highly significant difference ($p < 0.005$) suggested that coronary collaterals were unable to attenuate myocardial ischemia. But the same study demonstrated that those individuals with the most profound ST-segment changes during exercise, and therefore those with the collateral vessels, also had the most severe disease. Thus, nine of the 14 patients with ST-segment depression not exceeding 1 mm had one-vessel coronary disease, whereas nine of 19 patients with at least 2-mm ST-segment depression had three-vessel disease.

Tonkon et al.[223] used multifactorial analysis to define determinants of the exercise-induced ischemic electrocardiographic response in patients with coronary artery disease. They graded collateral quality by the extent of opacification of the collateral itself as well as the distal segment of the obstructed coronary artery. A score of 4 was equated with excellent collateralization. Ninety-one patients were in the study group. The quality of collateral vessels in patients with positive treadmill stress tests (collateral score 2.4 ± 0.2 per major vessel stenosis) was no different from that in patients with negative tests (collateral score 2.0 ± 0.3). However, patients with positive tests had more severe disease. The number of stenoses and their severity were both significantly higher in the patients with positive stress tests. When subsets of patients with specific coronary lesions were examined, there was again no apparent effect of collateral quality on the results of the stress test except in patients with isolated disease of the left anterior descending coronary artery. In the latter the collateral score was 3.6 ± 0.3 in those with positive excercise tests and 1.1 ± 0.6 in those with negative treadmill tests. Unfortunately, the degree of stenosis was not quantitated in these two subgroups. It is obvious that the initial conclusion from this study, as well as from the reports of Bartel,[3] Lavine,[66] and Helfant,[221] that those individuals with collateral vessels are likely to have more frequent and more intense myocardial ischemia during exercise cannot be accepted without reservation. All of these studies, as well as many of the other negative studies already cited, compare groups with and without collaterals that have differing degrees of coronary artery disease severity. It is expected that patients with more severe disease will have both more collaterals and more ischemia. These studies, therefore, cannot make valid conclusions about the functional value of collateral vessels.

Despite the obvious drawbacks of the above studies, several others have been more careful to compare patients with nearly equivalent disease. Helfant[62] analyzed the electrocardiographic response to exercise in patients with one-vessel disease and stenosis exceeding 90%. Seventy-nine percent of those with collaterals had positive Master's tests, whereas only 48% of those without these accessory channels had exercise-induced ischemia ($p < 0.05$). Regardless of whether the right coronary or left anterior descending artery was involved, those with collaterals appeared to have a greater chance of having a positive stress test. Tubau and colleagues[225] also evaluated exercise responses in patients with single-vessel disease and stenoses of at least 90%. Sixteen patients had and 21 did not have angiographically apparent collateral vessels. Treadmill time and the depth of ST-segment depression were similar in the two groups. It is unclear if the groups were truly comparable in these studies, since it is not known if the patients with collaterals had mainly vessel occlusions while the others had principally subtotal stenoses.

Studies by Harris,[219] Kaplan,[220] and Schwarz[68] have also concluded that collaterals are unable to modify the ischemic response to exercise successfully. Patients with multivessel disease and comparable severity and location of lesions were segregated into groups according to the presence or absence of collaterals. There appeared to be little effect of collaterals on the appearance of ST-segment shifts. However, the issues of jeopardized collaterals and collateral quality were not addressed in these reports, and therefore, the conclusions are again subject to serious reservation.

The incorporation of radioisotopic scanning techniques during exercise has permitted direct evaluation of myocardial perfusion and correlation with the presence of angiographically visualized collateral vessels. ^{201}Tl is the agent most commonly used for exercise scintigraphy. As described previously, uptake of this isotope by the myocardial cell is a flow-limited process.

Because uptake is an active process, cellular viability is a necessary prerequisite. Thus, irreversibly damaged or even transiently ischemic cells take up less[201]Tl, leaving a defect in the scintigraphic image. Therefore, this technique provides some information about the functional adequacy of the circulation. As detailed in Chapter 4, initial uptake and distribution of ^{201}Tl by the myocardium are proportional to blood flow. Infarcted tissue with very low blood flow, therefore, will not take up any isotope and will always appear as a defect or cold spot compared to the normal myocardium. Tissue that becomes ischemic during exercise because of inadequate blood flow will also take up less of the isotope injected during the exercise stress than normally perfused tissue, but during the hours following resolution of the ischemia the defect in these regions appears to fill in as the result of a complex process termed "redistribution." Infarcted tissue will continue to appear as a cold area (see Chapter 4). Careful correlative studies have demonstrated that specific scintigraphic perfusion regions correspond to defined segments of the angiographically identified coronary vasculature.[227,228] Thus, in contrast to the indirect electrocardiographic data, which lack the regional specificity required to evaluate collateral function during exercise, scintigraphy permits direct and accurate assessment of regional collateral perfusion and, by implication, functional adequacy, and permits confident correlation with coronary anatomy.

The majority of investigations using ^{201}Tl scintigraphy have concluded that collaterals can attenuate and in some subjects even prevent myocardial ischemia.[179,210,225,229−235] Kolibash and co-workers[210] studied 61 patients with angiographically visualized coronary collaterals. All had ^{201}Tl-exercise stress tests. Fifty-nine percent had no evidence of thallium perfusion in the distribution of the obstructed, collateralized vessel either at rest or during exercise, implying infarction. Thirty percent of the study group had normal resting scans, but exercise-induced defects. Thus, in these patients the collaterals could not prevent the development of myocardial ischemia during exercise. Finally, and perhaps of greatest interest, were six patients (16%) who had normal perfusion of the collateralized myocardium both at rest and during exercise. In these patients collateral flow was sufficient to maintain myocardial nutrition even during the stress of exercise. In Kolibash's more recent report,[179] nine myocardial areas in the distribution of totally occluded coronary arteries and without angiographically visualized collaterals had resting and exercise perfusion defects. One hundred and one additional myocardial segments perfused solely by collaterals were identified. However, despite the presence of collaterals 58 areas had abnormal resting perfusion, implying inadequate development of the accessory channels. As expected, perfusion during exercise was also abnormal in 53 of these regions (91%) (Figure 2-20). In contrast, 43 collateralized myocardial segments had normal resting perfusion, and in 29 (67%) there were also no perfusion defects during stress. The experience of Verani et al.[229] is similar. They evaluated 19 patients with coronary artery disease who had not had a prior myocardial infarction and identified seven myocardial areas in the distribution of totally occluded vessels that had normal thallium uptake during exercise. Six of these seven regions were supplied by good collaterals.

Wainwright et al.[231] identified 110 angiographically severe obstructive coronary lesions in a group of 65 patients, 53 of whom had complete occlusion of at least one vessel. Although all 110 lesions were severe enough to be collateralized, only 58% actually had visualized collaterals. All patients had ^{201}Tl-exercise tests. Regional count rates in the myocardium distal to the stenosis or occlusion were quantified and compared to count rates in normally perfused tissue. If the count rate in the abnormally supplied muscle was normal, then it was concluded that there was compete protection of the tissue. If the count rate was modestly decreased by 50−80%, then it was felt that the region was partially protected. But if the count rate was decreased by more than 80%, then it was concluded that the myocardium was not protected at all. Of patients with right coronary artery disease, 12 myocardial areas were completely protected and 10 of these 12 regions were supplied by collaterals graded as excellent by angiography. Twenty additional areas were partially protected, while six were unprotected. Although there was a smaller percentage of excellent collaterals in these latter two groups, the distribution of collateral grades was not significantly different in the three subgroups. In patients with disease of the left circumflex vessel, 14 areas were unprotected. Eleven of the 14 regions had no collateral perfusion, while the remaining three had only poor collaterals. Three additional regions were partially protected, and all were supplied by moderately good collaterals. One region with complete protection had excellent collaterals. No patient with left anterior descending disease had complete protection. But seven areas had partial protection and six of these had good collaterals. By contrast, 27 areas had no protection and 19 of these 27 regions had poor collateral supply. In an attempt to exclude the complicating effects of partial occlusions and myocardial scars, a subgroup of 17 patients with total vessel occlusions and no infarction was evaluated. There were 20 occlusions. Nine of 15 regions with collaterals had complete or partial protection, while all five vascular beds without collaterals had no protection.

Rigo and his colleagues[230] studied groups of patients with total coronary occlusions. All 15 myocardial regions without collaterals had abnormal exercise-induced scintigraphic images, whereas only 65 of 92 (71%) regions perfused by collaterals had abnormal scintigrams ($p < 0.05$). Because some of these myocardial areas were already infarcted and, therefore, had abnormal resting scintigraphic images with little change during exercise, these investigators separately evaluated patients with normal resting scintigrams in whom at least one myocardial region became abnormal during exercise. There were 13 diseased arteries without collaterals where the vessel was either totally occluded or the lesion represented the most severe stenosis in the heart. All regions took up ^{201}Tl abnormally during exercise. On the other hand, of 29 similarly diseased arteries with collateral vessels, the scintigraphic exercise study was abnormal in only 19 ($p < 0.05$). Rigo also recognized the importance of classifying collaterals as jeopardized or nonjeopardized. In 14 of 16 regions supplied by jeopardized collaterals, new stress-induced perfusion defects appeared, whereas 8 of 13 myocardial segments with nonjeopardized collateral vessels had normal scintigraphic images during exercise ($p < 0.025$).

Eng[234] evaluated exercise ^{201}Tl scintigrams in 31 patients with 41 totally occluded coronary arteries and no ventriculographic or scintigraphic evidence of infarction in the distribution of these vessels. All 41 occlusions were collateralized. During exercise, 19 of the 41 areas (46%) had normal perfusion. Thirteen of these 19 regions with normal exercise ^{201}Tl uptake were in patients in whom new scintigraphic defects appeared in myocardial regions perfused by adjacent diseased vessels. It is possible that if exercise had been permitted to continue beyond the point at which ischemia developed in these other areas, then the collateralized regions of interest might also have demonstrated perfusion deficits. However, there were also six regions that had normal perfusion during exercise and no evidence of exercise-induced perfusion defects elsewhere. Of interest, left anterior descending areas were much more likely to manifest perfusion deficits during exercise than either right coronary ($p < 0.025$) or left circumflex ($p < 0.05$) regions. Nonetheless, in some patients coronary collaterals appear to be an acceptable alternative to the obstructed native circulation even during stress.

Tubau's interesting study[225] in 22 patients with one-vessel disease and at least a 90% stenosis demonstrated that exercise-induced perfusion defects were more common in patients without (12 of 12, 100%) than with (4 of 10, 40%) collateral vessels ($p < 0.01$). Furthermore, more myocardial segments in patients without than with collaterals had abnormal thallium uptake ($p < 0.005$). Despite this demonstration of a functional role of the coronary collaterals, electrocardiographic monitoring during the stress test in these same patients revealed deeper ST-segment shifts and shorter exercise times in those with collaterals. Eng[234] also noted that there were ST-segment shifts during exercise in his patients with collateralized coronary occlusions and normal exercise scintigrams. Furthermore, Goldberg et al.[226] observed no effect of collaterals on exercise-induced ST-segment abnormalities despite very beneficial effects on left ventricular contraction patterns (see below). Thus, scintigraphic imaging and electrocardiographic monitoring must be evaluating different aspects of the ischemic process. It is unclear how to put this latter observation into proper perspective.

Most of these scintigraphic studies have evaluated ^{201}Tl distribution during exercise in two groups of patients: one with and the other without collaterals. Buda and colleagues[235] recorded scintigraphic images three weeks and again three months after myocardial infarction in the same individuals. In the follow-up studies scintigraphic defects were smaller despite higher rate-pressure products and, therefore, evidence of increased myocardial oxygen consumption. Although no angiographic studies were performed, it is reasonable to conclude that perfusion of the jeopardized myocardium improved during the nine-week interval between the two studies. Spontaneous recanalization of the coronary arterial lesion is possible, but collateral development is a more likely explanation.

Two reports by Iskandrian and colleagues[233,236] underscore the possibility that spurious conclusions may be related to faulty analytical techniques. Exercise ^{201}Tl scintigrams were studied to determine the effect of angiographically visualized coronary collaterals on myocardial perfusion. Iskandrian realized that patients with collaterals almost always had stenoses exceeding 90%. In the earlier study,[236] 44 of 45 patients with collaterals had exercise perfusion defects in the distribution of the collateralized vessel (Figure 2-24). Sixteen of 20 patients with comparable coronary lesions but no collaterals also had positive thallium tests. The authors concluded that there

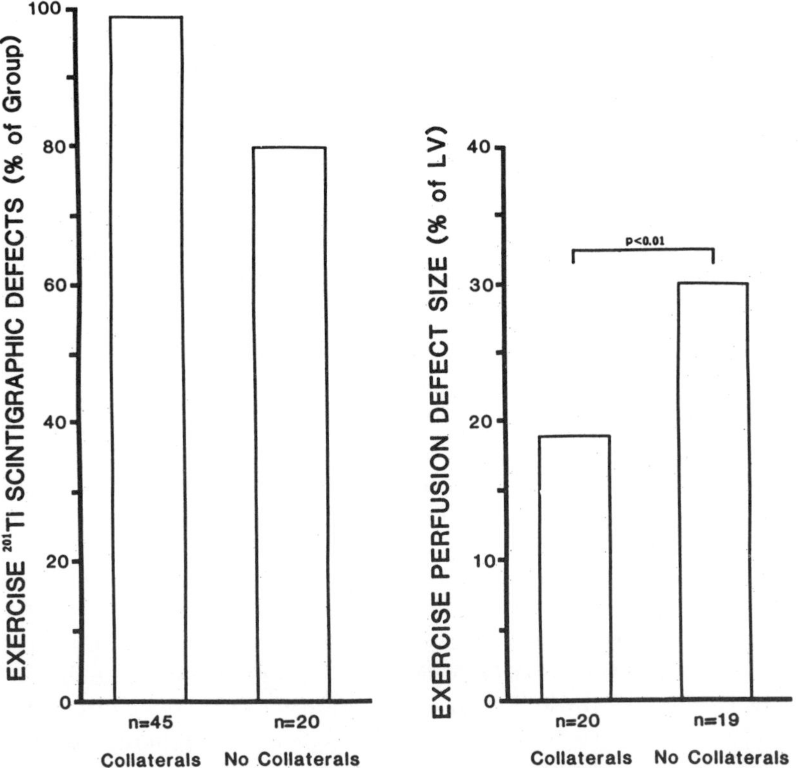

Figure 2-24 Effect of collaterals on exercise-induced ^{201}Tl scintigraphic defects in patients with coronary artery disease. When the scintigrams were analyzed subjectively (left), defects were evident in 80–100% of patients with and without collaterals, and it was concluded that collaterals did not protect the myocardium. However, in a second study by the same investigators (right), the scintigraphic defect size was quantitated. Patients with collaterals had significantly smaller defects than individuals with comparable single-vessel disease but no collaterals, and the authors concluded that these accessory vessels did attenuate myocardial ischemia during exercise. It is important to realize how much the method of data analysis can affect the ultimate conclusions. (Drawn from data presented by Iskandrian et al.[233,236])

was little evidence of protection by collateral vessels. However, in this study the scintigrams were analyzed subjectively. In the second study,[233] the perfusion scan defects were quantified, and the results were quite different. Of the 39 patients with single-vessel disease studied, there were 20 with and 19 without collaterals. The exercise perfusion scan was noted to be abnormal in 35 individuals. Subjective analysis of the scintigrams produced the same negative conclusion as the earlier study. But the size of the perfusion defect was quantified by measuring the perimeter of the cold spot and expressing it as a percentage of the entire left ventricular perimeter. Patients with collaterals had significantly smaller defects than those without accessory channels (19 ± 11% versus 30 ± 13%, $p < 0.01$). The subgroup with left anterior descending disease was large enough to be analyzed separately. Seven patients with collaterals had defects averaging 25 ± 16% of the left ventricular perimeter, significantly smaller than the size of the perfusion abnormalities in the nine individuals without collaterals (40 ± 9%, $p < 0.001$). Thus, by improving the method of analysis, Iskandrian et al. were able to conclude that collaterals do have a beneficial functional role in patients with coronary obstructive disease.

In addition to the dependence of early ^{201}Tl uptake during exercise on the presence of functioning collaterals, these accessory vessels also influence redistribution in the postexercise period.[229,232,237] Those areas with no or, at best, poor collaterals have little redistribution, while good collaterals insure partial and sometimes even complete redistribution. Because delayed distribution of ^{201}Tl, or redistribution, is a function of the mass of viable myocardium[238] (see Chapter 4), these data imply that coronary collaterals are associated with the maintenance of myocardial viability.

Goldberg et al.[226] used radionuclide ventriculograms to evaluate regional function of 141 noninfarcted left ventricular segments supplied by critically stenosed ($\geq 90\%$) coronary arteries in 125 patients. Thirty of 43 segments perfused by vessels receiving good collaterals contracted normally at rest, and 18 (60%) were still normal during maximal symptom-limited bicycle exercise. Of 98 segments perfused by narrowed arteries receiving either poor or no angiographically apparent collaterals, 77 contracted normally at rest, but only 17 (22%) of these continued to contract normally during exercise ($p < 0.001$). The contraction pattern of only 31% of segments supplied by good collaterals deteriorated during exercise, and 71% of these collaterals were jeopardized, whereas function of 73% of segments without good collaterals worsened ($p < 0.001$). These regional effects were echoed by measurements of global left ventricular function. For example, average ejection fraction fell minimally from 51% at rest to 46% during exercise in 18 patients with one-vessel disease and good collaterals. However, ejection fractions in the remaining 25 subjects with one-vessel disease but without good collaterals decreased more strikingly from 52% to 41% (p < 0.005). These benefical effects of collaterals are even more noteworthy when it is realized that 86% of the coronary arteries with good collaterals were totally occluded in contrast to only 15% of vessels with no or poor anastomotic channels ($p < 0.001$).

Hence, coronary collaterals can successfully attenuate and even prevent myocardial perfusion deficits and ischemia and left ventricular functional abnormalities. Radioisotopic imaging during exercise has provided important information about the functional adequacy of these accessory channels. The above studies have demonstrated the ability of the collateral to satisfy myocardial needs during the increased demand of exercise. Several reports, however, are not in agreement with this prevailing view.[6,239–241] Berger[6] reported on patients with obstructive lesions of their coronary arteries of at least 50%. There were 78 vessels with collaterals and 138 noncollateralized stenotic vessels. Myocardial segments with associated electrocardiographic Q waves had diminished thallium uptake during exercise, and the presence of collateral vessels did not influence the results. Because collaterals would not be expected to have much influence on already infarcted myocardium, the analysis was then limited to myocardial segments without associated Q waves. There were more segments with abnormal exercise-induced thallium uptake and fewer with normal uptake in the group with collaterals than in the individuals with noncollateralized vessels ($p < 0.001$). Furthermore, in abnormal segments the presence of collaterals did not affect the frequency of redistribution in the postexercise period. These investigators also ascertained that there was no difference in the conclusions if they segregated the collaterals into subgroups of jeopardized and nonjeopardized vessels. However, this study and its conclusions suffer from poor design. As already discussed, it is inappropriate to compare collateralized and noncollateralized hearts without assuring that the underlying disease of the coronary arteries is comparable. Berger's groups were clearly not similar. Of the arteries receiving collaterals, 73% were totally occluded, 23% had subtotal stenoses of at least 90%, and the remaining 4% had lesions between 80 and 90%. In contrast, only 6% of the noncollateralized vessels were totally occluded, 37% had subtotal lesions of at least 90%, 32% had stenoses of 70–89%, and 25% had mild 50–69% stenoses. Because of the significantly less severe disease in the noncollateralized group, one should not be surprised that these vessels had fewer perfusion abnormalities during exercise. Valid conclusions about collaterals cannot be made from this study. Furthermore, as graphically documented by the two studies of Iskandrian et al.[233,236] qualitative analysis of thallium scans may be misleading and should be replaced by quantitative measurements.

Verani et al.[239] also concluded that there was no correlation between the presence of angiographically visualized collaterals and the ^{201}Tl perfusion pattern during exercise. Fifteen of the 38 scans revealing perfusion defects were associated with good collaterals to the obstructed vessels, an incidence not different from that in patients with inadequate collaterals. Five of the ten false-negative scans occurred in patients with poor or no collaterals while the other five were recorded in patients with good collaterals. However, of the 15 patients with good collaterals and positive scans, seven had triple-vessel coronary artery disease and five others had significant disease ($\geq 50\%$) of two major coronary arteries. In contrast, only five of the other 23 patients with positive scans and either no, poor, or fair collateral channels had triple-vessel disease, while ten had two-vessel involvement. Therefore, the patients with collaterals again had worse underlying coronary disease. Furthermore, the high proportion of patients with triple-vessel disease in the group with collaterals raises the possibility that at least some of the collaterals may have been jeopardized. Among the five patients with false-negative scans and collaterals, four had triple-vessel disease and one had two diseased vessels. It is likely that collaterals, even if not well visualized by angiography, accounted for the absence of perfusion defects in these patients with severe disease. Of the five with normal exercise perfusion scans and no or poor collaterals, three had single-vessel disease and two had two diseased vessels. Therefore, the less severe disease in these patients alone may account for the lack of perfusion defects. The data from this study do not support the conclusion that collaterals have no functional role. On the contrary, the results suggest the opposite conclusion. Collaterals are able to prevent the appearance of regional flow abnormalities in 25% of exercising patients with triple-vessel disease, whereas in the absence of good collaterals, patients with less severe underlying coronary disease are likely to have exercise-induced perfusion defects.

The majority of these exercise studies confirm that collaterals can attenuate or even prevent myocardial ischemia during activities that substantially increase myocardial demand for oxygen and nutrients and, therefore, the requirement for coronary flow. But not all patients are protected. Because of the diminished reserve of these accessory channels, even when well developed, there will be circumstances in which the increased collateral flow will not satisfy the augmented needs, and ischemia will result. But even in these latter patients, the collaterals probably are important. Although it is not possible to prove this, their obliteration would probably make the induced ischemia more profound and widespread. The investigations described above are consistent with the previously developed theme that coronary collaterals are functionally important vessels.

X. Effect on Survival

Perhaps the ultimate test of collateral function is the evaluation of the effects of these accessory channels on patient survival. If collateral vessels improve left ventricular function at rest and during stress by increasing nutritional flow and attenuating or preventing the development of myocardial ischemia, then the limitation of ischemic events should also result in longer survival. The question of whether the coronary collateral circulation can alter the natural history of patients with coronary artery disease has been addressed. However, many of the clinical observations and longitudinal studies are difficult to interpret because of either their anecdotal nature or limited patient follow-up, the multiplicity of uncontrolled and unknown variables such as the severity and duration of disease and degree of left ventricular dysfunction, and unknown group risk factors and varied treatment modalities.

The effect of collaterals on survival is perhaps easiest to demonstrate in those patients with unusual or rare coronary artery abnormalities. Individuals with total proximal occlusion of all three major coronary arteries[39,69,86–88,163,242,243] or acquired occlusion of the main left coronary artery[86,88–96,161–167,244] clearly rely on extracardiac and/or intercoronary collateral vessels for continued perfusion of large portions of the ventricular muscle. Total obliteration of the coronary ostia in luetic aortitis except for occasional pinpoint openings has also been described,[245,246] and in one of the cases presented by Von Redwitz,[246] a prominent network of dilated vessels was seen to extend from the adventitia of the aorta and pulmonary artery to the nonoccluded segments of the coronary arteries. Survival of patients with an anomalous left coronary artery originating from the pulmonary artery is also dependent on development of an adequate coronary collateral circulation between the right coronary artery and peripheral vascular bed of the abnormally arising vessel.[247–250] Infants without collateral vessels usually die within the first few months of life, while those with collaterals usually survive infancy. However, the latter survivors may have evidence of myocardial ischemia later in childhood or as young adults. The early surgical approach in these patients, ligation of the anomalous coronary artery, presupposed adequate collateral supply from the right coronary artery to the distribution of the ligated left coronary artery, and most of these procedures were successful.

Spain's pathologic study[27] suggested that sudden coronary death may be related to failure of the development of a functional intercoronary collateral circulation. He and his colleagues performed postmortem injection studies in hearts of 105 men ranging in age from 35 to 55 years. Plastic spheres with diameters of 40–75 μm were injected into one coronary artery while the effluent was collected from the other main coronary artery. Identification of plastic spheres in the drainage enabled the investigators to determine which hearts had intercoronary anastomoses with dimensions exceeding 40 μm, the minimal diameter of the plastic beads. The collaterals were then opacified with coronary injections of barium sulphate-gelatin mass. Seventy-six of the 105 individuals had died suddenly in an accident, while 16 males with severe atherosclerotic coronary artery disease but no prior clinical symptoms had succumbed suddenly within 30 minutes of their initial symptoms. The final 13 patients had known obstructive disease of the coronary arteries and prior myocardial infarction. Of the group of 76 men who died in accidents, only four had evidence of severe atherosclerotic coronary disease on postmortem examination, and in none of the group was there evidence of myocardial infarction or enlarged intercoronay anastomoses (Figure 2-25). Only one (6.3%) of the group who died suddenly had demonstrable coronary collaterals; no heart had evidence of recent or old infarction. In the one case with collaterals, hypertension and cardiac hypertrophy may have influenced development of the anastomoses. Ten (76.9%) of the 13 hearts from patients with prior infarcts had anastomoses exceeding 40 μm which were especially

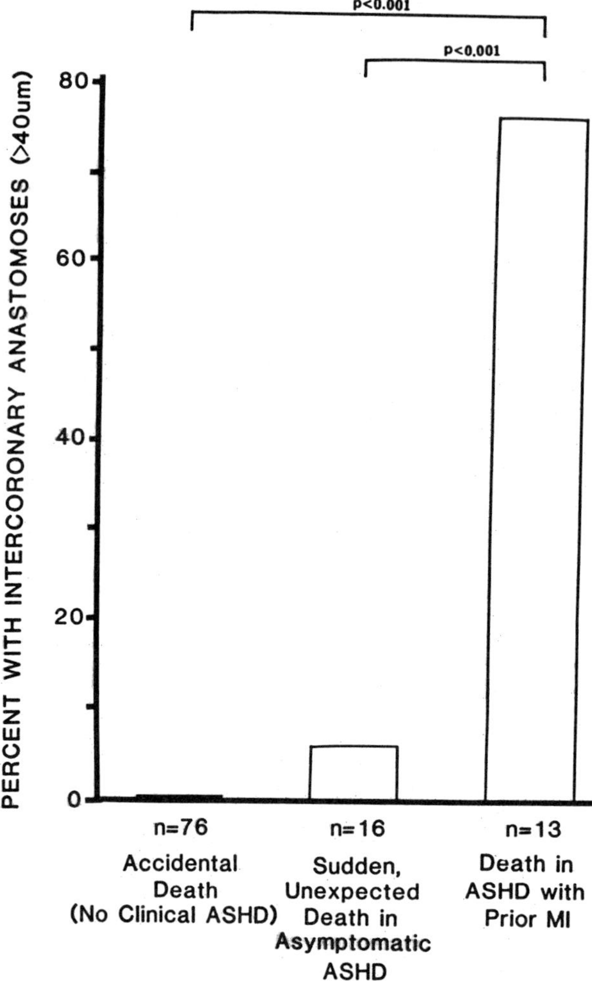

Figure 2-25   Coronary collaterals were abundant in patients who died of known atherosclerotic heart disease (ASHD), but were absent in accident victims without clinical ASHD, and were rare in individuals with asymptomatic ASHD who died suddenly within 30 minutes of their initial symptoms. Thus, the coronary collateral circulation was no better developed in patients with coronary artery disease and sudden unexpected death than in subjects with normal hearts who died in accidents. The failure of formation of an adequate intercoronary anastomotic network may have been one factor accounting for sudden death during a possible ischemc episode because of inability to attenuate or prevent hypoxia of critical myocardial regions. (Drawn from data presented by Spain et al.[27])

evident in the infarcted region. Thus, the coronary collateral circulation was no better developed in patients with coronary artery disease and sudden unexpected death than in subjects with normal hearts who died accidentally. The failure of formation of an adequate intercoronary anastomotic network may have been one factor accounting for sudden death during a possible ischemic episode in these patients because of inability to attenuate or prevent hypoxia of critical myocardial regions.

Others have also examined the hearts of patients with sudden death. Baroldi and Scomazzoni[15] attempted to compare the anastomotic networks in hearts from patients who died suddenly of "acute heart failure" and from hospitalized individuals with coronary artery disease who died of both cardiac and noncardiac causes. Although they concluded that the collateral circulations were similar in the two groups, the number of hearts without ventricular hypertrophy in the sudden death group was quite small, making statistical comparisons hazardous. Furthermore, incomplete description of the characteristics of the group who died suddenly also makes it difficult to compare these results with those of Spain et al.[27] Crawford et al.[251] also reported on sudden death in patients with coronary artery disease. They noted that 50% of hearts had inadequate anastomotic networks.

Weaver and co-workers[252] performed cardiac catheterization on 64 patients with coronary artery disease who had had "sudden coronary death" (ventricular fibrillation) outside the hospital but who had been successfully resuscitated. There were one or more collateral pathways in 49 patients (75%). But of 165 vessels with severe stenosis ($\geq$ 70% obstruction) or occlusion, only 39% had their distal vascular beds supplied by collaterals. After the cardiac catheterization 59 patients were followed for an average of 20.4 months. Fourteen had recurrent ventricular fibrillation and/or sudden death. Nine of these 14 (64%) and 32 of the 45 late survivors without recurrent episodes (71%) had coronary collaterals (p = NS). Although there were fewer collaterals perfusing areas distal to severe coronary lesions in the patients with their second episode of ventricular fibrillation and/or sudden death (15 of 49 vessels collateralized in the latter, versus 44 of 103 vessels collateralized in the survivors), this difference was not significant. It is instructive to note, however, that the survivors had less severe coronary artery disease. Thus, 22% of the long-term survivors had triple-vessel disease, whereas 64% of those with recurrent ventricular fibrillation and/or sudden death had lesions of all three major coronary arteries (p < 0.01). Patients with more severe disease and fewer collaterals, therefore, appeared to be at greater risk for sudden death.

The effect of collaterals on death following acute myocardial infarction is controversial. Miale and Bledsoe[24] correlated the extent of the coronary collateral circulation determined by postmortem angiography with the cause of death in patients with atherosclerotic coronary disease. Eighteen hearts had either no demonstrable or only 1+ anastomoses. Seven of these patients had had recent infarctions, and five died shortly after onset of symptoms (less than 24 hours in two, and three, five, and eight days in the other three). Nineteen hearts demonstrated numerous (3 or 4+) anastomoses. Of seven patients sustaining recent infarctions, three died at one, four, and seven days after the initial symptoms.

Herman and Gorlin[73] studied 16 patients with sudden coronary occlusion during or immediately after cardiac catheterization and concluded that preexisting collaterals were not a factor in the final outcome. Preexisting collaterals were present in six of the eight patients who developed immediate pump failure following acute coronary occlusion and died. In the eight survivors, two had preexisting collateral vessels and collaterals appeared in four others following the coronary occlusion. However, in a study of 20 patients undergoing emergency cardiac catheterization for refractory pump failure or persistent chest pain 2 to 23 days after onset of an acute myocardial infarction, Williams[78] concluded that the collateral circulation did play a favorable role in the preservation of left ventricular function and prognosis. Of six patients with good collateral channels, none had cardiogenic shock and all survived. In contrast, there were 14 patients with absent or inadequate collateral vessels, and ten developed cardiogenic shock, with eight succumbing. Comparison of those with and without adequate collateral vessels revealed no group differences in age, prevalence of prior infarctions, site of acute infarction, or presence of multivessel coronary disease. Therefore, in this selected group of patients with acute infarction, collaterals were identified as an important factor influencing survival.

Fulton[22] attempted to correlate coronary collateral development with duration of symptomatic ischemic heart disease before the demise of the individuals. He noted that the collateral patterns of those who died with an anginal history of less than three months were little different from the patterns of the normal heart. In this recently symptomatic group, thrombotic occlusion of a major coronary artery produced extensive infarction and death. By contrast, the collateral circulation was significantly better developed in patients with anginal histories of six months to two years prior to death, and large-scale anastomoses were numerous in those with longstanding symptoms of seven to fourteen years. Often in this latter group only widely scattered focal ischemic lesions in the inner zone of the left ventricle were apparent, and death was not always the direct result of coronary artery disease. Longer duration of symptomatic coronary artery disease was, therefore, associated with better collateral development, which in turn provided protection from coronary occlusion and death.

Clinical studies defining the role of the coronary collateral circulation in survival of individuals with chronic coronary artery disease are few in number and in general limited because of the small populations studied.[62,253,254] Webster, Moberg, and Rincon[253] have published data on a six- to eleven-year follow-up of a relatively large group of 468 patients with severe coronary artery disease ($\geq$ 80% obstruction) and normal or only moderately impaired left ventricular function. In patients with one-vessel disease and good collaterals, the cumulative six-year mortality rate was 15% regardless of age (Figure 2-26). In those with no or poor collaterals, the six-year mortality rate was 15% for those between 30 and 50 years, and 50% for older patients (51−70 years). This difference in the older patients was highly significant ($p < 0.00002$). For two-vessel disease, the six-year mortality rates were 38% in those with good collaterals and 54% in those with inadequate collaterals ($p < 0.04$). These results were the same in the younger and older patients. Patients with three-vessel disease had six-year mortality rates of 63% regardles of age or the presence of collateral vessels. Perhaps jeopardized collaterals accounted for the lack of effect in patients with severe disease of all three major coronary arteries. Webster attempted to eliminate all doubts about the effect of collaterals on prognosis by selecting a subgroup of patients with total occlusion of a single artery. Obviously, the collaterals could not be jeopardized in this form of coronary obstructive disease. Ten of 18 patients with inadequate collaterals died during the first six years of follow-up, whereas only five of 64 with

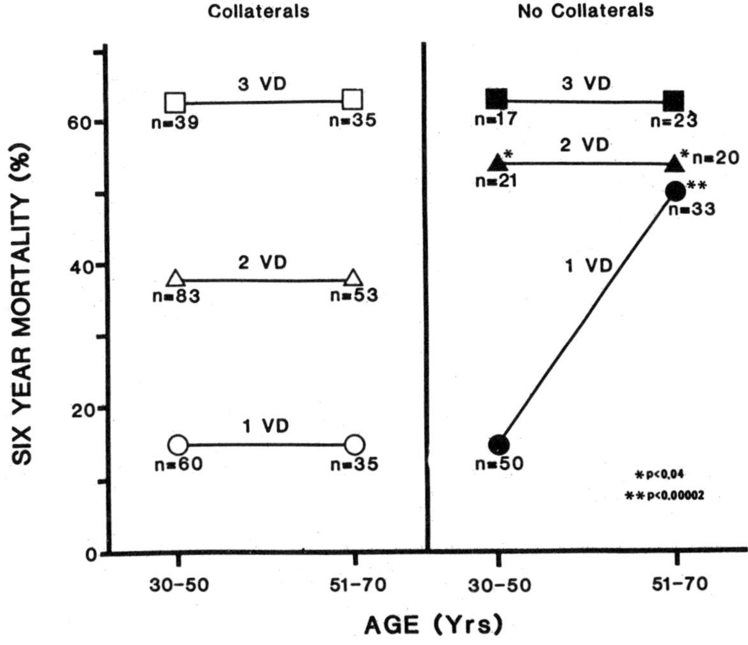

Figure 2-26   Six-year mortality data in patients with severe (≥ 80% obstruction) coronary artery disease and normal or only moderately impaired left ventricular function. Collaterals appeared to affect survival favorably in patients with two-vessel disease (VD) and older individuals with single-vessel disease. Statistical comparisons were made between subjects with and without collaterals. (Modified and printed with permission of Dun-Donnelly Publishing Corporation from Webster et al.[253])

good collaterals succumbed during the same period. These data demonstrate that collaterals provide protection and influence prognosis in chronic coronary artery disease.

Helfant and co-workers[62] followed 61 patients with and 58 patients without a coronary collateral circulation. All had severe single-vessel disease (≥ 90% obstruction). The duration of angina, electrocardiographic evidence of prior myocardial infarction, and left ventricular hemodynamics and contraction patterns were similar in both groups. There was no significant difference in mortality between those with and those without collaterals. However, the small number of patients in each group and the short follow-up (average 22.9 months) make these conclusions less meaningful than those of Webster et al.[253]

Platia and associates[254] studied 68 patients with at least 70% narrowing of the left anterior descending artery or left main coronary artery. The mean follow-up for these patients was 9.9 years. Fourteen of 24 (58%) patients with collaterals to the stenotic or obstructed vessel died during the follow-up period compared to 12 of the 44 (27%) without collateral channels. Actuarial survival analysis of these groups demonstrated a significantly higher mortality rate in the patients with collaterals ($p < 0.04$). At six years after coronary arteriography, the group with collaterals had a cumulative survival rate of 56%, whereas the patients without collateral vessels had a survival rate of 73%. One has the initial impression that collaterals had an adverse effect on prognosis. No data are supplied about the nature of the obstructive disease of the other coronary arteries, and no assessment of possible jeopardized collaterals was made. It may also be unfair to lump patients with disease of the left anterior descending artery together with those having stenoses of the left main coronary artery. Furthermore, it is likely that the patients with collaterals had more severe obstructive disease of the left anterior descending artery since 55% of patients with collaterals followed for at least eight years had complete occlusion of this vessel, whereas no one without collaterals had similar lesions. Finally, progression of coronary lesions over the prolonged follow-up period in individuals initially without collaterals may have stimulated collateral development, thus possibly obscuring perceived differences between the two groups. Therefore, the data do not permit evaluation of the presence of collateral channels as a possible independent prognostic variable.

Most of these clinical studies on survival are limited by small patient group size and short follow-up. Nonetheless, the preponderance of evidence suggests that collaterals are associated with longer survival in patients with chronic coronary artery disease as well as acute myocardial infarction. Pathologic studies have also implied that collaterals diminish the likelihood of dying suddenly. It is clear that collaterals are central to the continuing adequate function of hearts with proximal total occlusion of all major vessels or obstruction or anomalous origin of the main left coronary artery.Therefore, despite the shortcomings of the clinical observations, it is probably fair to conclude that coronary collaterals do have a salutary effect on survival.

References

1. Mason DT, Amsterdam EA, Miller RR, et al: Consideration of the therapeutic roles of pharmacologic agents, collateral circulation and saphenous vein bypass in coronary artery disease. *Am. J. Cardiol.* 28:608−613, 1971.
2. Miller RR, Amsterdam EA, Zelis R, et al: Determinants and functional significance of the coronary collateral circulation in ischemic heart disease. In *Cardiovascular Disease: New Concepts in Diagnosis and Therapy* (ed HI Russek). University Park Press, Baltimore, 1974, pp 75−83.
3. Bartel AG, Behar VS, Peter RH, et al: Graded exercise stress tests in angiographically documented coronary artery disease. *Circulation* 49:348−356, 1974.
4. Gorlin R: Coronary collaterals. *Major Probl. Intern. Med.* 11:59−70, 1976.
5. Williams DO, Amsterdam EA, Miller RR, and Mason DT: The role of the coronary collateral circulation in acute and chronic coronary artery disease. In *Advances in Heart Disease*, vol. 1 (ed DT Mason). Grune and Stratton, New York, 1977, pp 253−267.

6. Berger BC, Watson DD, Taylor GJ, et al: Effect of coronary collateral circulation on regional myocardial perfusion assessed with quantitative thallium-201 scintigraphy. *Am. J. Cardiol.* 46:365−370, 1980.

7. Schlesinger MJ: An injection plus dissection study of coronary artery occlusions and anastomoses. *Am. Heart J.* 15:528−568, 1938.

8. Blumgart HL, Schlesinger MJ, and Davis D: Studies on the relation of the clinical manifestations of angina pectoris, coronary thrombosis, and myocardial infarction to the pathologic findings: With particular reference to the significance of the collateral circulation. *Am. Heart J.* 19:1−91, 1940.

9. Blumgart HL, Schlesinger MJ, and Zoll PM: Angina pectoris, coronary failure and acute myocardial infarction: The role of coronary occlusions and collateral circulation. *JAMA* 116:91−97, 1941.

10. Zoll PM, Wessler S, and Blumgart HL: Angina pectoris: A clinical and pathologic correlation. *Am. J. Med.* 11:331−357, 1951.

11. Blumgart HL, and Zoll PM: Pathologic physiology of angina pectoris and acute myocardial infarction. *Circulation* 22:301−307, 1960.

12. Baroldi G, Mantero O, and Scomazzoni G: The collaterals of the coronary arteries in normal and pathologic hearts. *Circ. Res.* 4:223−229, 1956.

13. Baroldi G: Acute coronary occlusion as a cause of myocardial infarct and sudden coronary heart death. *Am. J. Cardiol.* 16:859−880, 1965.

14. Baroldi G: Myocardial infarct and sudden coronary heart death in relation to coronary occlusion and collateral circulation. *Am. Heart J.* 71:826−836, 1966.

15. Baroldi G, and Scomazzoni G: *Coronary Circulation in the Normal and the Pathologic Heart.* United States Government Printing Office, Washington, DC, 1967.

16. Baroldi G: Functional morphology of the anastomotic circulation in human cardiac pathology. *Meth. Achievm. Exp. Path.* 5:438−473, 1971.

17. Fulton WFM: Arterial anastomoses in the coronary circulation. I. Anatomical features in normal and diseased hearts demonstrated by stereoarteriography. *Scot. Med. J.* 8:420−434, 1963.

18. Fulton WFM: Arterial anastomoses in the coronary circulation. II. Distribution, enumeration and measurement of coronary arterial anastomoses in health and disease. *Scot. Med. J.* 8:466−474, 1963.

19. Fulton WFM: The time factor in the enlargement of anastomoses in coronary artery disease. *Scot. Med. J.* 9:18−23, 1964.

20. Fulton WFM: Anastomotic enlargement and ischaemic myocardial damage. *Br. Heart J.* 26:1−15, 1964.

21. Fulton WFM: The dynamic factor in enlargement of coronary arterial anastomoses, and paradoxical changes in the subendocardial plexus. *Br. Heart J.* 26:39−50, 1964.

22. Fulton WFM: *The Coronary Arteries: Arteriography, Microanatomy, and Pathogenesis of Obliterative Coronary Artery Disease.* Charles C Thomas, Springfield, IL, 1965, pp 72−128.

23. Ravin A, and Geever EF: Coronary arteriosclerosis, coronary anastomoses and myocardial infarction: A clinicopathologic study based on an injection method. *Arch. Intern. Med.* 78:125−138, 1946.

24. Miale JB, and Bledsoe A: Pathologic anatomy of coronary heart disease: Particular reference to cardiac muscle bundles. *Arch. Pathol.* 56:577−596, 1953.

25. Pitt B: Interarterial coronary anastomoses: Occurrence in normal hearts and in certain pathologic conditions. *Circulation* 20:816−822, 1959.

26. James TN, and Burch GE: Differences in naturally occurring arterial anastomoses of normal and pathological human hearts. (abstr) *Am. J. Med.* 27:313, 1959.

27. Spain DM, Bradess VA, Iral P, and Cruz A: Intercoronary anastomotic channels and sudden unexpected death from advanced coronary atherosclerosis. *Circulation* 27:12−17, 1963.

28. Allison RB, Rodriguez FL, Higgins EA Jr, et al: Clinicopathologic correlations in coronary atherosclerosis: Four hundred thirty patients studied with postmortem coronary angiography. *Circulation* 27:170−184, 1963.
29. Jones AM: The functional role of intercoronary anastomoses. *Acta Cardiol. (Suppl.)* 11:130−144, 1965.
30. Robbins SL, Solomon M, and Bennett A: Demonstration of intercoronary anastomoses in human hearts with a low viscosity perfusion mass. *Circulation* 33: 733−743, 1966.
31. Tsuchiya G: Postmortem angiographic studies on the intercoronary arterial anastomoses. Report I. Studies on intercoronary arterial anastomoses in adult human hearts and the influence on the anastomoses of strictures of the coronary arteries. *Jpn. Circ. J.* 34:1213−1220, 1970.
32. Kato T: A comparative study of the coronary arterial structure in the left ventricular free wall in infarcted and non-infarcted human hearts. *Jpn. Circ. J.* 40: 989−1003, 1976.
33. Hutchins GM, Miner MM, and Bulkley BH: Tortuosity as an index of the age and diameter increase of coronary collateral vessels in patients after acute myocardial infarction. *Am. J. Cardiol.* 41:210−215, 1978.
34. Schuster EH, and Bulkley BH: Ischemia at a distance after acute myocardial infarction: A cause of early postinfarction angina. *Circulation* 62:509−515, 1980.
35. DeWood MA, Spores J, Notske R, et al: Prevalence of total coronary occlusion during the early hours of transmural myocardial infarction. *N. Engl. J. Med.* 303:897−902, 1980.
36. Maseri A, Chierchia S, and L'Abbate A: Pathogenetic mechanisms underlying the clinical events associated with atherosclerotic heart disease. *Circulation* 62 (Suppl V):V-3−V-13, 1980.
37. Fulton WFM: Chronic generalized myocardial ischaemia with advanced coronary artery disease. *Br. Heart J.* 18:341−354, 1956.
38. Giese W: Die Anastomosen im Koronarkreislauf bei Koronarsklerose. *Dtsch. Med. Wochenschr.* 82:602−604, 1957.
39. Leary T, and Wearn JT: Two cases of complete occlusion of both coronary orifices. *Am. Heart J.* 5:412−423, 1930.
40. Saphir O, Priest WS, Hamburger WW, and Katz LN: Coronary arteriosclerosis, coronary thrombosis, and the resulting myocardial changes: An evaluation of their respective clinical pictures including the electrocardiographic records, based on the anatomical findings. *Am. Heart J.* 10:567−595, 762−792, 1935.
41. Moritz AR, and Beck CS: The production of a collateral circulation to the heart. II. Pathological anatomical study. *Am. Heart J.* 10:874−880, 1935.
42. Holyoke JB: Coronary arteriosclerosis and myocardial infarction as studied by an injection technic. *Arch. Pathol.* 39:268−273, 1945.
43. Blumgart HL: Coronary disease: Clinical-pathologic correlations and physiology. *Bull. N.Y. Acad. Med.* 27:693−710, 1951.
44. Yater WM, Welsh PP, Stapleton JF, and Clark ML: Comparison of clinical and pathologic aspects of coronary artery disease in men of various age groups: A study of 950 autopsied cases from the Armed Forces Institute of Pathology. *Ann. Intern. Med.* 34:352−392, 1951.
45. Lesbre J-P, Calazel P, Mériel P, and Salvador M: Le circulation coronaire. *Coeur Med. Interne* 6:455−476, 1967.
46. Baroldi G: Coronary heart disease: Significance of the morphologic lesions. *Am. Heart J.* 85:1−5, 1973.
47. Snow PJD, Jones AM, and Daber KS: Coronary disease: A pathological study. *Br. Heart J.* 17:503−510, 1955.
48. Campbell JS: Stereoscopic radiography of the coronary system. *Q. J. Med.* 22: 247−267, 1929.

49. Le Capon J, Chelloul N, and Roujeau J: Les anastomoses intercoronariennes. Valeur fonctionnelle et signification pathologique. *Sem. Hôp. Paris* 46:238–242, 1970.
50. Fulton WFM: Intercoronary anastomoses studied by postmortem stereoarteriography: Relationship to coronary occlusion and myocardial damage. In *Coronary Heart Disease: 3rd International Symposium Frankfurt* (eds M Kaltenbach, P Lichtlen, R Balcon, and W-D Bussmann). Georg Thieme, Stuttgart, 1978, pp 2–11.
51. Lee JT, Ideker RE, and Reimer KA: Myocardial infarct size and location in relation to the coronary vascular bed at risk in man. *Circulation* 64:526–534, 1981.
52. Jugdutt BI, Hutchins GM, Bulkley BH, and Becker LC: Similar relation between size of infarct and occluded bed in dog and man: Evidence for collateral protection. (abstr) *Clin. Res.* 29:212A, 1981.
53. Bean WB: Infarction of the heart. III. Clinical course and morphological findings. *Arch. Intern. Med.* 12:71–94, 1938.
54. Blumgart HL, Zoll PM, Paul MH, and Norman LR: The effect of experimental acute coronary occlusion on stimulation of intercoronary collateral anastomoses. *Trans. Assoc. Am. Phys.* 68:155–158, 1955.
55. Wessler S, Zoll PM, and Schlesinger MJ: The pathogenesis of spontaneous cardiac rupture. *Circulation* 6:334–351, 1952.
56. Schuster EH, and Bulkley BH: Expansion of transmural myocardial infarction: A pathophysiologic factor in cardiac rupture. *Circulation* 60:1532–1538, 1979.
57. James TN: Coronary circulation in acute myocardial infarction. *Br. Heart J.* 33(Suppl):138–144, 1971.
58. Rafflenbeul W, Urthaler F, Lichtlen P, and James TN: Quantitative difference in "critical" stenosis between right and left coronary artery in man. *Circulation* 62:1188–1196, 1980.
59. Miller R, Mason DT, Zelis R, et al: Determinants of the coronary collateral circulation in man: Development principally related to severity of regional atherosclerosis. (abstr) *Clin. Res.* 19:117, 1971.
60. Goldstein RE, Stinson EB, Scherer JL, et al: Intraoperative coronary collateral function in patients with coronary occlusive disease: Nitroglycerin responsiveness and angiographic correlations. *Circulation* 49:298–308, 1974.
61. Biffani G, Santoboni A, Vricella A, and Sabatini F: Il circolo collaterale coronarico nella cardiopatia arteriosclerotica. *G. Ital. Cardiol.* 8:1279–1285, 1978.
62. Helfant RH, Vokonas PS, and Gorlin R: Functional importance of the human coronary collateral circulation. *N. Engl. J. Med.* 284:1277–1281, 1971.
63. Hamby RI, Aintablian A, and Schwartz A: Reappraisal of the functional significance of the coronary collateral circulation. *Am. J. Cardiol.* 38:305–309, 1976.
64. Ramirez ML, and de la Reguera GF: Circulacion colateral coronaria: Importancia y significado en la cardiopatia isquemica. *Arch. Inst. Cardiol. Mex.* 53:397–405, 1983.
65. Miller RR, Mason DT, Salel A, et al: Determinants and functional significance of the coronary collateral circulation in patients with coronary artery disease. (abstr) *Am. J. Cardiol.* 29:281, 1972.
66. Lavine P, Filip Z, Najmi M, et al: Clinical and hemodynamic evaluation of coronary collateral vessels in coronary artery disease. *Am. Heart J.* 87:343–349, 1974.
67. Fuster V, Frye RL, Connolly DC, et al: Arteriographic patterns early in the onset of the coronary syndromes. *Br. Heart J.* 37:1250–1255, 1975.
68. Schwarz F, Flameng W, Ensslen R, et al: Effect of coronary collaterals on left ventricular function at rest and during stress. *Am. Heart J.* 95:570–577, 1978.
69. Schwarz F: Correlation between the degree of coronary artery obstruction and myocardial dysfunction. In *The Pathophysiology of Myocardial Perfusion* (ed W Schaper). North-Holland Biomedical Press, Amsterdam, 1979, pp 305–344.

70. Yasue H, Omote S, Takizawa A, et al: Comparison of coronary arteriographic findings during angina pectoris associated with S-T elevation or depression. *Am. J. Cardiol.* 47:539−546, 1981.
71. Webb WR, Parker FB Jr, and Neville JF Jr: Retrograde pressures and flows in coronary arterial disease. *Ann. Thorac. Surg.* 15:256−262, 1973.
72. Parker FB Jr, Neville JF Jr, Hanson EL, and Webb WR: Retrograde and antegrade pressures and flows in preinfarction syndrome. *Circulation* 50(Suppl II):II-122−II-125, 1974.
73. Herman MV, and Gorlin R: *In vivo* angiographic pathoanatomy of the acute syndromes of coronary heart disease. *Trans. Assoc. Am. Phys.* 85:231−246, 1972.
74. Neill WA, Ritzmann LW, and Selden R: The pathophysiologic basis of acute coronary insufficiency. Observations favoring the hypothesis of intermittent reversible coronary obstruction. *Am. Heart J.* 94:439−444, 1977.
75. Iskandrian AS, Tendler S, Mintz GS, et al: Significance of collateral circulation in patients with left main coronary artery disease. *Cathet. Cardiovasc. Diagn.* 4:135−141, 1978.
76. Neill WA, Wharton TP Jr, Fluri-Lundeen J, and Cohen IS: Acute coronary insufficiency—coronary occlusion after intermittent ischemic attacks. *N. Engl. J. Med.* 302:1157−1162, 1980.
77. Feldman RL, and Pepine CJ: Evaluation of coronary collateral circulation in conscious humans. *Am. J. Cardiol.* 53:1233−1238, 1984.
78. Williams DO, Amsterdam EA, Miller RR, and Mason DT: Functional significance of coronary collateral vessels in patients with acute myocardial infarction: Relation to pump performance, cardiogenic shock and survival. *Am. J. Cardiol.* 37:345−351, 1976.
79. Aygen M: Collateral circulation and regional myocardial function. *Bibl. Cardiol.* 36:136−140, 1977.
80. Cortina A, Prieto-Granda J, Torre F, and Pichard AD: Angiographic and functional correlation in patients with acute myocardial infarction. (abstr) *Am. J. Cardiol.* 49:947, 1982.
81. Ohgitani N: Time-delay of visualization of coronary collaterals after the onset of myocardial infarction. *Jpn. Circ. J.* 41:1277−1278, 1977.
82. Bertrand ME, Lefebvre JM, Laisne CL, et al: Coronary arteriography in acute transmural myocardial infarction. *Am. Heart J.* 97:61−69, 1979.
83. Pagenstecher: Weiterer Beitrag zur Herzchirurgie. Die Unterbindung der verletzten Arteria coronaria. *Dtsch. Med. Wochenschr.* 4:56−57, 1901.
84. Carleton RA, and Boyd T: Traumatic laceration of the anterior descending coronary artery treated by ligation without myocardial infarction: Report of a case with review of the literature. *Am. Heart J.* 56:136−142, 1958.
85. Fuster V, Frye RL, Kennedy MA, et al: The role of collateral circulation in the various coronary syndromes. *Circulation* 59:1137−1144, 1979.
86. Rathor AL, Gooch AS, and Maranhao V: Survival through conus artery collateralization in severe coronary heart disease. *Chest* 63:840−843, 1973.
87. Ensslen R, Schwarz F, Thormann J, and Schlepper M: Überleben und Kollateralzirkulation bei Koronararterienverschluss. *Herz Kreislaufforsch.* 9:20−24, 1977.
88. Goldberger AL, Costello DL, and Moores WY: Normal left ventricular function with total occlusion of right and left main coronary arteries. *Cathet. Cardiovasc. Diagn.* 6:185−190, 1980.
89. Frye RL, Gura GM, Chesebro JH, and Ritman EL: Complete occlusion of the left main coronary artery and the importance of coronary collateral circulation. *Mayo Clin. Proc.* 52:742−745, 1977.
90. Goldberg S, Grossman W, Markis JE, et al: Total occlusion of the left main coronary artery: A clinical, hemodynamic and angiographic profile. *Am. J. Med.* 64:3−8, 1978.

91. Greenspan M, Iskandrian AS, Segal BL, et al: Complete occlusion of the left main coronary artery. *Am. Heart J.* 98:83–86, 1979.

92. Valle M, Virtanen K, Hekali P, and Frick MH: Survival with total occlusion of the left main coronary artery. Significance of the collateral circulation. *Cathet. Cardiovasc. Diagn.* 5:269–275, 1979.

93. Barthe JE, Castells E, Ramos M, et al: Obstrucción completa del tronco común de la coronaria izquierda. Importancia de la circulación colateral. *Rev. Esp. Cardiol.* 34:537–540, 1981.

94. Sohi GS, and Flowers NC: Total occlusion of the left main coronary artery. *Vasc. Surg.* 15:409–414, 1981.

95. Zimmern SH, Rogers WJ, Bream PR, et al: Total occlusion of the left main coronary artery: The Coronary Artery Surgery Study (CASS) experience. *Am. J. Cardiol.* 49:2003–2010, 1982.

96. Choh JH, Wang T, Golbus GA, et al: Survival with total occlusion of left main coronary artery. *Texas Heart Inst. J.* 11:64–68, 1984.

97. Lage SC, Belotti G, Ramires JAF, et al: Influência da circulação colateral coronária na extensão do infarto agudo do miocárdio. *Arq. Bras. Cardiol.* 41:15–17, 1983.

98. Nohara R, Kambara H, Murakami T, et al: Collateral function in early acute myocardial infarction. *Am. J. Cardiol.* 52:955–959, 1983.

99. Schwarz F, Flameng W, and Thiedemann K-V: Vascular compensatory changes in obstructive coronary artery disease. In *Coronary Heart Disease: 3rd International Symposium Frankfurt* (eds M Kaltenbach, P Lichtlen, R Balcon, and W-D Bussmann). Georg Thieme, Stuttgart, 1978, pp 33–38.

100. Walter P, Schwarz F, Becker V, et al: Morphology of poorly contracting ventricle in patients with coronary artery disease. *Thorac. Cardiovasc. Surgeon* 28:177–183, 1980.

101. Schwarz F, Schaper J, Becker V, et al: Coronary collateral vessels: Their significance for left ventricular histologic structure. *Am. J. Cardiol.* 49:291–295, 1982.

102. Bodenheimer MM, Banka VS, Hermann GA, et al: The effect of severity of coronary artery obstructive disease and the coronary collateral circulation on local histopathologic and electrographic observations in man. *Am. J. Med.* 63:193–199, 1977.

103. Cosby RS, Giddings JA, See JR, and Mayo M: Clinicoarteriographic correlations in angina pectoris with and without myocardial infarction. *Am. J. Cardiol.* 30:472–475, 1972.

104. Cheng TO: Incidence of ventricular aneurysm in coronary artery disease: An angiographic appraisal. *Am. J. Med.* 50:340–355, 1971.

105. Manvi KN, and Ellestad MH: Elevated ST segments with exercise in ventricular aneurysm. *J. Electrocardiol.* 5:317–323, 1972.

106. Mullen DC, Posey L, Gabriel R, et al: Prognostic considerations in the management of left ventricular aneurysms. *Ann. Thorac. Surg.* 23:455–460, 1977.

107. Rowe GG: An angiographic and clinical study of coronary collateral circulation. *Basic Res. Cardiol.* 73:131–141, 1979.

108. Hamby RI, Hoffman I, Hilsenrath J, et al: Clinical, hemodynamic and angiographic aspects of inferior and anterior myocardial infarctions in patients with angina pectoris. *Am. J. Cardiol.* 34:513–519, 1974.

109. Martinez-Rios MA, DaCosta BCB, Cecena-Seldner FA, and Gensini GG: Normal electrocardiogram in the presence of severe coronary artery disease. *Am. J. Cardiol.* 25:320–324, 1970.

110. Knoebel SB, McHenry PL, Phillips JF, and Pauletto FJ: Coronary collateral circulation and myocardial blood flow reserve. *Circulation* 46:84–94, 1972.

111. Benchimol A, Harris CL, Desser KB, et al: Resting electrocardiogram in major coronary artery disease. *JAMA* 224:1489–1492, 1973.

112. Bourassa MG, Lespérance J, and David P: Considérations sur le rôle de la

circulation collatérale dans la maladie coronarienne. *Ann. Cardiol. Angéiol.* 23:473−478, 1974.

113. Dwyer EM, Coquia S, Greenberg H, and Pinkernell BH: Inferior myocardial infarction and right coronary artery occlusive disease: A correlative study. *Br. Heart J.* 37:464−470, 1975.

114. Schwarz F, Ensslen R, and Thormann J: Der Einfluss des Kollateralkreislaufes auf die totale und regionale Myokardfunktion bei koronarer Herzkrankheit. *Schweiz. Med. Wochenschr.* 106:1407−1412, 1976.

115. Ensslen R, Schwarz F, Thormann J, and Feige A: Die protektive Wirkung von Kollateralen auf die regionale linksventrikuläre Funktion bei koronarer Herzkrankheit. *Verh. Dtsch. Ges. Kreislaufforsch.* 42:327−330, 1976.

116. Berndt T, Shettigar UR, Lipton MJ, and Hultgren HN: Left anterior descending coronary artery obstruction: Clinical, electrocardiographic, and angiographic correlates. *Br. Heart J.* 38:633−640, 1976.

117. Wolf R, Engel H-J, Hundeshagen H, and Lichtlen P: Collateral myocardial blood flow at rest and after maximal arteriolar dilatation in patients with ischemic heart disease. In *Coronary Heart Disease: 3rd International Symposium Frankfurt* (eds M Kaltenbach, P Lichtlen, R Balcon, and W-D Bussmann). Georg Thieme, Stuttgart, 1978, pp 61−65.

118. Hamby RI: *Clinical-Anatomical Correlates in Coronary Artery Disease.* Futura Publishing Co., Mount Kisco, NY, 1979.

119. Vigorito C, De Caprio L, Poto S, et al: Protective role of collaterals in patients with coronary artery occlusion. *Internat. J. Cardiol.* 3:401−415, 1983.

120. Tuna N, and Amplatz K: The significance of coronary collateral circulation. Coronary arteriographic and electrovectorcardiographic correlations. (abstr) *Am. J. Cardiol.* 26:663, 1970.

121. McConahay DR, McCallister BD, Hallermann FJ, and Smith RE: Comparative quantitative analysis of the electrocardiogram and the vectorcardiogram: Correlations with the coronary arteriogram. *Circulation* 42:245−259, 1970.

122. Helfant RH, and Gorlin R: The coronary collateral circulation. *Ann. Intern. Med.* 77:995−997, 1972.

123. Miller R, Salel A, Bonanno J, et al: The functional significance of the coronary collateral circulation in man. (abstr) *Clin. Res.* 20:208, 1972.

124. Hecht HS, Aroesty JM, Morkin E, et al: Role of the coronary collateral circulation in the preservation of left ventricular function. *Radiology* 114:305−313, 1975.

125. Flameng W, Schwarz F, and Hehrlein FW: Intraoperative evaluation of the functional significance of coronary collateral vessels in patients with coronary artery disease. *Am. J. Cardiol.* 42:187−192, 1978.

126. Flameng W, Schwarz F, Hehrlein F, and Boel A: Functional significance of coronary collaterals in man. *Basic Res. Cardiol.* 73:188−199, 1978.

127. Flameng W, Schwarz F, Schaper W, and Hehrlein F: Functional significance of coronary collaterals. In *Coronary Heart Disease: 3rd International Symposium Frankfurt* (eds M Kaltenbach, P Lichtlen, R Balcon, and W-D Bussmann). Georg Thieme, Stuttgart, 1978, pp 67−72.

128. Oldham HN Jr, Rembert JC, Greenfield JC Jr, et al: Intraoperative relationships between aorto-coronary bypass graft blood flow, peripheral coronary artery pressure and reactive hyperemia. In *Primary and Secondary Angina Pectoris* (eds A Maseri, GA Klassen, and M Lesch). Grune and Stratton, New York, 1978, pp 363−371.

129. Reneman RS, and Spencer MP: The use of diastolic reactive hyperemia to evaluate the coronary vascular system. *Ann. Thorac. Surg.* 13:477−487, 1972.

130. Bittar N, Kroncke GM, Dacumos GC Jr, et al: Vein graft flow and reactive hyperemia in the human heart. *J. Thorac. Cardiovasc. Surg.* 64:855−859, 1972.

131. Greenfield JC Jr, Rembert JC, Young WG Jr, et al: Studies of blood flow

in aorta-to-coronary venous bypass grafts in man. *J. Clin. Invest.* 51: 2724–2735, 1972.

132. Kreulen TH, Kirk ES, Gorlin R, et al: Coronary artery bypass surgery: Assessment of revascularization by determination of blood flow and myocardial mass. *Am. J. Cardiol.* 34:129–135, 1974.

133. McKelvie RS, Kline RL, Black LL, et al: Influence of alternate sources of blood flow on the reactive hyperemia response in aorta-coronary saphenous vein bypass grafts in man. *J. Thorac. Cardiovasc. Surg.* 78:62–67, 1979.

134. Schwartz L, Froggatt G, Covvey HD, et al: Measurement of left anterior descending coronary arterial blood flow: Technique, methods of blood flow analysis and correlation with angiography. *Am. J. Cardiol.* 32:679–685, 1973.

135. Schwartz JN, Kong Y, Hackel DB, and Bartel AG: Comparison of angiographic and postmortem findings in patients with coronary artery disease. *Am. J. Cardiol.* 36:174–178, 1975.

136. Björk L, and O'Keefe A: Estimation of coronary artery stenosis: Limitations of present methods. *Acta Radiol. (Diagn.)* 17:777–780, 1976.

137. Galbraith JE, Murphy ML, and de Soyza N: Coronary angiogram interpretation: Interobserver variability. *JAMA* 240:2053–2056, 1978.

138. Conti CR, Pepine CJ, Feldman RL, and Nichols WW: The angiographic definition of critical coronary stenosis. *Acta Med. Scand.* 615(Suppl):9–17, 1978.

139. Conti CR, Pepine CJ, Feldman RL, et al: Angiographic definition of critical coronary artery stenosis. *Adv. Cardiol.* 26:100–109, 1979.

140. Arnett EN, Isner JM, Redwood DR, et al: Coronary artery narrowing in coronary heart disease: Comparison of cineangiographic and necropsy findings. *Ann. Intern. Med.* 91:350–356, 1979.

141. Staiger J, Adler CP, Dieckmann H, and Barmeyer J: Postmortem angiographic and pathologic-anatomic findings in coronary heart disease: A comparative study using planimetry. *Cardiovasc. Intervent. Radiol.* 3:139–143, 1980.

142. Waller BF, and Roberts WC: Amount of narrowing by atherosclerotic plaque in 44 nonbypassed and 52 bypassed major epicardial coronary arteries in 32 necropsy patients who died within 1 month of aortocoronary bypass grafting. *Am. J. Cardiol.* 46:956–962, 1980.

143. Isner JM, Kishel J, Kent KM, et al: Accuracy of angiographic determination of left main coronary arterial narrowing: Angiographic-histologic correlative analysis in 28 patients. *Circulation* 63:1056–1064, 1981.

144. Klocke FJ: Measurements of coronary blood flow and degree of stenosis: Current clinical implications and continuing uncertainties. *J. Am. Coll. Cardiol.* 1:31–41, 1983.

145. Björk L, Spindola-Franco H, Van Houten FX, et al: Comparison of observer performance with 16mm cinefluorography and 70mm camera fluorography in coronary arteriography. *Am. J. Cardiol.* 36:474–478, 1975.

146. Detre KM, Wright E, Murphy ML, and Takaro T: Observer agreement in evaluating coronary angiograms. *Circulation* 52:979–986, 1975.

147. Zir LM, Miller SW, Dinsmore RE, et al: Interobserver variability in coronary angiography. *Circulation* 53:627–632, 1976.

148. DeRouen TA, Murray JA, and Owen W: Variability in the analysis of coronary arteriograms. *Circulation* 55:324–328, 1977.

149. Fisher LD, Judkins MP, Lesperance J, et al: Reproducibility of coronary arteriographic reading in the Coronary Artery Surgery Study (CASS). *Cathet. Cardiovasc. Diagn.* 8:565–575, 1982.

150. Brown BG, Bolson E, Frimer M, and Dodge HT: Quantitative coronary arteriography: Estimation of dimensions, hemodynamic resistance, and atheroma mass of coronary artery lesions using the arteriogram and digital computation. *Circulation* 55:329–337, 1977.

151. Paulin S: Functional alterations in the coronary circulation as mirrored in the angiogram. *Cardiovasc. Intervent. Radiol.* 5:177−185, 1982.
152. Lewis BS, Bakst A, and Gotsman MS: Relationship between regional ventricular asynergy and the anatomic lesion in coronary artery disease. *Am. Heart J.* 88:211−218, 1974.
153. Bowyer A, and Asato H: Myocardial preservation correlated with coronary collateral vessel development in patients surviving proximal occlusion of the anterior descending artery. (abstr) *Chest* 74:331, 1978.
154. Kober G, Kuck H, Lentz RW, and Kaltenbach M: Angiographic evidence of collateral circulation and its effect on left ventricular function in coronary heart disease. In *Coronary Heart Disease: 3rd International Symposium Frankfurt* (eds M Kaltenbach, P Lichtlen, R Balcon, and W-D Bussmann). Georg Thieme, Stuttgart, 1978, pp 48−54.
155. Arie S, Solimene MC, Armelin E, et al: Circulação colateral como fator de proteção do miocárdio em portadores de insuficiência coronária crônica. *Arq. Bras. Cardiol.* 34:267−277, 1980.
156. Rousseau MF, Bertrand ME, Detry JMR, et al: Coronary collaterals and left ventricular function early after acute transmural myocardial infarction. *Eur. Heart J.* 3:223−229, 1982.
157. Aloan L, Truffa M, Anache M, et al: Circulação colateral e contratilidade ventricular em lesões da artéria descendente anterior. *Arq. Bras. Cardiol.* 31:167−171, 1978.
158. Sesto M, and Schwarz F: Regional myocardial function at rest and after rapid ventricular pacing in patients after myocardial revascularization by coronary bypass graft or by collateral vessels. *Am. J. Cardiol.* 43:920−928, 1979.
159. Betriu A, Castañer A, Sanz GA, et al: Angiographic findings 1 month after myocardial infarction: A prospective study of 259 survivors. *Circulation* 65:1099−1105, 1982.
160. Walker JK, Jones PRM, and Harding RH: Coronary collateral response and myocardial function. *Br. J. Radiol.* 54:731−735, 1981.
161. Crosby IK, Wellons HA Jr, and Burwell L: Total occlusion of the left coronary artery: Incidence and management. *J. Thorac. Cardiovasc. Surg.* 77:389−391, 1979.
162. Elayda MA, Mathur VS, Hall RJ, et al: Total occlusion of the left main coronary artery: Report of seven cases from 5312 cardiac catheterizations and review of the literature. *Texas Heart Inst. J.* 9:11−18, 1982.
163. Reul GJ, Morris GC Jr, Howell JF, et al: Coronary artery bypass in totally obstructed major coronary arteries. *Arch. Surg.* 102:373−379, 1971.
164. Kershbaum KL, Manchester JH, and Shelburne JC: Complete left coronary artery obstruction. *Chest* 64:539−540, 1973.
165. Sutherland RD, Allison W, Guynes WA, and Martinez HE: Complete obstruction of the left main coronary artery associated with congenital pulmonary valvular stenosis. *Chest* 69:238−239, 1976.
166. Trnka KE, Febres-Roman PR, Cadigan RA, et al: Total occlusion of the left main coronary artery: Clinical and catheterization findings. *Clin. Cardiol.* 3:352−355, 1980.
167. Esente P, Arquin PL, Giambartolomei A, and Gensini GG: Extreme protective action of coronary collateral vessels in complete occlusion of the left main coronary artery. *Am. J. Cardiol.* 50:1441−1442, 1982.
168. Levin DC, Sos TA, Lee JG, and Baltaxe HA: Coronary collateral circulation and distal coronary runoff: The key factors in preserving myocardial contractility in patients with coronary artery disease. *Am. J. Roentgenol.* 119:474−483, 1973.
169. Levin DC: Pathways and functional significance of the coronary collateral circulation. *Circulation* 50:831−837, 1974.

170. Banka VS, Bodenheimer MM, and Helfant RH: Determinants of reversible asynergy: Effect of pathologic Q waves, coronary collaterals, and anatomic location. *Circulation* 50:714–719, 1974.

171. Shah R, Bodenheimer M, Banka VS, and Helfant RH: The relationship between severity and extent of asynergy and the coronary collateral circulaton. (abstr) *Clin. Res.* 23:208A, 1975.

172. Kolibash AJ, Beaver BM, Fulkerson PK, et al: The relationship between abnormal echocardiographic septal motion and myocardial perfusion in patients with significant obstruction of the left anterior descending artery. *Circulation.* 56: 780–785, 1977.

173. Helfant RH, Bodenheimer MM, and Banka VS: Asynergy in coronary heart disease: Evolving clinical and pathophysiologic concepts. *Ann. Intern. Med.* 87:475–482, 1977.

174. Zeitler E: The collateral circulation. Correlation with the left ventricular function. *Ann. Radiol. (Paris)* 22:268–271, 1979.

175. Jang GC: The relation of inferior infarction to coronary distributional area and collateral vessels. (abstr) *Circulation* 60(Suppl II):II-160, 1979.

176. Peilen K, Goodyer AVN, and Langou RA: Role of coronary collaterals on left ventricular wall motion in patients with severe isolated single vessel coronary disease. (abstr) *Clin. Res.* 27:567A, 1979.

177. Nieminen MS, Valle M, Lassila E, et al: Global and regional left ventricular contractility and coronary collaterals in stable ischemic heart disease. *Clin. Cardiol.* 3:163–168, 1980.

178. Kupper W, and Bleifeld W: Coronary collateral circulation—"A functionless quirk?" (abstr) *Am. J. Cardiol.* 45:456, 1980.

179. Kolibash AJ, Bush CA, Wepsic RA, et al: Coronary collateral vessels: Spectrum of physiologic capabilities with respect to providing rest and stress myocardial perfusion, maintenance of left ventricular function and protection against infarction. *Am. J. Cardiol.* 50:230–238, 1982.

180. Helfant RH, Kemp HG, and Gorlin R: Coronary atherosclerosis, coronary collaterals, and their relation to cardiac function. *Ann. Intern. Med.* 73:189–193, 1970.

181. Miller RR, Zelis R, Mason DT, and Amsterdam EA: Relation of coronary collateral vessels to ventricular function in patients with equal extent of coronary artery disease. (abstr) *Circulation* 44(Suppl II):II-202, 1971.

182. Vismara LA, Miller RR, DeMaria AN, et al: Collateral circulation in chronic coronary disease: Effects on segmental left ventricular contractile function. (abstr) *Am. J. Cardiol.* 35:174, 1975.

183. Cohn PF, Maddox DE, Holman BL, and See JR: Effect of coronary collateral vessels on regional myocardial blood flow in patients with coronary artery disease: Relation of collateral circulation to vasodilatory reserve and left ventricular function. *Am. J. Cardiol.* 46:359–364, 1980.

184. Metzger J-P, LePailleur C, Delage B, and DiMatteo J: La circulation collatérale coronarienne: Étude anatomique et signification fonctionnelle. *Ann. Cardiol. Angéiol.* 25:491–496, 1976.

185. Markis JE, Joffee CD, Roberts BH, et al: Evolution of left ventricular dysfunction in coronary artery disease: Serial cineangiographic studies without surgery. *Circulation* 62:141–148, 1980.

186. Martinez-Rios MA, Humbolt G, Gil M, et al: Significado funcional de la circulacion colateral coronaria en obstrucciones univasculares (Parte la). *Arch. Inst. Cardiol. Méx.* 53:327–335, 1983.

187. da Luz PL, Cruz MdLA, Arie S, et al: Função ventricular regional e global em pacientes com infarto recente do miocárdio. *Arq. Bras. Cardiol.* 40:15–20, 1983.

188. Björk L: Angiographic demonstration of collaterals to the coronary arteries in patients with angina pectoris. *Acta Radiol. (Diagn.)* 8:305–309, 1969.

189. Bakst A, Lewis BS, and Gotsman MS: Isolated obstruction of the left anterior descending coronary artery. *S. Afr. Med. J.* 47:1534–1540, 1973.
190. Carroll RJ, Verani MS, and Falsetti HL: The effect of collateral circulation on segmental left ventricular contraction. *Circulation* 50:709–713, 1974.
191. Bourassa MG, Campeau L, and Lespérance J: Regression and appearance of coronary collaterals after aortocoronary bypass surgery. In *Coronary Heart Disease: 3rd International Symposium Frankfurt* (eds M Kaltenbach, P Lichtlen, R Balcon, and W-D Bussmann). Georg Thieme, Stuttgart, 1978, pp 40–47.
192. Rentrop P: Mortality and functional changes after intracoronary streptokinase infusion. (abstr) *Circulation* 66(Suppl II):II-335, 1982.
193. Schwarz F, Schuler G, Katus H, et al: Intracoronary thrombolysis in acute myocardial infarction: Correlations among serum enzyme, scintigraphic and hemodynamic findings. *Am. J. Cardiol.* 50:32–38, 1982.
194. Schuler G, Schwarz F, Hofmann M, et al: Thombolysis in acute myocardial infarction using intracoronary streptokinase: Assessment by thallium-201 scintigraphy. *Circulation* 66:658–664, 1982.
195. Rentrop P, Merx W, Mathey D, et al: Functional results of streptokinase-reperfusion in relation to collaterals and duration of symptoms. (abstr) *Circulation* 64(Suppl IV):IV-194, 1981.
196. Rentrop P, Blanke H, Karsch KR, et al: Changes in left ventricular function after intracoronary streptokinase infusion in clinically evolving myocardial infarction. *Am. Heart J.* 102:1188–1193, 1981.
197. Rogers WJ, Hood WP Jr, Mantle JA, et al: Return of left ventricular function after reperfusion in patients with myocardial infarction: Importance of subtotal stenoses or intact collaterals. *Circulation* 69:338–349, 1984.
198. Brindis RG, Brundage BH, Ullyot DJ, et al: Graft patency in patients with coronary artery bypass operation complicated by perioperative myocardial infarction. *J. Am. Coll. Cardiol.* 3:55–62, 1984.
199. Marcus ML, Doty DB, Hiratzka LF, et al: Decreased coronary reserve: A mechanism for angina pectoris in patients with aortic stenosis and normal coronary arteries. *N. Engl. J. Med.* 307:1362–1366, 1982.
200. Horwitz LD, Groves BM, Walsh RA, et al: Functional significance of coronary collateral vessels in patients with coronary artery disease. *Am. Heart J.* 104:221–225, 1982.
201. Braunwald E, Ross J Jr, and Sonnenblick EH: *Mechanisms of Contraction of the Normal and Failing Heart*, 2nd edition. Little, Brown and Company, Boston, 1976, pp 171–180.
202. Cannon PJ, Dell RB, and Dwyer EM Jr: Measurement of regional myocardial perfusion in man with ^{133}xenon and a scintillation camera. *J. Clin. Invest.* 51:964–977, 1972.
203. Gould KL, Hamilton GW, Lipscomb K, et al: Method for assessing stress-induced regional malperfusion during coronary arteriography: Experimental validation and clinical application. *Am. J. Cardiol.* 34:557–564, 1974.
204. Cannon PJ, Sciacca RR, Fowler DL, et al: Measurement of regional myocardial blood flow in man: Description and critique of the method using xenon-133 and a scintillation camera. *Am. J. Cardiol.* 36:783–792, 1975.
205. Cannon PJ, Schmidt DH, Weiss MB, et al: Studies of regional myocardial perfusion in patients with coronary atherosclerosis, using xenon-133 and a multiple crystal scintillation camera. In *The Metabolism of Contraction*, Vol. 10 of *Recent Advances in Studies on Cardiac Structure and Metabolism* (eds P-E Roy and G Rona). University Park Press, Baltimore, 1975, pp 501–523.
206. Schmidt DH, Weiss MB, Casarella WJ, Fowler DL, Sciacca RR, and Cannon PJ: Regional myocardial perfusion during atrial pacing in patients with coronary artery disease. *Circulation* 53:807–819, 1976.

207. Frick MH, Korhola O, Valle M, et al: Radiologically detected collaterals and regional myocardial flow responses to ischaemia in ischaemic heart disease. *Ann. Clin. Res.* 8:241–247, 1976.

208. Cannon PJ, Schmidt DH, Weiss MB, et al: Alterations of regional myocardial blood flow produced by atrial pacing. *Herz* 2:38–45, 1977.

209. Cannon PJ, Weiss MB, and Sciacca RR: Myocardial blood flow in coronary artery disease: Studies at rest and during stress with inert gas washout techniques. *Prog. Cardiovasc. Dis.* 20:95–120, 1977.

210. Kolibash AJ, Call TD, Tetalman MR, et al: Comparison of resting intracoronary particulate imaging and stress thallium-201 studies. *Radiology* 135:439–444, 1980.

211. Frick MH, Valle M, Korhola O, et al: Analysis of coronary collaterals in ischaemic heart disease by angiography during pacing induced ischaemia. *Br. Heart J.* 38:186–196, 1976.

212. Frick MH, Valle M, Korhola O, and Wiljasalo M: Selective coronary angiography during pacing-induced ischemia. In *Coronary Angiography and Angina Pectoris* (ed PR Lichtlen). Georg Thieme, Stuttgart, 1976, pp 51–54.

213. Holmberg S, Serzysko W, and Varnauskas E: Coronary circulation during heavy exercise in control subjects and patients with coronary heart disease. *Acta Med. Scand.* 190:465–480, 1971.

214. Bertrand ME, Carré A, Ginestet A, et al: Modifications du débit coronaire, des indices de contractilité, du métabolisme énergétique du coeur au cours de l'effort chez les sujets normaux. In *Les Épreuves d'Effort en Cardiologie.* Sandoz, Paris, 1975, pp 17–34.

215. Heiss HW, Barmeyer J, Wink K, et al: Studies on the regulation of myocardial blood flow in man. I.: Training effects on blood flow and metabolism of the healthy heart at rest and during standardized heavy exercise. *Basic Res. Cardiol.* 71: 658–675, 1976.

216. Demany MA, Tambe A, and Zimmerman HA: Correlation between coronary arteriography and the postexercise electrocardiogram. *Am. J. Cardiol.* 19:526–530, 1967.

217. McConahay DR, McCallister BD, and Smith RE: Postexercise electrocardiography: Correlations with coronary arteriography and left ventricular hemodynamics. *Am. J. Cardiol.* 28:1–9, 1971.

218. Martin CM, and McConahay DR: Maximal treadmill exercise electrocardiography: Correlations with coronary arteriography and cardiac hemodynamics. *Circulation* 46:956–962, 1972.

219. Harris CN, Kaplan MA, Parker DP, et al: Anatomic and functional correlates of intercoronary collateral vessels. *Am. J. Cardiol.* 30:611–614, 1972.

220. Kaplan MA, Harris CN, Aronow WS, et al: Inability of the submaximal treadmill stress test to predict the location of coronary disease. *Circulation* 47:250–256, 1973.

221. Helfant RH, Banka VS, DeVilla MA, et al: Use of bicycle ergometry and sustained handgrip exercise in the diagnosis of presence and extent of coronary heart disease. *Br. Heart J.* 35:1321–1325, 1973.

222. Froelicher VF, Thompson AJ, Longo MR Jr, et al: Value of exercise testing for screening asymptomatic men for latent coronary artery disease. *Prog. Cardiovasc. Dis.* 18:265–276, 1976.

223. Tonkon MJ, Miller RR, DeMaria AN, et al: Multifactor evaluation of the determinants of ischemic electrocardiographic response to maximal treadmill testing in coronary disease. *Am. J. Med.* 62:339–346, 1977.

224. Berman JL, Levin DA, and Cohn PF: Effect of coronary collaterals on exercise performance. (abstr) *Am. J. Cardiol.* 45:392, 1980.

225. Tubau JF, Chaitman BR, Bourassa MG, et al: Importance of coronary collateral

circulation in interpreting exercise test results. *Am. J. Cardiol.* 47:27–32, 1981.

226. Goldberg HL, Goldstein J, Borer JS, et al: Functional importance of coronary collateral vessels. *Am. J. Cardiol.* 53:694–699, 1984.

227. Lenaers A, Block P, Van Thiel E, et al: Segmental analysis of Tl-201 stress myocardial scintigraphy. *J. Nucl. Med.* 18:509–516, 1977.

228. Bailey I, Burrow R, Griffith LSC, and Pitt B: Localizing value of thallium 201 myocardial perfusion imaging in coronary artery disease. (abstr) *Am. J. Cardiol.* 39:320, 1977.

229. Verani MS, Jhingran S, Attar M, et al: Poststress redistribution of thallium-201 in patients with coronary artery disease, with and without prior myocardial infarction. *Am. J. Cardiol.* 43:1114–1122, 1979.

230. Rigo P, Becker LC, Griffith LSC, et al: Influence of coronary collateral vessels on the results of thallium-201 myocardial stress imaging. *Am. J. Cardiol.* 44:452–458, 1979.

231. Wainwright RJ, Maisey MN, Edwards AC, and Sowton E: Functional significance of coronary collateral circulation during dynamic exercise evaluated by thallium-201 myocardial scintigraphy. *Br. Heart J.* 43:47–55, 1980.

232. Cooper R, Puri S, Francis CK, and Spencer RP: Role of coronary artery disease and collateral circulation in redistribution of thallium-201. *Clin. Nucl. Med.* 5:292–298, 1980.

233. Iskandrian AS, Lichtenberg R, Segal BL, et al: Assessment of jeopardized myocardium in patients with one-vessel disease. *Circulation* 65:242–247, 1982.

234. Eng C, Patterson RE, Horowitz SF, et al: Coronary collateral function during exercise. *Circulation* 66:309–316, 1982.

235. Buda AJ, Dubbin JD, MacDonald IL, et al: Spontaneous changes in thallium-201 myocardial perfusion imaging after myocardial infarction. *Am. J. Cardiol.* 50:1272–1278, 1982.

236. Iskandrian AS, Segal BL, Haaz W, and Kane S: Effects of coronary artery narrowing, collaterals, and left ventricular function on the pattern of myocardial perfusion. *Cathet. Cardiovasc. Diagn.* 6:159–172, 1980.

237. Kondo M, Miyazaki S, Takahashi M, and Shimono Y: Assessment of viable myocardium within infarct zone by exercise thallium-201 scintigraphy. *Jpn. Circ. J.* 48:219–224, 1984.

238. Khaw BA, Strauss HW, Pohost GM, et al: Relation of immediate and delayed thallium-201 distribution to localization of iodine-125 antimyosin antibody in acute experimental myocardial infarction. *Am. J. Cardiol.* 51:1428–1432, 1983.

239. Verani MS, Marcus ML, Razzak MA, and Ehrhardt JC: Sensitivity and specificity of thallium-201 perfusion scintigrams under exercise in the diagnosis of coronary artery disease. *J. Nucl. Med.* 19:773–782, 1978.

240. Banka VS, Bodenheimer MM, Fouche CM, et al: Relationship between coronary collaterals and zonal ischemia in man. (abstr) *Circulation* 58 (Suppl II):II-134, 1978.

241. Agarwal JB, and Helfant RH: Functional importance of coronary collateral circulation. *Int. J. Cardiol.* 4:94–99, 1983.

242. Thorel C: Pathologie der Kreislauforgane. *Ergebn. Allg. Path.* 9:559–1116, 1903.

243. Bellet S, Gouley BA, and McMillan TM: Nourishment of the myocardium through Thebesian vessels: In a heart in which the large coronary arteries and veins were destroyed by tuberculous myocarditis. *Arch. Intern. Med.* 51:112–121, 1933.

244. Lim JS, Proudfit WL, and Sones FM Jr: Left main coronary arterial obstruction: Long-term follow-up of 141 nonsurgical cases. *Am. J. Cardiol.* 36:131–135, 1975.

245. Crooke GF: Ueber zwei seltene und aus verschiedenen Ursachen entstandene Fälle von rapider Herzlähmung. *Virchows Arch. (Path. Anat.)* 129:186–202, 1892.

246. Von Redwitz EF: Der Einfluss der Erkrankungen der Koronararterien auf die Herzmuskulatur mit besonderer Berücksichtigung der chronischen Aortitis. *Virchows Arch. (Path. Anat.)* 197:433–472, 1909.

247. Wesselhoeft H, Fawcett JS, and Johnson AL: Anomalous origin of the left coronary artery from the pulmonary trunk: Its clinical spectrum, pathology, and pathophysiology, based on a review of 140 cases with seven further cases. *Circulation* 38:403−425, 1968.

248. Perry LW, and Scott LP: Anomalous left coronary artery from pulmonary artery. Report of 11 cases; Review of indications for and results of surgery. *Circulation* 41:1043−1052, 1970.

249. Askenazi J, and Nadas AS: Anomalous left coronary artery originating from the pulmonary artery: Report on 15 cases. *Circulation* 51:976−987, 1975.

250. Grace RR, Angelini P, and Cooley DA: Aortic implantation of anomalous left coronary artery arising from pulmonary artery. *Am. J. Cardiol.* 39:608−613, 1977.

251. Crawford T, Dexter D, and Teare RD: Coronary-artery pathology in sudden death from myocardial ischaemia: A comparison by age-groups. *Lancet* 1:181−185, 1961.

252. Weaver WD, Lorch GS, Alvarez HA, and Cobb LA: Angiographic findings and prognostic indicators in patients resuscitated from sudden cardiac death. *Circulation* 54:895−900, 1976.

253. Webster JS, Moberg C, and Rincon G: Natural history of severe proximal coronary artery disease as documented by coronary cineangiography. *Am. J. Cardiol.* 33:195−200, 1974.

254. Platia EV, Grunwald L, Mellits ED, et al: Clinical and arteriographic variables predictive of survival in coronary artery disease. *Am. J. Cardiol.* 46:543−552, 1980.

CHAPTER THREE

Stimulation and Responses of the Coronary Collateral Circulation in Man

Coronary collateral vessels do exist in man and do play a functionally important role in ischemic myocardium. One might assume, therefore, that increased development of the coronary collateral circulation as well as increased utilization of already existing channels should benefit the heart. Indeed, much effort has been expended to determine those external stimuli that can either stimulate the formation of new collateral vessels or improve blood flow in functioning anastomotic connections. Salvage of ischemic myocardium following critical narrowing of a coronary artery will ultimately depend on the coronary collateral circulation. Hence, the ability to manipulate this accessory blood supply is an important goal.

I. Coronary Arterial Narrowing

A. Pathologic Studies

Although debate about the existence of coronary collaterals in normal hearts raged for many years, virtually all pathologists appreciated the abundance of coronary collaterals in hearts with obstructive disease of the coronary arteries and the obvious increase in luminal dimensions when compared to collateral vessels in normal hearts.[1-25] Whereas Fulton[10] noted that collaterals with diameters of 20−200 μm were abundant in normal hearts and larger vessels with diameters of 200−300 μm were occasionally seen, collaterals in hearts with coronary obstructive disease were commonly five- to tenfold wider,[12,16] and occasionally diameters were increased by a factor of 20.[12] Thus, 300−800 μm vessels were frequently observed in these pathologic hearts, and collateral diameters exceeded 1 mm in some cases.[10] Tsuchiya[21] and Baroldi[6,19] have also observed significantly larger collaterals in arteriosclerotic hearts, with some vessel diameters approaching 2 mm. Rodriguez and Robbins[15] reported maximal collateral diameters of 5 mm in their hearts with coronary artery disease.

In addition to the obvious increase in luminal diameter of collateral vessels in hearts with coronary arterial obstructive disease, increased length and tortuosity are also apparent.[7,25] Hutchins[25] hypothesized that flow along a collateral occurring after development of a critical stenosis in the recipient artery increases shear stress on the endothelium, resulting in compensatory relaxation of medial smooth muscle and dilatation of the vessel until the endothelial drag is returned to control values. Subsequent proliferation of the vessel wall results in radial as well as longitudinal growth. However, because of fixation of the two ends of the collateral channel, the vessel buckles. Thus, the observed tortuosity of the coronary collateral is really a reflection of its increased length.

Thus, it is apparent that the coronary collateral is both wider and longer in hearts with coronary obstructive disease. Some investigators have established a relationship between the severity of coronary arterial narrowing (and therefore possibly the degree of resulting myocardial ischemia) and the size of the collateral vessels.[11,17,18,20,21,24] Baroldi[17,18] calculated his anastomotic index derived from numbers of collaterals and average diameters (see Chapter 1) for both normal and pathologic hearts. In the latter the anastomotic index was little changed from that derived for normal hearts if the arterial lumen was narrowed by less than 60%. But the index was doubled for stenoses of 60 to 80%, and was increased manyfold to its maximal value in hearts with old complete occlusions of the coronary artery. Tsuchiya[21] noted that only 16% of hearts with stenoses compromising the coronary artery's lumen by less than 25% had collaterals with diameters exceeding 400 μm. The incidence was minimally higher (22%) in hearts with 25−50% stenoses. However, 71% of hearts with coronary arterial narrowing of at least 50% had these large collaterals. Hence, coronary collateral development appeared to be proportional to the severity of the arterial obstructive disease. Furthermore, there seemed to be a critical arterial narrowing (50−60% in these postmortem studies) beyond which collateral development was stimulated.

Baroldi's data[17,22,24] also support an association between the extent of coronary obstructive disease and collateral development. Compared to hearts with only one arterial obstruction, the anastomotic indices of hearts with three occlusions were twice as great. The index in hearts with three occlusions was approximately sevenfold higher than in normal hearts. Thus, extent as well as severity of coronary lesions appears to affect coronary collateral development.

Barmeyer[26,27] attempted to derive more physiologic data about collateral flow in postmortem hearts. He perfused the coronary vessels with a mixture of paraffin oil and diesel oil that had the same viscosity as blood. He first perfused a pair of coronary vessels simultaneously and then perfused each separately. The difference between the sum of flows through the individual vessels and the combined flow was felt to reflect the maximal collateral flow between the two vessels. Relative anastomotic flow was then derived by dividing this collateral flow by the combined two-vessel antegrade flow. In normal hearts this relative anastomotic flow was 25%, and it was 52%

in hearts with severe coronary obstructive disease (usually triple-vessel disease).[27] The anastomotic index was generally in the normal range for mild degrees of coronary atherosclerosis.[26,27] These data, therefore, also suggest stimulation of collateral development by coronary obstructive disease.

Attempts have been made to identify other factors that might have some influence on coronary collateral growth. Zoll et al.[3] concluded that collaterals were better developed following myocardial infarction. Whereas 58% of hearts with marked coronary artery narrowing but without occlusion and 68% of hearts with recent occlusions had collaterals, 96% of hearts with old occlusions demonstrated enlarged collateral vessels. Kato[23] also noted that large collaterals were more frequent in infarcted hearts. Both Jones[14] and Hutchins and colleagues[25] observed that collaterals became progressively larger as the interval between infarction and death increased. In contrast, however, neither Baroldi[17,24] nor Anitschkow et al.[11] could confirm any relationship between myocardial infarction or the mode of death, e.g., sudden death, and collateral development.

Fulton[13,16] believed that the duration of ischemic symptoms prior to the patient's demise affected collateral development. He noted that collateral dimensions were essentially those of a normal heart if patients died with less than three months of anginal complaints. However, if angina pectoris had been present for as long as 7 to 14 years, then many large-scale anastomoses were evident.

The enlarged collaterals found in hearts with coronary obstructive disease were not equally distributed between the three major coronary arteries. Both Tsuchiya[21] and Robbins et al.[28] noted that intercoronary collaterals were most frequent between the left anterior descending and right coronary arteries, while Kato[23] observed the anastomotic channels to be most prevalent between the left anterior descending and left circumflex arteries. The most common source of intracoronary collaterals was also the left anterior descending artery,[21,23] while the left circumflex artery was the second most commonly observed site of homocoronary anastomoses. Thus, of the three major coronary arteries, the left anterior descending coronary artery appears to be the most frequent collateral source as well as recipient.

B. Angiographic Studies

Despite the shortcomings of necropsy examinations, the above studies have clearly demonstrated that collateral vessels are better developed in hearts with coronary obstructive disease. Since the introduction of coronary angiography approximately 25 years ago, numerous observations, both primary and casual, have confirmed the stimulatory effect of coronary obstructions on collateral development. As described in Chapter 1, angiography has its own limitations. Nonetheless, the data seem clear and the conclusions obvious.

All investigators agree that there is a critical degree of coronary narrowing which is a prerequisite for the angiographic visualization of coronary collaterals. Some angiographers have claimed that the coronary lesion must compromise the luminal diameter by at least 50 to 60% before coronary collaterals may be expected,[21,29−33] while others have been able to visualize anastomotic vessels only after the coronary arterial narrowing has reached 70 to 75%.[34−42] However, the bulk of clinical studies insist that the stenosis must be subtotal (90−95%) before collateral vessels can be reliably demonstrated by angiographic techniques.[43−56] As explained previously (see Chapter 1), uncertainty regarding qualitative estimates of stenosis severity may account for some of the discrepancy between these studies. Stenoses less severe than this critical narrowing are rarely accompanied by collateral vessels, while more severe obstructions are uncommonly without collaterals (Figure 3−1).

Hecht and colleagues[37] also noted that the angiographic appearance of coronary collaterals was not solely dependent on stenosis severity. Distal runoff in the stenotic vessel was an equally important factor. Thus, collaterals were evident if a vessel was totally occluded or if its lumen was narrowed by at least 75% and circulation beyond the lesion was impaired. Vessels narrowed by less than 75% and arteries with more severe lesions but good filling distal to the stenosis were not collateralized. Therefore, coronary arteries with

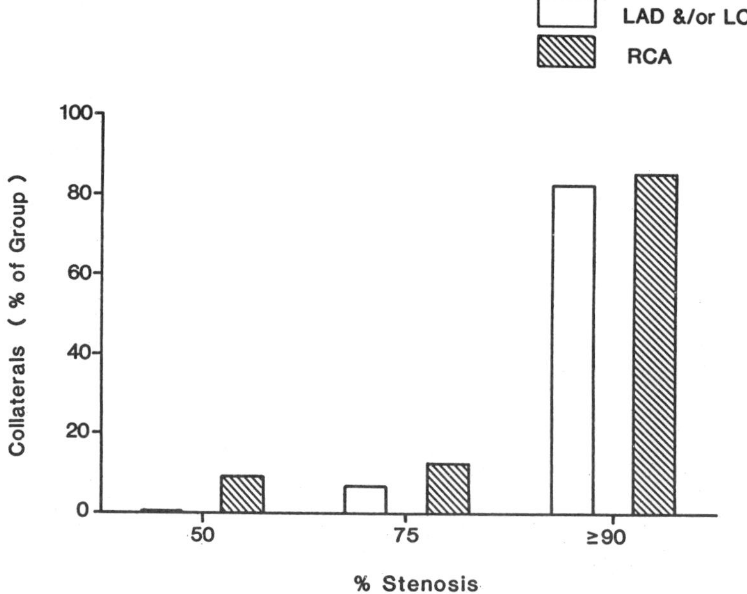

Figure 3−1   Effect of severity of coronary artery narrowing on angiographic visualization of coronary collaterals. There is a critical reduction in luminal dimensions below which collaterals are rarely visualized, and above which obstructions are uncommonly without collaterals. These data support the notion that coronary collaterals are a marker of severe coronary obstructive disease. (Drawn from data presented by Heinle et al.[31])

less severe stenoses might have collaterals whereas vessels with more marked narrowings might not. Adequacy of myocardial perfusion and not merely stenosis appeared to be the critical factor.

Angiographic visualization of a coronary collateral is dependent on establishment of a pressure gradient along its course. Intravascular pressure beyond a coronary lesion does not begin to decrease until the lumen is compromised by more than approximately 80%. Hence, it is expected that a critical narrowing of approximately 80% must be surpassed before coronary collaterals could be demonstrated by coronary angiography. Therefore, appearance of collaterals could be solely the consequence of favorable hemodynamic conditions rather than the result of stimulated development related to the myocardial effects of a critical coronary stenosis. However, angiographically visible collateral vessels in patients with coronary artery disease are typically larger than the anastomotic channels found in normal hearts. In some cases collateral diameters exceed 1 mm,[48] the size of small arterial branches. The causes of this striking vascular growth are as yet unclear, although a biochemical factor produced by myocardium has recently been isolated[57] (see below).

The presumed link between coronary artery disease and collateral development is strengthened by data documenting the relationship between angiographically evident collaterals and both the severity and extent of the coronary lesions. Numerous angiographers have described increasing collateralization as the coronary stenosis becomes more severe.[29,31−35,38,40,41,47,49,50,52,54,58] Schwarz et al.[38] evaluated the coronary arteriograms of 132 consecutive patients with obstructive coronary disease. In this group there were 19 vessels with stenoses compromising the luminal diameter by 75 to 84%, and only 5% were collateralized. Increasing stenosis severity increased the likelihood of collateralization. Collaterals to 19% of the 37 arteries with 85−94% stenoses were visualized. When the obstruction was either complete or subtotal (≥ 95%), as many as 82% of the 125 affected vessels received collaterals. Berger's data[41] are quite similar. Seventy-eight stenotic vessels among a selected study group of 97 patients having had both ^{201}Tl scintigraphy and coronary angiography were collateralized. Of these, 57 (73%) were totally obstructed, 18 (23%) had lesions obstructing the vessel's lumen by at least 90%, and 3 (4%) had 70−89% stenoses. No collateralized vessels had stenoses compromising the lumen by less than 70%. In contrast, the obstructive disease was significantly less severe ($p < 0.001$) in the 138 stenotic, noncollateralized vessels. Only eight (6%) were totally obstructed, and 51 (37%) had subtotal (≥ 90%) stenoses. Forty-five (32%) of the vessels without collaterals had stenoses in the 70−89% range, while the remaining 34 (25%) had only mild 50−69% reductions in luminal dimensions. Thus, patients with collaterals have more severe coronary obstructive disease. As already indicated (Chapter 2), this relationship has caused some investigators[41,59−63] to conclude that coronary collaterals are merely markers of the severity of the underlying coronary artery disease without any independent functional role.

As might be expected, totally obstructed vessels are frequently the recipients of coronary collaterals[32,33,37,40,41,47,50−52,54,55,64−67] (Figure 3−2). Virtually all studies have documented the presence of coronary collaterals in at least 70% of these patients,[32,33,37,40,41,47,50−52,54,55,64−67] while the majority of reports have noted large collateral channels supplying the distal segment of the occluded vessel in more than 90% of the study population with complete arterial occlusions.[32,33,37,40,47,50,52,55,65−67] In fact, Valle,[32] Rafflenbeul,[40] Bourassa,[47] and Flameng[65−67] have observed that all totally obstructed vessels are collateralized. It seems odd that a vessel with absent antegrade flow would not have some evidence of collateral flow because of the favorable pressure gradient between adjacent source arteries and the distal segment of the occluded vessel. Perhaps the inadequacies of angiographic visualization of coronary collaterals partially explain this paradox (see Chapter 1). It should be noted, however, that when visualized, the large collaterals in these patients or the functional evidence of complete opacification of the artery beyond the occlusion when the collaterals are not individually identified attest to the striking collateral stimulation and vascular growth that have already occurred.

Patients with coronary collaterals also appear to have more extensive

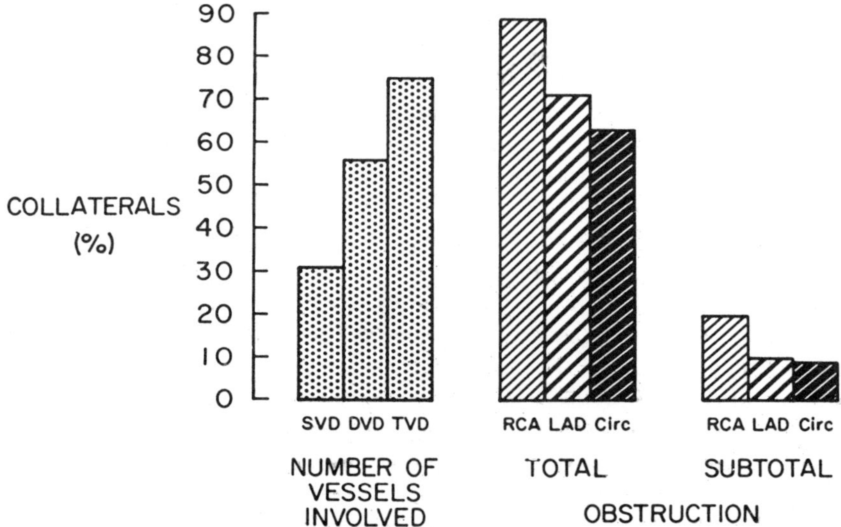

Figure 3−2   Effects of severity and extent of coronary artery obstructive disease on the presence of angiographically visible coronary collaterals. Patients with total occlusions of any of the three major coronary arteries are much more likely to have collaterals than those with subtotal lesions. Furthermore, collateralization is more evident as the number of major diseased vessels increases. SVD = single-vessel disease; DVD = double-vessel disease; TVD = triple-vessel disease; RCA = right coronary artery; LAD = left anterior descending coronary artery; Circ = left circumflex coronary artery. (Reprinted with permission of Futura Publishing Co. from Hamby.[54])

disease of the major coronary arteries.[29,34,39,54,58,68,69] In Hamby's experience[54] with 1,000 patients having coronary angiography, 31.0% of those with significant one-vessel disease had collaterals (Figure 3−2). The incidence of collaterals increased to 55.6% in patients with two-vessel disease, and again to 74.7% in three-vessel disease. Helfant[68] also demonstrated a progressive increase in the incidence of coronary collateralization as lesions involved more of the major coronary arteries (Figure 3−3). Miller[29] noted a similar trend. Fifty-three percent of patients with significant one-vessel disease had collaterals. Although the incidence was not different (47%) in two-vessel disease, it jumped to 84% in patients with three diseased vessels.

Hamby[58] used a scoring system based on both the severity and extent of coronary obstructive disease to quantitate the degree of coronary obstruction in any individual patient and permit comparison between patients. Each of the three major coronary arteries was assigned a grade from 0 to 6, and the total coronary score was the sum of the three grades. A normal vessel was given a grade of 0. A narrowing of 30 to 50% of the lumen's diameter was assigned a grade of 2, and a subtotal narrowing of more than 90% was equivalent to grade 4. Grade 5 was reserved for total occlusion with distal filling by collateral flow, and grade 6 for total occlusion with little or no distal filling. Thus, a subject with collaterals would have a lower score than a second with comparable disease but no collaterals. In Hamby's study, subjects with collaterals had a score of at least 10. In contrast, only 24.9% of those without anastomotic connections had comparable coronary scores. As the total coronary score rose, more patients had angiographically visible collaterals and fewer were collateral-free (Figure 3−4). Of interest is the observation that the

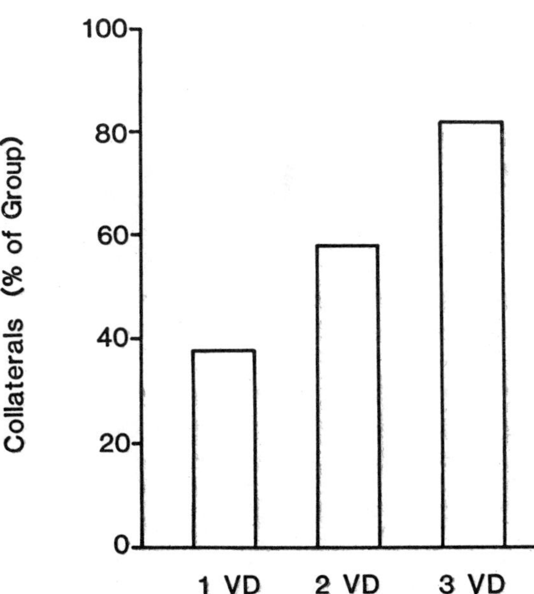

Figure 3−3   Coronary collaterals were visualized in increasing numbers of patients as more of the major coronary arteries became obstructed. 1, 2, 3, VD = one-, two-, three-vessel disease. (Drawn from data presented by Helfant et al.[68])

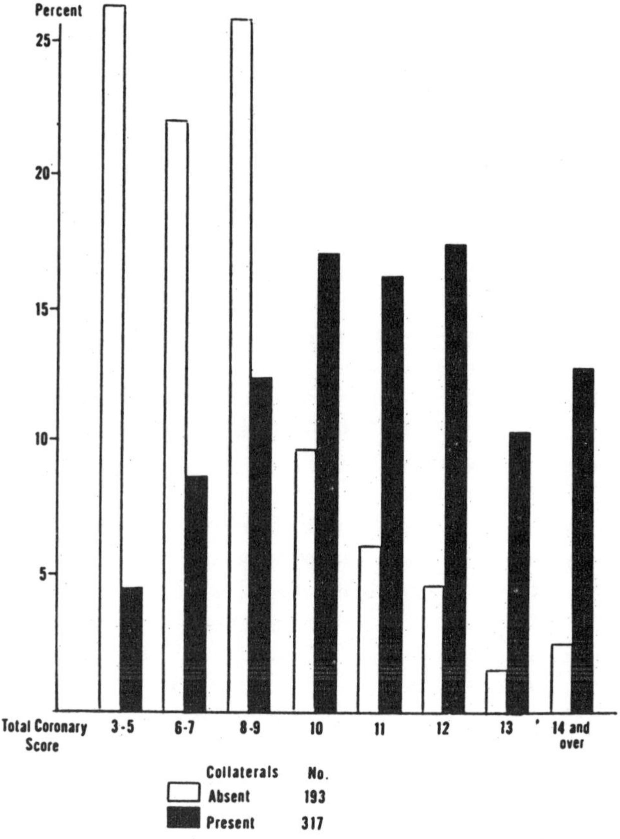

Figure 3—4   Frequency distribution of patients with and without coronary collateral vessels arranged according to the total coronary score (based on both the severity and extent of coronary obstructive disease). The occurrence of collaterals appears to be directly related to the total coronary score. Furthermore, as the coronary score increases, fewer individuals are collateral-free. (Reprinted with permission of F.A. Davis Co., from Hamby.[58])

number of patients with collaterals plateaued after the total coronary score reached 10. Thus, the presence of collaterals was directly related to both the extent and the severity of coronary artery disease.

Although coronary angiography may initially be performed for diagnostic purposes, some patients will have a second study months to years later to check for progression of symptoms or in compliance with some predetermined protocol. Regardless of the precise indication for the second angiogram, these serial studies[40,50,52,70−73] have resulted in unique insights into the rate of progression of coronary lesions in individual patients and its effect on collateral development. All of these investigations have noted significant progression (increase in stenosis severity of at least 20% or occurrence of complete occlusion) in a large proportion of the study population, and in these same patients either collaterals have become more evident or new collaterals have appeared. In one of the first reports, Bemis and colleagues[70] observed progression of obstructing lesions in 38 of 73 (52%) patients. No increase in collateralization or appearance of new anastomoses was ever observed unless progression had been documented. Thus, patients with stable coronary artery lesions had no change in collateral patterns. Kimbiris[71] evaluated 24 patients with progressive disease, of whom 62.5% had evidence of improved or new collateralization. Of 11 patients with stable disease for the same time interval, only one (9.1%) had new collaterals. Rafflenbeul[40] observed that 14 stenoses in 11 patients progressed between the first and second angiographic studies, and new or increased collaterals were seen in nine (64%). By contrast, only 5 of 39 (13%) vessels without change in the degree of stenosis had increased collateralization. Changes in collateralization have also been observed after occlusion of saphenous vein bypass grafts.[53,74] Graft occlusion shortly after attachment has almost always been associated with concomitant thrombosis of the native artery at the site of graft implantation. Bourassa[53,74] has noted that virtually all such patients have new collaterals to the distal artery. Hence, progression of coronary disease is associated with new or increased collateralization. The conclusion that collateral stimulation is definitely linked to progressive arterial narrowing is especially evident in individual patients with documented progression of disease where effects of other biological factors can largely be discounted.

Although coronary arterial obstruction may be a stimulus to collateral development, the stimulus may not be comparable for lesions of all major vessels. Rafflenbeul and colleagues[75] evaluated patients with the recent onset of angina pectoris. Thirteen patients with isolated stenoses of the right coronary artery had average decreases in luminal area of 63% (approximately equivalent to 39% reduction in diameter), while the 17 individuals with isolated lesions of the left anterior descending artery had mean area reductions of 78% (approximately equivalent to 53% reduction in diameter) ($p < 0.05$). Hence, less of a narrowing of the right coronary artery caused myocardial ischemia and symptoms. When patients with identical stenoses (78% area reduction) of the left anterior descending and right coronary arteries were compared, collaterals were visualized angiographically in 53% with right coronary artery disease and 29% with left anterior descending stenoses. This difference was not significant, but does suggest that comparable anatomic lesions of major coronary arteries may not have similar functional effects.

Gensini and da Costa,[44] Harris et al.,[35] Baldighi and associates,[30] Levine,[48] and Hamby[54] have all noted that the right coronary artery is the most common donor of collaterals, although Hecht and colleagues[37] felt that all coronary arteries participated equally in anastomotic pathways. The right coronary artery may also be the most frequent recipient of collaterals, while the left circumflex artery is the least frequent.[35,54] In Levin's report,[48] 70.5% of patients with subtotal (≥ 90%) stenoses of the right coronary artery received collaterals, whereas only 55.1% of critically stenosed left anterior and 43.8% of left circumflex arteries were collateralized. Collaterals to completely occluded right coronary, left anterior descending, and left circumflex arteries were visualized in 89, 71, and 62% of cases, respectively[54] (Figure 3−2). The left anterior descending artery is the least frequent collateral source.[35] It is odd that postmortem injection studies have identified the left anterior descending artery to be the most frequent donor as well as recipient of collaterals.[21,23,28]

Angiographically visible collaterals are more often intercoronary than intracoronary vessels.[30,36,44,48] The intercoronary variety may be two to three times more frequent.[30,36] For each of the three major coronary arteries some collateral pathways appear more frequently than others. Paulin,[76] Gensini and da Costa,[44] Jochem et al.,[34] and Levin[48] have catalogued the various collateral pathways. In obstructive disease of the right coronary artery, the most frequent collateral pathways are septal perforators linking the posterior descending and left anterior descending arteries, anastomoses between distal left circumflex and right coronary arteries, and links between the obtuse marginal branch of the circumflex artery and the posterior left ventricular branch of the right coronary artery. Other less common connections are intracoronary collaterals between conus branch or proximal acute marginal and more distal acute marginal branch, Kugel's artery, and anastomoses between the distal left anterior descending artery wrapping around the apex and the distal right coronary artery. The left anterior descending artery is most often collateralized by vessels arising from the acute marginal branch of the right coronary artery. The intracoronary pathway from a proximal to more distal septal perforator is also frequently observed. Two other slightly less common collateral pathways involve the obtuse marginal branch of the circumflex artery and the right coronary artery's conus branch. As previously noted, collaterals to the left circumflex artery are less frequent. When this vessel is collateralized, the left atrial circumflex, proximal obtuse marginal, and diagonal branch of the left anterior descending artery are the most common sources. (See Figures 1−18 to 1−20 for diagrams of pathways.)

Attempts to define other features in patients with ischemic heart disease that might influence or affect collateral development have been made. Increasing duration[29,39,51] and severity[29] of angina pectoris and prior myocardial infarction[39] have all been associated with increased collateral development. Ohgitani[50] noted that coronary collaterals were better developed in patients who had coronary angiography more than three months following myocardial infarction. When angiography was done in the initial three months after the infarction, only 15 of 26 (58%) individuals had visualized collaterals, and in only seven of these patients were the collaterals adequate to opacify the distal segment of the obstructed vessel. In contrast, angiography done beyond the first three months revealed collaterals in 18 of 23 (78%) of the subjects, and in 14 (78%) the collaterals were capable of adequately opacifying the distal portion of the diseased artery. Furthermore, within the initial three months collaterals were uncommonly visualized with any lesion other than a complete occlusion. Beyond three months, however, subtotal occlusions were also often well collateralized. These temporal factors further support the notion that coronary obstruction promotes collateral development. The longer a coronary lesion or ischemic stimulus is present, the more likely is collateral development and/or formation.

Heinle et al.[31] observed that lipoprotein abnormalities, glucose intolerance, hypertension, and obesity did not seem to affect the presence of coronary collaterals. On the other hand, Vigorita and his associates[77] documented richer collateralization in patients with adult-onset diabetes mellitus. However, the latter individuals also had more severe coronary obstructive disease than subjects who did not have diabetes mellitus.

C. Intraoperative and Cardiac Catheterization Studies

Neither pathologic nor in-vivo angiographic study can quantify collateral flow or capacity (see Chapter 1). Indices of collateral flow, retrograde flow and peripheral coronary pressure (see Chapters 1 and 4), measured at the time of open heart surgery in humans have been used to judge the amount of collateral flow and to make interpatient comparisons. Webb and his associates[45,46,49] and Goldstein et al.[78] have demonstrated a good correlation between the angiographic appearance of collaterals and the collateral indices. Thus, in patients without angiographically evident coronary collaterals, retrograde flow was less then 6 ml/min regardless of the severity of the stenosis.[46] The largest retrograde flows (up to 18 ml/min) were seen in those individuals with the best angiographic collaterals. Similarly, in Goldstein's patients[78] without collaterals, mean retrograde flow was 0.83 ml/min and the ratio of peripheral coronary pressure to aortic pressure averaged 0.24 (Figure 3—5). In patients with the best angiographic collaterals, both retrograde flow and the ratio of peripheral coronary to aortic pressure were significantly elevated ($p < 0.05$) to 15.7 ml/min and 0.5, respectively. Furthermore, calculated collateral resistance was 5.1 mmHg/ml/min in the latter group, significantly lower ($p < 0.05$) than the average value of 94 mmHg/ml/min in the group of subjects without visible collaterals (Figure 3—6). Intermediate angiographic collateral grades were associated with intermediate collateral index values.

Of course, the above evaluations have been performed during surgery with anesthetized subjects and other potentially unphysiologic conditions. Feldman and Pepine[79] reported coronary hemodynamic data obtained at the time of coronary angioplasty in conscious subjects. During the course of this procedure a balloon dilatation catheter is introduced into the stenotic coronary artery and advanced across the lesion. The balloon is then inflated, preventing further antegrade flow, and peripheral coronary pressure can be measured. In 19 patients with balloon catheters in the left anterior descend-

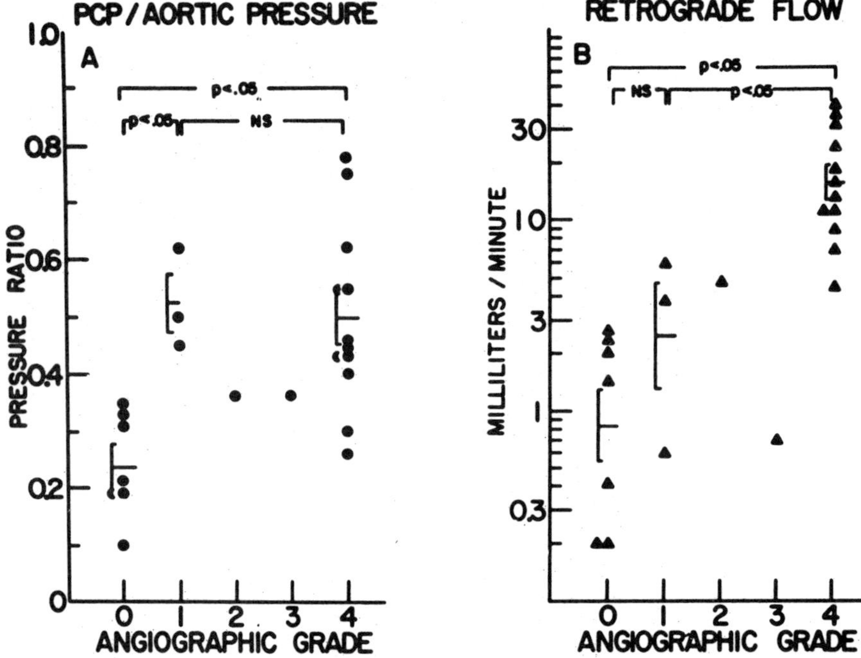

Figure 3-5   Relationship between angiographic grade of coronary collaterals and collateral indices, peripheral coronary pressure normalized for aortic pressure and retrograde flow. As the collaterals become more abundant and better visualized, both normalized peripheral coronary pressure and retrograde flow increase significantly. These data support the utilization of angiographic grading of coronary collaterals to estimate their functional adequacy. (Modified and printed with permission of the American Heart Association from Goldstein et al.[78])

ing coronary artery, a multithermistor catheter was introduced into the great cardiac vein to monitor venous flow from the perfusion territory of that same artery. Of the 19 patients, 6 had angiographic evidence of left anterior descending collateralization, while the remaining 13 did not. During acute coronary artery occlusion, peripheral coronary pressure was not different in the two groups (28 ± 11 and 29 ± 6 mmHg, respectively). Certainly, normalization of this distal pressure by aortic pressure would have yielded a better collateral index and might have revealed a distinction between the groups. However, residual great cardiac vein flow during balloon occlusion of the coronary artery was 62 ± 24 ml/min in those with collaterals, and only 40 ± 14 ml/min in the subjects without visualized anastomoses ($p < 0.05$). Therefore, collateral flow was most likely considerably greater in the former individuals. Accordingly, a calculated coronary collateral resistance index in those with collaterals was nearly half that in the patients without visualized collaterals (1.07 ± 0.25 versus 1.93 ± 0.55 mmHg/[ml/min], $p < 0.01$). Thus, again, the association between angiographic visualization of collaterals and collateral function is evident. This correlation provides credibility for many of

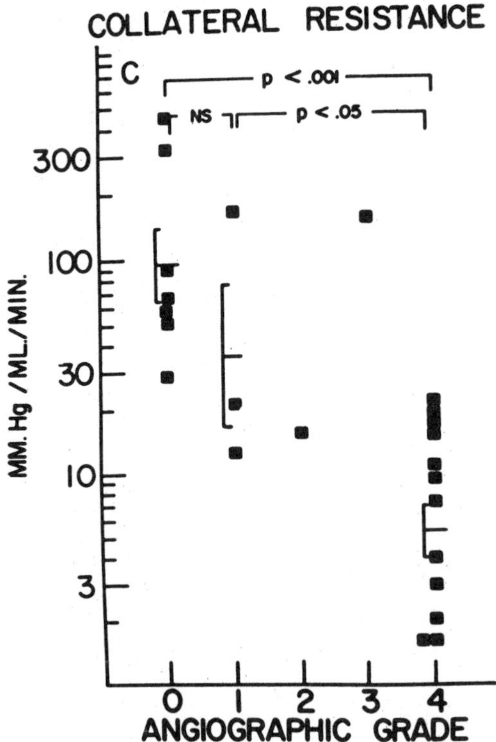

Figure 3—6 Calculated coronary collateral resistance falls precipitously as the angiographic collateral grade increases. Thus, the angiographic evaluation of collateral adequacy is an excellent index of collateral development. (Modified and printed with permission of the American Heart Association from Goldstein et al.[78])

the conclusions cited above based solely on angiographic evaluation of collateral adequacy. As noted in Chapter 2, however, radioisotopic flow techniques have, on occasion, demonstrated obvious discrepancies between angiographic appearance of collaterals and their functional adequacy.[80]

Webb[46] measured retrograde flow in groups of surgical patients with differing degrees of coronary stenosis. These measurements were made after transient occlusion of the native coronary artery and, therefore, after cessation of antegrade flow. Hence, any blood leaking from the incision in the coronary artery must have been flowing retrogradely from distal beds and must have been delivered by collaterals. Retrograde flow was lowest and ranged from 0—1 ml/min in patients with stenotic lesions narrowing the lumen by 50—70%. When the stenosis was 70 to 85%, retrograde flow averaged 1.3 ml/min (range 0—6 ml/min). Mean retrograde flow increased further to 2.2 ml/min (range 0—6 ml/min) with stenoses of 85 to 95%. Finally, with subtotal obstructions of > 95%, retrograde flow jumped to 7.0 ml/min (range 1.5—18 ml/min). The steady rise in retrograde flow in patients with advancing degrees of obstructive disease demonstrates the increase in collateral function that accompanies progressive narrowing of the coronary artery lumen. Since retrograde flow is measured with the native artery vented to the atmosphere, the hemodynamic conditions for collateral flow are optimal and favor maximal collateral flow in all individuals. Hence, the observation of increasing collateral flow with advancing stenosis severity is not merely the result of development of a favorable pressure gradient along the collateral vessel. Rather, the relationship between increasing luminal constriction and increasing collateral flow is one of cause and effect. Coronary obstruction really does stimulate collateral development.

Goldstein and his associates measured collateral indices in patients with normal coronary arteries who were undergoing aortic valve replacement[81] as well as in patients with significant coronary obstructive disease who were to receive saphenous vein bypass grafts.[78] In the former, retrograde flow from the left coronary artery averaged 2.4 ml/min and the ratio of peripheral coronary to aortic pressure was 0.19. Right coronary artery collateral indices were not different. As noted above, mean retrograde flow in patients with coronary artery disease but no collaterals was 0.83 ml/min while the pressure ratio averaged 0.24.[78] Thus, these collaterals had very limited capacity. On the other hand, when proximal coronary lesions resulted in stimulation of collateral development, retrograde flow was significantly increased to 15.7 ml/min and the pressure ratio was 0.5. Flameng[65-67] also measured the ratio of peripheral coronary pressure to aortic pressure. In Flameng's series, all patients with collaterals had complete arterial occlusions, while those without collaterals had subocclusive lesions. In patients with collaterals, the pressure ratio averaged 0.40, whereas individuals without collaterals had ratios of 0.19. Thus, again there was a relationship between increasing severity of coronary disease and increasing evidence of collateral function. These intraoperative and hemodynamic studies clearly support the impressions of the postmortem and angiographic evaluations, and remove any doubt that coronary obstructive disease results in stimulation of coronary collaterals.

D. Biochemical Studies

The mechanism of this stimulation of coronary collateral growth by coronary obstructive disease is unclear. It is tempting to believe that myocardial ischemia is somehow implicated. Presumably coronary lesions would produce critical decreases in antegrade myocardial perfusion, resulting in ischemia. This tissue ischemia would then trigger coronary collateral development, which would theoretically proceed until the ischemic stimulus had been abolished. The precise biophysical or biochemical stimulus is not yet known. Increased tangential wall stress and endothelial shear following establishment of a pressure gradient along the collateral and initiation of flow have been postulated as possible causes of collateral transformation, and diffusible substances that stimulate collateral growth in animals have been isolated (see Chapter 7). Recently, Kumar et al.[57] have identified a substance in human infarcted myocardium that is capable of stimulating vascular neogenesis in the chick chorioallantoic membrane.

Kumar[57] removed infarcted tissue within 48 hours of death from eight human hearts. Six of the patients had had recent infarcts. The tissue was homogenized, fractionated with Sephadex columns, and purified. Angiogenesis in chorioallantoic membranes was compared to the known vascular stimulatory effect of tumor angiogenesis factor (TAF) isolated from rat tumors. Five of the eight tissue extracts stimulated growth of new blood vessels that was indistinguishable from that produced by TAF. Furthermore, TAF and myocardial infarct angiogenesis factor (MIAF) were antigenically identical. The age of the dying patients did not appear to be important, but the age of the infarct was. Four of the five active samples were from infarcts that were one, one, seven, and ten days old, while the age of the fifth infarct causing vascular neogenesis was indeterminate. Of the three infarcts without effect, one was only half an hour old, one was felt to be "old," and the third had "new" and "old" infarct. Thus, very recent infarcts most likely have not had time to produce MIAF, while old infarcts are no longer active. Normal myocardium of man, dog, or rat does not have angiogenic activity. The authors estimated that only picogram quantities of the active factor were needed for the angiogenic response. They also speculated that MIAF may have been produced by monocytes or macrophages. These exciting observations clearly establish the plausibility of a collateral-stimulating biochemical transmitter that might be produced during periods of myocardial ischemia. It is obvious that additional investigations are necessary to characterize this new active substance further.

II. Hypoxia—Decreased Oxygen Uptake

Trying to understand the mechanism by which coronary obstructive disease and the resulting myocardial ischemia might promote collateral development, students of coronary physiology suggested that an imbalance between oxygen supply and demand was central to the stimulus. It was felt that limitation of oxygen delivery to the tissue might be the critical factor. Although coronary arterial stenosis is the most obvious means of limiting oxygen availability to the myocardium, diminished oxygen uptake from alveoli could be a possible second cause. Chronic pulmonary infection and fibrosis from tuberculosis and parenchymal destruction from emphysema and other chronic pulmonary ailments have been associated with enlarged coronary collateral vessels. Zimmerman[82] injected the coronary arteries of hearts of six patients with cor pulmonale and three with chronic severe pulmonary emphysema with a barium sulphate-latex mass. He observed a marked increase in the number of visible anastomotic connections. Zoll and colleagues[3] also studied the hearts of 15 patients with clinical histories of cor pulmonale after injecting the arteries with Schlesinger mass. Eleven of these hearts, or 73%, had intercoronary collaterals. This frequency was substantially higher than that of 9% which was observed in their normal hearts. Barmeyer[27] attempted to quantitate collateral capacity in two patients who had had severe pulmonary disease and markedly diminished arterial oxygen tensions by perfusing the coronary arteries with a mixture of paraffin and diesel oil (see above). The mean relative anastomotic flow, a reflection of postmortem flow through intercoronary collaterals, in these two hearts was 41.9%, whereas this index in normal hearts averaged 25.3%. Finally, Cheng[83] did coronary angiography in a 48-year-old male with chronic obstructive pulmonary disease and cor pulmonale whose arterial oxygen saturation was 56%. The coronary arteries were free of obstructive disease. However, following injection of contrast medium into the right coronary artery, the conus branch and subsequently the left anterior descending artery were opacified. Left coronary artery injection also led to visualization of the conus branch.

Hence, individuals with pulmonary disease and presumed low arterial oxygen saturations have large intercoronary collaterals. It is tempting to conclude that systemic hypoxia causes global myocardial ischemia, which in turn triggers collateral development. One provocative report[84] that individuals living at high altitudes where ambient oxygen tension is low also have large coronary collaterals would support this hypothesis and exclude the pulmonary disease process itself and other related issues as important causative factors.

III. Anemia

If coronary obstruction and pulmonary disease produce collateral stimulation because of hypoxia (either regional or systemic) and resulting myocardial ischemia, then other conditions interfering with oxygen delivery to the heart should have similar effects. Chronic anemia with a hemoglobin level of less than 70% of normal significantly impairs oxygen transport. Hearts from individuals with longstanding anemia also have large coronary collaterals.

Zoll[3] studied the coronary vasculature of hearts from chronically anemic individuals after injecting the coronary arteries with Schlesinger mass and taking radiographs of the unrolled specimens. There were 91 patients with otherwise normal hearts. Thirty-five (39%) of this group had large coronary collaterals, an incidence that was strikingly higher than that observed in normal hearts from nonanemic individuals, but considerably lower than the nearly 100% incidence in patients with longstanding coronary occlusion. Zimmerman[82] also observed large anastomotic connections in hearts from one patient with aplastic anemia and two with pernicious anemia. Baroldi[6,18,19] made plastic corrosion casts of the coronary vasculature and studied them after overlying myocardial tissue had been digested. In normal hearts collateral diameters generally ranged from 190 to 270 μm. In patients with anemia, both intra- and intercoronary collateral channels were more evident in all areas of the heart, and diameters were in the 200−320-μm range. Baroldi calculated an anastomotic index based on number and size of counted collateral vessels in histologic sections (see Chapter 1). In normal hearts, this index averaged 4.7, whereas in hearts from anemic patients the mean anastomotic index was 12.4.[19] Of these 18 hearts from anemic subjects studied by Baroldi, seven were from patients who also had had some form of pulmonary disease. However, after elimination of these seven, the anastomotic index averaged 13.7.

Pitt[85] sized coronary collaterals by perfusing one main coronary artery with wax spheres with diameters of 35−45 μm and 75−90 μm. He collected the effluent from the other main coronary artery. Any wax spheres that appeared in the effluent must have passed through collaterals. Wax spheres were recovered from the contralateral artery in only 6% of normal hearts. Pitt perfused only two hearts from individuals who had had hemoglobin levels under 70% of normal, but in both, spheres were found in the effluent from the other coronary artery.

Laurie and Woods[86] studied hearts from African Bantu tribesmen by injecting a lead phosphate-gelatin mass into the coronary arteries. There was a surprisingly high incidence of collaterals in hearts without coronary disease. In fact, 75% of normal hearts from patients older than four years had abundant collaterals. In contrast, only 23% of hearts with coronary obstructive disease had many demonstrated coronary collaterals. These observations were later confirmed by Pepler and Meyer,[87] who used similar investigative techniques. Coronary collaterals were present in 74% of otherwise normal Bantu hearts, but in only 38% of hearts from Europeans. There was no obvious explanation for this difference, and Pepler and Meyer suggested that frequent megaloblastic and iron-deficient anemias seen in the African natives could be the cause. However, in a follow-up report by Laurie and Woods,[88] Bantu tribesmen, Australian immigrants, and Canadian natives and immigrants all had similar evidence of coronary collaterals.

Barmeyer[26,27] measured relative anastomotic flow in patients with hemoglobin levels less than 8−9 g/100ml. This index of collateral capacity was 42.6%, again emphasizing the increased collateral development occurring in individuals with longstanding, severe anemia.

IV. Hypoxemia—Congenital Heart Disease, Right-to-Left Shunts

Cyanotic congenital heart disease also causes arterial oxygen desaturation and hypoxemia. If, as hypothesized, collateral stimulation is related to tissue hypoxemia, then right-to-left intracardiac shunts resulting in mixing of arterial and venous blood should also produce increased collateral diameters. Bloor and associates[89] injected wax spheres suspended in sodium chloride solution into one coronary artery of hearts randomly selected from the available pediatric autopsy material and hearts with known congenital anatomical defects. Four sphere sizes were used: 20−25 μm; 37−44 μm; 63−74 μm; and 100−120 μm. The effluent from a second coronary artery was collected and examined to determine the maximal diameter of spheres passing through intercoronary collaterals. In the randomly selected normal hearts, spheres with diameters as high as 74 μm were found in the effluent, but 100−120-μm spheres were never found. In contrast, the effluent of 11 of 21 hearts from patients who had been cyanotic contained 100−120-μm spheres. Of course, the intercoronary collaterals in these hearts might have been wide enough to pass considerably larger spheres. In this same study, hearts from patients with acyanotic heart disease were also found frequently to have collaterals through which 100−120-μm spheres passed. But it is not possible to compare the results in hearts from cyanotic and acyanotic individuals since the collateral diameters were not bracketed in these groups, and, therefore, maximal collateral sizes are not known. Furthermore, the acyanotic subjects were older at the time of demise than the cyanotic patients.

Zimmerman[82] used postmortem coronary injections of a barium sulphate-latex suspension to examine a heart from a young patient with cyanosis and polycythemia. Radiographs of the unrolled heart revealed an increased number of anastomotic connections when compared to similarly injected normal hearts.

These data in young patients with cyanotic heart disease further support the basic premise that myocardial ischemia, whether the result of systemic or regional hypoxemia, results in coronary collateral development. This concept has actually guided clinical attempts to promote comparable collateral growth.

V. Cardiac Hypertrophy

In cardiac hypertrophy the thickness of the walls of the chambers is increased. In at least one type of hypertrophy, that resulting from aortic stenosis, coronary vascular reserve is significantly diminished.[90] Thus, many cardiac stresses in individuals with aortic stenosis would be expected to result in myocardial demand outstripping supply with subsequent ischemia and potential stimulation of collateral growth. In fact, several studies have confirmed increased collateral development in hypertrophied hearts.[3,16,18,19,27,85] Diverse investigative techniques have all arrived at the same conclusion. Thus, radiography of hearts after intracoronary perfusion of radiopaque mass,[3,16] plastic casts of the coronary circulation,[18,19] intracoronary injections of wax spheres,[85] and determination of postmortem collateral capacity[27] have suggested that hypertrophied hearts with normal coronary arteries are more likely to have larger collateral vessels than normal hearts. Baroldi[19] calculated the anastomotic index of hypertrophied hearts to be 7.4, compared to 4.7 in normal hearts. Barmeyer[27] determined mean relative anastomotic flow in normal and hypertrophied hearts to be 25.3% and 36.1%, respectively. Furthermore, coronary collaterals were three to eight times more frequent in individuals with hypertrophied than normal hearts.[3,85]

Cardiac hypertrophy, like occlusive coronary artery disease, is associated with diminished coronary vascular reserve, which makes these hearts susceptible to repeated episodes of myocardial ischemia. This situation obviously contrasts with those conditions of pulmonary disease causing hypoxia, high-altitude living, anemia, or admixture of venous with arterial blood because of right-to-left shunts in which the hypoxic stimulus is constantly present. It is important to realize that the inciting stimulus need not be present continuously to promote collateral growth.

VI. Exercise

It is apparent from the preceding discussion that hypoxemia and myocardial ischemia are potent stimuli of collateral development. It is also obvious that these stimuli cannot easily be employed in man to promote collateral growth. Because of the apparent beneficial functional effects of coronary collaterals (see Chapter 2), many attempts have been made to find simple, safe methods that could be used clinically to accelerate collateral growth, especially in patients with coronary obstructive disease. Exercise has been examined as one possible stimulus. It was theorized that the diminished coronary reserve in patients with coronary occlusive disease would result in an imbalance between oxygen supply and demand during exercise and subsequent transient myocardial ischemia. This ischemia might in turn stimulate collateral development.

Several attempts have been made to define the benefits of an exercise program in patients with coronary obstructive disease.[91–103] In most programs the patients do light exerrcise—walking, jogging, bicycling, calisthenics—for 30 to 60 minutes on each of three days during the week. The duration of the program prior to clinical evaluation has usually been 3 to 13 months, but occasionally conditioning has continued for several years. After beginning training, the patients always feel better, take less nitroglycerin, and can do more work than before enrollment in the program. Following completion of a training program, heart rate, blood pressure, the pressure-rate double product, and even the triple product are lower for any level of exercise when performances before and after conditioning are compared. Decreased myocardial oxygen demand may thus account for the diminished frequency of angina pectoris.

Many have also searched for evidence that these exercise programs might enhance myocardial oxygen delivery by improving the coronary collateral circulation. Coronary angiography done before and after a training program has demonstrated remarkable increases in coronary collateralization in selected patients.[91,95,104] These anecdotal reports of increased collateral circulation resulting from supervised training programs prompted the design of prospective[95,96,105–109] and randomized[101] trials to document possible reproducible effects of training on the coronary collateral circulation. In all of these studies angiographic evaluation of the coronary collateral circulation before and after the exercise program revealed no significant change. In the few patients in whom collaterals appeared to be more abundant following completion of training, there was almost always progression of the severity of a proximal coronary obstruction which provided an alternate explanation for collateral development. The angiographic results in 56 patients compiled from several of these reports[95,96,101,105–107] are summarized in Figure 3–7. Only two and possibly a third of nine patients with enhanced collateralization did not have evidence of progressive obstructive disease of the coronary arteries. Lack of change of left ventricular ejection fraction and regional wall motion also confirmed absence of improvement of myocardial perfusion.

Other techniques have also been used to uncover possible salutary effects of exercise programs on the coronary collateral circulation. Nolewajka et al.[101] selectively injected macroaggregated albumin particles labeled with either ^{131}I or ^{99m}Tc into the right and left coronary arteries, respectively, to reveal the possible presence of undetected right-to-left or left-to-right collaterals, and Verani et al.[109] used ^{201}Tl scintigraphy during exercise to better

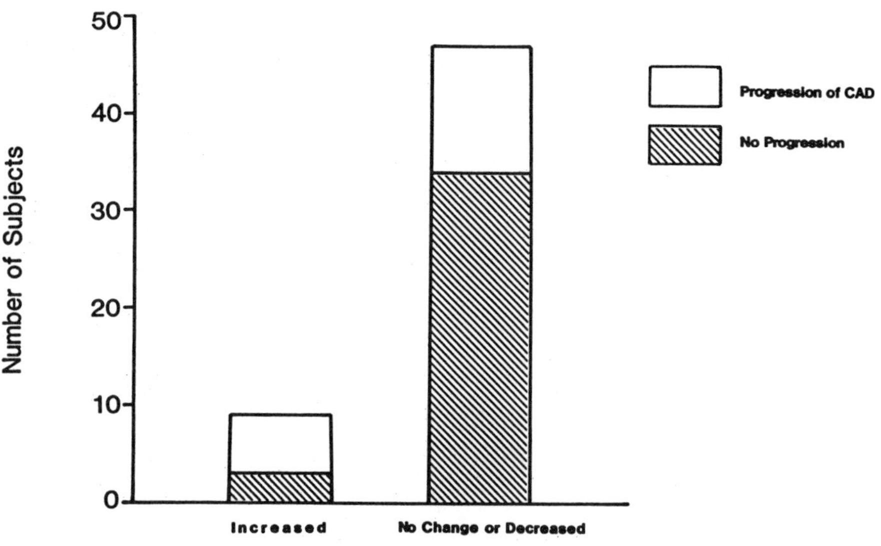

Figure 3–7   Angiographic evidence of coronary collateral development following completion of exercise program in 56 individuals with coronary artery disease. Because the data have been compiled from several different studies,[95,96,101,105–107] the training programs as well as durations are not identical for all subjects. Only a small proportion of the conditioned individuals had evidence of enhanced collateral formation following completion of training, but at least six of these nine also had progression of underlying coronary obstructive disease. Consequently, it is not possible to attribute the accelerated collateral development unequivocally to exercise except in two subjects and possibly a third.

define myocardial perfusion defects. Neither investigation uncovered evidence to support the development of collateral vessels during the course of the exercise program. Finally, Sim and Neill[107] noted that the threshold for angina pectoris during atrial pacing was unchanged after physical conditioning, and those patients with myocardial lactate production before training had similar production afterward as well.

Thus, neither angiographic visualization, radioisotopic evaluation, nor indices of collateral function can support the premise that exercise training in patients with coronary artery disease stimulates coronary collateral development. One must conclude from these data that exercise training affects only the demand side of the supply-demand relationship.

Despite the evidence that exercise does not affect blood supply to ischemic myocardium, there are several provocative reports that suggest or conclude otherwise. Sim and Neill[107] and Ferguson et al.[100,106] observed in many of their patients with coronary disease that heart rate and the heart rate-blood pressure double product during exercise were higher at the onset of angina pectoris following completion of the training protocol. In Ferguson's later study[100] total coronary blood flow was monitored with a coronary sinus thermodilution catheter at rest and during increasing exercise work loads until the onset of angina pectoris before and after a six-month training program. Although group changes revealed no differences after training, six of nine subjects exercised to higher double products before angina appeared following completion of the training protocol, and in these six, peak exercise coronary sinus blood flows were higher. Maximal myocardial oxygen consumption was also increased in four patients in whom these measurements were made. The higher myocardial blood flows and oxygen consumptions may simply be the result of increased work of the normal heart muscle. However, the increased exercise double products attained prior to appearance of anginal symptoms in the trained subjects suggest that some factor improved the functional capacity of the potentially ischemic myocardium despite increased metabolic demands.

Raffo et al.[102] used ST-segment depression rather than onset of angina pectoris as a more objective sign of exercise-induced myocardial ischemia. They also observed that the majority of their trained patients were able to exercise to a higher heart rate following the conditioning program before electrocardiographic changes became evident. Thus, in these patients a significantly higher workload was necessary to provoke myocardial ischemia. Ehsani and associates[103] observed that following a vigorous 12-month training program, subjects had a 22% higher double product at the time of initial ST-segment depression (0.1 mV) ($p < 0.001$). Furthermore, the extent of ST-segment displacement at the same double product was significantly less ($p < 0.02$) after training. The increased heart rate and double product necessary to provoke electrocardiographic evidence of ischemia suggest that the maximal myocardial oxygen consumption obtainable following training was increased. It follows that if myocardial oxygen consumption was higher in the trained subjects during some exercise stage before the onset of ST-segment shifts, then myocardial oxygen delivery must also have been increased to keep supply and demand in balance. This conclusion suggests the presence of a richer collateral network supplying the ischemic myocardium. With progressive increases in exercise load, even this increased collateral flow would become inadequate, and ischemia would become manifest, albeit at a higher workload and higher heart rate and double product. Of course, there are other possible explanations for the improved performance and apparent increase in myocardial oxygen consumption at the onset of electrocardiographic changes of myocardial ischemia following training. A myocardial biochemical adaptation, e.g., change in ATPase enzyme activity,[110,111] or chronic alteration of one of the other determinants of myocardial oxygen consumption, e.g., left ventricular wall thickness or contractility, might have resulted in a shift in the relationship of heart rate and double product to myocardial oxygen consumption. Similar values of these hemodynamic variables before and after training might then actually reflect different levels of myocardial demand, making direct meaningful comparisons of data obtained at the two times difficult at best and probably impossible.

A recent report by Froelicher et al.[112] described in detail five of a larger group of 16 patients who had trained for 3 to 12 months with arm and leg exercises and a walking/running program. Each subject had both ^{201}Tl scintigraphy and ^{99m}Tc multigated acquisition (MUGA) scans during exercise before and after physical conditioning. These five patients could perform more work following training, although the heart rate-blood pressure double products were unchanged at the onset of myocardial ischemia. However, the MUGA and ^{201}Tl scans demonstrated improved left ventricular function and myocardial perfusion following training. This study provides the most direct evidence available that training may increase the collateral blood supply in humans and hence perfusion of ischemic myocardium. Of the other 11 patients who completed the training program, one subject showed evidence of improved myocardial perfusion but without better left ventricular function, eight had no change, and two showed evidence of a deteriorating perfusion pattern.

Although the bulk of evidence in man suggests that exercise training does not result in an improvement in coronary collateral supply to ischemic myocardium, Froelicher's report is a striking departure from this consensus. One must examine the techniques used in these investigations critically. All studies except those of Verani et al.[109] and Froelicher et al.[112] have employed coronary angiography as the major, if not sole, means of demonstrating coronary collaterals. As already indicated, angiography does not result in opacification of all collaterals, and therefore the degree of collateralization is necessarily underestimated, although a decent correlation has been demonstrated between angiographic evaluation of collaterals and intraoperative measurement of collateral indices.[46,78,79] ^{201}Tl scintigraphy is a better technique for assessment of the functional adequacy of coronary collaterals. It is hoped that future studies will use this or other more sensitive techniques for the analysis of coronary collaterals. Perhaps then a more accurate evaluation of the effect of training on the coronary collateral circulation will be possible.

Another major drawback of studies purporting to study the collateral circulation before and after a training program is the exercise program itself. Most programs consist of simple exercises and calisthenics lasting for approximately one hour on each of three days every week for 3 to 12 months. The exercises are generally designed to have the patient perform at 60 to 80% of his or her maximal oxygen consumption or symptom-limited heart rate. Only Ehsani's exercise protocol[103] had subjects exercising at 70 to 80% of their maximal oxygen consumption, with two to three intervals of exercise requiring 80 to 90% of maximal oxygen consumption lasting two to five minutes and incorporated in the nearly one-hour-long exercise session. Because myocardial ischemia appears to be the most potent stimulus of collateral development[113] one would anticipate that exercise sufficient to elicit myocardial ischemia would have the best chance of stimulating collateral development. Since most of the exercise programs employed are specifically designed to avoid angina pectoris and myocardial ischemia, one must conclude that it would be unrealistic to expect physical conditioning as performed in these studies to have an easily detectable effect. Therefore, to determine whether exercise has the potential to stimulate development, it may be necessary to use animal models (see Chapter 7).

VII. Pharmacologic Agents

Many drugs with vasodilatory properties have been used in the treatment of patients with coronary artery disease. Some, like nitrates, have had enormous therapeutic efficacy and success, whereas others, like dipyridamole, have been distinctly less effective and possibly even deleterious. Many of these pharmacologic agents have multiple sites of action, and, therefore, elucidation of precise mechanisms for their clinical effects may not be possible. Definition of effects on the coronary collateral vasculature has proven to be quite difficult. For example, nitrates reduce preload by diminishing venous return, and afterload by increasing distensibility of large arteries.[114] These peripheral effects of nitrates will alter myocardial oxygen demand, resulting in secondary changes in coronary blood flow.[115] Furthermore, a decrease in arterial and hence coronary perfusion pressure will also result in an absolute fall in collateral flow. Thus, evaluation of the direct effect of administered agents on either coronary blood flow or coronary collateral function has been hampered by the necessity to consider their simultaneous effects on the peripheral circulation. Perhaps this difficulty explains in part conflicting reports on the action of nitroglycerin on coronary blood flow.[116–118] The effect of various drugs on the collateral circulation has been extensively studied in the experimental animal (see Chapter 7). However, because of methodologic limitations and restrictions, only limited studies have been reported in man (see below).

The coronary arterial bed can be divided functionally into two types of arteries: large conductance (or capacitance) extramural arteries and smaller intramural precapillary arteriolar resistance vessels[119,120] (Figure 3–8). Both

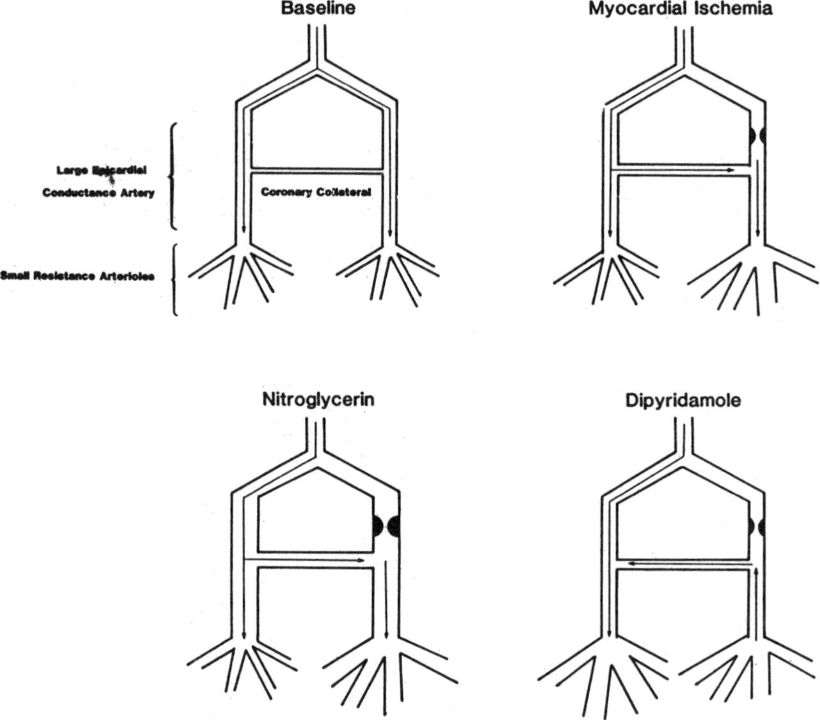

Figure 3–8   Schematic representation of coronary arterial bed and effects of myocardial ischemia, nitroglycerin, and dipyridamole. In the normal heart, coronary arteries can be divided into two functional components, large epicardial conductance arteries and smaller resistance arterioles. Each responds differently to exogenous stimuli. Coronary collaterals are present in the normal heart, but are thin-walled, nonfunctional conduits. After significant narrowing of a coronary artery, the ischemic stimulus results in autoregulation of the small resistance vessels, and consequently maximal vasodilatation. In addition, the stimulus initiates collateral transformation, which causes a striking increase in both wall thickness and dimensions. Nitroglycerin is principally a large-vessel dilator and probably also dilates developed collaterals. Dilatation of these segments of the vascular bed increases flow in the collateral channels to the ischemic myocardium. Dipyridamole mainly dilates small resistance arterioles. Dilatation of these latter vessels in the normal tissue causes a marked increase in flow and fall in distal coronary pressure. The fall in pressure at the source of collaterals may actually diminish collateral flow and perfusion of the ischemic myocardium. This deleterious effect is termed "coronary steal."

components determine the total coronary resistance in a given vascular bed, although the smaller resistance vessels are more important in this regard (see Chapter 7). In general, coronary dilators may have their principal effect on either the larger capacitance or smaller resistance vessels. The primary site of action of these agents largely determines their effects on the heart's collateral circulation.

A. *Nitrates*

Nitrates dilate the large epicardial conductance arteries in patients with and without obstructive coronary disease (Figure 3—8). Gensini[121] used computer analysis of coronary arteriograms before and after sublingual administration of isosorbide dinitrate and concluded that this agent caused an average 16% increase in coronary diameters, although the effect tended to be more marked in individuals with normal coronary arteries. Physiologic data also support the conclusion that nitrates preferentially dilate the large epicardial segments of coronary arteries rather than the smaller arteriolar resistance vessels.[122] Perhaps more important, Gensini[121] noted a dose-dependent increase in both the size and the number of angiographically visualized collateral channels in individuals with severe stenoses ($\geq$ 90%).

Cohn and associates[123] evaluated the effect of sublingual nitroglycerin on myocardial perfusion after injecting ^{133}Xe directly into the ostium of the left coronary artery. Radioisotopic washout was monitored with an Anger scintillation camera, and washout curves calculated for the first 40 seconds after injection in the distal quadrants overlying the left anterior descending and left circumflex arteries. Regional myocardial specific blood flow was represented as the mean of the two values. Patients were divided into three groups: (1) normal coronary arteries; (2) stenoses ($\geq$ 75%) of either the left anterior descending or left circumflex artery without angiographically visible collateral vessels; and (3) similar coronary obstructive disease with collaterals. The effects of nitroglycerin on mean blood pressure and heart rate-blood pressure double product were comparable in all groups. Although regional myocardial specific blood flow declined in each of the three groups following nitroglycerin administration, the decrease of 8 $\pm$ 6% in the subjects with coronary artery disease and collaterals was significantly less ($p < 0.05$) than that in either those with normal arteries (31 $\pm$ 5%) or the individuals with obstructive disease but no collaterals (23 $\pm$ 5%). This difference is perhaps magnified even further by the observation that the stenotic lesions were more severe in those with collateral channels. Nitroglycerin actually increased flow in a subgroup of patients with collaterals. In those with good collaterals (dense opacification of the coronary arterial segment distal to the obstruction from many small or several large collateral vessels) arising from nonjeopardized arteries, regional blood flow increased by 10 $\pm$ 7% (Figure 3—9). This effect was significantly different ($p < 0.001$) from the 23 $\pm$ 3% fall in flow in those individuals with poorer collaterals (faint or moderate opacification of

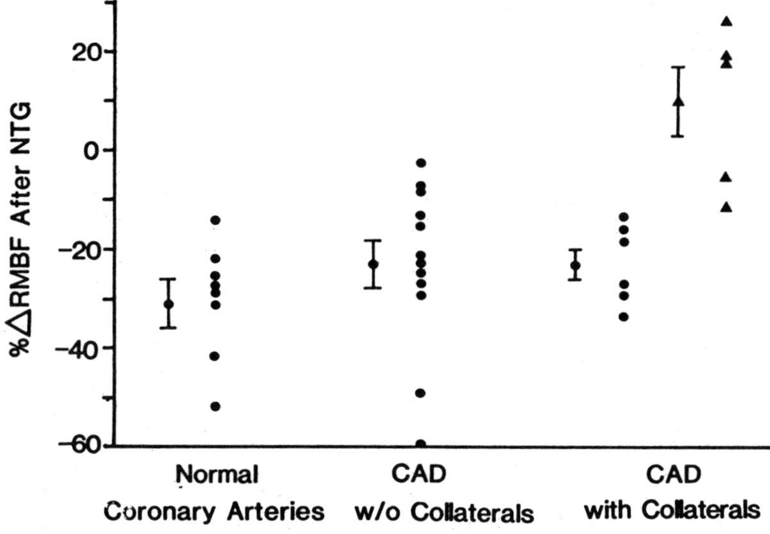

Figure 3–9   Regional myocardial blood flow (RMBF) measured with a ^{133}Xe washout technique before and after sublingually administered nitroglycerin (NTG) in normal patients and individuals with coronary artery disease (CAD). Nitroglycerin decreased blood flow in normal patients and patients with CAD but no angiographically visualized collaterals (CAD w/o collaterals). The response in patients with obstructive disease and collaterals (CAD with collaterals) was not uniform. In individuals with either compromised collaterals or collaterals that were not well visualized (●), nitroglycerin also caused regional flow to fall by 23 ± 3%. However, in the five subjects with unjeopardized, grade 3 or 4 collaterals (▲), average blood flow rose by 10 ± 7%. This change was significantly different from all other groups studied (*p* < 0.01 or 0.001). Therefore, nitroglycerin actually improved perfusion of well-collateralized myocardium despite the associated decrease in systemic blood flow. (Modified and printed with permission of Dun-Donnelly Publishing, from Cohn et al.[123])

the distal segment), some of which were also jeopardized. Hence, in spite of the systemic hypotensive effect of nitroglycerin and the anticipated secondary fall in myocardial perfusion, this agent actually improved regional myocardial blood flow in a selected group of individuals with well-developed collateral vessels.

Horwitz et al.[124] measured myocardial blood flow by monitoring regional washout curves after direct injection of ^{133}Xe into the subepicardium of ten patients at the time of thoracotomy. Patients usually had severe (> 75%) obstructive disease of the left anterior descending coronary artery, and the isotope was injected into myocardium in this vessel's perfusion territory. After the control curves had been recorded, a 0.4–mg nitroglycerin tablet was placed beneath the subject's tongue, and subepicardial injections of ^{133}Xe were repeated five minutes after dissolution of the pill. There was no consistent change in blood pressure during measurement of isotope washout after nitroglycerin administration since some patients were receiving intravenous phenylephrine infusions which were adjusted to maintain a constant systemic pressure. Disappearance curves were closely approximated by two exponential decays. The faster component was felt to represent residual antegrade flow in the stenotic vessel, while the slower curve was felt to be related to collateral blood flow. Nitroglycerin increased both the rapid and slow phases of flow. Average slow-phase flow increased from 12 to 15 ml/min/100g ($p < 0.05$). Hence, nitroglycerin improved perfusion of diseased myocardium.

Despite these provocative results, the effect of nitroglycerin on coronary collateral vessels cannot be proved unequivocally because of the possible confounding influence of residual antegrade flow through incompletely occluded arteries. Goldstein and colleagues[78] addressed the issue more directly by measuring the collateral indices retrograde flow and peripheral coronary pressure (see Chapters 1 and 4) after completion of the saphenous vein-coronary artery anastomosis in patients undergoing myocardial revascularization surgery. During these measurements, the native coronary artery is transiently occluded proximal to the anastomosis. Accordingly, pressure and flow measurements are reflections of collateral function in the absence of residual antegrade coronary flow. In these subjects, systemic nitroglycerin infusion caused a predictable decline in aortic pressure without consistent change in retrograde flow. Therefore, calculated coronary collateral resistance (aortic pressure/retrograde flow) fell by 28% ($p < 0.02$). Peripheral coronary pressure also declined after nitroglycerin administration ($p < 0.005$). However, because this latter collateral measurement is significantly affected by changes in perfusion pressure, the independent effect of simultaneous decrease in aortic pressure could not be discounted. Changes in peripheral coronary pressure therefore were normalized for changes in aortic pressure. This modified peripheral coronary pressure index, i.e., peripheral coronary pressure/aortic pressure, actually rose by 9.9% following nitroglycerin infusion ($p < 0.02$). These changes in coronary collateral resistance and peripheral coronary pressure index clearly suggest that nitroglycerin is able to dilate collateral pathways, resulting in augmentation of blood flow to potentially ischemic regions. To further document nitroglycerin's salutary action on collaterals, similar measurements of collateral indices were made after the potentially confusing systemic effects of the drug were attenuated. The reduction in aortic pressure following nitroglycerin injection was counteracted by adjustment of systemic blood flow during cardiopulmonary bypass. Now nitroglycerin produced consistent and often dramatic rises in retrograde coronary blood flow and an average 50% fall in coronary collateral resistance (Figure 3—10). Both absolute and relative peripheral coronary pressure tended to rise. This responsiveness to nitroglycerin was correlated with the duration of angina pectoris (Figure 2—3). Thus, none of seven patients with angina for less than six months had decreases in collateral resistance exceeding 30%, whereas nine of 21 subjects with angina for more than six months had falls in resistance at least as great as 30% ($p < 0.05$). In

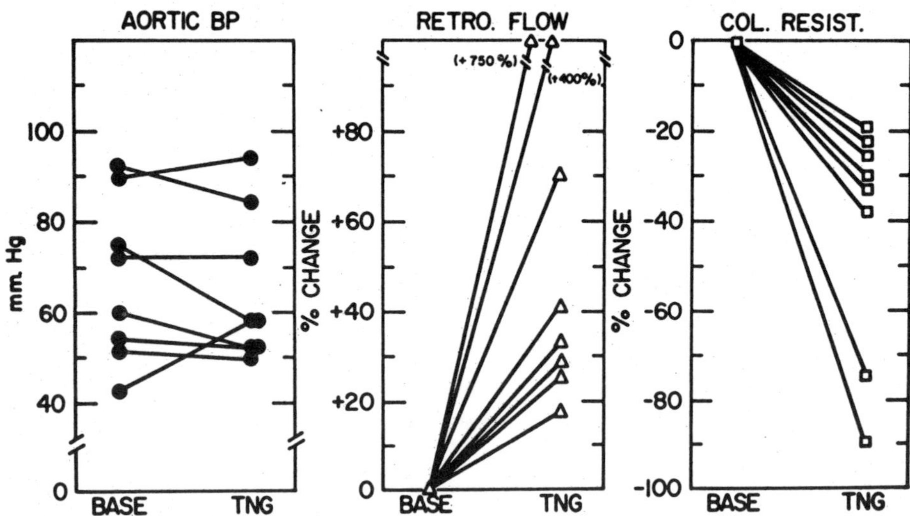

Figure 3−10   Effect of intravenous nitroglycerin (TNG) on retrograde flow and calculated collateral resistance (col. resist.) in patients at the time of saphenous vein bypass surgery when changes in aortic blood pressure (BP) were buffered by adjustment of systemic flow during cardiopulmonary bypass. Under these conditions, nitroglycerin elicited large increases in retrograde flow, and therefore falls in collateral resistance. (Reprinted with permission of the American Heart Association from Goldstein et al.[78])

fact, nitroglycerin had no effect on collaterals in patients without obstructive coronary disease.[81] Thus, these studies demonstrate that nitroglycerin can definitely augment collateral functional indices in man, and that this responsiveness to nitrates is positively correlated with increasing duration of ischemic symptoms.

The intraoperative studies of Klein et al.[125] support Goldstein's conclusions.[78,81] In Klein's patients, saphenous vein bypass graft flow was measured with an electromagnetic flow probe after both the distal anastomosis with the obstructed coronary artery and proximal anastomosis with the aorta had been completed. He reasoned that graft flow would be maximal if there were no other sources of blood to the distal arterial bed; conversely, flow would be minimal if other well-established sources, such as antegrade flow or collateral flow, were present. In these investigations, aortic pressure was maintained constant by adjusting the rate of blood infusion. Intravenous nitroglycerin decreased bypass graft flow in patients with severe obstructive disease (> 90%) and angiographically visible coronary collaterals. On the other hand, graft flow increased in those with comparable coronary disease but no collaterals to the grafted vessels. These data can be explained if it is accepted that nitroglycerin can dilate collateral vessels. In patients without collaterals, nitroglycerin dilated native conductance vessels distal to the graft. The severe proximal arterial lesion minimized the likelihood of increased antegrade coronary flow, and graft flows consequently increased. However, those patients with well-developed anastomotic pathways also had simultaneous dilatation of collateral channels. This second source of blood to the grafted vessel's distal bed competed with the antegrade flow from the graft itself with resultant net decrease in graft flow.

Wald[126] evaluated changes in regional myocardial blood flow in patients with 99–100% obstructions of the right coronary artery and angiographically visible collaterals from the left anterior descending artery by injecting human albumin macroaggregates labeled with either ^{99m}Tc or ^{131}I into the left coronary artery to measure resting flow and flow after nitroglycerin injection. The left coronary artery nitroglycerin bolus injections were small enough (60 μg) to insure absence of systemic effects. Nitroglycerin caused a significant fall in the proportion of total left coronary perfusion delivered by collaterals to the myocardium previously supplied by a normal right coronary artery. These observations are clearly contrary to the conclusions of others cited above.[78,81,123–125] However, in seven of Wald's eight patients, the left anterior descending artery, which gave rise to the collateral vessels, was itself the site of obstructive lesions (> 50%). As already noted by Cohn,[123] flow from compromised donor coronary arteries through collaterals to distal portions of recipient vessels may not be able to be enhanced. In fact, administration of vasodilators in the presence of a stenotic donor artery may produce a coronary steal with absolute decrease in collateral flow (see Chapter 7).

Despite the above evidence, studies continue to appear that demonstrate that nitroglycerin decreases total coronary blood flow and perfusion to ischemic regions,[127,128] thus supporting this drug's peripheral effects as the clinically important mechanism of action. These latter investigations, however, usually have not controlled for the systemic hypotensive effect of the nitrate, thereby making the drug's direct coronary effects and their importance virtually impossible to elucidate. The study by Ganz and Marcus[129] attempted to define more precisely the relative importance of the direct coronary and peripheral vascular effects of nitroglycerin. They delivered the drug alternately into the coronary arterial circulation and systemically in patients with pacing-induced angina pectoris. Although intracoronary injections of nitroglycerin (0.075 mg) increased coronary sinus blood flow, no patients experienced relief of angina. In contrast, systemic infusion of 0.2 mg resulted in falls in arterial blood pressure and coronary sinus blood flow and relief of the chest pain. Thus, in this investigation the peripheral vascular and not the coronary effects of nitroglycerin appeared to account for the agent's antianginal action. However, analysis of the coronary anatomy of these patients perhaps explains the lack of direct coronary effect of the injected nitrate. Infusion into the critically stenosed artery whose distal bed would have already been maximally dilated by the increased metabolic state induced by atrial pacing would not have been expected to cause additional vasodilatation and improved perfusion of ischemic myocardium. Fifteen stenotic vessels received collaterals. However, the source artery had a stenosis compromising at least 76% of its lumen in nine cases, and one vessel had a 50–75% narrowing. Only five vessels had less than 50% obstructions. Therefore, in most of these patients nitroglycerin injection into the coronary artery giving rise to the collaterals could have caused a detrimental coronary redistribution or steal (see Chapter 7), resulting in further fall in blood flow to the ischemic tissue. Hence, this study cannot completely exclude the possibility that nonjeopardized collaterals could be dilated by nitroglycerin, resulting in increased perfusion of ischemic myocardium and relief of angina pectoris.

During the early phase of an acute myocardial infarction, ST-segment elevation, the characteristic electrocardiographic sign of myocardial injury and ischemia, is commonly seen. Intravenous nitroglycerin infusion can significantly reduce the magnitude of these precordial ST-segment shifts.[130–132] Of course, these observations imply at least partial restoration of the balance between myocardial oxygen supply and demand by the nitrate. Because intravenous nitroglycerin decreased arterial pressure, and therefore afterload, in all of these clinical studies, it is not possible to determine whether its salutary effect on ischemic myocardium was the result of this peripheral vasodilatation, or whether an independent action on coronary collaterals was also operative. Borer[131] investigated this possibility by simultaneously infusing phenylephrine in the patients to restore arterial pressure to pre-nitroglycerin levels. Under these conditions there was further diminution in the summation of individual precordial lead ST-segment elevations. These latter data strongly suggest that nitroglycerin also has a direct cardiac salutary effect, presumably by dilating coronary collaterals and improving perfusion of ischemic tissue.

It is apparent that nitrates have direct beneficial effects on the coronary collateral circulation of man. Schematic representation of the coronary circulation and the effect of nitroglycerin is seen in Figure 3–8. Beyond critical coronary lesions, the ischemic myocardial stimulus causes small resistance vessels to dilate, but the larger conductance arteries are relatively unaffected. Nitroglycerin dilates both epicardial and collateral vessels. Dilatation of the stenosed vessel would not have any effect on flow unless somehow the geometry of the stenosis were favorably altered. However, dilatation of the normal epicardial and collateral vessels would increase blood flow to the already maximally dilated vascular bed of the diseased coronary vessel, thus attenuating or relieving myocardial ischemia.

B. Dipyridamole

Dipyridamole is a pyrimidine derivative which is a powerful vasodilator of both the coronary and peripheral arterial beds. As depicted in Figure 3–8, this pharmacologic agent, in contrast to nitroglycerin, dilates principally the smaller resistance vessels which are located more peripherally in the arterial tree than the large conductance arterial segments observed on the surface of the heart[119] (see Chapter 7). Because of the different sites of action of nitroglycerin and dipyridamole, one might anticipate different clinical responses to the two agents. In fact, as a consequence of dipyridamole's marked dilatation of the coronary resistance vessels, a coronary steal is theoretically possible (Figure 3—8) (see Chapter 7). Because precapillary arteriolar resistance vessels in the ischemic region are already maximally dilated, dipyridamole cannot alter vascular tone or further improve perfusion of that territory. It can, however, dilate arterioles in nonischemic zones, thus decreasing total coronary vascular resistance. Collateral blood flow originally directed to the ischemic vascular bed would instead be shunted toward the newly dilated, nonischemic bed. The resulting diminution of tissue perfusion may precipitate or exacerbate myocardial ischemia.

Dipyridamole has been used clinically. Initially it was promoted as a therapeutic agent for patients with angina pectoris because of its coronary vasodilating properties. However, controlled studies revealed that it was ineffective in relieving angina.[133–136] Furthermore, numerous observations, some anecdotal and others representing a more extensive experience with the drug, have documented that dipyridamole may actually cause angina.[127,137–145] Dipyridamole, administered either orally or intravenously, may also precipitate ischemic electrocardiographic abnormalities[134,143] or redistribution of myocardial flow away from already underperfused regions.[127,142–144,146] These rheologic and clinical effects of dipyridamole may be related in part to the previously described coronary steal effect. Of course, apparent flow redistribution documented with thallium scintigraphy might also be related to greater dipyridamole-induced flow increases in normal regions than in ischemic areas as opposed to absolute decreases in flow to the underperfused myocardium.

Lichtlen and his co-workers[127,147] measured ^{133}Xe myocardial washout rates after intracoronary injection of the radioisotope in patients with isolated obstructive disease (> 50%) of one major coronary branch. Rate constants were calculated by monoexponential analysis of the washout slopes registered at the many matrix points of the scintillation camera. Flows were determined by the Kety-Schmidt formula and averaged in selected myocardial areas. Regional flows were then correlated with the coronary arteriogram so that both normal and poststenotic coronary flows were known. In these patients, ^{133}Xe clearance from poststenotic vascular beds increased following intravenous dipyridamole infusion. However, as discussed later in relation to animal studies (see Chapter 7), contamination of the field of interest by even small areas of normally perfused myocardium with intact vasodilatory reserve can result in flow increases following dipyridamole administration which are wrongly attributed to the collateral circulation. Furthermore, because the coronary lesions were not complete obstructions, the myocardium in the artery's vascular territory is perfused by both residual antegrade flow as well as collateral flow. Hence, in these situations it is possible that dipyridamole might have increased the former without affecting the latter. Because of these theoretical limitations and methodologic difficulties, the actual effect of dipyridamole on collateral flow is probably best determined in an animal model (see Chapter 7).

A preliminary report of a 3½-year study of the long-term effects of oral dipyridamole administered according to a double-blind protocol has demonstrated that this pharmacologic agent can promote coronary collateral development.[148] Longevity was assessed, and postmortem hearts were injected with a modified Schlesinger technique. Mortality from acute coronary occlusion was significantly less, patient longevity longer, and intercoronary anastomotic channels more numerous in individuals treated with dipyridamole. This evidence that repeated coronary vasodilatation will stimulate collateral-vessel growth has been confirmed in animal models (see Chapter 7). Perhaps the success of chronic exercise and even myocardial ischemia in promoting the growth of coronary collateral channels is in part related to the ability of these stimuli to effect repeated coronary arterial dilation.

C. Nitroprusside

Nitroprusside can dilate both large conductance vessels and smaller resistance arterioles (see Chapter 7). It is another vasodilator that has been infused intravenously in patients with both chronic congestive heart failure[149] and acute myocardial infarction and heart failure or shock.[150] In both clinical settings nitroprusside significantly decreases aortic pressure and left ventricular end-diastolic or pulmonary capillary wedge pressure. Accompanying the decreases in preload and afterload are significant increases in cardiac output in those individuals in whom it is initially depressed. Despite these beneficial hemodynamic changes, the effect of nitroprusside on ischemic myocardium and blood flow to myocardium perfused by stenotic arteries is controversial.

In patients with acute anterior myocardial infarction, Chiariello[132] noted that nitroprusside in doses causing mean falls in aortic and pulmonary wedge pressures of 26 and 7 mmHg, respectively, further raised ST segments in precordial leads by an average of 2.4 ± 0.3 mm. In contrast, sublingual nitroglycerin in these same subjects caused similar hemodynamic alterations, but lowered ST segments by 1.4 ± 0.4 mm in each monitored lead. In support of the significance of these observations, Mann[151] noted that nitroprusside decreased systemic blood pressure and regional myocardial blood flow determined from ^{133}Xe washout curves in patients with significant (> 75% stenosis) coronary artery disease both with and without angiographically visible collateral vessels. In two patients with a single stenotic collateralized artery, myocardial flow in the ischemic and normal distal quadrants was analyzed independently. In both individuals there was a greater reduction in blood flow following nitroprusside in the distal quadrant of the stenotic vessel's area of perfusion than in the distal quadrant of the normal vessel's territory. When similar patients were given nitroglycerin and identical techniques used to measure myocardial blood flow, blood pressure also fell (perhaps not as much as with nitroprusside) but flow significantly increased in patients with nonjeopardized collaterals (Figure 3—9). Thus, these studies strongly suggest a fundamental difference between nitroglycerin and nitroprusside. Nitroprusside, like dipyridamole, may principally dilate small resistance arterioles and, therefore, may initiate a flow redistribution, which could account for the deleterious effects on myocardial blood flow and ischemia. Of course, drug-mediated hypotension may also contribute to deleterious changes in blood flow to underperfused myocardium (see Chapter 7).

Other reports have not always confirmed the above observations. The changes following nitroprusside infusion in ST-segment elevation caused by myocardial infarction may be variable,[152,153] with increases in some patients and decreases in others. The direction and magnitude of the alterations seemed to be related to the extent of drug-related change in heart rate and double product. Miller[154] noted that ST-segment depression during atrial pacing in individuals with coronary artery disease was significantly attenuated if the subjects had been pretreated with nitroprusside. He, as well as Feldman,[155] observed no change in coronary blood flow following nitroprusside infusion, although coronary sinus or great cardiac vein thermodilution catheters were used for this purpose. These data are confusing. Possible small differences in systemic hemodynamic effects in the various investigations or minor differences in the patient populations may account for the variability of results. For these reasons, investigations in experimental animals where variables can be controlled more rigidly are useful in defining the precise effects on the collateral circulation of this and other drugs.

Perhaps the variability of results may be related to the ablity of nitroprusside to dilate both large and small coronary arteries (see Chapter 7). Dilatation of the former would be beneficial in the patient with ischemic heart disease, whereas dilation of the latter might have deleterious effects. It is conceivable that the balance between the effects on large and small vessels may be different in different individuals, and that the net effect on the large and small vessels determines the drug's actual in-vivo action.

D. Nifedipine

Nifedipine, a calcium-channel antagonist, is currently used widely in the treatment of both exercise-induced angina pectoris and spontaneous coronary spasm. It reduces smooth-muscle tone and dilates peripheral as well as coronary arteries.[156] Its effect on coronary collateral vessels is less certain. Existing evidence suggests that nifedipine dilates distal coronary arteriolar resistance vessels and not proximal capacitance vessels (see Chapter 7). One recent report, however, has noted that nifedipine can increase the diameter of the proximal coronary artery in conscious dogs.[157] But unlike dipyridamole, another small vessel dilator, nifedipine does not exhaust coronary vascular reserve since further increases in coronary flow (e.g., during exercise) can occur after administration of this agent.[158]

Nifedipine prevents pacing-induced angina pectoris[128,158,159] and may improve lactate metabolism of the stressed heart.[128] It increases total coronary flow,[128] and also may increase or at least maintain perfusion of myocardium in the vascular territory of stenotic arteries despite drug-induced declines in arterial pressure.[127,146,158−160] It should be noted, however, that in a minority of subjects nifedipine may actually decrease poststenotic myocardial blood flow.[127] The drug's antianginal action cannot confidently be attributed to possible increases in perfusion of ischemic myocardium because of concomitant falls in afterload resulting in lowered myocardial oxygen consumption. Furthermore, drug effects on collaterals cannot be separated from possible changes in antegrade flow in subtotally occluded arteries, and therefore the cause of the demonstrated increases in poststenotic myocardial flow cannot be clarified. These clinical studies cannot truly define the effect of nifedipine on coronary collaterals. As noted previously, investigations in animal models are necessary to derive accurate data (see Chapter 7).

VIII. Aortic Counterpulsation

Mechanical devices such as the intraaortic balloon unload the left ventricle by expanding during diastole and accelerating runoff of arterial blood into the peripheral capillary beds. Thus, systolic ejection of the left ventricle is into a relatively empty arterial reservoir, and less energy is expended in stretching the elastic arterial walls. Studies in humans have demonstrated that myocardial oxygen consumption declines as a consequence of the fall in left ventricular work.[161,162] The increase in aortic diastolic pressure might also be expected to increase blood flow to ischemic beds. Although these same studies have evaluated the response of coronary blood flow during aortic counterpulsation, the techniques for flow measurement were unable to separate possible differences in response of normal and ischemic tissue. Hence, the effect of counterpulsation on collateral perfusion cannot be deduced.

Williams et al.[163] studied the effect of aortic counterpulsation on regional blood flow in six patients with high-grade (75−100%) stenoses of either the main left or left anterior descending coronary artery. These investigators placed the tip of a thermodilution catheter in the great cardiac vein, a tributary of the coronary sinus which drains the blood from the perfusion territory of the left anterior descending coronary artery. Although these investigators were thereby able to evaluate changes in regional myocardial flow, the presence of subtotal occlusions in many of the individuals in the study population does not enable one to decide whether flow changes might have been related to changes in antegrade and/or collateral flow.

More recently, Fuchs and colleagues[164] addressed the question once again. They also placed the tip of a thermodilution catheter in the great cardiac vein. Their study population consisted of seven patients with unstable angina pectoris who had greater than 90% stenoses of the left anterior descending coronary artery. Although flow measurements in this heterogeneous group would suffer from the same objections raised above, four of the seven had 100% proximal occlusions. In these four individuals, systolic aortic pressure fell from 113 ± 10.2 to 103.5 ± 9.7 mmHg, while diastolic pressure rose dramatically from 82.0 ± 7.0 to 104.8 ± 13.2 mmHg ($p < 0.05$). Great cardiac vein flow rose from 50.2 ± 11.4 to 63.0 ± 10.6 ml/min ($p < 0.02$) (Figure 3-11). Thus, in these patients, where perfusion of the left anterior descending territory was completely dependent on collaterals, increases in aortic diastolic pressure increased flow through the anastomotic channels.

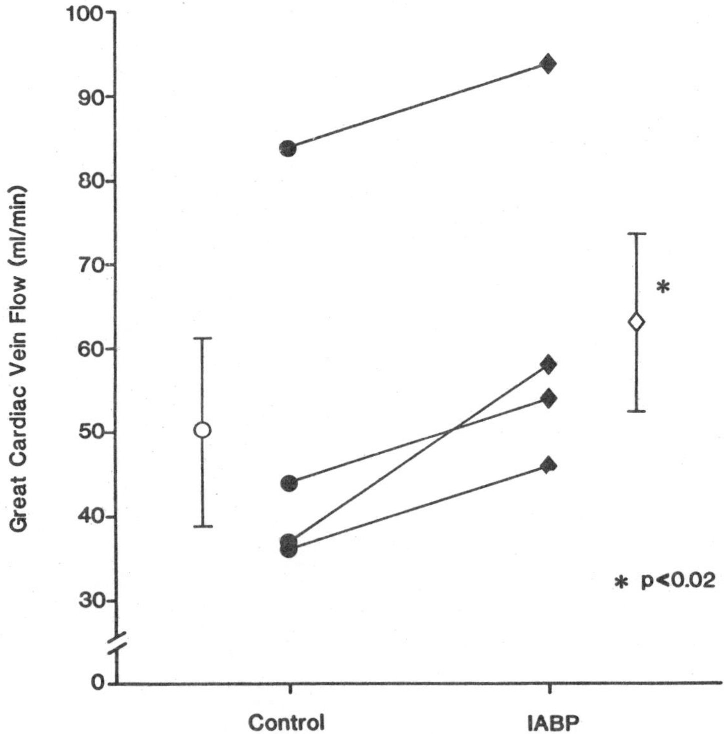

Figure 3−11   Intraaortic balloon pumping (IABP) and its effect on perfusion of ischemic myocardium in four patients with total occlusion of the left anterior descending coronary artery. Collateral blood flow was evaluated by selectively measuring efflux from the great cardiac vein which drains the myocardium once perfused by a patent left anterior descending artery. IABP increased aortic diastolic and hence coronary perfusion pressure. Collateral flow in these individuals increased by approximately 25% ($p < 0.02$). (Drawn from data presented by Fuchs et al.[164])

IX. Surgical Interventions

A. Right-to-Left Shunt

The role of chronic depression of oxygen saturation of arterial blood on coronary collateral development has intrigued many investigators. Chronic hypoxemia and resulting diminished myocardial oxygenation have been considered to represent the most important stimuli of collateral formation in patients with coronary occlusive disease. Accordingly, Day and Lillehei[165] attempted to lower arterial oxygen saturation and theoretically increase the stimulus to collateral development by diverting desaturated blood into the arterial circulation. They surgically created a side-to-side anastomosis between the pulmonary artery and left atrium in one patient who had debilitating symptoms of coronary artery disease. Arterial oxygen saturation was decreased to 86%. Postoperatively the patient enjoyed substantial relief of angina pectoris and his nitroglycerin consumption was markedly diminished. Furthermore, he was able to return to strenuous work. Unfortunately, the coronary collateral circulation was not directly evaluated in this patient. Although the clinical data strongly suggest that the surgical procedure significantly attenuated myocardial ischemia, the well-known placebo effect of an operative intervention on the subjective evaluation of frequency and severity of anginal pains could also have accounted for the dramatic improvement of the patient's clinical condition.

B. Cardiopexy and Pericardial Adhesions

Because of Beck's pioneering work in the research laboratory (see Chapter 7) and in the clinical arena (see below), myocardial revascularization became an important premise in the treatment of patients with coronary obstructive disease. Techniques, often ingenious, were devised to supply the heart with a new source of blood. One of the simplest procedures was instillation of substances into the pericardial space to induce the formation of pericardial adhesions. Because of the closeness of the pericardial vascular supply with its potential connections to multiple mediastinal arterial systems, it was hoped that granulation tissue induced to develop within the pericardial space would form a vascular connection and hence bridge between coronary and pericardial and therefore other mediastinal arterial systems. Thompson and Raisbeck[166] sprinkled talc over the epicardial surface of the heart. This irritant created numerous pericardial adhesions which successfully obliterated the pericardial space. In one patient who died three weeks after surgery, one of the engorged pericardial vessels was injected with india ink. The dye could be traced into the myocardial vessels. Similar anastomoses between pericardial vessels and vessels of the myocardium and mediastinal structures were observed in many other subjects after talc poudrage.[167] In order to prove that the vessels in the pericardial granulation tissue were continuous with coronary arteries and mediastinal arterial systems, Plachta and colleagues[168] perfused arteries with a radiopaque mass to facilitate tracing of the connecting channels. The injectate also contained trichrome stain, which was intended to stain and highlight vascular endothelium so that continuity between arterial systems could be assured. Injection into pericardial vessels led to the appearance of dye in intercoronary vascular channels as well as in the coronary sinus. Histologic examination of the granulation tissue revealed vessels as large as 650 μm. Free communications between extracardiac collaterals and intracardiac channels through newly formed vessels in the bridging granulomatous tissue were present in abundant numbers. Connections to the mediastinum, pleurae, roots of the lungs, and diaphragm had been formed in many specimens. Thus, arterial blood from the vasa vasorum of the pulmonary artery and aortic root, intercostal and bronchial arteries, pericardial and esophageal branches of the thoracic aorta, superior phrenic and pericardiophrenic arteries, and the anterior mediastinal, thymic, pericardial, and sternal branches of the internal mammary artery was available to the coronary circulation.

Cardiopexy, thus, resulted in the formation of numerous extracardiac collateral vessels. Thompson and co-workers [166–169] reported consistently good short- and long-term clinical results with abolition or at least attenuation of ischemic symptoms, as well as a projected trend toward increased survival.[167] However, the clinical follow-up of these patients consisted of only subjective evaluations. Therefore, despite the success with which talc poudrage stimulated the formation of extracoronary collateral channels, the clinical efficacy of the procedure was never adequately proved.

C. Attachment of Other Tissues or Foreign Substances to Cardiac Surface

To increase further the likelihood of development of collaterals between extracardiac structures and coronary vessels, numerous tissues with attached vascular pedicles, free tissue grafts, or foreign substances were sutured to the cardiac surface, usually after mechanical abrasion or chemical treatment of the epicardium and addition of talc, asbestos, or other irritant to promote adhesions. Thus, pectoral muscle,[170–173] omentum,[174–176] mediastinal and pericardial fat pads[172,173,177–185] and lung[186,187] have been successfully transplanted to the epicardial surface. In these procedures the transplanted tissue's vascular supply was preserved. In the Beck I operation, the coronary sinus was narrowed in addition to epicardial abrasion, sprinkling of asbestos in the pericardial sac, and suturing of pericardial or mediastinal fat to the epicardial surface.[177–179,181–185] Injection of a barium sulphate-gelatin mass into the coronary arteries of at least one postmortem specimen following pectoral muscle grafting produced filling of the graft vessels through 10 to 12 large anastomotic channels easily visualized without magnification.[172,173] In patients with prior omentopexy, injection of the abdominal aorta[174] or superior mesenteric artery[175] demonstrated evidence of rich vascular ingrowth from the graft into the myocardium. In O'Shaughnessy's specimens,[174] india ink even appeared in the heart's chambers after being injected into the abdominal aorta.

Vineberg[188–190] sutured isolated pieces of omentum to the hearts of individuals with ischemic symptoms. Because of the well-recognized ability of the omentum to form adhesions, he felt that this tissue, even when divorced from its native blood supply, would increase formation of pericardial adhesions and hence form a better bridge between coronary and extracardiac vessels. Favaloro,[191] however, abandoned free omental grafting because he was unable to obtain any angiographic evidence of new collateral formation.

In selected patients, Vineberg[188,192] sutured strips of Ivalon sponge to the epicardial surface. This inert material, like strips of omentum, was intended to promote the growth of vessels within the pericardial space to link the pericardial and myocardial arterial systems. Examination of hearts from patients who have undergone this procedure did reveal numerous blood vessels in the interstices of the sponge, and some of these vessels could be followed into the myocardium.

Clinical follow-up of patients subjected to any of these procedures uncovered uniformly dramatic improvement in exercise tolerance and frequency and severity of anginal pains. Several reports also suggested that survival might have been favorably affected.[179,181,184] However, as already indicated for the cardiopericardiopexy procedure, the recognized ability of these operations to promote formation of transepicardial collateral channels does not imply that the channels are physiologically significant. In the clinical setting there were no objective evaluations of the efficacy of these interventions. A long-lasting symptomatic effect was also not consistently observed. Hence, after a relatively short period of intense interest, this approach to revascularization of the heart was abandoned.

D. Internal Mammary Artery Ligation

As previously described (see Chapter 1), the coronary arterial system has numerous anastomotic connections with vasa vasorum of the great vessels and vascular networks of many mediastinal structures. In 1942 Fieschi[193] demonstrated vascular links between the internal mammary artery and parietal pericardium through the pericardiophrenic artery, as well as anastomoses with arterioles in the epicardial fat and myocardium. Battezzati and colleagues[194] injected india ink and methylene blue into the internal mammary artery at the level of the second intercostal space near the origin of the pericardiophrenic artery in cadavers. They observed an extensive vascular network in the parietal pericardium, and in two subjects they also saw dye in the vascular rami of the myocardium and in the epicardial fat.

Because of this anatomic evidence of anastomoses between the internal mammary artery and coronary arterial system, it was proposed that ligation of the internal mammary artery beyond the origin of the pericardiophrenic branch would result in diversion of blood normally flowing down the distal internal mammary artery into the pericardiophrenic artery and thence into the myocardial circulation. This proposed technique of myocardial revascularization had great appeal because of the procedure's simplicity. It was done under local anesthesia and required only a few minutes. Initial reports of clinical results, as for the other procedures for the relief of angina pectoris described above, were very enthusiastic.[194–203] In a large proportion of operated patients, relief of anginal pains was immediate and subjects claimed they could perform activities they were unable to perform preoperatively because of pain.

Despite the early enthusiastic reception of internal mammary artery ligation, some investigations cast serious doubt on the efficacy of this simple procedure. Fish[204] followed 24 patients for approximately two months after bilateral ligation of the internal mammary arteries. Although clinical improvement was excellent immediately following operation, angina pectoris returned within 60 days in 18 patients. Only four patients continued to claim moderate and two slight improvement. Adams[205] reported his experience with four patients who had this procedure. In two of the patients the ligation was performed in a two-stage procedure. Both internal mammary arteries were isolated and encircled with sutures but not ligated. These two patients became asymptomatic. There was no further change when the vessels were ligated two and five days later, respectively. Of the two remaining patients, one had less pain because of diminished physical exertion, while the other experienced no improvement. This last patient died shortly after the surgical procedure. Because of these disappointing results and the suspicion that internal mammary artery ligation was itself not responsible for the relief of symptoms, Adams studied the pericardiophrenic artery anatomy in three fresh cadavers. He noted that this vessel was variable in size and even existence. Furthermore, he perfused the aortic root with an aqueous solution after ligation of the great vessels arising at the arch and the distal aorta. The pericardiophrenic artery was severed and its effluent collected in a receptacle. There was no increase in flow when the internal mammary artery was ligated. Of course, these postmortem studies could not be directly extrapolated to living humans, but did suggest that the presumed physiologic basis for the operative procedure might not be sound.

Double-blind prospective trials of the efficacy of internal mammary artery ligation were reported by Dimond et al.[206] and Cobb and colleagues.[207] In both studies neither the physician evaluating the patients' progress nor the patients themselves knew whether the internal mammary arteries had actually been ligated or whether a simple sham operation in which the arteries had only been isolated had been performed. The results of the two trials were quite complementary. There was no difference in symptoms,[206] nitroglycerin consumption,[207] exercise-induced electrocardiographic changes,[207] or exercise tolerance[207] between those with and those without internal mammary artery ligations. Finally, neither surgical procedure affected the ischemic response to exercise observed in the preoperative state.[206] Thus, these objective investigations were unable to detect any benefit of internal mammary artery ligation.

Rowe[208] measured cardiac output and total coronary blood flow (nitrous oxide saturation technique with catheter in coronary sinus) after isolation of both internal mammary arteries and again after ligation. Cardiac output and the coronary arteriovenous oxygen difference were unchanged. Coronary blood flow increased negligibly from 79 to 82 ml/min/100g left ventricle. These measurements certainly suggest that the surgery did not have grossly detectable effects on left ventricular hemodynamics or perfusion. Of course, possible changes in flow distribution would not have been detected. Four of the five subjects claimed immediate symptomatic relief. However, with longer follow-up angina pectoris returned in three, and the severity of symptoms gradually progressed. Two patients died. Again, ligation of internal mammary arteries had no documented objective benefits, and even its subjective benefits were not long-lasting.

Glover, one of the original proponents and strong enthusiasts of bilateral ligation of the internal mammary arteries,[196,200,201] reevaluated his opinion of the procedure several years after his initial report was published.[209] He followed 219 patients for one to two and a half years after surgery, and observed that 63% had had at least some relief of anginal pains. However, he was very impressed with his own animal experiments (see Chapters 5 and 7) which demonstrated definite anastomoses between coronary and internal mammary arteries but no increase in myocardial blood flow following ligation of the latter. Glover concluded that the clinical benefits of internal mammary artery ligation consisted solely of relief of anginal pain by either a psychosomatic, neurogenic, or possible other, as yet undefined, mechanism.

Although the procedure of bilateral internal mammary artery ligation was devised to stimulate the development of extracardiac coronary collaterals and hence furnish the heart with an alternate blood supply, it is highly unlikely that mere obstruction of distal outflow of these vessels could have resulted in significant increases in flow through more proximal branches, namely the pericardiophrenic arteries. This operation was subsequently proved to be without physiologic basis or objective value. Any observed subjective clinical improvement was likely to be psychogenic in origin, and the procedure was abandoned. This history serves to reemphasize the necessity for objective criteria for evaluation of procedures designed to benefit patients with ischemic heart disease.

E. Arterialization of the Coronary Sinus

In his continuing effort to supply the diseased heart with a new source of blood, Beck proposed introducing arterial blood into the coronary sinus. Because the coronary sinus and its tributaries are continuous with the capillary bed, Beck reasoned that arterial blood pumped into the coronary sinus would flow retrogradely through the veins into the capillary bed where oxygen exchange could take place. To encourage the retrograde flow of arterial blood, Beck proposed constricting or even occluding the coronary sinus near its ostium. Arterialization of the coronary sinus, or the Beck II operation, in man was first reported by Beck in 1948.[210] Subsequently, he[177,178,211] and Bailey[212,213] performed this operation in many individuals with ischemic heart disease. This revascularization procedure was generally done in two stages. During the first phase a vein graft was anastomosed between the aorta and coronary sinus, thus effectively creating an arteriovenous fistula. Three weeks later the second phase, consisting of narrowing of the coronary sinus, was completed. This latter step insured retrograde passage of arterial blood into the coronary sinus, but also diminished the amount of shunting between the arterial and venous circuits and therefore the possibility of high output failure or ventricular volume overload. However, because of the procedure's difficulty and the necessity for two stages, coronary sinus arterialization did not acquire widespread popularity. Furthermore, pumping of arterial blood into the coronary sinus provided a new source of oxygenated blood for the ischemic myocardium for only a finite interval. As in experimental animals (see Chapter 7), the arterialized coronary sinus gradually lost contact with the capillary bed. In one postmortem specimen from an individual who had undergone a Beck II operation, none of the blood injected into the coronary sinus appeared in any of the coronary arteries.[178] In contrast, blood injected into one coronary artery freely issued from the ostium of a second artery. Thus, this procedure did promote the formation of intercoronary collateral vessels, an observation also previously made in experimental animals (see Chapter 7). These new collaterals might have resulted in beneficial redistribution of already existing coronary arterial flow, but certainly could not have been the source of a new blood supply. Therefore, despite the expected excellent clinical follow-up of patients with this operation, it too was soon abandoned.

F. Internal Mammary Artery Implantation

More physiologic attempts to bring a new source of blood to beleaguered myocardium were championed by Vineberg and his surgical colleagues. He advocated making a superficial tunnel in the anterior wall of the left ventricle and then pulling the isolated internal mammary artery through the tunnel and securing it in place. Thus, a systemic artery was brought into close contact with ischemic myocardium. Vineberg's careful examinations in dogs demonstrated the eventual development of anastomotic connections between the implanted internal mammary artery and the adjacent coronary arterioles (see Chapter 7). On the basis of these observations Vineberg proposed the use of this procedure in patients suffering from severe myocardial ischemia and angina pectoris.[180,188] Sewell slightly modified the operation and implanted the internal mammary vein as well as adjacent connective tissue and chest wall muscle along with the artery as a single pedicle.[214,215] Despite this and other changes (Smith implanted distal ends of saphenous veins or nylon artery grafts into the myocardium after anastomosing the proximal ends to the descending thoracic aorta[216]), Vineberg's pioneering work became the basis of revascularization surgery for nearly 15 years until early in the 1970s when internal mammary artery implantation was abandoned for the more direct saphenous vein bypass graft surgery with its immediate revascularization of ischemic tissue.

Internal mammary artery implantation, like its predecessors in the field of myocardial revascularization, generated much debate regarding its value and effect. Numerous clinical reports documented relief or improvement of symptoms in from 50 to 90% of operated patients.[180,188−191,214,215,217−235] Vineberg[188] and Sewell[219,220,223] recognized that symptomatic benefits would not be immediate, and they documented gradual improvement in clinical results during the first six to nine months after surgery. These investigators commented that clinical improvements should not be expected until collaterals between the new source artery and the recipient coronary arterial bed had had time to form. Nonetheless, because of false hopes raised by glowing clinical reports following other alleged revascularization procedures that were in time attributed solely to their psychological rather than physiologic effects, more objective evidence to support the beneficial value of arterial implantation into left ventricular myocardium was required before others would accept the therapeutic value of the procedure.

Postmortem injection studies[190,217,218,221,228,235] and coronary casting[219] adequately demonstrated numerous collateral connections between the implanted internal mammary artery and coronary arterial bed. These pathologic studies were supported by numerous clinical reports documenting passage of radiopaque contrast medium from the surgically implanted internal mammary artery to the coronary bed during routine in-vivo cineangiography of the subclavian or internal mammary artery.[190,191,215,218−228,231,232,234−241] Some angiographic studies demonstrated proximal occlusion of all major coronary arteries, with the only patent vessel in the heart being the implanted artery.[235] In some patients the anastomoses were fine vessels which when opacified formed a myocardial blush, while in others large collaterals could be identified which permitted retrograde filling of major coronary arteries with the injected contrast medium. In several reports the adequacy of collateralization from the internal mammary artery and therefore the degree of myocardial revascularization were correlated with the patient's symptomatic response to the operation.[224,226,233] In Kemp's series,[233] 11 of 13 patients with patent arterial implants anastomosing with the coronary vasculature had clinical improvement, whereas symptoms in seven of ten with occluded implants were unchanged. These results were further amplified by the detailed data of Groves[226] in which the adequacy of revascularization was assessed by assigning one of four grades to the angiographic appearance of the collaterals between the internal mammary artery and coronary vasculature. There was an unmistakable trend for better clinical results as angiographic determinations of collateral adequacy improved.

Claims that internal mammary artery implantation limited recurrence of myocardial infarction[228,232] and improved survival[222,224,228,232,235,241,242] also buoyed assertions that this operation provided major clinical benefits. In Gorlin's experience,[228] the rate of recurrent infarction after an average 18-month follow-up period was half that in an apparently comparable control group (5% versus 10%). Furthermore, survival at six and twelve months was significantly better ($p < 0.05$) in operated patients than in medically treated patients from the same institution.[228] This difference (92% versus 86%) was maintained after two and three years of observation. Sewell[242] noted that longevity improved as the number of collateral connections between the implanted artery and coronary circulation increased.

Gorlin and colleagues[221,225,228,233] evaluated myocardial metabolism at rest and during isoproterenol infusion before and again approximately one year after surgery. The myocardium normally extracts lactate. However, when conditions, such as coronary artery lesions, limit oxygen supply to the myocardium, the heart must switch to anaerobic metabolism, and lactate becomes a byproduct that spills out into the venous blood draining the ischemic tissue. The technique of stressing the heart with either atrial pacing or isoproterenol infusion and measuring coronary venous lactate levels attempts to identify hearts that can become ischemic and, therefore, in which myocardial perfusion cannot meet demands. Gorlin noted that approximately 75% of patients with successful arterial implants had improved lactate metabolism, and many of these subjects converted from lactate production during stress before surgery to lactate extraction afterwards. Kemp[233] correlated clinical response to surgery with changes in lactate metabolism in 13 patients with patent arterial implants which successfully collateralized the coronary arteries and ten others with occluded implants. Of 11 subjects with successful operations who had been lactate producers before surgery, eight extracted lactate during isoproterenol infusion during the postoperative follow-up. Two additional patients with patent implants extracted lactate both before and after arterial implantation. All but two of these 13 subjects experienced striking clinical improvement. On the other hand, one lactate-producing patient with a closed graft became an extractor after surgery, while two others converted from extraction to production. Lactate metabolism was unchanged in the others. Seven of this group of ten patients did not experience any clinical improvement. These data imply that successful internal mammary artery implantation improved myocardial metabolism by preventing anaerobic oxidation during periods of increased tissue oxygen demands. One would assume that the most likely explanation is improved regional myocardial perfusion.

Indications that revascularization following internal mammary artery implantation had beneficial effects are also found in many of the exercise stress test follow-up studies.[218,222,230,232,243,244] Exercise tolerance and/or stress electrocardiograms improved in many of the surgical survivors, especially those with evidence of good revascularization.[230]

Kay et al.[245] evaluated left ventricular function before and again one year following surgery, and claimed that myocardial revascularization with internal mammary arteries improved stroke volume and cardiac output. There was no change in left ventricular end-diastolic pressure. However, because some of the patients receiving arterial implants also had left ventricular aneurysmectomy, it is not possible to determine how much improvement in cardiac output might actually be related to the former procedure.

Finally, several investigators attempted to measure blood flow through the implanted artery.[221,225,227,228,245,246] Gorlin[221,225,228] injected ^{85}Kr into the origin of the internal mammary artery and monitored the rate of isotope clearance from the myocardium. Flow through the implanted vessels often exceeded 50 ml/min/100 g, and frequently clearance from the internal mammary artery was the same as that from the rest of the myocardium when the radioactive tracer was injected directly into a coronary artery. Kay[227,245, 246] described a cineangiographic technique for the measurement of the velocity of the radiographic contrast medium in the internal mammary artery, and then converted these values into absolute flows. Flows ranging from 5 to 78 ml/min in the implanted arteries were reported.[245] These values should be contrasted with in-situ internal mammary artery flows measured directly with an electromagnetic flowmeter of 25−40 ml/min, flows of 40−70 ml/min when the severed artery was permitted to bleed freely, and flows of 5−7 ml/min immediately after implantation of the artery into the myocardium. Although these flows agree closely with those reported by Gorlin,[221,225,228] significant uncertainties about the methodology (see below) make cineangiography an unreliable technique for flow measurement.

The reports summarized above clearly concluded that internal mammary artery implantation often resulted in the formation of large transepicardial collateral channels linking the implanted systemic artery and the coronary arterial system. These anastomotic vessels effectively revascularized ischemic myocardium with subsequent clinical improvement, increased exercise capacity, improved survival, and restored myocardial function. However, a second group of investigators doubted the efficacy of this revascularization procedure and presented other data to support their contention.

Dart et al.[240] concluded that there was no correlation between the degree of coronary artery opacification following injection of contrast medium into the implanted internal mammary artery and either symptoms of angina pectoris, postoperative myocardial infarction, or late cardiac deaths. Six of 11 patients with occluded implants, 22 of 66 with low-grade myocardial revascularization, and 17 of 41 with high-grade revascularization all experienced clinical improvement. This lack of correlation between collateral adequacy as judged by angiography and the degree of clinical improvement was also noted by others.[230,231,234,241,247] Langston[234] observed that 17 of 20 surgical survivors acknowledged postoperative clinical improvement, but only 3 of 21 internal mammary artery implants in this group resulted in good myocardial revascularization. This disturbing lack of correlation between symptomatic response and angiographic pattern of the new collaterals may perhaps be related to technical difficulties encountered during performance of the angiograms. Dart[240] demonstrated that the intensity and extent of coronary artery opacification during angiography were dependent on the pressure with which the contrast agent was injected into the internal mammary artery and the position of the catheter tip. Thus, high injection pressures and/or catheter wedging produced much more dramatic visualization of the coronary arterial system than if lower pressure or a more proximal catheter position had been used. Because of difficulty in standardization of the angiographic procedure, Dart concluded that visualization of coronary collaterals and anastomoses between the internal mammary artery and coronary bed and estimation of their size and extent should not be equated with functional adequacy. These considerations also account for the likely unreliability of cineangiographic estimates of internal mammary artery flow.[227,245,246]

When Sethi[247] compared actuarial survival curves for surgical patients with curves for medically treated individuals, he noted no difference. Because this retrospective comparison could have been biased, Takaro and others from the Veterans Administration Hospital system began a prospective, randomized trial where patients accepted for study were assigned to either medical or surgical groups according to a specific protocol.[248] The study was abandoned after enrollment of only 146 patients because of the greater appeal of direct surgical revascularization with aortocoronary saphenous vein grafts. Commenting on the preliminary observations, however, Takaro noted that there was no difference in the cumulative survival for the medical and surgical groups.

Neither exercise performance[230,234] nor left ventricular function[234,239] was improved by arterial implantation in groups of surgical patients. If initially positive, the exercise stress test generally continued to reveal evidence of myocardial ischemia following surgery. In only a few patients with excellent revascularization did an initially positive test become negative after surgery.[230] McCallister[239] documented the infrequency with which left ventricular hemodynamics normalized after successful surgery, while Langston[234] demonstrated that left ventricular function at rest and during exercise actually tended to deteriorate in the surgical patient.

Dart[249] had a unique opportunity to measure flow in implanted internal mammary arteries with an electromagnetic flowmeter at the time of thoracotomy in individuals undergoing a left dorsal sympathectomy for continued or recurrent angina pectoris. All 13 patients had had their original arterial implantation two to five years before the attempted sympathectomy. The average flow was 8.1 ml/min (range 4−19 ml/min). In those with low-grade revascularization, flow averaged 5.9 ml/min (range 4−10 ml/min), whereas average flows of 10.7 ml/min (range 6−19 ml/min) were recorded in individuals with angiographic evidence of high-grade revascularization. These flows are considerably lower than those recorded by Gorlin.[221,225,228] It must be recognized, however, that all of Dart's patients had either recurrent angina or little evidence of symptomatic relief following the initial surgery. It is possible that individuals with higher flows would have been less symptomatic, and therefore would not have required a second operation.

Thus, internal mammary artery implantation, like other revascularization procedures, engendered considerable controversy. It was clear that insertion of a systemic artery into ischemic myocardium could lead to formation of numerous collateral vessels, although the process would realistically require months. Perhaps early occlusion of the graft and poor collateral formation in individuals with patent grafts were related to arterial implantation into insufficiently ischemic tissue. The search for the true value of this surgery was abruptly abandoned in the early 1970s when saphenous vein bypass grafting became popular. This latter procedure had the distinct advantage of providing immediate revascularization of ischemic areas. Arterial implantation became another historical milestone in the field of myocardial revascularization.

X. Collateral Regression and/or Disappearance: Roles of Aortocoronary Bypass Surgery and Spontaneous Resolution of Coronary Obstruction

Whereas the process of collateral stimulation and development occurs over a period of many months in response to regional myocardial hypoperfusion or ischemia, the disappearance of collaterals following successful aortocoronary bypass graft operations occurs rapidly. Disappearance of both inter- and intracoronary collaterals after bypass surgery has been well documented.[32,53,250−259] Postoperative angiography within two to three weeks of the revascularization procedure in patients with patent grafts commonly demonstrates disappearance of collateral vessels that were readily opacified before surgery.[53,251,253,257] Bourassa[53,253] has shown that if the saphenous vein grafts should then become occluded by the time of the second postoperative angiographic procedure at one year, the same collateral pathways present before surgery reappear.

Patency of grafts to arteries supplied by collaterals before surgery has typically been associated with either complete disappearance of those collaterals or at least a pronounced decrease in their number and in the extent of collateral filling.[32,53,250-259] Persistence of collaterals or appearance of new channels may imply occlusion, stenosis, or other malfunction of the venous graft. Whereas graft occlusion is almost always accompanied by at least persistence of old and often appearance of new collaterals, angiographic visualization of collaterals after surgery should not be interpreted to signify certain graft occlusion. Levin and co-workers[259] have noted that disease of the distal segment of the grafted artery which impedes runoff may result in persistent or new collaterals in the presence of a still patent graft. Furthermore, collaterals may even persist following successful revascularization. In these individuals selective angiography of the patent grafts demonstrates flow reversal in the collateral channels. The contrast agent flows in a direction opposite to that noted in the preoperative study from the successfully grafted artery into the preexisting collateral channels and thence into stenotic coronary arteries that were the sources of these same collateral vessels before surgery. Therefore, the successfully grafted artery may in turn become a collateral source for ungrafted, diseased vessels. As a new source of myocardial blood, it may also give rise to new collateral vessels not previously identified.

Despite the above data, the fate of collaterals no longer seen following successful revascularization is not truly known. The term "regression" implies disuse atrophy, but there is no evidence that this occurs in man. After aortocoronary bypass procedures, blood is pumped at systemic pressures into the distal segment of the grafted vessel, effectively abolishing any pressure gradient beyond the arterial obstruction that had previously been part of the stimulus to collateral development. This same pressure gradient also determines the volume and direction of flow of blood (and injected contrast agent) along the collateral into the diseased vessel. Abolition of the pressure gradient along the collateral from the normal source vessel to the newly grafted artery effectively terminates flow and the possibility that the collateral can be opacified during routine coronary angiography. Grüntzig's data[260] from patients undergoing percutaneous transluminal coronary angioplasty support these conclusions. Coronary angiography immediately after balloon dilatation of the stenosis revealed complete disappearance of collaterals in 13 of 26 vessels with collaterals present before the procedure, a less prominent collateral circulation in ten, and unchanged collaterals in three. The fate of the collaterals was directly linked to the success of the dilatation. The experience of Kimbiris and his colleagues[73] is similar. In Siepser's case[261] of traumatic fistula between the right coronary artery and right atrium, collaterals to the distal right coronary artery from the left anterior descending artery disappeared after continuity between the proximal and distal portions of the damaged artery was reestablished. Conversely, sudden creation of a pressure gradient between two coronary vascular beds by either wedging of an angiographic catheter into a coronary artery prior to injection of contrast agent[262] or coronary spasm[263-270] causes abrupt appearance of collateral vessels which then disappear during repeat angiography after the catheter is pulled back or the spasm is resolved. Therefore, angiographic appearance and disappearance of coronary collaterals are dynamic events that may depend principally on the presence of pressure gradients. After successful revascularization it is not known whether any structural changes occur to the collateral wall during periods when flow is minimal. Hence, absence of angiographic visualization of collaterals known to be present before surgery might better be termed "disappearance" rather than "regression." In experimental animals some changes in collateral function have been documented to occur during periods when blood no longer has to flow through previously developed collaterals (see Chapter 5).

Disappearance of collaterals does not occur only after successful revascularization, although this latter setting is certainly the most common. Spontaneous regression of coronary obstructive lesions has been documented with serial angiograms by several investigators.[40,50,271,272] In each of these reports collaterals present when a coronary artery was critically narrowed disappeared when the stenosis became less severe. Roth's patient,[271] a 46-year-old male with exertional angina, had a markedly positive exercise stress test with 5 mm of ST-segment depression and an abnormal ^{201}Tl exercise scintigram. The left anterior descending artery was subtotally occluded with many right-to-left collaterals. One year later the patient had become asymptomatic, and repeat exercise stress testing and radionuclide study were normal. The lesion of the left anterior descending artery had substantially regressed, and collaterals could no longer be visualized. Thus, reperfusion, whether spontaneous or surgically induced, can lead to disappearance of collaterals.

XI. Miscellaneous Conditions

A. Congenital Heart Disease

As previously discussed (see above), collateral dimensions in patients with cyanosis and congenital right-to-left shunts are larger than in other pediatric patients without heart disease.[82,89] These data helped to confirm the primary importance of tissue hypoxemia as a stimulus of collateral development, and may have even prompted Day and Lillehei[165] to create surgically a shunt from the pulmonary artery to the left atrium in the hopes that this procedure would promote collateral growth and thus relieve the individual's ischemic symptoms. Although the patient's exercise tolerance was dramatically improved following the operation, no objective data relating to collateral development were available.

Survival is often dependent on the development of an adequate intercoronary collateral circulation in patients with anomalous origin of the left coronary artery from the pulmonary artery.[273–278] In this condition the right coronary artery is usually dilated and tortuous, and arises normally from the aorta. The aberrant left coronary artery arises from the pulmonary artery, and is typically thin walled and veinlike. The left ventricular wall supplied by the right coronary artery is either normal or hypertrophied,[279] but the territory supplied by the left coronary artery is usually dilated and fibrotic and sometimes aneurysmal.[273,275,276,278,280] Papillary muscle scarring is frequently seen, and may cause clinically apparent mitral insufficiency.[273,276,278] Coronary collaterals connecting the right coronary artery and anomalous left coronary artery may be apparent on gross inspection of the cardiac surface. The most common collateral pathways in these hearts are the Circle of Vieussens, the septal perforating arteries, and the continuation of the right coronary artery around the apex to the terminations of the left anterior descending and circumflex arteries.[278] In some hearts an abundant intramural vascular network may link the ventricular lumen with epicardial coronary arteries in the perfusion territory of the anomalous left coronary artery, and these vessels may act as endomural collaterals.[273,280]

The pathophysiology of this anomaly was initially suggested by Brooks[281] in 1885 when he described two hearts with anomalous left coronary arteries. The potential role of the intercoronary collaterals has been well described since this early report.[273,278] During fetal and early neonatal development the pressure is higher in the pulmonary artery than in the aorta and the right coronary artery normally arising from the aortic root. Thus, blood will flow antegradely from the pulmonary artery into the anomalous left coronary artery. As pulmonary resistance and pressure fall in the neonate, antegrade flow in the anomalous vessel will diminish. When aortic pressure eventually exceeds pulmonary artery pressure, flow will reverse in the aberrant coronary artery. Blood will then flow from the normal right coronary artery through intercoronary anastomotic channels into the low-pressure anomalous artery. part of this collateral blood supply will pass retrogradely along the anomalous vessel into the pulmonary artery. Hence the anomalous vessel becomes a functional arteriovenous fistula. The rest of the oxygenated blood will flow into the peripheral coronary vascular bed to perfuse left ventricular myocardium. The ratio of distribution of blood to the peripheral vascular bed and to the pulmonary artery will be determined by hemodynamic conditions. Exercise or other stimulus that increases pulmonary flow or lowers pulmonary artery pressure may cause a steal syndrome. By diversion of more blood into the pulmonary artery, less will be available for supply of the left ventricular myocardium with possible resultant ischemia.

Infants without collateral vessels usually die within the first few months of life, while those with collaterals typically survive infancy.[273–278] However, in spite of development of an extensive coronary collateral circulation, ischemia and infarction frequently occur, resulting in myocardial scarring and even premature death.[273–278,280] Surgical management has included simple ligation of the proximal portion of the anomalous left coronary artery, saphenous vein bypass graft to the left coronary artery after division of its connection with the pulmonary artery, and autotransplantation of the artery from the pulmonary artery to aorta.[274,275,277,278,282] Obviously, the collaterals would continue to function only in those patients having isolated proximal ligation of the anomalous vessel without attempt to provide an alternative antegrade arterial blood supply.

Retrocardiac collateral vessels are also more numerous in various congenital cardiac disorders (see Chapter 1). Anastomoses between bronchial and coronary arteries are prominent in individuals with cyanotic heart disease (tetralogy of Fallot, pulmonary atresia, double outlet right ventricle),[283,284] coarctation of the aorta,[285] and supravalvular aortic stenosis.[286,287] The collaterals arise from the atrial branch of the left circumflex, right, and/or main left coronary artery, and may be as large as the main circumflex branch of the left coronary artery.[283] In-vivo angiographic studies have documented that the direction of blood flow in these individuals is from the coronary arteries into dilated bronchial vessels.[283,284,286,287] In subjects with cyanotic heart disease, blood flow is diverted from the relatively high-pressure coronary arterial circuit into bronchial vessels which themselves communicate with high-capacitance, low-pressure pulmonary arteries. In patients with either aortic coarctation or supravalvular aortic stenosis, the intracoronary systolic pressure is significantly higher than the pressure in the bronchial arteries that originate from the descending thoracic aorta distal to the obstruction. Thus, a coronary-bronchial artery gradient is established which results in preferential blood flow away from the coronary bed. Diversion of arterial blood away from the myocardium could theoretically cause ischemic symptoms, a so-called steal syndrome (see Chapter 1).

Zureikat[284] observed coronary-bronchial collateral vessels in 5 of 23 subjects with cyanotic congenital heart disease, but in none of the 44 patients with a noncyanotic congenital disorder. Four of the five had tetralogy of Fallot, while the fifth had double outlet right ventricle. Although hypoxemic episodes are commonly noted in patients with tetralogy of Fallot, it is of interest that none of the four in this series with coronary-bronchial collateral channels had such episodes. On the other hand, five of the remaining 14 patients with tetralogy and no coronary-bronchial vessels had hypoxemic spells. It is possible that the coronary-bronchial collaterals were able to provide enough blood to the lungs to abort or attenuate the hypoxemia, which would ordinarily result from the periodic sudden increases in resistance of the right ventricular outflow tract and increased right-to-left shunting observed in these patients.

B. Acromegaly

A provocative report of a 68-year-old acromegalic man with triple-vessel coronary disease raises the issue of the effect of growth hormone on myocardial neovascularization.[288] As expected, this patient had intercoronary collaterals. But the collaterals were remarkably large, thick walled, and tortuous. Goldberg and his co-authors commented on the striking appearance of these anastomotic vessels, and suggested that their unusual size might be related to increased circulating levels of growth hormone. Of course, this speculation cannot be proved, but evidence does support a role for growth hormone in the neovascularization of the retina in diabetic patients.[289]

References

1. Blumgart HL, Schlesinger MJ, and Zoll PM: Angina pectoris, coronary failure and acute myocardial infarction: The role of coronary occlusions and collateral circulation. *JAMA* 116:91–97, 1941.
2. Prinzmetal M, Simkin B, Bergman HC, and Kruger HE: Studies on the coronary circulation. II. The collateral circulation of the normal human heart by coronary perfusion with radioactive erythrocytes and glass spheres. *Am. Heart J.* 33:420–442, 1947.
3. Zoll PM, Wessler S, and Schlesinger MJ: Interarterial coronary anastomoses in the human heart, with particular reference to anemia and relative cardiac anoxia. *Circulation* 4:797–815, 1951.
4. Zoll PM, Wessler S, and Blumgart HL: Angina pectoris: A clinical and pathologic correlation. *Am. J. Med.* 11:331–357, 1951.
5. Miale JB, and Bledsoe A: Pathologic anatomy of coronary heart disease: Particular reference to cardiac muscle bundles. *Arch. Pathol.* 56:577–596, 1953.
6. Baroldi G, Mantero O, and Scomazzoni G: The collaterals of the coronary arteries in normal and pathologic hearts. *Circ. Res.* 4:223–229, 1956.
7. James TN, and Burch GE: Differences in naturally occurring arterial anastomoses of normal and pathological human hearts. (abstr) *Am. J. Med.* 27:313, 1959.
8. James TN: *Anatomy of the Coronary Arteries*. Harper and Row, Hagerstown, MD, 1961.
9. Fulton WFM: Arterial anastomoses in the coronary circulation. I. Anatomical features in normal and diseased hearts demonstrated by stereoarteriography. *Scot. Med. J.* 8:420–434, 1963.
10. Fulton WFM: Arterial anastomoses in the coronary circulation. II. Distribution, enumeration and measurement of coronary arterial anastomoses in health and disease. *Scot. Med. J.* 8:466–474, 1963.
11. Anitschkow NN, Wolkoff KG, Kikaion EE, and Pozharisski KM: Compensatory adjustments in the structure of coronary arteries of the heart with stenotic atherosclerosis. *Circulation* 29:447–455, 1964.
12. Fulton WFM: The dynamic factor in enlargement of coronary arterial anastomoses, and paradoxical changes in the subendocardial plexus. *Br. Heart J.* 26:39–50, 1964.
13. Fulton WFM: The time factor in the enlargement of anastomoses in coronary artery disease. *Scot. Med. J.* 9:18–23, 1964.
14. Jones AM: The functional role of intercoronary anastomoses. *Acta Cardiol. (Suppl.)* 11:130–144, 1965.
15. Rodriguez FL, and Robbins SL: Postmortem angiographic studies on the coronary arterial circulation: Intercoronary arterial anastomoses in adult human hearts. *Am. Heart J.* 70:348–364, 1965.
16. Fulton WFM: *The Coronary Arteries: Arteriography, Microanatomy, and Pathogenesis of Obliterative Coronary Artery Disease*. Charles C Thomas, Springfield, IL, 1965.
17. Baroldi G: Acute coronary occlusion as a cause of myocardial infarct and sudden coronary heart death. *Am. J. Cardiol.* 16:859–880, 1965.
18. Baroldi G: Myocardial infarct and sudden coronary heart death in relation to coronary occlusion and collateral circulation. *Am. Heart J.* 71:826–836, 1966.

19. Baroldi G, and Scomazzoni G: *Coronary Circulation in the Normal and the Pathologic Heart.* United States Government Printing Office, Washington, DC, 1967.
20. LeCapon J, Chelloul N, and Roujeau J: Les anastomoses inter-coronariennes. Valeur fonctionnelle et signification pathologique. *Sem. Hôp. Paris* 46:238−242, 1970.
21. Tsuchiya G: Postmortem angiographic studies on the intercoronary arterial anastomoses. Report I. Studies on intercoronary arterial anastomoses in adult human hearts and the influence on the anastomoses of strictures of the coronary arteries. *Jpn. Circ. J.* 34:1213−1220, 1970.
22. Baroldi G: Functional morphology of the anastomotic circulation in human cardiac pathology. *Meth. Achievm. Exp. Path.* 5:438−473, 1971.
23. Kato T: A comparative study of the coronary arterial structure in the left ventricular free wall in infarcted and non-infarcted human hearts. *Jpn. Circ. J.* 40: 989−1003, 1976.
24. Baroldi G: Coronary stenosis: Ischemic or nonischemic factor? *Am. Heart J.* 96:139−143, 1978.
25. Hutchins GM, Miner MM, and Bulkley BH: Tortuosity as an index of the age and diameter increase of coronary collateral vessels in patients after acute myocardial infarction. *Am. J. Cardiol.* 41:210−215, 1978.
26. Barmeyer J: Messung der Durchflusskapazität interkoronarer Anastomosen bei normalen pathologischen Herzen mit Hilfe der postmoralen Perfusion der Koronararterien. *Verh. Dtsch. Ges. Kreisslaufforsch.* 34:381−385, 1968.
27. Barmeyer J: Postmortem measurement of intercoronary anastomotic flow in normal and diseased hearts: A quantitative study. *Vasc. Surg.* 5:239−248, 1971.
28. Robbins SL, Solomon M, and Bennett A: Demonstration of intercoronary anastomoses in human hearts with a low viscosity perfusion mass. *Circulation* 33: 733−743, 1966.
29. Miller R, Mason DT, Zelis R, et al: Determinants of the coronary collateral circulation in man: Development principally related to severity of regional atherosclerosis. (abstr) *Clin. Res.* 19:117, 1971.
30. Baldighi G, Grugni A, Campiglio P, et al: Aspetti morfologici delle anastomosi coronariche nel vivente. *Minerva Med.* 63:4085−4098, 1972.
31. Heinle RA, Levy RI, and Gorlin R: Effects of factors predisposing to atherosclerosis on formation of coronary collateral vessels. *Am. J. Cardiol.* 33:12−16, 1974.
32. Valle M, Wiljasalo M, Frick MH, et al: Collateral circulation before and after coronary artery reconstruction. *Ann. Clin. Res.* 7:251−257, 1975.
33. Kober G, Kuck H, Lentz RW, and Kaltenbach M: Angiographic evidence of collateral circulation and its effect on left ventricular function in coronary heart disease. In *Coronary Heart Disease: 3rd International Symposium Frankfurt* (eds M Kaltenbach, P Lichtlen, R Balcon, and W-D Bussmann). Georg Thieme, Stuttgart, 1978, pp 48−54.
34. Jochem W, Soto B, Karp RB, et al: Radiographic anatomy of the coronary collateral circulation. *Am. J. Roentgenol.* 116:50−61, 1972.
35. Harris CN, Kaplan MA, Parker DP, et al: Anatomic and functional correlates of intercoronary collateral vessels. *Am. J. Cardiol.* 30:611−614, 1972.
36. Rabkin IK, Abugov AM, and Shabalkin BV: Assessment of collateral circulation according to selective coronarography. *Kardiologiia* 13(11): 15−19, 1973.
37. Hecht HS, Aroesty JM, Morkin E, et al: Role of the coronary collateral circulation in the preservation of left ventricular function. *Radiology* 114:305−313, 1975.
38. Schwarz F, Ensslen R, and Thormann J: Der Einfluss des Kollateralkreislaufes auf die totale und regionale Myokardfunktion bei koronarer Herzkrankheit. *Schweiz. Med. Wochenschr.* 106:1407−1412, 1976.
39. Biffani G, Santoboni A, Vricella A, and Sabatini F: Il circolo collaterale coronarico nella cardiopatia arteriosclerotica. *G. Ital. Cardiol.* 8:1279−1285, 1978.

40. Rafflenbeul W, Smith LR, Rogers WJ, et al: Quantitative coronary arteriography: Coronary anatomy of patients with unstable angina pectoris reexamined 1 year after optimal medical therapy. *Am. J. Cardiol.* 43:699−707, 1979.

41. Berger BC, Watson DD, Taylor GJ, et al: Effect of coronary collateral circulation on regional myocardial perfusion assessed with quantitative thallium-201 scintigraphy. *Am. J. Cardiol.* 46:365−370, 1980.

42. Nieminen MS, Valle M, Lassila E, et al: Global and regional left ventricular contractility and coronary collaterals in stable ischemic heart disease. *Clin. Cardiol.* 3:163−168, 1980.

43. Sheldon WC: On the significance of coronary collaterals. *Am. J. Cardiol.* 24: 303−304, 1969.

44. Gensini GG, and da Costa BCB: The coronary collateral circulation in living man. *Am. J. Cardiol.* 24:393−400, 1969.

45. Gensini GG, Esente P, Delmonico JE Jr, et al: Coronary collaterals and coronary backflow recordings in patients with coronary artery disease. A double blind angiographic-surgical correlation. (abstr) *Am. J. Cardiol.* 31:134, 1973.

46. Webb WR, Parker FB Jr, and Neville JF Jr: Retrograde pressures and flows in coronary arterial disease. *Ann. Thorac. Surg.* 15:256−262, 1973.

47. Bourassa MG, Lespérance J, and David P: Considérations sur le rôle de la circulation collatérale dans la maladie coronarienne. *Ann. Cardiol. Angéiol.* 23:473−478, 1974.

48. Levin DC: Pathways and functional significance of the coronary collateral circulation. *Circulation* 50:831−837, 1974.

49. Parker FB Jr, Neville JF Jr, Hanson EL, and Webb WR: Retrograde and antegrade pressures and flows in preinfarction syndrome. *Circulation* 50(Suppl. II):II-122−II-125, 1974.

50. Ohgitani N: Time-delay of visualization of coronary collaterals after the onset of myocardial infarction. *Jpn. Circ. J.* 41:1277−1278, 1977.

51. Aygen M: Collateral circulation and regional myocardial infarction. *Biblthca. Cardiol.* 36:136−140, 1977.

52. Neill WA, Ritzmann LW, and Selden R: The pathophysiologic basis of acute coronary insufficiency. Observations favoring the hypothesis of intermittent reversible coronary obstruction. *Am. Heart J.* 94:439−444, 1977.

53. Bourassa MG, Campeau L, and Lespérance J: Regression and appearance of coronary collaterals after aortocoronary bypass surgery. In *Coronary Heart Disease: 3rd International Symposium Frankfurt* (eds M Kaltenbach, P Lichtlen, R Balcon, and W-D Bussmann). Georg Thieme, Stuttgart, 1978, pp 40−47.

54. Hamby RI: *Clinical-Anatomical Correlates in Coronary Artery Disease.* Futura Publishing Co., Mount Kisco, NY, 1979.

55. Fuster V, Frye RL, Kennedy MA, et al: The role of collateral circulation in the various coronary syndromes. *Circulation* 59:1137−1144, 1979.

56. Iskandrian AS, Segal BL, Haaz W, and Kane S: Effects of coronary artery narrowing, collaterals, and left ventricular function on the pattern of myocardial perfusion. *Cathet. Cardiovasc. Diagn.* 6:159−172, 1980.

57. Kumar S, West D, Shahabuddin S, et al: Angiogenesis factor from human myocardial infarcts. *Lancet* 2:364−368, 1983.

58. Hamby RI: Angina pectoris: A clinical-electrocardiographic-angiographic correlative study in 510 patients. *Cardiovasc. Clin.* 8(3):79−109, 1977.

59. Mason DT, Amsterdam EA, Miller RR, et al: Consideration of the therapeutic roles of pharmacologic agents, collateral circulation and saphenous vein bypass in coronary artery disease. *Am. J. Cardiol.* 28:608−613, 1971.

60. Miller RR, Amsterdam EA, Zelis R, et al: Determinants and functional significance of the coronary collateral circulation in ischemic heart disease. In *Cardiovascular Disease: New Concepts in Diagnosis and Therapy* (ed HI Russek). University Park Press, Baltimore, 1974, pp 75−83.

61. Bartel AG, Behar VS, Peter RH, et al: Graded exercise stress tests in angiographically documented coronary artery disease. *Circulation* 49:348−356, 1974.
62. Gorlin R: Coronary collaterals. *Major Probl. Intern. Med.* 11:59−70, 1976.
63. Williams DO, Amsterdam EA, Miller RR, and Mason DT: The role of the coronary collateral circulation in acute and chronic coronary artery disease. In *Advances in Heart Disease*, Vol. 1 (ed DT Mason). Grune and Stratton, New York, 1977, pp 253−267.
64. Hamby RI, Aintablian A, and Schwartz A: Reappraisal of the functional significance of the coronary collateral circulation. *Am. J. Cardiol.* 38:305−309, 1976.
65. Flameng W, Schwarz F, and Hehrlein FW: Intraoperative evaluation of the functional significance of coronary collateral vessels in patients with coronary artery disease. *Am. J. Cardiol.* 42:187−192, 1978.
66. Flameng W, Schwarz F, Hehrlein F, and Boel A: Functional significance of coronary collaterals in man. *Basic Res. Cardiol.* 73:188−199, 1978.
67. Flameng W, Schwarz F, Schaper W, and Hehrlein F: Functional significance of coronary collaterals. In *Coronary Heart Disease: 3rd International Symposium Frankfurt* (eds M Kaltenbach, P Lichtlen, R Balcon, and W-D Bussmann). Georg Thieme, Stuttgart, 1978, pp 67−72.
68. Helfant RH, Kemp HG, and Gorlin R: Coronary atherosclerosis, coronary collaterals, and their relation to cardiac function. *Ann. Intern. Med.* 73:189−193, 1970.
69. Bopp P, Fournet PC, Simonin P, et al: La coronarographie sélective percutanée: À propos de 600 examens. *Arch. Mal. Coeur* 68:591−597, 1975.
70. Bemis CE, Gorlin R, Kemp HG, and Herman MV: Progression of coronary artery disease: A clinical arteriographic study. *Circulation* 47:455−464, 1973.
71. Kimbiris D, Lavine P, Van Den Broek H, et al: Devolutionary pattern of coronary atherosclerosis in patients with angina pectoris: Coronary arteriographic studies. *Am. J. Cardiol.* 33:7−11, 1974.
72. Markis JE, Joffee CD, Roberts BH, et al: Evolution of left ventricular dysfunction in coronary artery disease: Serial cineangiographic studies without surgery. *Circulation* 62:141−148, 1980.
73. Kimbiris D, and Segal BL: Coronary disease progression in patients with and without saphenous vein bypass surgery. *Am. Heart J.* 102:811−818, 1981.
74. Bourassa MG, Goulet C, and Lespérance J: Progression of coronary arterial disease after aortocoronary bypass grafts. *Circulation* 48(Suppl. III):III-127−III-131, 1973.
75. Rafflenbeul W, Urthaler F, Lichtlen P, and James TN: Quantitative difference in "critical" stenosis between right and left coronary artery in man. *Circulation* 62:1188−1196, 1980.
76. Paulin S: Interarterial coronary anastomoses in relation to arterial obstruction demonstrated in coronary arteriography. *Invest. Radiol.* 2:147−159, 1967.
77. Vigorita VJ, Moore GW, and Hutchins GM: Absence of correlation between coronary arterial atherosclerosis and severity or duration of diabetes mellitus of adult onset. *Am. J. Cardiol.* 46:535−542, 1980.
78. Goldstein RE, Stinson EB, Scherer JL, et al: Intraoperative coronary collateral function in patients with coronary occlusive disease: Nitroglycerin responsiveness and angiographic correlations. *Circulation* 49:298−308, 1974.
79. Feldman RL, and Pepine CJ: Evaluation of coronary collateral circulation in conscious humans. *Am. J. Cardiol.* 53:1233−1238, 1984.
80. Kolibash AJ, Bush CA, Wepsic RA, et al: Coronary collateral vessels: Spectrum of physiologic capabilities with respect to providing rest and stress myocardial perfusion, maintenance of left ventricular function and protection against infarction. *Am. J. Cardiol.* 50:230−238, 1982.
81. Goldstein RE, Michaelis LL, Morrow AG, and Epstein SE: Coronary collateral

function in patients without occlusive coronary artery disease. *Circulation* 51:118−125, 1975.

82. Zimmerman HA: The coronary circulation in patients with severe emphysema, cor pulmonale, cyanotic congenital heart disease, and severe anemia. *Dis. Chest* 22:269−273, 1952.

83. Cheng TO: Arteriographic demonstration of intercoronary arterial anastomosis in a living man without coronary artery disease. *Angiology* 23:76−88, 1972.

84. Gregg DE, and Fisher LC: Blood supply to the heart. In *Handbook of Physiology: Section 2: Circulation*, Vol. II. American Physiological Society, Washington, DC, 1963, p 1570.

85. Pitt B: Interarterial coronary anastomoses: Occurrence in normal hearts and in certain pathologic conditions. *Circulation* 20:816−822, 1959.

86. Laurie W, and Woods JD: Anastomosis in the coronary circulation. *Lancet* 2:812−816, 1958.

87. Pepler WJ, and Meyer BJ: Interarterial coronary anastomoses and coronary arterial pattern: A comparative study of South African Bantu and European hearts. *Circulation* 22:14−24, 1960.

88. Laurie W, and Woods JD: Interarterial coronary anastomoses in three race groups. *Lancet* 1:13−17, 1962.

89. Bloor CM, Keefe JF, and Browne MJ: Intercoronary anastomoses in congenital heart disease. *Circulation* 33:227−231, 1966.

90. Marcus ML, Doty DB, Hiratzka LF, et al: Decreased coronary reserve: A mechanism for angina pectoris in patients with aortic stenosis and normal coronary arteries. *N. Engl. J. Med.* 307:1362−1366, 1982.

91. Hellerstein HK, Horsten TR, Goldbarg A, et al: The influence of active conditioning upon subjects with coronary artery disease: Cardiorespiratory changes during training in 67 patients. *Can. Med. Assoc. J.* 96:758−759, 1967.

92. Frick MH, and Katila M: Hemodynamic consequences of physical training after myocardial infarction. *Circulation* 37:192−202, 1968.

93. Detry J-M, and Bruce RA: Effects of physical training on exertional S-T-segment depression in coronary heart disease. *Circulation* 44:390−396, 1971.

94. Redwood DR, Rosing DR, and Epstein SE: Circulatory and symptomatic effects of physical training in patients with coronary-artery disease and angina pectoris. *N. Engl. J. Med.* 286:959−965, 1972.

95. Conner JF, LaCamera F Jr, Swanick EJ, et al: Effects of exercise on coronary collateralization—Angiographic studies of six patients in a supervised exercise program. *Med. Sci. Sports* 8:145−151, 1976.

96. Kennedy CC, Spiekerman RE, Lindsay MI Jr, et al: One-year graduated exercise program for men with angina pectoris: Evaluation by physiologic studies and coronary arteriography. *Mayo Clin. Proc.* 51:231−236, 1976.

97. Clausen JP, and Trap-Jensen J: Heart rate and arterial blood pressure during exercise in patients with angina pectoris: Effects of training and of nitroglycerin. *Circulation* 53:436−442, 1976.

98. Clausen JP: Circulatory adjustments to dynamic exercise and effect of physical training in normal subjects and in patients with coronary artery disease. *Prog. Cardiovasc. Dis.* 18:459−495, 1976.

99. Ari EB, Kellermann JJ, Lapitod C, et al: Effect of prolonged intensive training on cardiorespiratory response in patients with angina pectoris. *Br. Heart J.* 40: 1143−1148, 1978.

100. Ferguson RJ, Côté P, Gauthier P, and Bourassa MG: Changes in exercise coronary sinus blood flow with training in patients with angina pectoris. *Circulation* 58:41−47, 1978.

101. Nolewajka AJ, Kostuk WJ, Rechnitzer PA, and Cunningham DA: Exercise and human collateralization: An angiographic and scintigraphic assessment. *Circulation* 60:114−121, 1979.

102. Raffo JA, Luksic IY, Kappagoda CT, et al: Effects of physical training on myocardial ischaemia in patients with coronary artery disease. *Br. Heart J.* 43: 262−269, 1980.

103. Ehsani AA, Heath GW, Hagberg JM, et al: Effects of 12 months of intense exercise training on ischemic ST-segment depression in patients with coronary artery disease. *Circulation* 64:1116−1124, 1981.

104. Kattus AA, and MacAlpin RN: Role of exercise in discovery, evaluation, and management of ischemic heart disease. *Cardiovasc. Clin.* 1(2):255−279, 1969.

105. Kattus AA, and Grollman J: Patterns of coronary collateral circulation in angina pectoris: Relation to exercise training. In *Changing Concepts in Cardiovascular Disease* (eds HI Russek and BL Zohman). Williams & Wilkins Co, Baltimore, 1972, pp 352−376.

106. Ferguson RJ, Petitclerc R, Choquette G, et al: Effect of physical training on treadmill exercise capacity, collateral circulation and progression of coronary disease. *Am. J. Cardiol.* 34:764−769, 1974.

107. Sim DN, and Neill WA: Investigation of the physiological basis for increased exercise threshold for angina pectoris after physical conditioning. *J. Clin. Invest.* 54:763−770, 1974.

108. Barmeyer J: Physical activity and coronary collateral development. *Adv. Cardiol.* 18:104−112, 1976.

109. Verani MS, Hartung GH, Hoepfel-Harris J, et al: Effects of exercise training on left ventricular performance and myocardial perfusion in patients with coronary artery disease. *Am. J. Cardiol.* 47:797−803, 1981.

110. Bhan AK, and Scheuer J: Effects of physical training on cardiac actomyosin adenosine triphosphatase activity. *Am. J. Physiol.* 223:1486−1490, 1972.

111. Bhan AK, and Scheuer J: Effects of physical training on cardiac myosin ATPase activity. *Am. J. Physiol.* 228:1178−1182, 1975.

112. Froelicher V, Jensen D, Atwood JE, et al: Cardiac rehabilitation: Evidence for improvement in myocardial perfusion and function. *Arch. Phys. Med. Rehabil.* 61:517−522, 1980.

113. Schaper W: *The Collateral Circulation of the Heart.* North-Holland Publishing Company, Amsterdam, 1971.

114. Mason DT, and Braunwald E: The effects of nitroglycerin and amyl nitrite on arteriolar and venous tone in the human forearm. *Circulation* 32:755−766, 1965.

115. Lochner W: Present basis of coronary therapy. In *2nd International Adalat Symposium: New Therapy of Ischemic Heart Disease* (eds W Lochner, W Braasch, and G Kroneberg). Springer-Verlag, Berlin, 1975, pp 2−10.

116. Bernstein L, Friesinger GC, Lichtlen PR, and Ross RS: The effect of nitroglycerin on the systemic and coronary circulation in man and dogs: Myocardial blood flow measured with Xenon[133]. *Circulation* 33:107−116, 1966.

117. Carson RP, Wilson WS, Nemiroff MJ, and Weber WJ: The effects of sublingual nitroglycerin on myocardial blood flow in patients with coronary artery disease or myocardial hypertrophy. *Am. Heart J.* 77:579−584, 1969.

118. Parker JO, West RO, and Di Giorgi S: The effect of nitroglycerin on coronary blood flow and the hemodynamic response to exercise in coronary artery disease. *Am. J. Cardiol.* 27:59−65, 1971.

119. Winbury MM, Howe BB, and Hefner MA: Effect of nitrates and other coronary dilators on large and small coronary vessels: An hypothesis for the mechanism of action of nitrates. *J. Pharmacol. Exp. Therap.* 168:70−95, 1969.

120. McGregor M: The nitrates and myocardial ischemia. *Circulation* 66:689−692, 1982.

121. Gensini GG: Coronary circulation in patients with and without coronary artery disease and the effects of chewable isosorbide dinitrate. *G. Ital. Cardiol.* 5:714−723, 1975.

122. Lichtlen P, Halter J, and Gattiker K: The effect of isosorbiddinitrate on coronary

blood flow, coronary resistance and left ventricular dynamics under exercise in patients with coronary artery disease. *Basic Res. Cardiol.* 69:402−421, 1974.

123. Cohn PF, Maddox D, Holman BL, et al: Effect of sublingually administered nitroglycerin on regional myocardial blood flow in patients with coronary artery disease. *Am. J. Cardiol.* 39:672−678, 1977.

124. Horwitz LD, Gorlin R, Taylor WJ, and Kemp HG: Effect of nitroglycerin on regional myocardial blood flow in coronary artery disease. *J. Clin. Invest.* 50:1578−1584, 1971.

125. Klein RC, Grehl TM, Stengert KB, and Mason DT: Evaluation of the effects of systemic nitroglycerin on perfusion of ischemic myocardium in coronary heart disease assessed intraoperatively by antegrade blood flow through intact saphenous vein bypass grafts. *Am. Heart J.* 101:292−299, 1981.

126. Wald RW, Sternberg L, Feiglin DHI, and Morch JE: Effect of intracoronary glyceryl trinitrate on perfusion distribution in the collateralised human myocardium. *Br. Heart J.* 44:175−178, 1980.

127. Lichtlen PR, Engel H-J, and Hundeshagen H: Regional myocardial blood flow in normal and poststenotic areas after nitroglycerin, betablockade (atenolol), coronary dilatation (dipyridamole), and calcium antagonism (nifedipine). *Herz* 2: 81−86, 1977.

128. Stone DL, Stephens JD, and Banim SO: Coronary haemodynamic effects of nifedipine: Comparison with glyceryl trinitrate. *Br. Heart J.* 49:442−446, 1983.

129. Ganz W, and Marcus HS: Failure of intracoronary nitroglycerin to alleviate pacing-induced angina. *Circulation* 46:880−889, 1972.

130. Flaherty JT, Reid PR, Kelly DT, et al: Intravenous nitroglycerin in acute myocardial infarction. *Circulation* 51:132−139, 1975.

131. Borer JS, Redwood DR, Levitt B, et al: Reduction in myocardial ischemia with nitroglycerin or nitroglycerin plus phenylephrine administered during acute myocardial infarction. *N. Engl. J. Med.* 293:1008−1012, 1975.

132. Chiariello M, Gold HK, Leinbach RC, et al: Comparison between the effects of nitroprusside and nitroglycerin on ischemic injury during acute myocardial infarction. *Circulation* 54:766−773, 1976.

133. Foulds T, and MacKinnon J: Controlled double-blind trial of "Persantin" in treatment of angina pectoris. *Br. Med. J.* 2:835, 1960.

134. Kinsella D, Troup W, and McGregor M: Studies with a new coronary vasodilator drug: Persantin. *Am. Heart J.* 63:146−151, 1962.

135. Newhouse MT, and McGregor M: Long term dipyridamole therapy of angina pectoris. *Am. J. Cardiol.* 16:234−237, 1965.

136. Sbar S, and Schlant RC: Dipyridamole in the treatment of angina pectoris: A double-blind evaluation. *JAMA* 201:865−867, 1967.

137. Hilger HH: Experimentelle Prüfung der Wirkung von Coronardilatatoren am Menschen. *Naunyn Schmiedeberg Arch. Pharm.* 263:168−184, 1969.

138. Mantero O, and Conti F: A paradoxical clinical response to dipyridamole. In *Pharmacological and Clinical Approach to the Detection and Evaluation of New Circulatory Drugs* (ed. A Bertelli). North-Holland Publishing, Amsterdam, 1969, pp 118−123.

139. Hilger HH: The influence of coronary vasodilators on coronary blood flow in man. *Brux. Med.* 50:557−565, 1970.

140. Wilcken DEL, Paoloni HJ, and Eikens E: Evidence for intravenous dipyridamole (Persantin) producing a "coronary steal" effect in the ischaemic myocardium. *Aust. N.Z. J. Med.* 1:8−14, 1971.

141. Tauchert M, Behrenbeck DW, Hötzel J, and Hilger HH: Ein neuer pharmakologischer Test zur Diagnose der Koronarinsuffizienz. *Dtsch. Med. Wochenschr.* 101:35−37, 1976.

142. Gould KL, Westcott RJ, Albro PC, and Hamilton GW: Noninvasive assessment of coronary stenoses by myocardial imaging during pharmacologic coronary vaso-

dilatation. II. Clinical methodology and feasibility. *Am. J. Cardiol.* 41:279—287, 1978.

143. Albro PC, Gould KL, Westcott RJ, et al: Noninvasive assessment of coronary stenoses by myocardial imaging during pharmacologic coronary vasodilatation. III. Clinical Trial. *Am. J. Cardiol.* 42:751—760, 1978.

144. Demangeat JL, Constantinesco A, Mossard JM, et al: Evaluation of myocardial perfusion and left ventricular function by ^{201}Tl scintigraphy after dipyridamole. *Eur. J. Nucl. Med.* 6:491—503, 1981.

145. Josephson MA, Brown BG, Hecht HS, et al: Noninvasive detection and localization of coronary stenoses in patients: Comparison of resting dipyridamole and exercise thallium-201 myocardial perfusion imaging. *Am. Heart J.* 103:1008—1018, 1982.

146. Lichtlen P, Engel HJ, Amende I, et al: Mechanisms of various antianginal drugs. Relationship between regional flow behavior and contractility. In *3rd International Adalat Symposium: New Therapy of Ischemic Heart Disease* (eds AD Jatene and PR Lichtlen). Excerpta Medica, Amsterdam, 1976, pp 14—29.

147. Wolf R, Engel H-J, Hundeshagen H, and Lichtlen P: Collateral myocardial blood flow at rest and after maximal arteriolar dilatation in patients with ischemic heart disease. In *Coronary Heart Disease: 3rd International Symposium Frankfurt* (eds M Kaltenbach, P Lichtlen, R Balcon, and W-D Bussmann). Georg Thieme, Stuttgart, 1978, pp 61—65.

148. Roberts LN, Villanueva M, Babacan BC, and Mason GP: A study of the effect of dipyridamole on the coronary circulation in man. (abstr) *Can. Med. Assoc. J.* 98:113, 1968.

149. Guiha NH, Cohn JN, Mikulic E, et al: Treatment of refractory heart failure with infusion of nitroprusside. *N. Engl. J. Med.* 291:587—592, 1974.

150. Franciosa JA, Guiha NH, Limas CJ, et al: Improved left ventricular function during nitroprusside infusion in acute myocardial infarction. *Lancet* 1:650—654, 1972.

151. Mann T, Cohn PF, Holman BL, et al: Effect of nitroprusside on regional myocardial blood flow in coronary artery disease: Results in 25 patients and comparison with nitroglycerin. *Circulation* 57:732—738, 1978.

152. Brown TM, Matthews OP, and Walter PF: Assessment of the effect of vasodilator therapy upon hemodynamics and ischemic injury in acute anterior myocardial infarction. (abstr) *Am. J. Cardiol.* 37:123, 1976.

153. Armstrong PW, Boroomand K, and Parker JO: Nitroprusside in acute myocardial infarction: Correlative effects on hemodynamics and precordial mapping. (abstr) *Circulation* 54 (Suppl. II):II-76, 1976.

154. Miller RR, Vismara LA, Williams DO, et al: Effects of ventricular unloading by nitroprusside on myocardial energetics and coronary blood flow in patients with ischemic heart disease. (abstr) *Circulation* 52(Suppl. II):II-217, 1975.

155. Feldman RL, Whittle JL, Pepine CJ, and Conti CR: Comparison of effects of nitroprusside and nitroglycerin on coronary collateral function. (abstr) *Circulation* 62(Suppl. III):III-127, 1980.

156. Fleckenstein A: On the basic pharmacological mechanism of nifedipine and its relation to therapeutic efficacy. In *3rd International Adalat Symposium: New Therapy of Ischemic Heart Disease* (eds AD Jatene and PR Lichtlen). Excerpta Medica, Amsterdam, 1976, pp 1—13.

157. Vatner SF, and Hintze TH: Effects of a calcium-channel antagonist on large and small coronary arteries in conscious dogs. *Circulation* 66:579—588, 1982.

158. Lichtlen PR, Engel H-J, Wolf R, and Pretschner P: Regional myocardial blood flow in patients with coronary artery disease after nifedipine. In *International Adalat Panel Discussion: New Experimental and Clinical Results* (eds PR Lichtlen, E Kimura, and N Taira). Excerpta Medica, Amsterdam, 1979, pp 69—85.

159. Engel H-J, Wolf R, Hundeshagen H, and Lichtlen PR: Different effects of nitroglycerin and nifedipine on regional myocardial blood flow during pacing induced angina pectoris. *Eur. Heart J.* 1(Suppl. B):53—58, 1980.

160. Lichtlen P: Coronary and left ventricular dynamics under nifedipine in comparison to nitrates, beta-blocking agents and dipyridamole. In *2nd International Adalat Symposium: New Therapy of Ischemic Heart Disease* (eds W Lochner, W Braasch, and G Kroneberg). Springer Verlag, Berlin, 1975, pp 212−224.

161. Mueller H, Ayres SM, Conklin EF, et al: The effects of intra-aortic counterpulsation on cardiac performance and metabolism in shock associated with acute myocardial infarction. *J. Clin. Invest.* 50:1885−1900, 1971.

162. Leinbach RC, Buckley MJ, Austen WG, et al: Effects of intra-aortic balloon pumping on coronary flow and metabolism in man. *Circulation* 43(Suppl. I):I-77−I-81, 1971.

163. Williams DO, Korr KS, Gewirtz H, and Most AS: The effect of intraaortic balloon counterpulsation on regional myocardial blood flow and oxygen consumption in the presence of coronary artery stenosis in patients with unstable angina. *Circulation* 66:593−597, 1982.

164. Fuchs RM, Brin KP, Brinker JA, et al: Augmentation of regional coronary blood flow by intra-aortic balloon counterpulsation in patients with unstable angina. *Circulation* 68:117−123, 1983.

165. Day SB, and Lillehei CW: Experimental basis for a new operation for coronary artery disease: A left atrial-pulmonary artery shunt to encourage the development of interarterial intercoronary anastomoses. *Surgery* 45:487−495, 1959.

166. Thompson SA, and Raisbeck MJ: Cardio-pericardiopexy; The surgical treatment of coronary arterial disease by the establishment of adhesive pericarditis. *Ann. Intern. Med.* 16:495−520, 1942.

167. Thompson SA, and Plachta A: Fourteen years' experience with cardiopexy in the treatment of coronary artery disease. *J. Thorac. Surg.* 27:64−71, 1954.

168. Plachta A, Thompson SA, and Speer FD: Pericardial and myocardial vascularization following cardiopericardiopexy: Magnesium silicate technique. *Arch. Pathol.* 59:151−161, 1955.

169. Thompson SA, and Raisbeck MJ: The surgical rehabilitation of the coronary cripple. *Ann. Intern. Med.* 31:1010−1018, 1949.

170. Beck CS: Further data on the establishment of a new blood supply to the heart by operation. *J. Thorac. Surg.* 5:604−611, 1936.

171. Beck CS: Coronary sclerosis and angina pectoris: Treatment by grafting a new blood supply upon the myocardium. *Surg. Gynecol. Obstet.* 64:270−272, 1937.

172. Beck CS: The coronary operation. *Am. Heart J.* 22:539−544, 1941.

173. Feil H, and Beck CS: Coronary sclerosis and angina pectoris: Report of thirty patients treated by the Beck operation. *J. Thorac. Surg.* 10:529−540, 1941.

174. O'Shaughnessy L: Surgical treatment of cardiac ischaemia. *Lancet* 1:185−194, 1937.

175. Strieder JW: Discussion of coronary sclerosis and angina pectoris. *J. Thorac. Surg.* 10:540, 1941.

176. Mason GA: Myocardial ischaemia and its surgical relief. *Lancet* 1:359−367, 1951.

177. Beck CS, and Leighninger DS: Operations for coronary artery disease. *JAMA* 156:1226−1233, 1954.

178. Beck CS, and Leighninger DS: Operations for coronary artery disease. *Ann. Surg.* 141:24−37, 1955.

179. Beck CS, and Leighninger DS: Scientific basis for the surgical treatment of coronary artery disease. *JAMA* 159:1264−1271, 1955.

180. Vineberg A, Munro DD, Cohen H, and Buller W: Four years' clinical experience with internal mammary artery implantation in the treatment of human coronary artery insufficiency including additional experimental studies. *J. Thorac. Surg.* 29:1−32, 1955.

181. Leighninger DS: A laboratory and clinical evaluation of operations for coronary artery disease. *J. Thorac. Surg.* 30:397−410, 1955.

182. Beck CS, and Brofman BL: The surgical management of coronary artery disease: Background, rationale, clinical experiences. *Ann. Intern. Med.* 45:975−988, 1956.

183. Beck CS: Symposium on coronary artery disease: Blood supply to ischaemic myocardium distal to the occlusion of a coronary artery. *Dis. Chest* 31:243–252, 1957.
184. Brofman BL: Surgical treatment of coronary artery disease: Medical management and evaluation of results. *Dis. Chest* 31:253–264, 1957.
185. Beck CS, Leighninger DS, Brofman BL, and Bond JF: Some new concepts of coronary heart disease: Results after surgical operation. *JAMA* 168:2110–2117, 1958.
186. Carter BN: Discussion of revascularization of the heart. *Ann. Surg.* 128:861–862, 1948.
187. Harken DE, Black H, Dickson JF III, and Wilson HE III: De-epicardialization: A simple, effective surgical treatment for angina pectoris. *Circulation* 12:955–962, 1955.
188. Vineberg A: Experimental background of myocardial revascularization by internal mammary artery implantation and supplementary technics, with its clinical application in 125 patients: A review and critical appraisal. *Ann. Surg.* 159:185–207, 1964.
189. Vineberg AM, Shanks J, Pifarré R, et al: Myocardial revascularization by omental graft without pedicle: Experimental background and report on 25 cases followed 6 to 16 months. *J. Thorac. Cardiovasc. Surg.* 49:103–126, 1965.
190. Vineberg A: Revascularization of the right and left coronary arterial systems: Internal mammary artery implantation, epicardiectomy and free omental graft operation. *Am. J. Cardiol.* 19:344–353, 1967.
191. Favaloro RG, Effler DB, Groves LK, et al: Myocardial revascularization by internal mammary artery implant procedures: Clinical experience. *J. Thorac. Cardiovasc. Surg.* 54:359–368, 1967.
192. Vineberg A., and Deliyannis TD: The sponge operation for myocardial revascularization: An experimental study. *Can. Med. Assoc. J.* 78:610–612, 1958.
193. Fieschi D: Criteri anatomo fisiologici per intervento chirurgico lieve in malati di Infarto di Cuore e di Angina Pectoris. *Arch. Ital. Chir.* 63:303–312, 1942.
194. Battezzati M, Tagliaferro A, and De Marchi G: La legatura delle due arterie mammarie interne nei disturbi di vascolarizzazione del miocardio: Nota preventiva relativa ai primi dati sperimentali e clinici. *Minerva Med.* 46:1178–1188, 1955.
195. De Marchi G, Battezzati M, and Tagliaferro A: Influenze della legatura delle arterie mammarie interne sulla insufficienza miocardica. *Minerva Med.* 47:1184–1195, 1956.
196. Glover RP, Davila JC, Kyle RH, et al: Ligation of the internal mammary arteries as a means of increasing blood supply to the myocardium. *J. Thorac. Surg.* 34:661–678, 1957.
197. Maccarini PA, and Frezza S: La rivascolarizzazione del cuore nelle cardiopatie anossiche, infartuali e non infartuali mediante legatura delle arterie mammarie interne. *G. Clin. Med.* 38:1201–1214, 1957.
198. Jelinek R, and Quitzow G: Beitrag zur chirurgischen Behandlung der Angina pectoris. *Wien. Klin. Wochenschr.* 70:3–6, 1958.
199. Knighton JE: Internal mammary artery ligation in cardiac disease. *J. La. State Med. Soc.* 110:251–256, 1958.
200. Glover RP, Kitchell JR, Kyle RH, et al: Experience with myocardial revascularization by division of the internal mammary arteries. *Dis. Chest* 33:637–657, 1958.
201. Kitchell JR, Glover RP, and Kyle RH: Bilateral internal mammary artery ligation for angina pectoris: Preliminary clinical considerations. *Am. J. Cardiol.* 1:46–50, 1958.
202. Battezzati M, Tagliaferro A, and Cattaneo AD: Clinical evaluation of bilateral internal mammary artery ligation as treatment of coronary heart disease. *Am. J. Cardiol.* 4:180–183, 1959.
203. Matoba S, Kitamura K, Yamakawa K, and Anazawa Y: Clinical evaluation of

internal mammary artery ligation as a treatment of coronary heart disease. *Jpn. Heart J.* 2:473−486, 1961.

204. Fish RG, Crymes TP, and Lovell MG: Internal-mammary-artery ligation for angina pectoris: Its failure to produce relief. *N. Engl. J. Med.* 259:418−420, 1958.

205. Adams R: Internal-mammary-artery ligation for coronary insufficiency: An evaluation. *N. Engl. J. Med.* 258:113−115, 1958.

206. Dimond EG, Kittle CF, and Crockett JE: Evaluation of internal mammary artery ligation and sham procedure in angina pectoris. (abstr) *Circulation* 18:712−713, 1958.

207. Cobb LA, Thomas GI, Dillard DH, et al: An evaluation of internal-mammary-artery ligation by a double-blind technic. *N. Engl. J. Med.* 260:1115−1118, 1959.

208. Rowe GG, Maxwell GM, Castillo CA, et al: Evaluation of the effect of bilateral internal-mammary-artery ligation on cardiac output and coronary blood flow. *N. Engl. J. Med.* 261:653−655, 1959.

209. Glover RP, Kitchell JR, Davila JC, and Barkley HT Jr: Clinical and experimental study of bilateral internal mammary artery ligation (Bimal) for the relief of angina pectoris. (abstr) *Circulation* 20:701−702, 1959.

210. Beck CS: Revascularization of the heart. *Ann. Surg.* 128:854−861, 1948.

211. Beck CS, Hahn RS, Leighninger DS, and McAllister FF: Operation for coronary artery disease. *JAMA* 147:1726−1731, 1951.

212. Bailey CP, Truex RC, Angulo AW, et al: The anatomic (histologic) basis and efficient clinical surgical technique for the restoration of the coronary circulation. *J. Thorac. Surg.* 25:143−168, 1953.

213. Bailey CP, Geckeler GD, Truex RC, et al: Arterialization of the coronary sinus. *JAMA* 151:441−449, 1953.

214. Sewell WH: A basic physiological approach to myocardial revascularization. *Conn. Med.* 27:76−78, 1963.

215. Sewell WH: Physiological background, coronary arteriography, and the pedicle operation for coronary arterial insufficiency. *J. Natl. Med. Assoc.* 55:299−305, 1963.

216. Smith S, Beasley M, Hodes R, et al: Auxiliary myocardial vascularization by prosthetic graft implantation. *Surg. Gynecol. Obstet.* 104:263−268, 1957.

217. Vineberg A, and Walker J: Six months' to six years' experience with coronary artery insufficiency treated by internal mammary artery implantation. *Am. Heart J.* 54:851−862, 1957.

218. Bigelow WG, Basian H, and Trusler GA: Internal mammary artery implantation for coronary heart disease: A clinical follow-up study one to eight years after operation. *J. Thorac. Cardiovasc. Surg.* 45:67−78, 1963.

219. Sewell WH, and Sealy WC: Coronary cinearteriography and pedicle operation in diagnosis and treatment of coronary insufficiency. *Surgery* 55:99−104, 1964.

220. Sewell WH, Sones FM Jr, Fish RG, et al: The pedicle operation for coronary insufficiency: Technique and preliminary results. *J. Thorac. Cardiovasc. Surg.* 49:317−329, 1965.

221. Gorlin R, and Taylor WJ: Selective revascularization of the myocardium by internal-mammary-artery implant. *N. Engl. J. Med.* 275:283−290, 1966.

222. Bigelow WG, Aldridge HE, and MacGregor DC: Internal mammary implantation (Vineberg operation) for coronary heart disease: Cineangiography and long-term follow up. *Ann. Surg.* 164:457−464, 1966.

223. Sewell WH: Results of 122 mammary pedicle implantations for angina pectoris. *Ann. Thorac. Surg.* 2:17−30, 1966.

224. Sewell WH: Evaluation of vascular implants for coronary insufficiency. *Ann. Thorac. Surg.* 3:439−445, 1967.

225. Taylor WJ, and Gorlin R: Objective criteria for internal mammary artery implantation. *Ann. Thorac. Surg.* 4:143−149, 1967.

226. Groves LK: Discussion of objective criteria for internal mammary artery implantation. *Ann. Thorac. Surg.* 4:149−150, 1967.

227. Kay EB, and Suzuki A: Myocardial revascularization by bilateral internal mammary artery implantation: Experimental and clinical data. *Am. J. Cardiol.* 22: 227–234, 1968.
228. Gorlin R: Myocardial revascularization by internal mammary artery implantation. *Bull. N.Y. Acad. Med.* 44:994–1011, 1968.
229. Yates AK: Myocardial revascularization: A review. *Guys Hosp. Rep.* 118:21–29, 1969.
230. Kassebaum DG, Judkins MP, and Griswold HE: Stress electrocardiography in the evaluation of surgical revascularization of the heart. *Circulation* 40:297–313, 1969.
231. Balcon R, Leaver D, Ross D, et al: Clinical evaluation of internal mammary-artery implantation. *Lancet* 1:440–443, 1970.
232. Saksena DS, and Liddle HV: Late results of myocardial revascularization. *Ann. Thorac. Surg.* 10:132–137, 1970.
233. Kemp HG, Manchester JH, Amsterdam EA, et al: Internal mammary artery implantation: Effect on myocardial lactate utilization. *Circulation* 41(Suppl. II):II-55–II-62, 1970.
234. Langston MF Jr, Kerth WJ, Selzer A, and Cohn KE: Evaluation of internal mammary artery implantation. *Am. J. Cardiol.* 29:788–792, 1972.
235. Vineberg A: Evidence that revascularization by ventricular-internal mammary artery implants increases longevity: Twenty-four year, nine month follow-up. *J. Thorac. Cardiovasc. Surg.* 70:381–394, 1975.
236. Effler DB, Groves LK, Sones FM Jr, and Shirey EK: Increased myocardial perfusion by internal mammary artery implant: Vineberg's operation. *Ann. Surg.* 158: 526–534, 1963.
237. Effler DB, Sones FM Jr, Groves LK, and Suarez E: Myocardial revascularization by Vineberg's internal mammary artery implant: Evaluation of postoperative results. *J. Thorac. Cardiovasc. Surg.* 50:527–531, 1965.
238. Sewell WH: Comparison of single and triple pedicle implantation for myocardial revascularization. *Ann. Thorac. Surg.* 8:274–280, 1969.
239. McCallister BD, Richmond DR, Saltups A, et al: Left ventricular hemodynamics before and 1 year after internal mammary artery implantation in patients with coronary artery disease and angina pectoris. *Circulation* 42:471–477, 1970.
240. Dart CH Jr, Kato Y, Scott SM, et al: Internal thoracic (mammary) arteriography: A questionable index of myocardial revascularization. *J. Thorac. Cardiovasc. Surg.* 59:117–127, 1970.
241. Razavi M, Heupler FA, Germanovich E, et al: Long-term clinical and angiographic results in bilateral internal mammary artery implants. (abstr) *Circulation* 46(Suppl. II):II-208, 1972.
242. Sewell WH: Relationships between coronary deaths and collateral from mammary artery pedicles. *Ann. Thorac. Surg.* 9:301–306, 1970.
243. Bloomer WE: Discussion of comparison of single and triple pedicle implantation for myocardial revascularization. *Ann. Thorac. Surg.* 8:280–281, 1969.
244. Kemp GL, Ellestad MH, Beland AJ, and Allen WH: The maximal treadmill stress test for the evaluation of medical and surgical treatment of coronary insufficiency. *J. Thorac. Cardiovasc. Surg.* 57:708–713, 1969.
245. Kay EB, Demaney M, Tambe AA, et al: Internal mammary artery revascularization: Fact or fantasy? *Chest* 64:227–234, 1973.
246. Kay EB, McLaughlin EE, and Suzuki A: Preliminary studies on postoperative volume flows after bilateral internal mammary artery implantation. *Am. J. Cardiol.* 22:235–241, 1968.
247. Sethi GK, Scott SM, and Takaro T: Myocardial revascularization by internal thoracic arterial implants: Longterm follow-up. *Chest* 64:235–240, 1973.
248. Takaro T: Discussion of evidence that revascularization by ventricular-internal mammary artery implants increases longevity: Twenty-four year, nine month follow-up. *J. Thorac. Cardiovasc. Surg.* 70:394, 1975.

249. Dart CH Jr, Scott S, Fish R, and Takaro T: Direct blood flow studies of clinical internal thoracic (mammary) arterial implants. *Circulation* 41(Suppl. II):II-64−II-71, 1970.

250. Rösch J, Dotter CT, and Starr A: Selektive Koronararteriographie und aortenkoronare Gefäss-Bypass-Plastik. *Fortschr. Geb. Rontgenstr. Nuklearmed Erganzungsband* 116:607−616, 1972.

251. Valle M: Postoperative coronary angiography. *Acta Radiol. Suppl.* 333:1−67, 1973.

252. Glassman E, Spencer FC, Krauss KR, et al: Changes in the underlying coronary circulation secondary to bypass grafting. *Circulation* 50(Suppl. II):II-80−II-83, 1974.

253. Bourassa MG, Solignac A, Goulet C, and Lespérance J: Regression and appearance of coronary collaterals in humans during life. *Circulation* 50(Suppl. II): II-127−II-134, 1974.

254. DiLuzio V, Roy PR, Sowton E, and Dow J: Fate of coronary collateral circulation after aorto-coronary saphenous vein bypass grafts. *Br. Heart J.* 37:397−400, 1975.

255. Frick MH, Harjola P-T, and Valle M: Effect of aorto-coronary grafts and native vessel patency on the occurrence of angina pectoris after coronary bypass surgery. *Br. Heart J.* 37:414−419, 1975.

256. McLaughlin PR, Berman ND, Morton BC, et al: Saphenous vein bypass grafting: Changes in native circulation and collaterals. *Circulation* 52(Suppl. I):I-66−I-70, 1975.

257. See JR, Marlon AM, Feikes HL, and Cosby RS: Effect of direct revascularization surgery on coronary collateral circulation in man. *Am. J. Cardiol.* 36:734−738, 1975.

258. Uflacker R, and Enge I: The bahavior of collateral circulation after coronary artery bypass surgery. *Cardiovasc. Radiol.* 1:225−227, 1978.

259. Levin DC, Beckmann CF, Sos TA, and Sniderman K: The effect of coronary artery bypass on collateral circulation. *Radiology* 141:317−322, 1981.

260. Grüntzig A, Pyle R, Goebel N, and Schlumpf M: The fate of collaterals after percutaneous transluminal coronary angioplasty (PTCA). (abstr) *Circulation* 62(Suppl. III):III-161, 1980.

261. Siepser SL, Kaltman AJ, Mills N, et al: Coronary collateral flow after traumatic fistula between right coronary artery and right atrium. *N. Engl. J. Med.* 287:754−756, 1972.

262. Kattus A: Relation of coronary events to spasm of coronary arteries, precariousness of obstructive lesions and availability of collateral channels. In *Current Topics in Coronary Research: Advances in Experimental Medicine and Biology,* Vol. 39 (eds CM Bloor and RA Olsson). Plenum Press, New York, 1973, pp 219−233.

263. Specchia G, Bramucci E, Angoli L, et al: Spontaneous and provoked coronary artery spasm: Are they the same? *Eur. J. Cardiol.* 8:581−588, 1978.

264. Awdeh MR: Coronary arterial spasm and collateral circulation. *Chest* 74:237, 1978.

265. Maseri A, Severi S, de Nes M, et al: "Variant" angina: One aspect of a continuous spectrum of vasospastic myocardial ischemia. Pathogenetic mechanisms, estimated incidence and clinical and coronary arteriographic findings in 138 patients. *Am. J. Cardiol.* 42:1019−1035, 1978.

266. Benacerraf A, Castillo-Fenoy A, Tonnelier M, and Wagniart P: Le test au maléate de méthyl-ergométrine au cours de la coronarographie dans les douleurs thoraciques spontanées. *Arch. Mal. Coeur* 72:39−47, 1979.

267. de Servi S, Specchia G, Angoli L, et al: Coronary arterial spasm in angina at rest associated with transient ST-segment changes. *Clin. Cardiol.* 3:54−60, 1980.

268. Metzger JP, Bor J, Rojano-Guzman A, et al: Spasme coronaire provoqué, revascularisation immédiate par suppléance hétérocoronarienne: Apport de la scintigraphie myocardique. *Arch. Mal. Coeur* 73:307−312, 1980.

269. Hattori R, Nosaka H, and Nobuyoshi M: Two cases with spontaneous spasm of left main trunk. *Br. Heart J.* 47:249−252, 1982.

270. Garfein OB, and Feit A: Dynamic intercoronary collateral flow in a patient with variant angina and coronary artery spasm. *Am. J. Med.* 72:463–466, 1982.
271. Roth D, and Kostuk WJ: Noninvasive and invasive demonstration of spontaneous regression of coronary artery disease. *Circulation* 62:888–896, 1980.
272. Kramer JR, Kitazume H, Proudfit WL, et al: Progression and regression of coronary atherosclerosis: Relation to risk factors. *Am. Heart J.* 105:134–144, 1983.
273. Wesselhoeft H, Fawcett JS, and Johnson AL: Anomalous origin of the left coronary artery from the pulmonary trunk: Its clinical spectrum, pathology, and pathophysiology, based on a review of 140 cases with seven further cases. *Circulation* 38:403–425, 1968.
274. Dalton ML Jr, Arrington JO Jr, and King SM: Surgical treatment of adult-type anomalous origin of the left coronary artery from the pulmonary artery. *Ann. Thorac. Surg.* 7:333–340, 1969.
275. Perry LW, and Scott LP: Anomalous left coronary artery from pulmonary artery: Report of 11 cases; review of indications for and results of surgery. *Circulation* 41:1043–1052, 1970.
276. Askenazi J, and Nadas AS: Anomalous left coronary artery originating from the pulmonary artery: Report on 15 cases. *Circulation* 51:976–987, 1975.
277. Grace RR, Angelini P, and Cooley DA: Aortic implantation of anomalous left coronary artery arising from pulmonary artery. *Am. J. Cardiol.* 39:608–613, 1977.
278. LaPorta AJ, Suy-Verburg RM, Stalpaert G, et al: The spectrum of clinical manifestations of anomalous origin of the left coronary artery and surgical management. *J. Pediatr. Surg.* 14:225–227, 1979.
279. Bland EF, White PD, and Garland J: Congenital anomalies of the coronary arteries: Report of an unusual case associated with cardiac hypertrophy. *Am. Heart J.* 8:787–801, 1933.
280. Gouley BA: Anomalous left coronary artery arising from the pulmonary artery (adult type). *Am. Heart J.* 40:630–637, 1950.
281. Brooks H St J: Two cases of an abnormal coronary artery of the heart, arising from the pulmonary artery, with some remarks upon the effect of this anomaly in producing cirsoid dilatation of the vessels. *Trans. Acad. Med. Ire.* 3:447–449, 1885.
282. Chaitman BR, Bourassa MG, Lespérance J, and Grondin P: Anomalous left coronary artery from pulmonary artery: An eight year angiographic follow-up after saphenous vein bypass graft. *Circulation* 51:552–555, 1975.
283. Björk L: Anastomoses between the coronary and bronchial arteries. *Acta Radiol. (Diagn.)* 4:93–96, 1966.
284. Zureikat HY: Collateral vessels between the coronary and bronchial arteries in patients with cyanotic congenital heart disease. *Am. J. Cardiol.* 45:599–603, 1980.
285. Viamonte M Jr, Petelenz T, and Viamonte M: Radiologic study of extracoronary arteries in living humans with special attention to coarctation of the aorta. *South. Med. J.* 66:1403–1406, 1973.
286. Beuren AJ, Schulze C, Eberle P, et al: The syndrome of supravalvular aortic stenosis, peripheral pulmonary stenosis, mental retardation and similar facial appearance. *Am. J. Cardiol.* 13:471–483, 1964.
287. DoValle PV, Barcia A, Bargeron LM Jr, et al: Angiographic study of supravalvular aortic stenosis and associated lesions: Report of five cases and review of literature. *Ann. Radiol.* (Paris) 12:779–796, 1969.
288. Goldberg E, Berger M, and Garber M: Extensive coronary collateral formation in a patient with untreated acromegaly. *Angiology* 34:306–310, 1983.
289. Lundbaek K, Christensen NJ, Jensen VA, et al: Diabetes, diabetic angiopathy, and growth hormone. *Lancet* 2:131–133, 1970.

CHAPTER FOUR

Coronary Collaterals in Experimental Animals: Techniques for Quantitation and Choice of Animal Model

I. Limitations of Clinical Studies

Review of the available clinical studies leaves little doubt about the existence of coronary collaterals in normal myocardium and their enlargement in subjects with obstructive disease of the coronary arteries. It is equally obvious, though, that there is no consensus regarding the functional significance of these vessels. As previously discussed, many of the studies purporting to prove that coronary collateral channels are merely markers of the severity of the underlying coronary disease,[1-6] and as such are unable to preserve myocardial integrity and/or function, can be criticized because of poor patient selection for the groups being compared, resulting in unavoidable bias. Increased attention to the degree of stenosis of the coronary lesions and the angiographic quality of the collateral vessels will undoubtedly produce more homogeneous groups and more valid comparisons in the future.

One may wonder, however, if the use of collateral vessels as a marker differentiating two otherwise seemingly comparable groups of subjects might not be self-defeating. If the degree of collateralization truly reflects the severity of the coronary obstructive disease, then the patient with more advanced coronary artery disease would theoretically have the more developed collateral network. Therefore, the group with collaterals may at one time have had more intense myocardial ischemia, resulting in stimulation and development of a collateral network than the group with allegedly comparable obstructive disease and no collaterals. Intuitively, one would expect worse cardiac function in the group with more intense ischemia. Hence, the observation of even equivalent myocardial functional states in the two groups would then actually imply that the collateral channels have a functionally beneficial role. Therefore, selection of the initial groups based on comparability of all variables except the presence of collaterals might again be introducing a bias that would drastically affect the conclusions.

Most clinical studies attempting to define the functional role of coronary collaterals have depended on the radiographic appearance of the vessels. Perhaps the inadequacies of angiographic visualization of collateral channels is truly the principal cause of the disagreement concerning their value. Present radiologic techniques are unable to visualize opacified vessels with diameters smaller than 100 μm, and most clinical equipment used for routine cardiac catheterization studies cannot unequivocally identify vessels two and even three times as large as this minimum. Despite the positive correlations of angiographic appearance of coronary collaterals and functional indices measured in the operating room at the time of saphenous vein bypass graft surgery,[7-9] one wonders if some patients without apparent collateral channels merely have many vessels that are smaller than the resolving capacity of the equipment. Furthermore, angiography detects mainly epicardial vessels and provides little information about endomural and even subendocardial collateral channels. Thus, a better indicator of collateral presence would be useful. Quantitation of collateral flow following intracoronary injection of either dissolved radioactive gases such as ^{133}xenon[10-12] or ^{85}krypton[13] or particles tagged with an appropriate radioisotope[14,15] is becoming more popular. One recent study[15] has demonstrated that evidence of collateralization not obtainable with typical angiographic equipment can be confidently determined by intracoronary injection of radioactive particles, thus further emphasizing the inadequacies of radiographic identification of coronary collaterals. However, except in the situation of total coronary occlusion, most of these techniques necessarily measure some combination of normal antegrade and collateral flows, and therefore may not yield specific information about the collateral channels. Selective injection into the right and left coronary arteries of macroaggregated albumin labeled with different isotopes can in part determine the magnitude of collateral flow in the presence of persistent antegrade flow.[15] But because it is extremely difficult, and perhaps impossible, to resolve all of these difficulties in the clinical setting, and because adequate control of factors that influence collateral development and function is equally difficult, experimental animals have been used extensively in the study of coronary collateral vessels.

In the more controlled environment of the animal laboratory, it has been possible to approach more closely the answer to the possible significance of the collateral circulation. The physiology of collateral development, the changes in collateral structure occurring in acutely ischemic myocardium, the magnitude of the beneficial effects of the collateral vessels, and the extent to which these channels can be affected by pharmacologic or mechanical interventions have all been defined. Although results in the experimental animal cannot be applied directly to man, the information has helped us improve our understanding of the role of the collateral vessel.

II. Indices and Measurements of Collateral Flow

Study of the dynamic collateral circulation requires that assessment of flow and its changes be made. Numerous direct and indirect methods of measurement have been devised, but none is free of reservations and potential sources of error. In his monograph, Schaper[16] has reviewed the usefulness of many of these indices. To understand many of the animal studies, as well as some of the clinical ones, it is important to be familiar with these indices of collateral flow.

A. Histologic Techniques

Initial studies of collaterals relied solely on measurement of size and number from either pathologic specimens or specially prepared radiographs.[17–19] To better quantitate collateral capacity, Fulton[20] derived an anastomotic index. With laborious techniques, he counted the anastomoses present and then graded them according to caliber—10–40 μm, 40–100 μm, etc. An anastomotic score was then based on the number of anastomoses in each category. Using Poisseuille's law relating flow to dimensions of a conduit, Fulton calculated an index of total flow, or capacity, by multiplying this score by the fourth power of the mean radius. This index was felt to be proportional to the capacity of the collateral bed. Menick et al.[21] compared this index in dogs to retrograde flow (rate of blood flowing retrogradely through the cannulated distal portion of an occluded coronary artery into a graduated receiving vessel; see below) normalized for aortic pressure, a traditional collateral index. Although the calculated regression equation relating these two variables had a high correlation coefficient $(r = 0.87)$, there are few experimental points, and the distribution of published data points along the regression line suggests that the significance of the relationship hinges on only one of these points. Because of the time-consuming methods involved and the inability to assess temporal changes in collateral flow with this technique, this index has limited applicability.

B. Retrograde Flow

One of the earliest physiologic collateral indices described was retrograde flow.[22] Following coronary occlusion, the coronary artery distal to the obstruction was cannulated. When the cannula was opened to atmospheric pressure, the rate of blood flowing from the coronary bed along the distal coronary artery and through the rent in the vessel wall into the collection vessel was termed retrograde flow. Because there could be no antegrade flow, it was reasoned that this blood must have reached the ischemic coronary bed and subsequently the cannulated vessel via collateral channels. Therefore, retrograde flow was originally considered by Anrep and Häusler[22] to be an index of collateral flow. Although this index has been used innumerable times in the past 55 years, its relationship to actual collateral flow is uncertain.

It was initially assumed that retrograde flow overestimated the actual collateral flow nourishing the ischemic myocardium.[23] Since peripheral coronary pressure beyond an acute occlusion averages 15 to 20 mmHg, Gregg and other investigators reasoned that when the occluded vessel was opened to atmospheric pressure decreasing intracoronary pressure at the cannulation site to 0 mmHg, the blood carried by the collaterals would take the path of least resistance and flow retrogradely to the cannula. An electrical analog of the presumed flow circuit is illustrated in Figure 4-1A. This model assumes that the collaterals are all prearteriolar vessels, and predicts that flow is preferentially diverted to the low-resistance cannula. In the face of a constant driving pressure, effective removal of the peripheral vascular resistance which was in series with the collateral resistance would result in an increase in flow along these collateral vessels, which would then be shunted to the cannulated vessel and collected. Hence, retrograde flow would exceed true collateral flow.

This view was challenged by Prinzmetal[24] who believed retrograde flow underestimated blood supply to the ischemic region. Following intravenous injection of ^{32}P-labeled erythrocytes, he noted that radioactivity appeared in the acutely ischemic myocardium beyond a coronary occlusion, thus documenting the presence of a collateral circulation. However, because the level of radioactivity was not constantly increasing in this region, Prinzmetal felt that venous channels must be draining blood away from the region. He argued that this venous drainage would result in at least some collateral blood escaping collection in the retrograde flow determination.

Eckstein favored Gregg's argument, and insisted that retrograde flow overestimated true collateral flow by 10%.[25] Because collateral flow runs antegradely against a peripheral coronary pressure of approximately 15 mmHg, whereas retrograde flow is collected at a pressure of 0 mmHg, Eckstein felt that blood would flow preferentially along the path with the steepest gradient. He believed the two flows could be equated with a simple mathematical equation: *capillary flow = retrograde flow* · [1 − (PCP/Ao)], where *Ao* = aortic pressure and *PCP* = peripheral coronary pressure with the cannula closed. Thus, for a *PCP* of 15 mmHg and an *Ao* of 100 mmHg, capillary flow is 85% of that registered when *PCP* = 0. When Eckstein used an experimental flow model with *Ao* = 100 mmHg and *PCP* = 15 mmHg, capillary flow was actually 94% of that occurring when *PCP* was 0, thus causing him to approximate the average overestimation of retrograde flow as 10%. Recent theoretical "load line" analysis by Wyatt et al.[26] arrived at an identical mathematical expression for capillary flow, and their experimental results in animals suggested that the modified expression, *collateral flow = retro-*

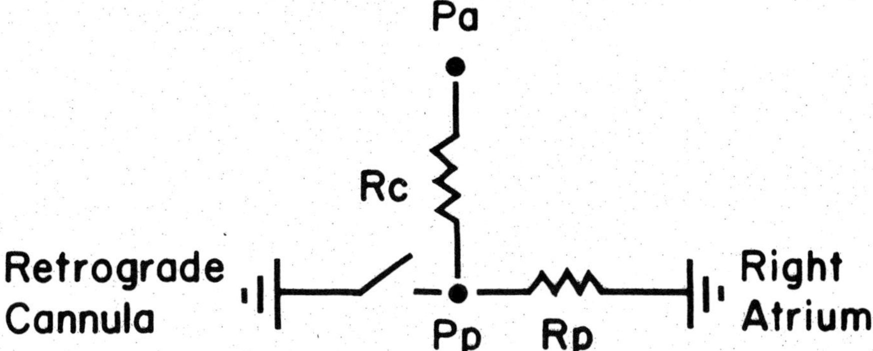

Figure 4-1A Electrical analog of coronary circulation assuming prearteriolar locus of all collateral vessels. The driving pressure for collateral flow is mean aortic pressure, Pa. Collateral blood would normally flow first through the collateral network (Rc) and then through the arteriolar bed of the occluded vessel (Rp) to perfuse the ischemic myocardium. All collateral flow would be diverted from the myocardium when the retrograde cannula was opened forcing pressure in the obstructed vessel beyond the occlusion (Pp) to zero. (Reprinted with permission of Academic Press from Downey et al.[35])

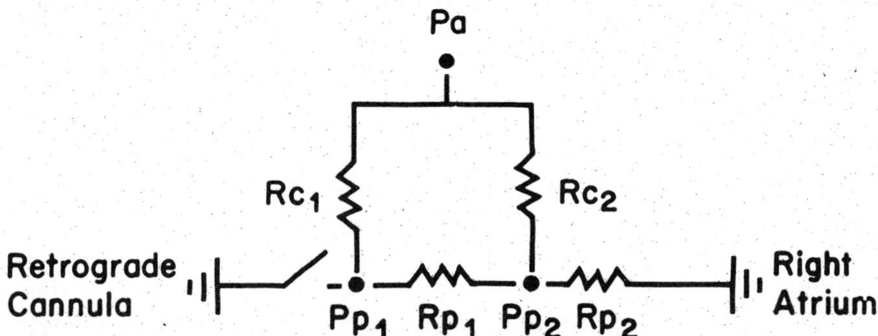

Figure 4-1B Electrical analog of coronary circulation assuming some collaterals (Rc$_1$) are prearteriolar (as in Figure 5-1A) while others (Rc$_2$) connect to the vascular bed of the occluded artery beyond some of the arteriolar resistance vessels of the peripheral bed (Rp$_1$) but proximal to others (Rp$_2$). In this situation only a fraction of the collateral flow would be diverted when the retrograde cannula was opened. The driving pressure for collateral flow is aortic pressure, Pa. (Reprinted with permission of Academic Press from Downey et al.[35])

grade flow · [1 – (PCP/0.8 Ao)], was a very close approximation of collateral flow measured by an independent technique (radioactive microspheres; see below).

But the other side was championed by Levy and co-workers[27] who used ^{86}Rb clearance to quantitate collateral flow. To measure coronary flow following coronary occlusion, myocardial uptake of ^{86}RbCl (see below) was determined by infusing this agent intravenously for one minute followed by removal of the heart. Retrograde flow was consistently less than the ischemic myocardial flow calculated from the ^{86}Rb uptake data. Furthermore, ^{86}Rb uptake by the ischemic myocardium continued even while retrograde flow was being collected, thus documenting that the collateral vessels could simultaneously supply both antegrade flow passing through the capillaries to the ischemic muscle and retrograde flow exiting from the cannula. With the coronary artery open to atmospheric pressure during the collection of retrograde flow, ^{86}Rb clearance in the ischemic area was as high as 50−60% of that measured when the vessel was clamped. These data supported the idea that there was collateral flow that was not sampled by the retrograde flow technique, thus accounting for the conclusion that retrograde flow underestimated true collateral flow.

Levy's conclusion was criticized because of the suggestion that Rb extraction increases at low flow rates.[28,29] Furthermore, the results were attacked by Bloor and Roberts,[30] who felt that Levy et al.[27] had mistakenly included the residual intravascular ^{86}Rb content present at the time of heart extirpation as part of the myocardial pool, thus resulting in a systematic overestimation of tissue flow. To rectify this situation, Bloor and Roberts used ^{131}I−PVP to label myocardial blood volume and ^{3}H$_2$O to measure myocardial blood flow. They were then able to correct the myocardial isotope content for the amount of isotope contained intravascularly, and demonstrated striking agreement between ischemic myocardial flow and retrograde flow.

Despite the evidence cited above, continuing evaluation of the retrograde flow index and comparison with independent determinations of collateral flow suggest retrograde flow may actually be an underestimate of coronary collateral flow. Rees,[31] Cibulski and co-workers,[32,33] and Downey et al.[34,35] have all documented continuing antegrade flow to ischemic myocardium during collection of retrograde flow. Downey used radioactive microspheres (see below) to measure flow to myocardium beyond chronically occluded coronary arteries[35] and noted that myocardial flow during retrograde flow collection was 67% of that when there was no flow diversion. When collateral flow was determined by observing the increase in antegrade flow in one vessel upon acute occlusion of the contralateral artery,[33] or by determining the rate of ^{85}Kr clearance from the ischemic zone,[32,33] retrograde flow in the normal dog was 40−47% as great as true collateral flow, although in the dog with a chronic coronary occlusion, retrograde flow was 200−600% greater than true collateral flow. Thus, retrograde flow underestimates collateral flow in the animal with an acute coronary occlusion, and is 35−40% of total anastomotic flow (sum of concomitantly measured antegrade capillary and retrograde arterial flows). On the other hand, it overestimates collateral flow in hearts with chronic coronary occlusions where it represents 90% of total anastomotic flow.[32] Further evidence that retrograde flow underestimates collateral flow because of an unmeasured, antegrade component is found in the work of Schulz et al.[36,37] After cannulating and establishing arterial perfusion of the left anterior descending coronary artery (LAD), 5×10^6 25−μm latex microspheres in gum arabic were embolized into the distal LAD. This procedure virtually blocked the entire peripheral LAD vascular bed, causing antegrade flow to decrease from 0.82 to 0.07 ml/min/g. Therefore, any collateral flow entering the LAD following embolization would have little opportunity to flow antegradely, and would flow retrogradely when the LAD cannula was opened to atmospheric pressure. Following blockade of the peripheral LAD bed, retrograde flow increased threefold, and even this post-embolization retrograde flow may be low because of potential obstruction of some of the collateral pathways with the latex microspheres. These observations suggest that the electrical analog in Figure 4-1B is a more accurate model of the coronary collateral circulation. The blood collected during retrograde flow measurements passes directly through large intercoronary prearteriolar channels without having passed through a capillary bed. This is consistent with the observation that retrogradely flowing blood has the same oxygen content as arterial blood.[38,39] The remainder of the collateral flow enters the ischemic vascular bed at the arteriolar level through much smaller vessels. By applying certain assumptions, it can be calculated that these vessels join the peripheral vascular bed of the occluded coronary artery at a point where the bed's more proximal vessels account for two-thirds of the vasculature's total peripheral resistance.[35] Thus, the collateral flow entering at this point continues in an antegrade direction.

In an attempt to define the origins of retrograde flow further, several investigators have clamped the normal coronary arteries adjacent to the occluded vessel and noticed reductions of retrograde flow to nearly zero.[39−41] Downey et al.[34] studied the transmural origin of the blood contributing to the retrograde flow. In dogs with acute coronary ligations there was always less concentration of the injected ^{42}K, ^{86}Rb, or radioactive microspheres in the endocardial and mid-myocardial samples than in the epicardium. Following opening of the retrograde flow cannula (retrograde flow approximately 3.5 ml/min), however, the transmural gradient was reversed. Now isotope uptake in the outer two layers decreased more (−74%) than in the inner layer (−30%). These experiments thus suggest that retrograde flow is mainly a reflection of collateral flow to the outer third of the left ventricular wall. In an earlier study, Cibulski and co-workers[42] had arrived at slightly different conclusions. They cannulated the left circumflex coronary artery (LCf) both proximally and distally to a large marginal branch. Retrograde flow from the proximal cannula was measured before and after ligation of all visible epicardial collaterals, while the distal LCf was perfused with arterial blood through the distal cannula. In dogs with chronic coronary occlusions, the eipcardial ligations decreased retrograde flow by 85%, demonstrating, as did Downey et al.,[34] that retrograde flow was derived mainly from epicardial vessels. However, in the dog with an acute coronary occlusion, further ligation of epicardial collateral vessels decreased retrograde flow by only 30%, suggesting that intramural anastomoses are the major source of retrograde flow and, therefore, the collateral circulation in this model.

This evidence suggests that retrograde flow cannot be equated with collateral coronary flow. However, Cibulski et al.[32] found a significant relationship between collateral flow measured by ^{85}Kr clearance and retrograde flow. More recently, Kirk[43,44] has also found a good correlation between microsphere measurements of collateral flow in dogs with acute coronary occlusions and retrograde flow determinations. He attempted to exclude all normal myocardium that might be contaminating ischemic zone tissue and artifactually raising the measured flows, and concluded that retrograde and ischemic tissue flows were nearly equal. This same study documented marked and equal diminution of inner and outer layer flows during the collection of retrograde flow. Kirk has asserted that the studies of Downey[34] and others purporting to demonstrate that antegrade flow continues while retrograde flow is being collected are flawed by inadvertent inclusion of normally perfused tissue with the collateral-dependent myocardium. His feeling that retrograde flow is a reliable reflection of collateral flow has been echoed by Wyatt and colleagues.[26] In contrast to the studies of Schulz et al.[36,37] these latter investigators[26] did not find any change in retrograde flow when the distal microvasculature of the occluded coronary artery was blocked by embolization of large microspheres. The explanation for the differing results is not apparent. It is clear that there is no consensus regarding the relationship of retrograde flow to true collateral flow, at least following acute coronary occlusion. But changes in retrograde and collateral flow are directionally similar.

Numerous investigators have shown a direct relationship between retrograde flow and aortic or coronary perfusion pressure.[22,38,40,45,46] In one study, only changes in diastolic, and not systolic, aortic pressure were noted to affect retrograde flow.[46] Some investigators normalize retrograde flow by dividing by aortic pressure to facilitate comparisons between interventions and animals. Retrograde flow decreases as the left ventricular end-diastolic pressure increases,[38] presumably because of increased myocardial tissue pressure affecting flow in the thin-walled collateral conduits. Finally, heart rate is inversely related to retrograde flow[46] because of the dependence of collateral and therefore retrograde flow on the duration of diastole.

C. Peripheral Coronary Pressure

Peripheral coronary pressure is another indirect collateral index that refers to the intracoronary pressure distal to a coronary occlusion. Because of the absence of antegrade flow, it was felt that the residual arterial pressure reflected filling of the distal vascular bed by blood being delivered by collateral channels. Increased collateral flow would then result in greater filling of the vascular bed and a higher peripheral pressure. Following acute coronary occlusion, the pressure pulse in the distal artery averages 34/22 mmHg, whereas following chronic occlusion it increases to approximately 75/45 mmHg[40] (Figure 4-2). The significance of this measurement following acute coronary occlusion in the experimental animal has been questioned. Gregg, Green, and Wiggers[47] observed that the steep major rise of the peripheral coronary pressure pulse occurred prior to the development of maximal aortic pressure and was instead synchronous with the development of left ventricular pressure. Furthermore, clamping of the other coronary arteries

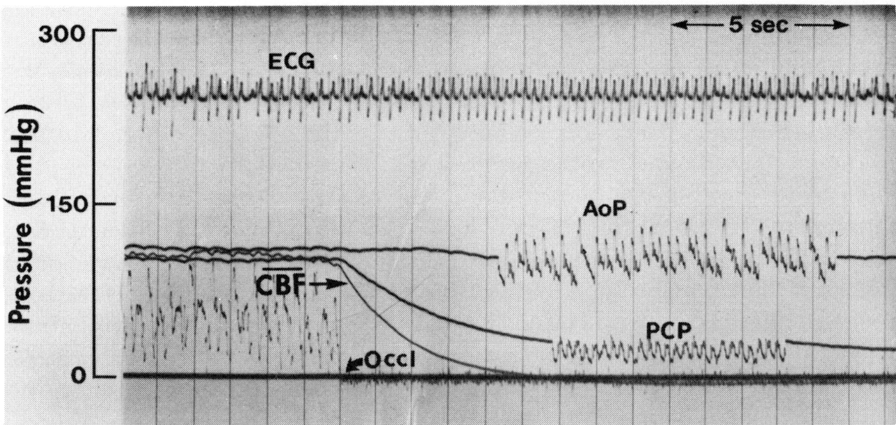

Figure 4-2A   Aortic pressure (AoP), coronary blood flow (CBF), and coronary pressure beyond a balloon occluder (PCP) before and after abrupt balloon inflation and resulting coronary occlusion (Occl) in a dog. Before coronary occlusion blood is flowing through the artery at a rate of 42 ml/min and there is virtually no pressure differential between driving aortic pressure and distal coronary pressure. However, following inflation of the balloon, coronary flow falls to zero and PCP declines to 20−25% of aortic pressure (25 versus 110 mmHg).

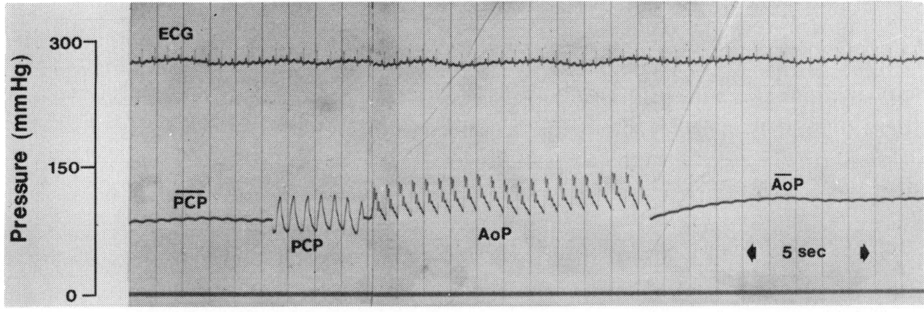

Figure 4-2B   Aortic pressure (AoP) and coronary pressure (PCP) beyond a chronic coronary occlusion (at least two months). In this dog, PCP was 83% of aortic pressure (88 versus 106 mmHg).

produced no phasic changes in the pressure wave and only changes in magnitude that were best explained by concurrent alterations in the dynamics of ventricular contraction. They concluded that the peripheral coronary pressure in the setting of acute coronary occlusion was determined mainly by intramural intraventricular tension and was not related to transmission of pressure from collateral channels. Bloor and White[48] and Selmonosky and Ellison[49] also felt that peripheral coronary pressure was not a reliable collateral index. They considered changes in peripheral coronary pressure in acute preparations to be reflections of changes in extravascular resistance. During acute coronary occlusion the distal bed of the occluded vessel has little inflow, and therefore represents an intramyocardial space subject to the forces of myocardial contraction. Thus, the peripheral pulsatile wave following acute coronary occlusion resembles that of the left ventricular chamber. Premature ventricular contractions unable to open the aortic valve and generate an aortic pulse pressure still result in a pulsatile peripheral coronary pressure.[49] Acute coronary occlusion results in noncontractile myocardium with subsequent diminution of extravascular resistance and fall in peripheral coronary pressure. As contractility increases, peripheral coronary pressure also increases. Schaper[16] has attempted to avoid some of these objections by using diastolic peripheral coronary pressure as the collateral index, but Rees[31] has found a poor correlation between this pressure and collateral flow measured in other ways.

After several days of coronary occlusion the pressure trace in the distal coronary artery more closely resembles an aortic pressure wave.[48] In dogs with chronic coronary occlusions, peripheral coronary pressure is markedly decreased when adjacent coronary arteries or visible epicardial collaterals are ligated.[41] Scheel et al.[50] also noted the absence of a linear relationship between peripheral coronary pressure and collateral flow immediately following coronary occlusion, which they postulated was related to the markedly increased resistance of the collateral vasculature and the autoregulatory vasodilatation of the arterioles in the ischemic bed. However, following the ischemic phase when the coronary vasculature reverts to a constant flow system, decreases in collateral resistance will be directly reflected as a rise in peripheral coronary pressure (Figure 4-3). Thus, peripheral coronary pressure appears to be a more reliable collateral index in the animal with a chronic, as opposed to an acute, coronary occlusion.

Schaper and Winkler[51] noted the marked influence of aortic pressure and peripheral coronary vascular resistance on the peripheral coronary pressure measurement independent of changes in collateral flow. To avoid the confounding effects of changes in systemic pressure, they have advocated use of a corrected collateral index in which peripheral coronary pressure is normalized by dividing by aortic pressure. To eliminate the influence of peripheral vasomotion and autoregulation, they suggest that measurements be made only after maximal vasodilation of the peripheral resistance vessels has been accomplished. Under these conditions, they have found the peripheral coronary pressure index to be a reliable estimate of collateral function in hearts with chronic coronary occlusions.

D. Myocardial Clearance with Inert Gases

Although retrograde flow and peripheral coronary pressure have historical importance and are still occasionally used, they have largely been replaced by one of several techniques that are able to evaulate collateral flow

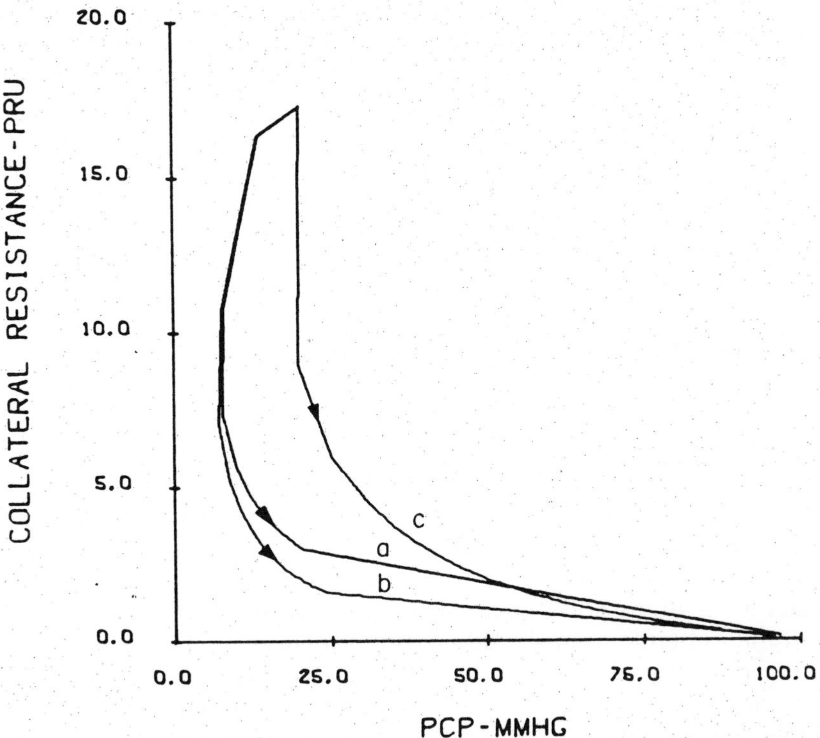

Figure 4-3 Relationship between collateral resistance and peripheral coronary pressure (PCP) following coronary occlusion (common point in upper left corner). Arrows point in the direction of increasing time. This mathematical derivation which was based on experimental data obtained in dogs was made using different assumptions about the behavior of the peripheral coronary bed: (a) autoregulation (see Chapter 5) and increasing peripheral resistance during ischemia; (b) autoregulation and no increase in peripheral resistance during ischemia; (c) non-autoregulating peripheral coronary bed. Under the more physiologic conditions (a or b) the relationship is nonlinear until sufficient collateral development occurs to make the myocardium nonischemic. Thereafter, PCP and collateral resistance are linearly related, and an increase in collateral development is directly reflected as a rise in PCP. (Reprinted with permission of Dr. Dietrich Steinkopff Verlag from Scheel et al.[50])

more directly. Clearance techniques using inert gases such as [85]Kr and ^{133}Xe have achieved great popularity. When dissolved in saline, the gases may be injected into either the coronary artery directly, the myocardium, or the left ventricular chamber. These isotopes emit low-energy gamma rays, and washout curves are recorded either by monitoring the efflux of radioisotope from the coronary sinus or by counting precordially.[52] Because the gases diffuse into the alveoli and are exhaled, there is essentially no recirculating radioisotope after the first passage through the pulmonary circulation. The $t_{1/2}$ of the washout is calculated from a semilogarithmic plot of the falling myocardial radioactivity as a function of time, and then the Kety-Schmidt formula[53] is used to calculate myocardial flow. In hearts without coronary obstructions, flow is homogeneous, clearance of the isotope from the heart is complete in approximately three minutes, and the washout is exponential for most of the slope.[54] Despite the absence of identifiable compartments, rapid uptake of the indicator by epicardial fat[55] does result in tailing off of the washout curve, which could affect flow determinations.[56,57]

Theoretical and practical difficulties might limit the usefulness of this technique in hearts with coronary occlusions. Distribution of the indicator is flow dependent; well-perfused areas will therefore contain more indicator and consequently, washout will be more heavily influenced by these regions and less by the poorly perfused areas. Hence, overestimation of average myocardial flow will occur.[31,57–59] Accurate determination of myocardial flow requires more time for the isotope to diffuse into low-flow areas and to wash out of these same regions. Clearance is often not complete for up to 20 minutes, and the curve is not monoexponential. In this situation, the washout of radioactivity from the heart is represented by a composite curve which can be divided into contributing compartments by graphic analysis. There are at least two parts of the curve: the initial faster washout related to flow in normal myocardium, and the following slower washout related to collateral flow in the ischemic tissue.[60] Although the second compartment probably does represent the slower collateral flow, this part of the washout with a significantly prolonged $t_{1/2}$ is subject to multiple errors including the effects of isotope washout from epicardial fat and the inclusion of radioactive counts from extracardiac tissue, especially the lungs, and the right atrium, which contains recirculating tracer before its elimination by the lungs. The latter difficulties can be avoided by using a focused collimator and positioning the crystal over the desired myocardial region in the open-chest animal. Some of the other problems can be obviated by not injecting the isotope into a coronary artery that perfuses both normal and ischemic tissue. If the ^{133}Xe solution is injected directly into the occluded coronary artery distal to the occlusion and flushed in with a small volume of saline, then collateral flow can easily be determined from the almost monoexponential curve. In this fashion the effect of interventions on collateral flow may be monitored by observing whether they affect the washout curve (Figure 4-4).

The position of the precordial counter may be critical and can influence the counting rate.[57] More recent use of multiple precordial scintigraphic probes permits simultaneous recording of individual washout curves over several different areas of the heart,[11,12,61] and also eliminates part of the problem of multiple myocardial compartments influencing a single washout curve.

For the calculation of myocardial and collateral flows from washout curves, it is necessary to know the blood-myocardial partition coefficient or ratio of solubilities of the injected dissolved gas in blood and muscle. It is assumed that ischemic and normal myocardial tissue have the same partition coefficient and that fibrosis does not have a significant effect.[62] It is

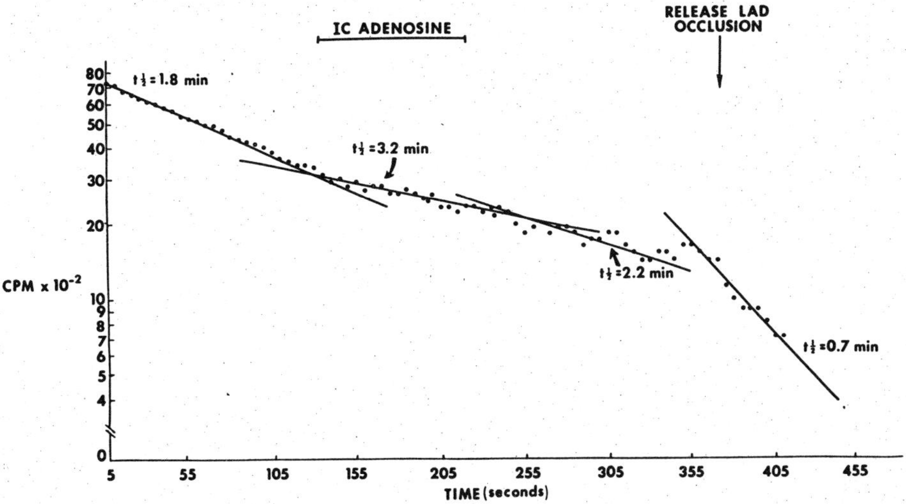

Figure 4-4   Continuously recorded ^{133}Xe washout curve in one experimental animal during several interventions. The left anterior descending (LAD) coronary artery was initially ligated, and the isotope then injected into the distal portion of the occluded vessel. ^{133}Xe clearance was measured before, during, and after administration of intracoronary (IC) adenosine, and after release of the LAD occlusion. The count rate recorded from the precordial area is presented semilogarithmically. The half-time ($t_{1/2}$) for each part of the experiment is indicated. During adenosine infusion into the left circumflex coronary artery the $t_{1/2}$ increased significantly. According to the Kety-Schmidt equation, this change is inversely proportional to the change in blood flow and documents a coronary steal (see Chapter 7). Following release of the occlusion, the $t_{1/2}$ fell to one-third of its prerelease value, indicating reperfusion. Thus, the various phases of the washout curve provide on-line information about the effects of interventions. (Reprinted with permission of Dun-Donnelly Publishing Corp., from Cohen MV, et al: Coronary steal: Its role in detrimental effect of isoproterenol after acute coronary occlusion in dogs. *Am. J. Cardiol.* 38:880−888, 1976.)

unlikely that this assumption is entirely correct, but the inaccuracies that are introduced do not appear to have a significant effect.

E. ^{86}RbCl

^{86}RbCl has also been widely employed in the evaluation of coronary collateral blood flow. The rubidium isotope is a potassium analog that is diffusible and actively enters the myocardial cell. It is usually introduced as an intravenous bolus injection. Extraction of this tracer from the blood by the myocardium is dependent on the rate of blood flow through the capillary bed, capillary surface area, and permeability of the capillary and cellular membranes.[63] If the ^{86}Rb permeability of the capillary and cellular membranes and therefore the isotope extraction are great in comparison to capillary blood flow, then the tracer exchange becomes a flow-limited process and can be used to measure myocardial blood flow. Fractional uptake of the ^{86}Rb tracer by the myocardium corresponds to the fractional distribution of cardiac output if the extraction ratio of the tracer by the heart is the same as the overall extraction ratio of the total body.[64] Then, coronary blood flow/ cardiac output = myocardial ^{86}Rb uptake/total body isotope uptake.

This method of quantitating myocardial flow is based on the assumption that uptake of ^{86}Rb is a flow-dependent process. However, various considerations may invalidate this assumption. For example, tissue extraction of the tracer is higher at lower flows.[65-68] These reports complement earlier studies[28,69] demonstrating that ^{86}Rb extraction became limited at higher flow rates (Figure 4-5). At high flows extraction becomes limiting because the ^{86}Rb ion is lipid insoluble and its movement into the myocardial cell is dependent on active transport. Furthermore, ionic backflux[66,67] which is a function of

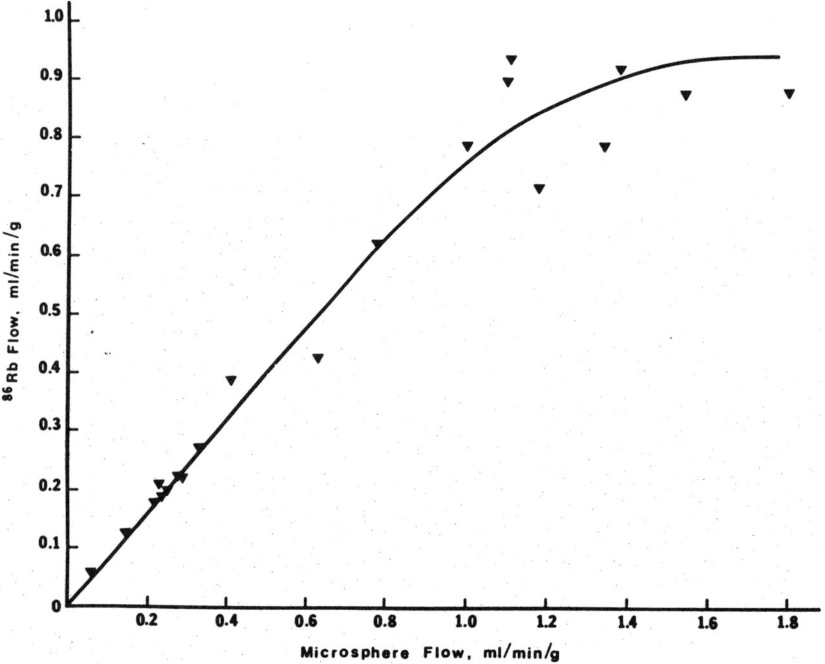

Figure 4-5   Graph of simultaneously determined ^{86}Rb and microsphere myocardial blood flows in normal and ischemic regions of the left ventricle. Dogs were prepared by ligating the left anterior descending coronary artery and injecting radioactive microspheres and [86]RbCl together into the left atrium. At low perfusion rates the relationship between flows determined with the two markers is linear, but at higher microsphere flows, ^{86}Rb flow appears to reach a plateau. This observation is consistent with the known dependence of ^{86}Rb extraction on flow. (Reprinted with permission of the American Physiological Society from Cohen.[68])

the previous extraction, recirculation which depends on the extraction of other capillary beds, and intracellular reservoirs which depend on the integrity of the sarcolemmal membrane which is itself affected by ischemic processes[70] also influence the net ^{86}Rb uptake by the myocardium. Because of these considerations of backflux and incomplete extraction, relative ^{86}Rb content in normal myocardial tissue should be less than that of a tracer that is completely trapped, such as particulate microspheres (see below). In ischemic tissue, inactivation of the Na^+-K^+ membrane pump should severely impair the reservoir function of the myocardial cell,[70] further affecting the myocardial ^{86}Rb content. A recent comparison[68] of myocardial blood flows in ischemic and normally perfused tissue with ^{86}Rb and radioactive microspheres has been made. In contrast to the theoretical objections concerning the use of ^{86}Rb to quantitate flows in ischemic tissues, ^{86}Rb was found to be a reliable tracer for the quantitation of ischemic flows. The ratio of ^{86}Rb/microsphere flows was close to unity (approximately 0.85), and the correlation coefficient of the linear regression relating microsphere and ^{86}Rb flows in ischemic myocardium (flows 10–37% of normal) averaged 0.933.[68] Moir[69] also had concluded that under hypoxic conditions ^{86}Rb extraction and clearance were still related to flow rate and that the cellular transport mechanism for ^{86}Rb remained nonlimiting in spite of the incident metabolic abnormalities.

Unlike the technique using ^{133}Xe or ^{85}Kr, use of ^{86}Rb permits quantitation of blood flow to any region of the heart, including the endocardium and epicardium. However, the heart must be excised, the myocardium cut into pieces, and the radioactivity of each piece counted in a γ spectrometer. Hence, only one flow determination is possible. Because of continuing backflux and extraction of the rubidium by the myocardium, the interval between isotope injection and heart removal becomes important. In a series of experiments in dogs with LAD occlusions, ^{86}Rb and radioactive microspheres were injected simultaneously and the hearts removed either 40 seconds or 2.5 minutes after the injection (Cohen, unpublished observation). In the former group, the reference arterial sample was collected for 40 seconds until the heart was fibrillated with intravenous KCl, whereas the reference sample was collected for 60 seconds in the latter group, ending 1.5 minutes before excision of the heart. As noted in Table I, the time interval had a significant effect on the ratio of ^{86}Rb/microsphere flows in the normal areas ($p < 0.05$), but not in the ischemic regions.

Endocardial/epicardial flow ratios using ^{86}Rb as the tracer typically exceed 1.0. Although the results are probably real, Gillespie and Love[71] have pointed out that ^{86}Rb diffuses into the epicardial layers of a heart placed in a bath containing the radioisotope, while the isotope also diffuses from an intraventricular solution into the left ventricular myocardium. Since flow-related uptake of the isotope generally greatly exceeds the amount diffusing into the myocardium during the short period between isotope injection and heart removal, this theoretical difficulty can usually be ignored.

Table I

COMPARISON OF ^{86}Rb AND MICROSPHERE FLOWS IN NORMAL AND ISCHEMIC MYOCARDIAL AREAS

Dog	Sacrifice Time*	$\dfrac{^{86}Rb\ Flow_N}{Microsphere\ Flow_N}$	$\dfrac{^{86}Rb\ Flow_I}{Microsphere\ Flow_I}$
1	2½ min	0.81	0.91
2	2½ min	0.82	0.82
3	2½ min	0.78	0.88
4	2½ min	0.85	0.95
5	2½ min	0.67	0.82
6	2½ min	0.57	0.76
Average		0.75 ± 0.04**	0.86 ± 0.03***
7	40 sec	0.61	0.76
8	40 sec	0.59	0.78
9	40 sec	0.49	0.77
10	40 sec	0.68	1.06
Average		0.59 ± 0.04	0.84 ± 0.07***

*Interval between injection of radioisotopes and arrest of heart. **Mean ± SEM. ***Statistical comparison of ratios in ischemic and normal regions: $p < 0.02$. I = ischemic myocardium; N = normal myocardium.

F. $^{201}TlCl$

As described in Chapter 1, the thallium cation, a potassium analog, is a useful agent for determining the distribution of myocardial blood flow with the use of a gamma camera. This radiopharmaceutical agent appears to concentrate in myocardium in a manner similar to that of potassium or rubidium, and distribution is proportional to flow. Because an active transport mechanism is involved, myocardial cellular metabolism and structural integrity of the cell membrane are prerequisites for cellular uptake. Therefore, ischemia and conditions of low flow reduce uptake and produce a cold spot. Imaging after ^{201}Tl administration has been used for delineation of myocardial perfusion defects both at rest and during exercise stress.

Following intravenous injection of ^{201}Tl in normal dogs, myocardial activity reaches 80% of peak activity within one minute.[72] Maximal activity is achieved within 10 to 30 minutes.[72-74] Thereafter activity decreases monoexponentially with an effective half-life of 7.2 hours.[72,75] Initial myocardial distribution of ^{201}Tl activity is linearly related to regional myocardial blood flow.[76-78] This relationship has been established for a wide range of flows, including the low flows following coronary occlusion[76-78] and high flows of exercise.[77]

Redistribution of isotope in ischemic and infarcted myocardium is more complex. Khaw et al.[79] used ^{125}I-cardiac-specific antimyosin F_{ab} antibodies which localize in necrotic myocytes. ^{201}Tl was injected either at the same time as the antibody and the heart excised 36 hours later, or 23 hours after the antibody injection and 1 hour before animal sacrifice. In both cases there was an inverse linear relationship between antimyosin-F_{ab} uptake and ^{201}Tl distribution. These observations indicate that the delayed distribution of ^{201}Tl is a function of the distribution of viable myocardium, and is no longer simply proportional to regional blood flow.

As already noted, ^{201}Tl uptake and distribution are decreased in low-flow ischemic areas, which results in cold spots. With resolution of the ischemic process, the cold spot is gradually obliterated. Continuing loss of thallium from the normal area and less rapid loss from or actual accumulation by the previously ischemic area account for this filling in of the original defect.

To record ^{201}Tl scintigrams, a gamma camera equipped with an all-purpose collimator is positioned over the heart. A 15% energy window centered at 77 Kev is generally used to collect the scintigraphic data. Radioactive counts are acquired in a suitable matrix on a computer. Scans may be interpreted qualitatively by visual inspection. However, more recently multiple computer techniques have been developed to analyze the scans quantitatively without bias. Quantitative methods employ either circumferential profiles[80] or profile slices across the ventricle.[81,82] Most investigators advocate the use of background correction and employ the interpolated background subtraction method originally developed by Goris et al.[83] and later modified by Watson and colleagues.[81] Importantly, these quantitative methods detect an initial defect, as well as determine the rate of ^{201}Tl loss from normal, infarcted, and ischemic regions.

G. Radioactive Microspheres

Because of the technical and theoretical problems encountered with ^{86}Rb, a particulate radioactive tracer was developed. Microspheres are small spherules made of an ion exchange copolymer such as styrene-divinyl copolymer. The spheres are not compact but have a lattice structure. After exposure to sulfonic acid, the copolymer becomes negatively charged and can then attract cations such as ^{46}Sc, ^{51}Cr, ^{85}Sr, ^{113}Sn, and ^{141}Ce, which pass into the spaces within the lattice. Or, if the copolymer is positively charged, anions such as ^{125}I will be attracted. Then, with patented processes the spherules are either coated with a polymeric resin (New England Nuclear, North Billerica, MA) or heated until the copolymer becomes carbonized (3M Co., St. Paul, MN). Thus, the radioactive ion is trapped within the lattice by a combination of physical, chemical, and electrostatic forces. Although microspheres ranging in size from 9 to 50 μm have been used, the most popular size is 15 ± 1 μm.

These particulate tracers have many advantages that make them ideal for the evaluation of coronary and collateral flows. When injected into either the left atrium or the left ventricle, they are carried with the blood stream and are trapped in the precapillary vessels of all organs, including the heart. Injection of up to ten million spheres at one time in the dog has little hemodynamic effect, and thus the safety margin is appreciable. In the conscious rat, almost 100% of the microspheres are trapped by tissues within 20 seconds of cessation of the microsphere injection.[84] Several studies have demonstrated negligible (0.05−1.0%) recovery of 15-μm microspheres in the coronary sinus following left atrial injection in the dog as well,[85−89] although during conditions causing vasodilatation, significant numbers of 9-μm microspheres may be recovered on the right side of the heart after they have passed through either arteriovenous shunts or the capillary bed.[89] In addition, shunting of 9-μm microspheres is increased as coronary perfusion pressure is raised.[90] Thus, 4% of injected spheres with this diameter are shunted at perfusion pressures of 100 mmHg, whereas 10% are recovered in the coronary sinus effluent at pressures of 200 mmHg. One careful investigation has evaluated the extent of microsphere loss from the heart within the first few minutes following injection directly into the coronary arteries, over the next two hours, and finally after as many as five weeks in chronically instrumented dogs.[91] Total myocardial loss when 9-μm spheres had been injected averaged 13.8 ± 10.6% (mean ± SD), and the magnitude of the loss increased as the interval between injection and animal sacrifice was prolonged. On the other hand, only 3.3 ± 4.6% of 15-μm spheres were lost, and there was no relationship between the amount of loss and time from injection. In some dogs the diameters of spheres escaping from the myocardium and lodging in the lungs were examined. Ninety-eight percent were less than 10.3 μm in diameter, and the maximum diameter observed regardless of the nominal size injected was 12.5 μm.[91] The experience of Murdock and Cobb[92] with 9-μm spheres was somewhat different. They injected a mixture of 9-μm and 15-μm radioactive microspheres with different labels into conscious dogs three days prior to sacrifice. The ratio of blood flow determined with 9-μm spheres to that measured with 15-μm particles three days before sacrifice was slightly greater than 1.0. Therefore, there could not have been preferential loss of the smaller spheres from the myocardium during the three days following injection.

Because microspheres tend to clump, it is necessary to add small quantities of a surfactant (e.g., Tween-80) to the suspension and to agitate the suspended beads in an ultrasonic bath prior to injection. Adequate sphere dispersion may be checked by microscopic examination of an aliquot of the suspension. Consigny et al.[91] studied histologic sections of myocardium following several injections of microspheres. Eighty-four percent of the microspheres located in the sections were solitary. Occasional short chains of two to six beads were felt to represent addition of microspheres from subsequent injections to a microsphere already lodged in an arteriole in which blood was still flowing.

The organ content of microsphere radioactivity is proportional to the number of trapped spherules, which is in turn proportional to the fraction of cardiac output received by this organ. Thus, the same expression previously presented to calculate ^{86}Rb flows is also used for microspheres. Usually a timed reference arterial sample is collected during the microsphere injection and for a variable period thereafter. In this situation, coronary blood flow = $(CPM_M/CPM_R)(F_R)$, where CPM_M and CPM_R = radioactive counts in the myocardium and arterial reference sample, and F_R = pump withdrawal rate of the arterial reference sample.[85]

Use of the microsphere technique permits measurement of coronary and collateral flow under different experimental conditions in the same animal, since a differently labeled radioactive microsphere can be injected each time. Before or just after removal of the heart, the ischemic region should be demarcated either by injection into the occluded coronary artery of a dye such as Evans blue, which binds to albumin and therefore remains in the vascular compartment,[68] or by performing postmortem arteriography to outline the vascular bed of the occluded vessel.[93,94] Simple delineation of a postocclusion cyanotic area or selection of the ischemic area based on anatomy of superficial branches risks inclusion of appreciable amounts of normal tissue. Even when the stained (Evans blue) ischemic myocardium is separated from the nonstained tissue by meticulously following the serpiginous border between the two regions, there still may be significant contamination of the stained tissue by nonischemic myocardium and subsequent overestimation of the true collateral flow.[68,95] After the heart is removed, it is generally sliced into several 0.5–1.0-cm-thick rings from apex to base. After separation of the ischemic and nonischemic zones, the regions are cut into several transmural pieces, each of which is subdivided into two to four pieces from endocardium to epicardium. The radioactivity of each piece is determined in a multichannel γ spectrometer, and computer techniques are employed to correct the raw counts for overlap and decay and calculate myocardial flows.

Because of counting statistics, microspheres flows are reliable only if the tissue samples contain more than 400 microspheres.[87] Since usually $2–6 \times 10^6$ microspheres are injected each time, this lower limit of spheres is generally not a problem unless very small pieces are cut from the ischemic zone. Because of the finite sphere size there have been questions of the reliability of microsphere distribution within the ischemic region. However, theoretical fears that 15-μm microsphere distribution might be significantly affected by geometrical factors, such as relative diameters of microspheres and vessels and presence of axial streaming,[65,88,96] resulting in exaggerated distribution to high-flow regions, have not been substantiated[68] (Figure 4-5). In experiments in dogs with occluded coronary arteries where ^{86}Rb and radioactive microspheres were injected simultaneously into the left atrium, no segment of the ischemic myocardium that contained ^{86}Rb was free of microspheres. Therefore, the geometry of undeveloped collateral channels is adequate to permit passage of 15-μm particles, which can be used to assess collateral flow in dogs.

The difference between coronary flows determined with left atrial injections of radioactive microspheres and with external flow probes averages –3.6%.[87] However, the range of the difference was –35% to +25% with 10 of 50 differences exceeding 20%. The cause of this discrepancy may be the spatial and temporal myocardial flow heterogeneity described by Sestier and co-workers.[97] When microspheres with different radioactive labels were injected simultaneously, the coefficient of variation was 6.5 ± 1.0%. Spatial variation was assessed by examining flows in adjacent small myocardial pieces, and in these experiments the coefficient of variation was 21.7%. Finally, temporal heterogeneity was evaluated by making several microsphere injections at 20-second intervals. The coefficient of variation was 11.1%. The data suggested a periodicity of flow cycles of 30–90 seconds. Variability of flows is also affected by the site of microsphere injection. The microsphere technique is reliable only if the injected spheres are evenly dispersed in the blood ejected from the left ventricle. Left atrial injections in dogs[87] and rats[98] have been shown to yield more dependable results and less marked differences in the distribution of microspheres in cardiac muscle than injections into the left ventricle. Presumably, left ventricular injections may result in streaming and incomplete mixing.

Chronic experiments can easily be performed with microsphere injections before and after some prolonged intervention. Several cautions are necessary, however, when an occluded coronary artery results in myocardial infarction. Since this technique presents data as flow/g tissue, the mass of the piece of tissue is an important variable. In a given experiment it may be important to know the flow to an ischemic region immediately after coronary occlusion, thus prompting injection of a radioactive microsphere. During the early course of myocardial infarction the ischemic area becomes edematous, increasing the weight of the tissue with effective dilution of the lodged microspheres and resultant underestimation of the flow if the heart is removed during this early period.[99] On the other hand, resorption of necrotic tissue after several weeks will result in a diminution of ischemic mass and effective microsphere concentration. Therefore, if the heart were excised and postocclusion flow measured with microspheres injected shortly after coronary obstruction were determined at this later time, flow would be overestimated.[99] It is possible to correct the early underestimation if preocclusion flow is determined with an additional microsphere injection.[99] If the preocclusion flow in the ischemic area is the same as nonischemic area flow, the degree of underestimation of collateral flow can be calculated by determining the actual deviation of the preocclusion flow in the ischemic region from the expected level and applying this correction factor to flows measured in the same area after coronary occlusion. Of course, this analysis presupposes that rates of loss of microspheres injected before and after occlusion are identical. Correction of later overestimation is also possible, although additional theoretical drawbacks make this more problematical.[99] In addition, several investigators have suggested that microspheres may be physically lost from the necrotic tissue after several days,[100–103] further complicating the use of microspheres after coronary occlusion. Ten hours after Lekven and Andersen[103] occluded a coronary artery, they observed that 26% of the 15-μm microspheres injected before ligation were lost from the ischemic tissue. Because they were unable to detect any edema of the ischemic muscle, actual microsphere migration was felt to be the cause. Jugdutt et al.[102] estimated that 40% of flow underestimation in the early postocclusion period represented only an apparent loss of microspheres which was related to tissue edema and inflammation. But the remainder of the underestimation was felt to be caused by actual migration of spheres out of the tissue. Thus, in dogs with myocardial necrosis, microspheres were found in lungs and regional lymph nodes. None was found in extracardiac tissues if there was no infarction. Preliminary results obtained by Consigny et al.,[91] however, suggest that actual microsphere loss from necrotic myocardium up to 48 hours following coronary occlusion is insignificant, and they suggest that difficulties with microsphere flow determinations during this early postocclusion period can be explained solely by intramyocardial edema formation. Murdock and Cobb[92] confirmed that real and/or apparent microsphere loss occurred by 24 hours after coronary occlusion, although none was apparent at six hours. At 24 hours, mainly epicardial flows less than 0.35 ml/min/g were underestimated. By three days the endocardium was also affected. By six days after occlusion the maximum microsphere loss was 22.2.%. In general, the greatest apparent microsphere loss occurred in those regions with the lowest blood flows. Davenport et al.[104] also concluded that it was the diminished blood flow and not the process of infarction that accounted for the underestimation of postocclusion flows. Despite the precise cause, it should be acknowledged that in the setting of coronary occlusion with edema, necrosis, and fibrosis, microsphere flow determinations may be inaccurate.

The microsphere technique also permits one to determine the endocardial/epicardial flow ratio. In normal dogs the ratio for the left ventricle ranges from approximately 1.1 to 1.3 when determined with 15-μm microspheres. This ratio is significantly higher when larger spheres are used[85,86,88] because of more axial streaming with the larger spheres and less tendency to be diverted to the branching arteriole going to the epicardium. Thus, the endo/epi ratio is 1.43 for 20−22-μm spheres and 2.7 for 51−61-μm microspheres.[85]

H. Other Techniques

There are other less frequently employed methods of evaluating collateral flow. Some investigators have implanted thermocouples in the myocardium and measured changes in heat clearance.[105] However, the presence of the probe itself in the tissue may distort flow patterns, especially in areas of low flow, and at best the probe monitors changes in flow in only small anatomic areas. Therefore this technique has never gained wide acceptance. Elliot et al.[106] directly measured collateral flow by chronically implanting a flow probe around a branch of an occluded coronary artery. However, the flow probe was able to record flows in only a few of the experimental animals.

Hood's group has adapted a radioautographic method to assess regional blood flow.[107,108] After infusing 1 mCi of ^{14}C-antipyrine, animals were sacrificed and radioautograms prepared from 20-μm full-thickness myocardial sections. Photodensitometric scanning of the radiographs then permitted quantification of regional and transmural blood flow distributions.

Of all of the described techniques used for the measurement of coronary and collateral blood flows, radioactive microspheres appear to be the best tracer. If attention is paid to a few precautions, collateral flows can be measured reliably and reproducibly with these spherules.

Although they are not measurements of collateral flow, indices of myocardial function may be used to assess the adequacy of the residual blood flow. Wiggers and Green[109] used strain gauges sewn to the myocardial surface to monitor contractile force, and believed this functional evaluation of the effects of collateral flow was more important than actual quantitation of the flow changes. Thus, interventions increasing collateral flow should enhance regional myocardial function[110] (Figure 4-6). More recently, pairs of ultrasonic crystals embedded within the myocardial wall have been used to monitor changes of segmental myocardial length and wall thickness within the ischemic region.[111,112]

III. Animal Model

A. Coronary Artery Anatomy

The choice of an appropriate animal model is often difficult. The investigator hopes to maximize convenience and ease of handling while at the same time choosing a species that approaches its human counterpart as closely as possible. Although the monkey or baboon would perhaps be the logical choice for these types of experiments, problems of cost and availability have dictated that other species be used. The two most commonly employed animal models are the pig and the dog. The pig has three major coronary arteries supplying the left ventricular myocardium, a situation analogous to that in man. The right and main left coronary arteries originate from the root of the aorta, and, as in man, the left coronary artery bifurcates into the left anterior descending and left circumflex arteries. The latter gives rise to marginal branches, and terminates in small branches on the posterior wall. The right coronary artery of the pig gives rise to the posterior descending artery which provides the principal blood supply to the left ventricle's posterior wall. The porcine heart thus is right dominant. This anatomy is quite similar to that of the human heart, which displays right dominance in 86% of cases.[113]

The dog, on the other hand, has only two principal coronary arteries, the left anterior descending and left circumflex arteries, bringing blood to the left ventricular myocardium. The main left coronary artery usually bifurcates

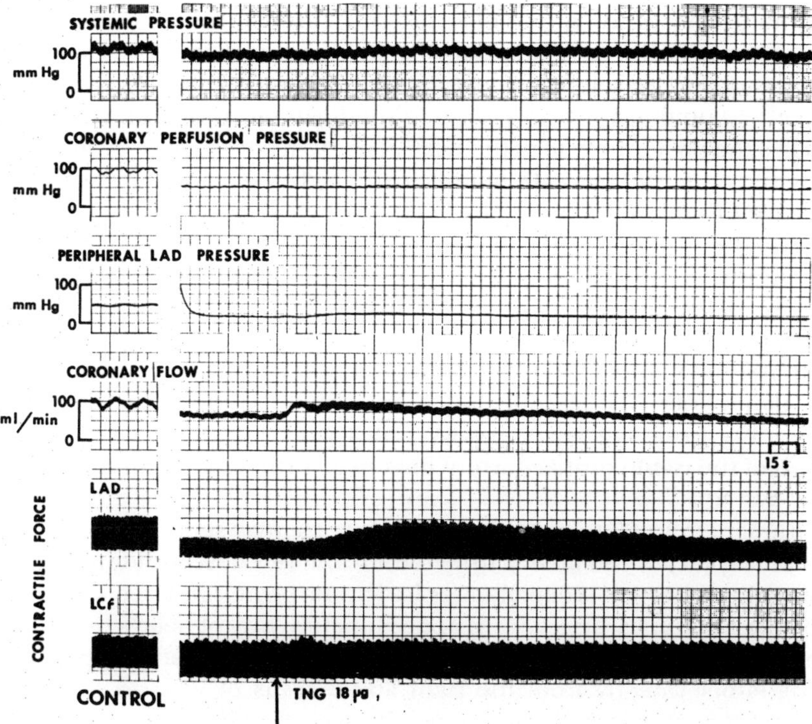

Figure 4-6   Effect of intracoronary nitroglycerin (TNG) on the peripheral left anterior descending (LAD) pressure and contractile force in the LAD and left circumflex (LCf) areas. The experimental animal had had embolization and occlusion of the LAD four weeks earlier. A small catheter was inserted into the distal LAD for measurement of pressure, and isometric strain gauge arches were sewn to the epicardium in an orientation parallel to the superficial fibers. The strain gauge arch measures myocardial contractile force which is dependent on local metabolic processes and therefore coronary flow. As demonstrated, a modest diminution of coronary perfusion pressure affected the contractile process and force development in the collateral-dependent LAD region but not in the normally perfused LCf myocardium. LAD contractile force fell to approximately 60% of the basline value and was restored by intracoronary nitroglycerin which also raised peripheral LAD pressure and presumably collateral blood flow to the ischemic myocardium. Thus, functional measurements are dynamic, respond to interventions affecting flow, and can be used as indices of ischemia and the adequacy of perfusion. (Reprinted with permission of the American Society for Clinical Investigation from Cohen et al.[110])

close to its origin from the aorta into these branches. In a minority of canine hearts (13–14%), a third branch (angular branch) may also arise from the main left coronary artery.[114,115] In this position it closely resembles the intermediate artery (ramus medianus or third primary division of the left coronary artery) present in 20 to 33% of human hearts.[113] In dogs, however, this angular branch is usually the first anterior ventricular branch of the left anterior descending coronary artery. The length of the left coronary artery prior to its bifurcation is quite variable, and at times (5% of specimens) the LAD and LCf vessels originate separately from the left sinus of Valsalva.[116] The left circumflex artery gives rise to the posterior descending artery and supplies the posterior wall of the heart. The right coronary artery terminates before the crux, and basically supplies only right ventricular myocardium. A similar left dominant system is present in only 12% of human hearts.[113]

Because of these major differences in canine and porcine topography, the pattern of blood supply to the interventricular septum and potential collateral pathways are different.[116,117] In dogs with left coronary dominance, the septum is supplied solely from the left coronary artery, and, therefore, only potential homocoronary collaterals are present. But in the pig, with its right dominance, the septum has a dual blood supply. The left anterior descending from the left coronary artery and the posterior descending branch of the right coronary artery thus may form an intercoronary anastomotic system.

In man, from 60 to 100% of the interventricular septum is supplied by multiple septal arteries arising from the left anterior descending artery, while the remaining portion is usually supplied by the posterior descending branch of the right coronary artery.[118] In approximately 12% of hearts the descending septal artery (ramus crista supraventricularis or superior septal artery), arising either directly from the right aortic sinus of Valsalva or as a very proximal branch of the right coronary artery, also contributes blood to the septum.[119] In the dog, the septum is supplied entirely by the left coronary artery.[117] One large septal artery in the dog accounts for perfusion of the major portion of the interventricular septum.[114–117] Blair[116] reported that the septal artery arose from the distal stem of the main left coronary artery at the point of bifurcation into its two major branches in 55% of cases. In 36% of hearts it originated from the proximal anterior descending artery, and less commonly from the main left coronary artery (5%) or left circumflex vessel (4%). This anatomic variation has important consequences if one wants to isolate and perfuse the entire left coronary system of the dog by introduction of a cannula into the main left coronary artery through its ostium in the aorta. The septal artery penetrates the septum at its anterosuperior angle and terminates in the posterior-inferior angle after giving off numerous branches that supply nearly three-quarters of the septum. The remaining portion of the septum is perfused by branches from the left anterior descending artery and terminal posterior descending branch of the left circumflex vessel.[114,116] Supply of the interventricular septum in the pig is quite similar to that in the human heart with a right dominant circulation.[117] Whereas dogs do not have descending septal arteries, and these vessels appear in only 12% of clinical material, as many as 66% of porcine hearts have this vascular supply.[117,119] The descending septal artery supplies a variable portion of the interventricular septum, but forms yet another vascular network that is a potential source of collateral channels.

Branches from the major coronary arteries give rise to a variable number of extramural vessels overlying adjacent portions of the heart.[114–116,120–122] These branches often resemble those noted in human hearts. Whereas in man a separate and distinct conus artery frequently (51%) arises from its own ostium in the right sinus of Valsalva,[123] this pattern is variable in the dog.[114–116] The canine conus artery arises from either the proximal right coronary artery or the right coronary sinus and forms a vascular ring with a left conus branch arising from the proximal left anterior descending artery and overlying the base of the right ventricle.[115,116]

The blood supply to the canine atria has been thoroughly studied by Meek and co-workers.[120] Both the right coronary and left circumflex arteries give rise to three atrial vessels designated as right or left anterior, intermediate, and posterior atrial vessels (ramus atrialis dexter or sinister anterior, intermedius, and posterior). The right intermediate branch anastomoses with each of the three major left auricular branches, and in 85% of the hearts supplies the sinoatrial node. In 84% of Halpern's series[121] of injected dog hearts the dorsal right atrial artery was the source of the cristal artery which perfused the sinus node. This artery is probably the same as Meek's right intermediate branch. In the remaining 15% of hearts the left anterior atrial vessel perfuses the sinus node. In contrast, in man the sinus node artery arises as a proximal branch of either the right coronary artery (60%) or left circumflex vessel (40%).[113]

If the sole prerequisite for choice of an experimental model were the distribution of the major coronary arteries, then the pig would be used for all investigations. However, the successful study of collaterals is not dependent on the anatomy of the major vessels supplying the myocardium. Rather, the size of the preformed collaterals and the ease and success with which collaterals can enlarge greatly determine whether a given species is an appropriate model.

B. Coronary Collateral Anatomy and Distribution

Collateral pathways in the dog are largely determined by the topography of the epicardial vessels. Epicardial arteries with adjacent vascular beds tend to form anastomoses. The most common collateral interconnection developing in the left dominant circulation of the dog is the homocoronary (intracoronary) type between vessels derived from the anterior descending and circumflex arteries. Collateral pathways observed by Blair[116] in the normal canine heart included interconnection of the terminal branch of the left anterior descending artery and the posterior descending branch of the left circumflex artery around the apex (in 75% of hearts), and anastomosis between the anterior epicardial left ventricular branch of the left anterior descending vessel and medial branch of the left circumflex artery (in 63% of hearts). Other frequently observed intracoronary collateral pathways are located within the interventricular septum. The main septal artery connects with septal perforators from the posterior (branch of the left circumflex artery) and left anterior descending arteries.[116,117] Intercoronary anastomoses may occur between the acute marginal branch and terminal portion of the right coronary artery and the right ventricular epicardial branches of the left anterior descending artery, and also between terminal vessels of the right coronary artery and distal vessels of the left circumflex artery.[114,116,124] The pulmonary conus branches of the left anterior descending and right coronary arteries also freely anastomose, thus forming another potential intercoronary pathway,[116] analogous to the Circle of Vieussens in human hearts (see Chapter 1). Vascular bridges or bypass collaterals around an obstructed vessel are the least common collateral network observed in dogs. Finally, interarterial atrial anastomoses also occur in dogs.[120,121] Intercoronary networks connecting right (from right coronary artery) and left (from left circumflex artery) atrial branches, usually located over the posterior atrial wall in the vicinity of the pulmonary veins, are evident. Typically the intermediate[120] or dorsal[121] right atrial artery, a branch of the right coronary artery, curves over the dorsal and lateral parts of the right atrium to enter and course through the crista terminalis. This cristal branch supplies the sinus node and also sends branches around the superior caval funnel where they anastomose with similar branches from the anterior (ventral) left atrial branch of the left circumflex coronary artery, forming an arterial vascular ring. Atrial arteries may also form homocoronary connections with adjacent atrial vessels.

The anatomy of the collateral circulation of the pig is in many respects similar to man's.[117,125−128] An extensive fine anastomotic network within the intramuscular (endomural) region has been observed, together with arborization of vessels into both the papillary and trabecular muscles. Vessels penetrating the endocardial layer are derived from perforating branches from the surface of the heart. The trabecular muscles contain long slender arteries that terminate in a fine vascular meshwork. This vascular supply interconnects with similar adjacent arterial networks to form an endocardial anastomotic system. A similar vascular system is found in the papillary muscles of both ventricles, thus establishing an interconnecting arcade which together with the trabecular structures forms an extensive endocardial anastomotic network.[125,126] To some extent this resembles the subendocardial plexus of the human heart. In the porcine heart, numerous myocardial regions have dual blood supply, thus creating potential intercoronary anastomoses, e.g., in the interventricular septum (left anterior and posterior descending arteries), anterior left ventricular papillary muscle (left anterior descending and circumflex arteries), and papillary muscles of the right ventricle and moderator band (left anterior and posterior descending arteries).[126−128] Thus, in the pig, with its right dominant circulation, there are several potential sites of intercoronary collaterals. Other collateral interconnections include the conus arteries (right coronary and anterior descending arteries), collateral bridging of the left anterior and posterior descending arteries around the apex, and intracoronary anastomoses between muscular and marginal branches of the circumflex and left anterior descending arteries. Bypass or bridging collaterals characterized by fine vessels spanning obstructions in native vessels have also been observed.[129,130]

Early studies of the coronary collateral circulation of the pig and dog employed the technique of simultaneous pressurized injection of the lead-agar Schlesinger mass into all main coronary arteries.[17] Whereas 100-μm-diameter anastomoses were demonstrated in normal dog hearts, pig hearts were felt to have virtually no intercoronary anastomoses exceeding 40 μm.[131] These results were later confirmed by the same investigators who studied the hearts of 161 pigs.[132] Only three animals had evidence of collateral formation, and in two of these, merely fine collateral twigs were observed. However, as previously noted, the results of these studies by Schlesinger and his co-workers underestimate the true incidence of collateral channels in the normal heart. Modifications of the technique by Robbins and Rodriguez[126] demonstrated that 75% of pigs had large intercoronary arterial anastomoses. In contrast, Reiner et al.[133] also injected a barium sulphate-gelatin mixture separately into the right and left coronary arteries of neonatal pigs, and were unable to detect any opacification of the contralateral coronary system when injection was made into one coronary artery. Additional studies by Bellman and Frank,[125] James,[134] and Schaper[16,127,128,135] have described in detail the dimensions, location, and structure of the collateral vessels in the porcine and canine heart both before and after chronic coronary artery occlusion.

When Bellman and Frank[125] injected radiopaque mass into a trunk or branch of either of the three coronary arteries of the dog, the contrast material appeared in surface branches of one or both of the other coronary systems. The mass was also seen to pass retrogradely up the other coronary arteries and reflux from the aortic ostia. The pattern of arborization and opacification of terminal branches in the dog hearts was noted to be similar to that seen following LAD injection of human hearts. Similar studies in 19 pigs revealed intercoronary collaterals in 14. However, in only one of the latter animals was there the free passage of contrast mass seen in either the dog or man and in seven there was only minimal penetration of mass into one or two fine twigs of the adjacent coronary systems. Patterson and Kirk[136] also injected a barium sulphate-gelatin mass into a coronary artery of canine and porcine hearts and then cleared the myocardial tissue to enhance visualization of the injected vessels. Whereas coronary networks adjacent to that of the injected vessel were commonly opacified in the dog, there was negligible filling of neighboring vessels in the pig hearts, and any visualized interconnections were very fine.

The suggestion that the collateral systems in pig and dog hearts might be quite different was confirmed by further radiographic and histologic analysis. Canine anastomoses are numerous and generally epicardial in location,[127,128,135] although endocardial connections do exist.[125] The pig, on the other hand, has virtually no epicardial connections, and only sparse endocardial and endomural connections,[125,127,128] although Robbins and Rodriguez identified endocardial anastomoses up to 0.3 mm diameter at or near the tips of the papillary muscles with formation of miniature interconnecting arcades.[126] Although the histologic structure of pig and dog collaterals is similar to man's,[135] the coronary collateral architecture of the human heart is different from that of either of these models. Unlike the pig, man has numerous, often large endocardial, endomural, and epicardial collaterals,[127,128,134,135,137,138] although the superficial collaterals may not actually reach the epicardial surface as in the dog.[125,137] Human collaterals range from 20 to 200 μm in diameter and sometimes are as large as 500 μm.[137,138] A well-developed endocardial plexus of intercommunicating channels of 100−200 μm present in human hearts distinguishes man's collateral vasculature from that of the dog.[137]

The canine and porcine collateral systems thus have obvious differences. In the normal dog heart collaterals are numerous and located mainly in the epicardial layer, whereas porcine collaterals are sparse and if anything are concentrated toward the endocardium. Qualitative estimates of the extent of the collateral circulations of these two species are supported by quantitative measurements. Following coronary artery occlusion, flow does not fall to zero, and residual flow represents the collateral flow to the ischemic myocardium beyond the occlusion. Eckstein[139] cannulated a coronary artery in both dogs and pigs and measured peripheral coronary pressure and retrograde flow. The distal coronary pressure was significantly higher in the dogs. Furthermore, retrograde flow in pigs ranged from 0.3 to 0.6 ml/min, whereas dogs had flows of 0.4 to 17.1 ml/min. In the pigs studied by Patterson and Kirk, retrograde flows were 0.2 ± 0.1 ml/min.[136] Schaper's studies confirm that canine retrograde flows average 5 to 10% of normal antegrade flows, whereas retrograde flows in pigs range from 0.25 to 0.75%.[140] More direct measurements of collateral flow using ^{86}RbCl were made by Winbury et al.[141] In the pig ^{86}Rb uptake in the central ischemic zone following acute LAD occlusion was decreased to 3−9% of normal levels, while uptake was approximately 25% of normal in ischemic canine myocardium. Studies with radioactive microspheres permit precise measurement of ischemic tissue blood flow as well as evaluation of regional flow to the inner and outer halves of the left ventricular wall. In one series the residual collateral flow following LCf occlusion in mongrel dogs averaged 8.6% of preocclusion coronary flow.[142] Presumably because of genetic predisposition, collateral flows appeared to be higher in beagles and averaged 18.5% of control flows following LCf occlusion and 31.5% of control after LAD occlusion.[142] In normal canine myocardium the ratio of flows to the inner and outer layers of the left ventricular wall (endo/epi ratio) is consistently greater than 1.0.[142,143] Following coronary occlusion, this flow ratio decreased to 0.5 in beagles[142] and 0.24 in Becker's greyhounds.[143] Although both endocardial and epicardial flows fell, the decrease in endocardial flow was more marked. This observation correlates nicely with the principal epicardial location of the coronary collaterals in the dog and the endocardial location of most of the infarct. Average myocardial blood flow in the domestic pig is 1.28 ml/min/g and decreases to 0.01 ml/min/g in the central ischemic region following LAD occlusion.[144] Similar low flows following coronary occlusion in the pig have been measured by others.[73,136,145–148] The less ischemic surrounding myocardium has slightly higher flows of 0.17 ml/min/g.[144] Despite these very low flows, the decrease in transmural flow appears to be uniform, and the endo/epi ratio remains approximately 1.0 or higher.[136,144–147] Thus, it is not surprising that infarcts in pigs are usually large, with equivalent endocardial and epicardial involvement.[127,147]

A few investigators have studied the collateral circulation of nonhuman primates, but the paucity of studies does not permit one to conclude whether their collateral system is closer to that of the pig or dog. In one study in the baboon, postmortem retrograde flow from one coronary artery while the rest of the coronary arterial bed was perfused with saline at 150 mmHg averaged 0.08 ml/min/100g (2.2 ± 0.3 ml/min/100g in dogs), and the anastomotic index was 10% of the value for dogs.[149] Pathologic studies one month following coronary occlusion revealed only endocardial anastomoses and resultant transmural infarcts. In the rhesus monkey, ameroid constrictors on the left circumflex coronary artery produced large, virtually transmural infarcts.[150] In a few animals there was a thin margin of surviving myocardium at the epicardial surface. Perfusion of the coronary arteries with a barium sulphate-gelatin mass revealed infrequent and small collaterals, usually in the atria. Ventricular collaterals were intramural. In other species of monkeys central ischemic flows from 5 minutes to 24 hours after occlusion of the left anterior descending coronary artery were generally less than 0.05 ml/min/g.[151] In these animals infarcts were again transmural, with only some possible subepicardial sparing. These observations are surprisingly similar to those reported for the pig. A second study in the baboon found somewhat higher residual flows of 5 to 15% of normal in the central ischemic area,[152] while Weisse and colleagues noted that ischemic flows in the baboon were as high as 25% of normal with a greater fall in the endocardial than epicardial half of the left ventricular wall.[153] It is possible that normally perfused myocardium was inadvertently included with the truly ischemic tissue. These latter results are strikingly similar to those obtained in the dog following acute coronary ligation.

Despite the qualitative differences of transmural collateral distribution and quantitative differences of collateral density in the pig and dog, collateral histology is similar.[135] Unstimulated collateral channels are most like small precapillary arterioles, and have the usual endothelial enzymes and innervation with myelinated and nonmyelinated nerve fibers. Microscopic examination of the collateral vessel reveals a single endothelial layer bounded by an internal elastic membrane. The tunica media consists of a single circular or spiral layer of smooth-muscle cells.[16] After coronary occlusion, a dramatic transformation process occurs that ultimately results in conversion of this thin-walled vessel into an arteriole with a thick muscular media. The luminal diameter increases twentyfold, while the vascular volume increases by a factor of 173.[135] Immediately following LAD ligation in the dog, only 0.7% of

15-μm radioactive spherules injected into the LCf are collected in the retrograde LAD flow.[154] However, three to six weeks following occlusion, 18.7% of 35-μm spheres are recovered, and the recovery is increased to 40% after seven to twelve weeks. Thus, the diameter of the canine collateral vessel increases from 40 μm to 0.4 mm at three weeks and to 0.8 mm six months following coronary occlusion.[155] In the dog the greatest increase in collateral capacity is seen in the epicardial layer, although the capacity or conductance of the intramyocardial collaterals doubles.[42] This increase in collateral size is evident in the pig as well as in the dog. Six months following right coronary artery (RCA) occlusion in the pig, the diameters of the largest collateral vessels and the large RCA branches are equivalent.[156] Similar results have been noted following LAD occlusion.[157] In contrast to the dog, collateral density increases in the subendocardial and endomural layers.

To investigate the physiology and functional significance of collateral channels, it would be prudent to choose an animal model that has the capacity to form such collaterals readily. Furthermore, examination of the effect of acute interventions on collateral flow will be unsuccessful unless enough coronary anastomoses are already present at the time of coronary occlusion. Although prolonged studies attempting to examine the prophylactic effect of drugs or procedures on the collateral circulation might be well suited for the pig, it appears that the dog is a better model for acute and short-term studies that seek to evaluate changes in collateral flow.

References

1. Mason DT, Amsterdam EA, Miller RR, et al: Consideration of the therapeutic roles of pharmacologic agents, collateral circulation and saphenous vein bypass in coronary artery disease. *Am. J. Cardiol.* 28:608−613, 1971.
2. Bartel AG, Behar VS, Peter RH, et al: Graded exercise stress tests in angiographically documented coronary artery disease. *Circulation* 49:348−356, 1974.
3. Gorlin R: Coronary Collaterals. *Major Probl. Intern. Med.* Vol. 11:59−70, 1976.
4. Williams DO, Amsterdam EA, Miller RR, and Mason DT: The role of the coronary collateral circulation in acute and chronic coronary artery disease. In *Advances in Heart Disease*, Vol. 1 (ed DT Mason). Grune and Stratton, New York, 1977, pp 253−267.
5. Zeitler E: The collateral circulation. Correlation with the left ventricular function. *Ann. Radiol.* 22:268−271, 1979.
6. Berger BC, Watson DD, Taylor GJ, et al: Effect of coronary collateral circulation on regional myocardial perfusion assessed with quantitative thallium-201 scintigraphy. *Am. J. Cardiol.* 46:365−370, 1980.
7. Gensini GG, Esente P, Delmonico JE Jr, et al: Coronary collaterals and coronary backflow recordings in patients with coronary artery disease. A double blind angiographic-surgical correlation. (abstr) *Am. J. Cardiol.* 31:134, 1973.
8. Webb WR, Parker FB Jr, and Neville JF Jr: Retrograde pressures and flows in coronary arterial disease. *Ann. Thorac. Surg.* 15:256−262, 1973.
9. Goldstein RE, Stinson EB, Scherer JL, et al: Intraoperative coronary collateral function in patients with coronary occlusive disease: Nitroglycerin responsiveness and angiographic correlations. *Circulation* 49:298−308, 1974.
10. Smith SC Jr, Gorlin R, Herman MV, et al: Myocardial blood flow in man: Effects of

coronary collateral circulation and coronary artery bypass surgery. *J. Clin. Invest.* 51:2556−2565, 1972.

11. Cannon PJ, Dell RB, and Dwyer EM Jr: Regional myocardial perfusion rates in patients with coronary artery disease. *J. Clin. Invest.* 51:978−994, 1972.

12. Cannon PJ, Sciacca RR, Fowler DL, et al: Measurement of regional myocardial blood flow in man: Description and critique of the method using xenon-133 and a scintillation camera. *Am. J. Cardiol.* 36:783−792, 1975.

13. Sullivan JM, Taylor WJ, Elliott WC, and Gorlin R: Regional myocardial blood flow. *J. Clin. Invest.* 46:1402−1412, 1967.

14. Kolibash AJ, Tetalman MR, Olsen JO, et al: Intracoronary radiolabeled particulate imaging. *Sem. Nucl. Med.* 10:178−186, 1980.

15. Kolibash AJ, Call TD, Tetalman MR, et al: Comparison of resting intracoronary particulate imaging and stress thallium-201 studies. *Radiology* 135:439−444, 1980.

16. Schaper W: *The Collateral Circulation of the Heart.* North-Holland Publishing Co., Amsterdam, 1971.

17. Schlesinger MJ: An injection plus dissection study of coronary artery occlusions and anastomoses. *Am. Heart J.* 15:528−568, 1938.

18. Blumgart HL, Schlesinger MJ, and Davis D: Studies on the relation of the clinical manifestations of angina pectoris, coronary thrombosis, and myocardial infarction to the pathologic findings: With particular reference to the significance of the collateral circulation. *Am. Heart J.* 19:1−91, 1940.

19. Zoll PM, Wessler S, and Blumgart HL: Angina pectoris: A clinical and pathologic correlation. *Am. J. Med.* 11:331−357, 1951.

20. Fulton WFM: *The Coronary Arteries: Arteriography, Microanatomy, and Pathogenesis of Obliterative Coronary Artery Disease.* Charles C. Thomas, Springfield, IL, 1965, pp 72−128.

21. Menick FJ, White FC, and Bloor CM: Coronary collateral circulation: Determination of an anatomical anastomotic index of functional collateral flow capacity. *Am. Heart J.* 82:503−510, 1971.

22. Anrep GV, and Häusler H: The coronary circulation. I. The effect of changes of the blood-pressure and of the output of the heart. *J. Physiol.* 65:357−373, 1928.

23. Gregg DE: *Coronary Circulation in Health and Disease.* Lea & Febiger, Philadelphia, 1950, pp 187−192.

24. Prinzmetal M, Bergman HC, Kruger HE, et al: Studies on the coronary circulation. III. Collateral circulation of beating human and dog hearts with coronary occlusion. *Am. Heart J.* 35:689−717, 1948.

25. Eckstein RW: The ineffectiveness of cortisone on functional coronary interarterial anastomoses. *Circ. Res.* 2:466−470, 1954.

26. Wyatt D, Lee J, and Downey JM: Determination of coronary collateral flow by a load line analysis. *Circ. Res.* 50:663−670, 1982.

27. Levy MN, Imperial ES, and Zieske H Jr: Collateral blood flow to the myocardium as determined by the clearance of rubidium[86] chloride. *Circ. Res.* 9:1035−1043, 1961.

28. Love WD, and Burch GE: Influence of the rate of coronary plasma flow on the extraction of Rb[86] from coronary blood. *Circ. Res.* 7:24−30, 1959.

29. Nolting D, Mack R, Luthy E, et al: Measurement of coronary blood flow and myocardial rubidium uptake with Rb[86]. (abstr) *J. Clin. Invest.* 37:921, 1958.

30. Bloor CM, and Roberts LE: Effect of intravascular isotope content on the isotopic determination of coronary collateral blood flow. *Circ. Res.* 16:537−544, 1965.

31. Rees JR: The myocardial collateral circulation. *Br. Heart J.* 31:1−4, 1969.

32. Cibulski AA, Lehan PH, and Timmis HH: Retrograde flow technique vs. krypton-85 clearance technique for estimation of myocardial collaterals. *Am. J. Physiol.* 223:1081−1087, 1972.

33. Cibulski AA, Lehan PH, and Hellems HK: The relationship of coronary collat-

eral inlet flow and retrograde flow in mongrel dogs. *Am. Heart J.* 86:485−494, 1973.

34. Downey HF, Bashour FA, Stephens AJ, et al: Transmural gradient of retrograde collateral blood flow in acutely ischemic canine myocardium. *Circ. Res.* 35:365−371, 1974.

35. Downey HF, Crystal GJ, and Bashour FA: Functional significance of microvascular collateral anastomoses after chronic coronary artery occlusion. *Microvasc. Res.* 21:212−222, 1981.

36. Schulz FW, Raff WK, Meyer U, and Lochner W: Messung der Kollateraldurch-blutung am Hundeherzen mit Hilfe der selektiven Embolisierung eines Coro-nargefässes. *Pflügers Arch. Ges. Physiol.* 341:243−256, 1973.

37. Diemer HP, Wichmann J, and Lochner W: Coronary collateral flow: Effect of drugs and perfusion pressure. *Basic Res. Cardiol.* 72:332−343, 1977.

38. Kattus AA, and Gregg DE: Some determinants of coronary collateral blood flow in the open-chest dog. *Circ. Res.* 7:628−642, 1959.

39. Hammond GL, Juca ER, and Austen WG: The nature of intercoronary arterial flow in the normal heart. *Am. Heart J.* 78:559−568, 1969.

40. Gregg DE, Thornton JJ, and Mautz FR: The magnitude, adequacy and source of the collateral blood flow and pressure in chronically occluded coronary arteries. *Am. J. Physiol.* 127:161−175, 1939.

41. Cibulski AA, Lehan PH, Griffin JC, and Timmis HH: Functional capacity of major anastomoses in chronically ischemic canine hearts. *Am. Heart J.* 84:787−793, 1972.

42. Cibulski AA, Lehan PH, and Timmis HH: Contribution of intramyocardial collater-als to anastomotic flow in mongrel dogs. *J. Cardiovasc. Surg.* 14:275−281, 1973.

43. Kirk ES, Hirzel HO, and Sonnenblick EH: The role of necrosis and ischemia in altering coronary vasculature following acute coronary occlusion: Positive and negative feedback mechanisms. In *Primary and Secondary Angina Pectoris* (eds A Maseri, GA Klassen, and M Lesch). Grune and Stratton, New York, 1978, pp 311−321.

44. Kirk ES: Equivalence of retrograde blood flow and collateral flow following acute coronary occlusion. (abstr) *Circulation* 62 (Suppl. III): III-66, 1980.

45. Gundel WD, Brown BG, and Gott VL: Coronary collateral flow studies during variable aortic root pressure waveforms. *J. Appl. Physiol.* 29:579−586, 1970.

46. Brown BG, Gundel WD, Gott VL, and Covell JW: Hemodynamic determinants of retrograde arterial coronary flow following acute coronary occlusion. (abstr) *Circulation* 46 (Suppl. II):II-100, 1972.

47. Gregg DE, Green HD, and Wiggers CJ: Phasic variations in peripheral coronary resistance and their determinants. *Am. J. Physiol.* 112:362−373, 1935.

48. Bloor CM, and White FC: Functional development of the coronary collateral circulation during coronary artery occlusion in the conscious dog. *Am. J. Pathol.* 67:483−500, 1972.

49. Selmonosky CA, and Ellison RG: The role of the coronary collateral circulation in the pressure changes distal to an acute coronary occlusion. *Surgery* 71:283−289, 1972.

50. Scheel KW, Granger HJ, Brody DA, and Keller FW: Mechanisms of collateral development and hemodynamics of gradual coronary occlusion. *Basic Res. Cardiol.* 69:338−360, 1974.

51. Schaper W, and Winkler B: Determinants of peripheral coronary pressure in coronary artery occlusion. In *Primary and Secondary Angina Pectoris* (eds A Maseri, GA Klassen, and M Lesch). Grune and Stratton, New York, 1978, pp 351−361.

52. Rudolph W, Mayer L, and Bohnstengel R: Performance and results of myocardial blood flow measurements using radioactive noble gases. *J. Nucl. Biol. Med.* 16:248−253, 1972.

53. Kety SS, and Schmidt CF: The nitrous oxide method for the quantitative determi-

nation of cerebral blood flow in man: Theory, procedure and normal values. *J. Clin. Invest.* 27:476−483, 1948.

54. Rees JR, and Redding VJ: Anastomotic blood flow in experimental myocardial infarction: A new method, using [133]xenon clearance, for repeated measurements during recovery. *Cardiovasc. Res.* 1:169−178, 1967.

55. Shaw DJ, Pitt A, and Friesinger GC: Autoradiographic study of the [133]xenon disappearance method for measurement of myocardial blood flow. *Cardiovasc. Res.* 6:268−276, 1971.

56. Bassingthwaighte JB, Strandell T, and Donald DE: Estimation of coronary blood flow by washout of diffusible indicators. *Circ. Res.* 23:259−278, 1968.

57. Maseri A: Pathophysiological, diagnostic and methodological problems in the study of myocardial blood flow in ischaemic heart disease. *J. Nucl. Biol. Med.* 16:259−266, 1972.

58. Klocke FJ, and Wittenberg SM: Heterogeneity of coronary blood flow in human coronary artery disease and experimental myocardial infarction. *Am. J. Cardiol.* 24:782−790, 1969.

59. Baltaxe HA, Formanek G, Loken M, and Amplatz K: Clinical limitations to use of xenon for measurement of myocardial blood flow. *Invest. Radiol.* 4:317−322, 1969.

60. Johansson B, Linder E, and Seeman T: Collateral blood flow in the myocardium of dogs measured with krypton[85]. *Acta Physiol. Scand.* 62:263−270, 1964.

61. Bonte FJ, Parkey RW, Stokely EM, et al: Radionuclide determination of myocardial blood flow. *Sem. Nucl. Med.* 3:153−163, 1973.

62. Pachinger OM, Tillmanns HT, and Bing RJ: Coronary blood flow assessment with xenon and rubidium. *Sem. Nucl. Med.* 3:131−138, 1973.

63. Renkin EM: Transport of potassium-42 from blood to tissue in isolated mammalian skeletal muscles. *Am. J. Physiol.* 197:1205−1210, 1959.

64. LeBlanc AD, Riley RC, and Robinson RG: Simultaneous measurement of total and nutritional coronary blood flow in dogs. *Circulation* 49:338−347, 1974.

65. Yipintsoi T, Dobbs WA Jr, Scanlon PD, et al: Regional distribution of diffusible tracers and carbonized microspheres in the left ventricle of isolated dog hearts. *Circ. Res.* 33:573−587, 1973.

66. Bassingthwaighte JB, and Yipintsoi T: Organ blood flow, wash-in, washout, and clearance of nutrients and metabolites. *Mayo Clin. Proc.* 49:248−255, 1974.

67. Tancredi RG, Yipintsoi T, and Bassingthwaighte JB: Capillary and cell wall permeability to potassium in isolated dog hearts. *Am. J. Physiol.* 229:537−544, 1975.

68. Cohen MV: Quantitation of collateral and ischemic flows with microspheres and diffusible indicator. *Am. J. Physiol.* 234:H487−H495, 1978.

69. Moir TW: Measurement of coronary blood flow in dogs with normal and abnormal myocardial oxygenation and function: Comparison of flow measured by a rotameter and by Rb[86] clearance. *Circ. Res.* 19:695−699, 1966.

70. Conn HL Jr: Effects of digitalis and hypoxia on potassium transfer and distribution in the dog heart. *Am. J. Physiol.* 184:548−552, 1956.

71. Gillespie WJ, and Love WD: Gradients in the regional rates of myocardial rubidium-86 clearance in tranquilized dogs. *Circ. Res.* 20:606−615, 1967.

72. Okada RD, Jacobs ML, Daggett WM, et al: Thallium-201 kinetics in nonischemic canine myocardium. *Circulation* 65:70−77, 1982.

73. Schwartz JS, Ponto R, Carlyle P, et al: Early redistribution of thallium-201 after temporary ischemia. *Circulation* 57:332−335, 1978.

74. Gerwitz H, Maksad AK, Most AS, et al: The effect of transient ischemia with reperfusion on thallium clearance from the myocardium. *Circulation* 61:1091−1097, 1980.

75. Beller GA, Watson DD, Ackell P, and Pohost GM: Time course of thallium-201 redistribution after transient myocardial ischemia. *Circulation* 61:791−797, 1980.

76. Pohost GM, Zir LM, Moore RH, et al: Differentiation of transiently ischemic from infarcted myocardium by serial imaging after a single dose of thallium-201. *Circulation* 55:294−302, 1977.

77. Nielsen AP, Morris KG, Murdock R, et al: Linear relationship between the distribution of thallium-201 and blood flow in ischemic and nonischemic myocardium during exercise. *Circulation* 61:797−801, 1980.

78. Chu A, Murdock RH Jr, and Cobb FR: Relation between regional distribution of thallium-201 and myocardial blood flow in normal, acutely ischemic, and infarcted myocardium. *Am. J. Cardiol.* 50:1141−1144, 1982.

79. Khaw BA, Strauss HW, Pohost GM, et al: Relation of immediate and delayed thallium-201 distribution to localization of iodine-125 antimyosin antibody in acute experimental myocardial infarction. *Am. J. Cardiol.* 51:1428−1432, 1983.

80. Burow RD, Pond M, Schafer AW, and Becker L: "Circumferential profiles": A new method for computer analysis of thallium-201 myocardial perfusion images. *J. Nucl. Med.* 20:771−777, 1979.

81. Watson DD, Campbell NP, Read EK, et al: Spatial and temporal quantitation of plane thallium myocardial images. *J. Nucl. Med.* 22:577−584, 1981.

82. Berger BC, Watson DD, Taylor GJ, et al: Quantitative thallium-201 exercise scintigraphy for detection of coronary artery disease. *J. Nucl. Med.* 22:585−593, 1981.

83. Goris ML, Daspit SG, McLaughlin P, and Kriss JP: Interpolative background subtraction. *J. Nucl. Med.* 17:744−747, 1976.

84. Ishise S, Pegram BL, Yamamoto J, et al: Reference sample microsphere method: Cardiac output and blood flows in conscious rat. *Am. J. Physiol.* 239:H443−H449, 1980.

85. Domenech RJ, Hoffman JIE, Noble MIM, et al: Total and regional coronary blood flow measured by radioactive microspheres in conscious and anesthetized dogs. *Circ. Res.* 25:581−596, 1969.

86. Fortuin NJ, Kaihara S, Becker LC, and Pitt B: Regional myocardial blood flow in the dog studied with radioactive microspheres. *Cardiovasc. Res.* 5:331−336, 1971.

87. Buckberg GD, Luck JC, Payne DB, et al: Some sources of error in measuring regional blood flow with radioactive microspheres. *J. Appl. Physiol.* 31:598−604, 1971.

88. Utley J, Carlson EL, Hoffman JIE, et al: Total and regional myocardial blood flow measurements with 25 μ, 15 μ, 9 μ, and filtered 1−10 μ diameter microspheres and antipyrine in dogs and sheep. *Circ. Res.* 34:391−405, 1974.

89. Marshall WG, Boatman GB, Dickerson G, et al: Shunting, release, and distribution of nine and fifteen micron spheres in myocardium. *Surgery* 79:631−637, 1976.

90. Crystal GJ, Boatwright RB, Downey HF, and Bashour FA: Shunting of microspheres across the canine coronary circulation. *Am. J. Physiol.* 236:H7−H12, 1979.

91. Consigny PM, Verrier ED, Payne BD, et al: Acute and chronic microsphere loss from canine left ventricular myocardium. *Am. J. Physiol.* 242:H392−H404, 1982.

92. Murdock RH Jr, and Cobb FR: Effects of infarcted myocardium on regional blood flow measurements to ischemic regions in canine heart. *Circ. Res.* 47:701−709, 1980.

93. Jugdutt BI, Hutchins GM, Bulkley BH, and Becker LC: Myocardial infarction in the conscious dog: Three-dimensional mapping of infarct, collateral flow and region at risk. *Circulation* 60:1141−1150, 1979.

94. Jugdutt BI, Becker LC, and Hutchins GM: Early changes in collateral blood flow during myocardial infarction in conscious dogs. *Am. J. Physiol.* 237:H371−H380, 1979.

95. Kirk ES, and Hirzel HO: Critical role of coronary collateral blood flow in the pathophysiology of myocardial infarction. In *Coronary Heart Disease: 3rd International Symposium Frankfurt* (eds M Kaltenbach, P Lichtlen, R Balcon, and W-D Bussmann). Georg Thieme, Stuttgart, 1978, pp 11−20.

96. Fung Y-C: Stochastic flow in capillary blood vessels. *Microvasc. Res.* 5:34−48, 1973.

97. Sestier FJ, Mildenberger RR, and Klassen GA: Role of autoregulation in spatial and temporal perfusion heterogeneity of canine myocardium. *Am. J. Physiol.* 235: H64−H71, 1978.

98. Wicker P, and Tarazi RC: Importance of injection site for coronary blood flow determinations by microspheres in rats. *Am. J. Physiol.* 242:H94−H97, 1982.

99. Reimer KA, and Jennings RB: The changing anatomic reference base of evolving myocardial infarction: Underestimation of myocardial collateral blood flow and overestimation of experimental anatomic infarct size due to tissue edema, hemorrhage and acute inflammation. *Circulation* 60:866−876, 1979.

100. White FC, Sanders M, and Bloor CM: Regional redistribution of myocardial blood flow after coronary occlusion and reperfusion in the conscious dog. *Am. J. Cardiol.* 42:234−243, 1978.

101. Capurro NL, Goldstein RE, Aamodt R, et al: Loss of microspheres from ischemic canine cardiac tissue: An important technical limitation. *Circ. Res.* 44:223−227, 1979.

102. Jugdutt BI, Hutchins GM, Bulkley BH, and Becker LC: The loss of radioactive microspheres from canine necrotic myocardium. *Circ. Res.* 45:746−756, 1979.

103. Lekven J, and Andersen KS: Migration of 15 micron microspheres from infarcted myocardium. *Cardiovasc. Res.* 14:280−287, 1980.

104. Davenport N, Goldstein RE, Bolli R, and Epstein SE: Blood flow to infarct and surviving myocardium: Implications regarding the action of verapamil on the acutely ischemic dog heart. *J. Am. Coll. Cardiol.* 3:956−965, 1984.

105. Grayson J, and Mendel D: Myocardial blood flow in the rabbit. *Am. J. Physiol.* 200:968−974, 1961.

106. Elliot EC, Khouri EM, Snow JA, and Gregg DE: Direct measurement of coronary collateral blood flow in conscious dogs by an electromagnetic flowmeter. *Circ. Res.* 34:374−383, 1974.

107. Malsky PM, Vokonas PS, Paul SJ, et al: Autoradiographic measurement of regional blood flow in normal and ischemic myocardium. *Am. J. Physiol.* 232:H576−H583, 1977.

108. Vokonas PS, Malsky PM, Paul SJ, et al: Radioautographic studies in experimental myocardial infarction: Profiles of ischemic blood flow and quantification of infarct size in relation to magnitude of ischemic zone. *Am. J. Cardiol.* 42:67−75, 1978.

109. Wiggers CJ, and Green HD: The ineffectiveness of drugs upon collateral flow after experimental coronary occlusion in dogs. *Am. Heart J.* 11:527−541, 1936.

110. Cohen MV, Downey JM, Sonnenblick EH, and Kirk ES: The effects of nitroglycerin on coronary collaterals and myocardial contractility. *J. Clin. Invest.* 52:2836−2847, 1973.

111. Gallagher KP, Kumada T, Koziol JA, et al: Significance of regional wall thickening abnormalities relative to transmural myocardial perfusion in anesthetized dogs. *Circulation* 62:1266−1274, 1980.

112. Tomoike H, Franklin D, Kemper WS, et al: Functional evaluation of coronary collateral development in conscious dogs. *Am. J. Physiol.* 241:H519−H524, 1981.

113. Hamby RI: *Clinical-Anatomical Correlates in Coronary Artery Disease.* Futura Publishing Co., Mt. Kisco, 1979, pp 11−77.

114. Pianetto MB: The coronary arteries of the dog. *Am. Heart J.* 18:403−410, 1939.

115. Kazzaz D, and Shanklin WM: The coronary vessels of the dog demonstrated by colored plastic (vinyl acetate) injections and corrosion. *Anat. Rec.* 107:43−59, 1950.

116. Blair E: Anatomy of the ventricular coronary arteries in the dog. *Circ. Res.* 9:333−341, 1961.

117. Bertho E, And Gagnon G: A comparative study in three dimension of the blood supply of the normal interventricular septum in human, canine, bovine, porcine, ovine and equine heart. *Dis. Chest* 46:251−262, 1964.

118. James TN, and Burch GE: Blood supply of the human interventricular septum. *Circulation* 17:391−396, 1958.
119. Rodriguez FL, Robbins SL, and Banasiewicz M: The descending septal artery in human, porcine, equine, ovine, bovine, and canine hearts. A postmortem angiographic study. *Am. Heart J.* 62:247−259, 1961.
120. Meek WJ, Keenan M, and Theisen HJ: The auricular blood supply in the dog. I. General auricular supply with special reference to the sino-auricular node. *Am. Heart J.* 4:591−599, 1929.
121. Halpern MH: Arterial supply to the nodal tissue in the dog heart. *Circulation* 9:547−554, 1954.
122. Craig RL, and Learned BB: Patterns of the anterior descending branch of the left coronary artery in the dog. *Am. Heart J.* 48:455−458, 1954.
123. Schlesinger MJ, Zoll PM, and Wessler S: The conus artery: A third coronary artery. *Am. Heart J.* 38:823−836, 1949.
124. Mital RN: Intercoronary anastomoses and the right ventricle in dogs. *Indian Heart J.* 23:288−291, 1971.
125. Bellman S, and Frank HA: Intercoronary collaterals in normal hearts. *J. Thorac. Surg.* 36:584−603, 1958.
126. Robbins SL, and Rodriguez FL: Postmortem angiographic studies on the coronary arterial circulation: Intercoronary arterial anastomoses in normal young adult pig hearts. *Vasc. Dis.* 1:226−232, 1964.
127. Schaper W, Jageneau A, and Xhonneux R: The development of collateral circulation in the pig and dog heart. *Cardiologia* 51:321−335, 1967.
128. Schaper W, Flameng W, and DeBrabander M: Comparative aspects of coronary collateral circulation. In *Comparative Pathophysiology of Circulatory Disturbances: Advances in Experimental Medicine and Biology*, Vol. 22 (ed CM Bloor). Plenum Press, New York, 1972, pp 267−276.
129. Kong Y, Chen JTT, Zeft HJ, et al: Natural history of experimental coronary occlusion in pigs: A serial cineangiographic study. *Am. Heart J.* 77:45−54, 1969.
130. Ramo BW, Peter RH, Ratliff N, et al: The natural history of right coronary arterial occlusion in the pig: Comparison with left anterior descending arterial occlusion. *Am. J. Cardiol.* 26:156−161, 1970.
131. Blumgart HL, Zoll PM, Freedberg AS, and Gilligan DR: The experimental production of intercoronary arterial anastomoses and their functional significance. *Circulation* 1:10−27, 1950.
132. Paul MH, Norman LR, Zoll PM, and Blumgart HL: Stimulation of interarterial coronary anastomoses by experimental acute coronary occlusion. *Circulation* 16:608−614, 1957.
133. Reiner L, Vrbanovic D, and Madrazo A: Interarterial coronary anastomoses in neonatal pigs. *Proc. Soc. Exp. Biol. Med.* 106:732−734, 1961.
134. James TN: Anatomy of the coronary arteries in health and disease. *Circulation* 32:1020−1033, 1965.
135. Schaper W: Pathophysiology of coronary circulation. *Prog. Cardiovasc. Dis.* 14:275−296, 1971.
136. Patterson RE, and Kirk ES: Analysis of coronary collateral structure, function, and ischemic border zones in pigs. *Am. J. Physiol.* 244:H23−H31, 1983.
137. Baroldi G: Myocardial infarct and sudden coronary heart death in relation to coronary occlusion and collateral circulation. *Am. Heart J.* 71:826−836, 1966.
138. Fulton WFM: Intercoronary anastomoses studied by postmortem stereoarteriography: Relationship to coronary occlusion and myocardial damage. In *Coronary Heart Disease: 3rd International Symposium Frankfurt* (eds M Kaltenbach, P Lichtlen, R Balcon, and W-D Bussmann). Georg Thieme, Stuttgart, 1978, pp 2−11.
139. Eckstein RW: Coronary interarterial anastomoses in young pigs and mongrel dogs. *Circ. Res.* 2:460−465, 1954.

140. Schaper W, Schaper J, Xhonneux R, and Vandesteene R: The morphology of intercoronary anastomoses in chronic coronary artery occlusion. *Cardiovasc. Res.* 3:315−323, 1969.
141. Winbury MM, Losada M, Kissil D, et al: Pentaerythritoltetranitrate and dipyridamole on cardiac nutritive flow and blood content. *Am. J. Physiol.* 220:1558−1563, 1971.
142. Wüsten B, Flameng W, and Schaper W: The distribution of myocardial flow. Part I: Effects of experimental coronary occlusion. *Basic Res. Cardiol.* 69:422−434, 1974.
143. Becker LC, Ferreira R, and Thomas M: Mapping of left ventricular blood flow with radioactive microspheres in experimental coronary artery occlusion. *Cardiovasc. Res.* 7:391−400, 1973.
144. Fedor JM, McIntosh DM, Rembert JC, and Greenfield JC Jr: Coronary and transmural myocardial blood flow responses in awake domestic pigs. *Am. J. Physiol.* 235:H435−H444, 1978.
145. Millard RW: Changes in cardiac mechanics and coronary blood flow of regionally ischemic porcine myocardium induced by diltiazem. *Chest* 78 (Suppl):193−199, 1980.
146. Millard RW: Induction of functional coronary collaterals in the swine heart. *Basic Res. Cardiol.* 76:468−473, 1981.
147. Fujiwara H, Ashraf M, Sato S, and Millard RW: Transmural cellular damage and blood flow distribution in early ischemia in pig hearts. *Circ. Res.* 51:683−693, 1982.
148. Sjoquist P-O, Duker G, and Almgren O: Distribution of the collateral blood flow at the lateral border of the ischemic myocardium after acute coronary occlusion in the pig and the dog. *Basic Res. Cardiol.* 79:164−175, 1984.
149. Crozatier B, Ross J Jr, Franklin D, et al: Myocardial infarction in the baboon: Regional function and the collateral circulation. *Am. J. Physiol.* 235:H413−H421, 1978.
150. Buss DD, Hyde DM, and Steffey EP: Coronary collateral development in the rhesus monkey (Macaca mulatta). *Basic Res. Cardiol.* 78:510−517, 1983.
151. LaVallee M, and Vatner SF: Regional myocardial blood flow and necrosis in primates following coronary occlusion. *Am. J. Physiol.* 246:H635−H639, 1984.
152. Lubbe WF, Peisach M, Pretorius R, et al: Distribution of myocardial blood flow before and after coronary artery ligation in the baboon. Relation to early ventricular fibrillation. *Cardiovasc. Res.* 8:478−487, 1974.
153. Weisse AB, Kearney K, Narang RM, and Regan TJ: Comparison of the coronary collateral circulation in dogs and baboons after coronary occlusion. *Am. Heart J.* 92:193−200, 1976.
154. Blum RL, Alpern H, Jaffe H, et al: Determination of interarterial coronary anastomosis by radioactive spherules. Effect of coronary occlusion and hypoxemia. *Am. Heart J.* 79:244−249, 1970.
155. DeBrabander M, and Schaper W: Quantitative histology of the canine coronary collateral circulation in localized myocardial ischemia. *Life Sci.* 10:857−868, 1971.
156. Pifarré R, Yokoyama T, Ilano AC, and Hufnagel CA: Experimental evaluation of acute occlusion of the right coronary artery. *Am. J. Surg.* 112:3−6, 1966.
157. Pifarré R, and Hufnagel CA: An experimental study comparing the acute occlusion of the anterior descending and the left circumflex coronary arteries. *J. Thorac. Cardiovasc. Surg.* 51:761−766, 1966.

Coronary Collaterals and Luminal Communications in Experimental Animals after Recent and Chronic Coronary Occlusion: Changes in Histology and Flow

I. Histologic Transformation Following Coronary Occlusion

The coronary collateral vessel in the undiseased heart is a thin-walled conduit that is an initially unused pathway. Once it is recruited because of failure of the original vessel to permit normal flows, this collateral channel undergoes a striking histologic and anatomic transformation which increases the vessel's significance as an alternate route of supply to the ischemic heart. Thus, the thin-walled conduit in time becomes a thick-walled arteriole. Our understanding of the histologic transformation of the collateral vessel is largely due to the labors of Schaper and co-workers.[1–10] These investigators implanted ameroid constrictors around one or more coronary arteries of dogs. This constrictor consists of a small, hollowed horseshoe-shaped device containing a hygroscopic material. As the central core of the constrictor swells, the encircled coronary artery is gradually narrowed and finally occluded. The time to occlusion is variable, but in Schaper's studies, it is usually two to three weeks. At various intervals following occlusion the heart was excised by Schaper and his colleagues, and the coronary arteries injected with a Micropaque suspension in 9% gelatin. The anastomoses could then be identified and cut out for histologic examination. Hearts were also excised and maintained with an isolated heart perfusion apparatus. ^{3}H-thymidine, a DNA precursor readily taken up by actively reproducing cells, was injected into the perfusate. After one to three hours, histologic sections were prepared and autoradiograms done to gain insight into the dynamics of collateral growth.

The developing collateral channel can actually be subdivided into three sections. The stem is the subbranch of the coronary artery from which the collateral vessel originates. The midzone is that part of the collateral between the stem and reentry which demonstrates the most obvious and dramatic growth transformation, perhaps because of its very small initial diameter (average 40 μm). Finally, the reentry is the subbranch of the occluded coronary artery in which the collateral vessel terminates.

Although pronounced changes are not identified in the stem and reentry parts of the collateral vessel, the changes that do occur in the stem which is surrounded by normal tissue imply that it is not merely the presence of ischemic tissue that results in collateral transformation. Rather, it is likely to be some physical stimulus such as tangential wall stress or one or more biochemical mediators. The transformation of the midzone segment occurs in three distinct phases. The initial phase consists of a rapid increase in luminal dimensions without appreciable change in the vascular wall and occurs during the first days following coronary occlusion. During the next three or four days, the second phase is characterized by cellular proliferation which

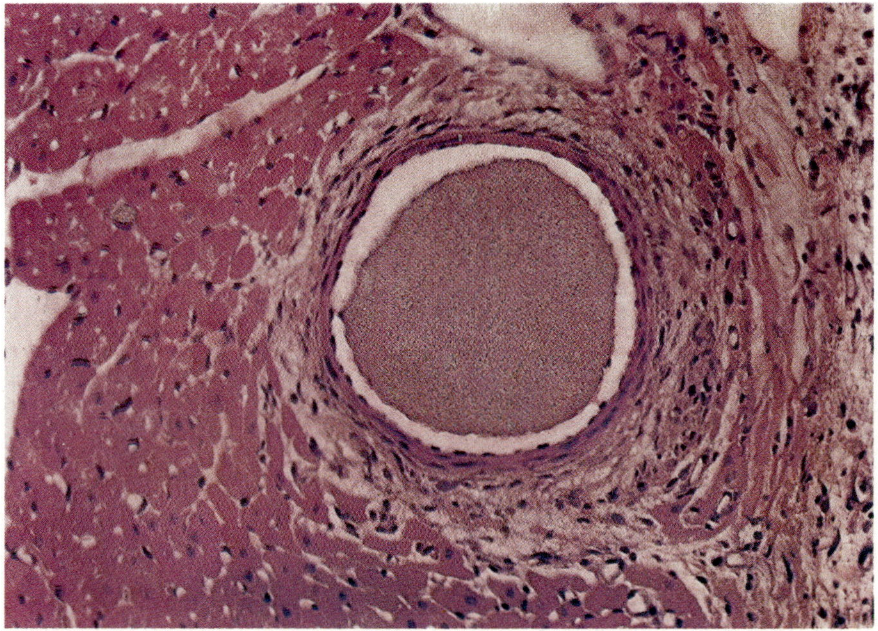

Figure 5-1A   Microscopic section of a dog coronary collateral vessel three to four weeks after implantation of an ameroid constrictor, and therefore approximately one week after coronary occlusion. The perivascular edema and inflammation are typical for this stage of development. However, the media is still composed of only one layer of smooth muscle cells. This is the appearance of an "acute" collateral. Hematoxylin-eosin stain, ×106. (Reprinted with permission of North-Holland Publishing Company from Schaper.[5])

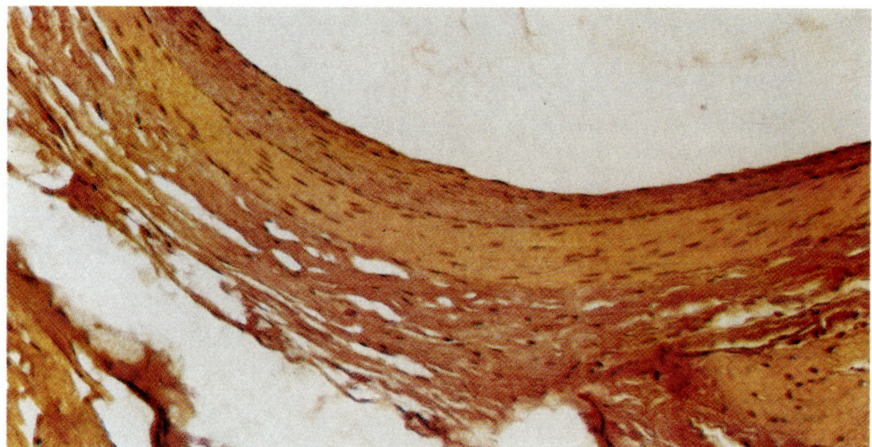

Figure 5-1B   Vascular wall of coronary collateral approximately three months after coronary artery occlusion in the dog. By this time the thickness of the wall has normalized and two different smooth muscle layers can be seen, one circular layer and one subintimal layer of longitudinal smooth muscle with cells running parallel to the longitudinal axis of the blood vessel. Fragments of the old disrupted internal elastic membrane are visible and displaced towards the media. In most cases these remnants demarcate the border between the two layers of smooth muscle. Weigert elastica-Van Gieson stain, ×270. (Reprinted with permission of North-Holland Publishing Company from Schaper.[5])

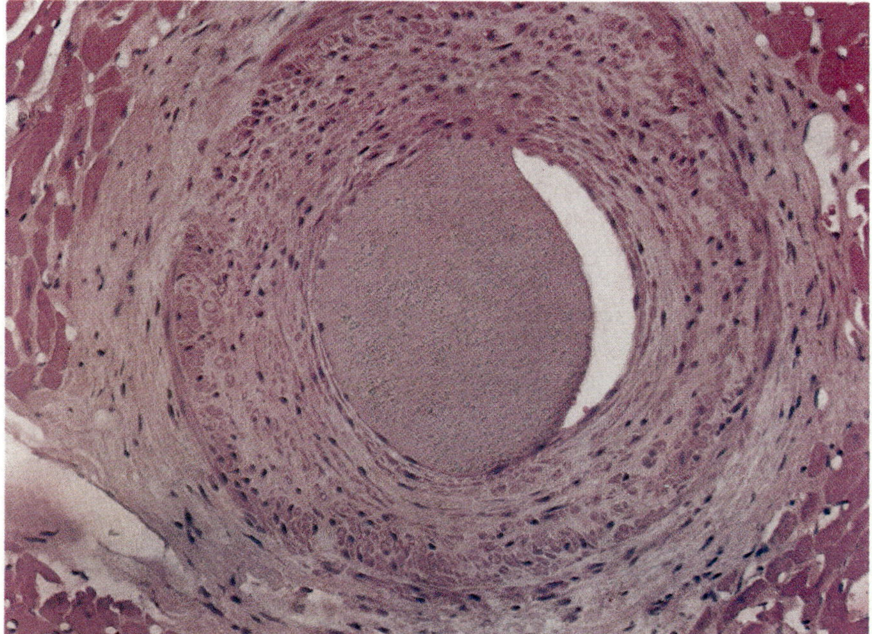

Figure 5-1C   Striking subintimal proliferation in a canine coronary collateral vessel several months after coronary occlusion. Almost no circular smooth muscle is visible. This type of transformed coronary collateral probably degenerates and becomes obliterated. Hematoxylin-eosin stain, ×106. (Reprinted with permission of North-Holland Publishing Company from Shaper.[5])

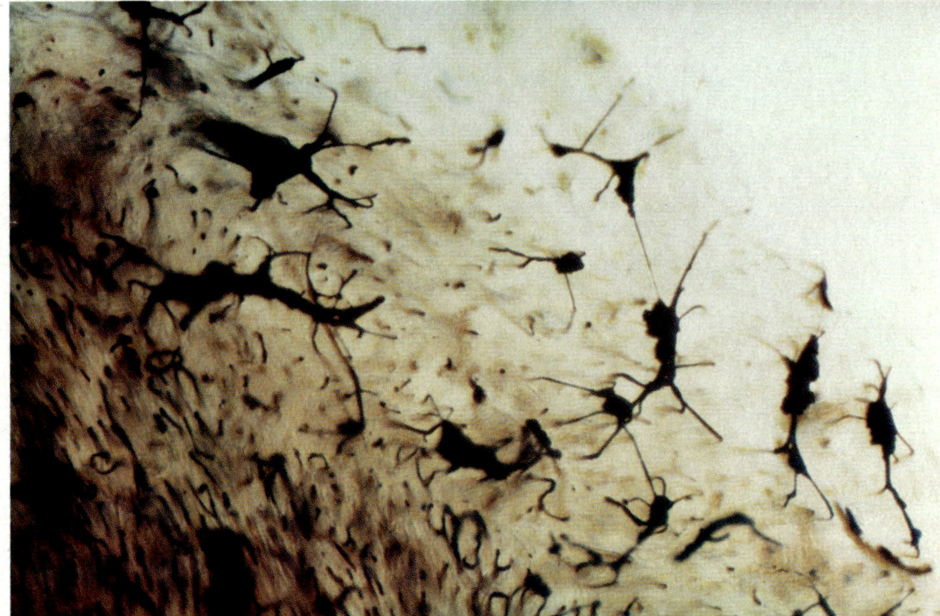

Figure 5-11   Subendocardial sinusoidal vessels in normal dog heart seen following silicone rubber perfusion of the left anterior descending coronary artery. The tissue has been cleared to visualize the microvasculature. Multiple large vascular spaces filled with silicone rubber (appearing black) with numerous interconnected branches are evident (magnification ×110). (Courtesy of Stephen M. Factor, M.D., Department of Pathology, Albert Einstein College of Medicine.)

further increases luminal dimensions. Finally, the third phase, which may actually last for months, involves a striking increase in the thickness of the vascular wall while little additional alteration of the luminal dimensions occurs. Because of this triple-phase transformation, a thin-walled 40 μm conduit is converted into a 1-mm thick-walled arteriole.

Immediately after coronary artery occlusion there are multiple factors that produce dilatation of the collateral vessel. There is a large pressure gradient across the collateral from the stem to the reentry which was not present prior to critical coronary artery narrowing. This intravascular pressure results in mechanical distension of the collateral. Pharmacologic dilatation related to the accumulation of adenosine and vasodilatory metabolites in the ischemic myocardium may also be important. This dilatation increases tangential wall stress, perhaps an important stimulus to further remodeling of the collateral channel. Because of the vessel's mechanical and possible pharmacologic dilatation, the thin wall of the collateral is overstretched, resulting in significant damage. The internal elastic membrane becomes fragmented and blood cells infiltrate into the vessel wall, which becomes edematous. The few medial smooth-muscle cells normally present are also stretched and become pale and swollen. This initial phase is purely passive, in contrast to the second and third phases in which active cellular proliferation occurs. During the second phase of the radial growth, all of the available cellular material is used to increase luminal dimensions of a seemingly maximally stretched vessel. Labeling studies with ^{3}H-thymidine demonstrate that the first cellular mitoses are seen 24 hours after coronary occlusion, and this appearance is independent of the duration or severity of stenosis prior to occlusion. The greatest degree of mitotic activity is usually observed several days later, although Yabe et al.[11] have detected continuing high levels of DNA synthesis for at least one month following coronary occlusion. Mitoses are seen in all cellular elements: endothelial cells, smooth muscle cells, and fibroblasts. In this early stage a rapid increase in density of endothelial cells leads to longitudinal bulges and infolding, resulting in "microstenoses" of the lumen. These luminal irregularities produce turbulent flow and eddy currents, and the orientation of cells along the axis of flow becomes chaotic.

After the maximal luminal diameter is obtained, the third phase of wall remodeling begins. Although the precise physiocochemical stimuli regulating this process are unknown, it is likely that tangential wall stress[5,12] plays some role in accordance with the Laplace relationship, $T\alpha[(P\cdot r)/h]$ where T=wall tension or stress, P = intravascular pressure, r = vessel radius, and h = wall thickness. In the acutely dilated vessel where the diameter is maximal and the wall thickness minimal, wall stress is exceptionally high. To normalize this stress, wall thickness must increase. Mitoses become especially numerous in the smooth-muscle layer. However, the dividing cells initially appear in a random, disorderly arrangement. Within six weeks after coronary occlusion, two distinct smooth-muscle layers can be detected. There is a normal circular or spiral layer separated by the remnants of the old elastic lamina from a subintimal longitudinal smooth-muscle layer in which the muscle cells are oriented parallel to the long axis of the vessel. Formation and development of this subendothelial muscle layer are usually self-limiting processes. However, continued development of the longitudinal muscle layer may eventually result in obliteration of the lumen and may account for the collateral vessel degeneration with smooth-muscle necrosis, and leakage of blood-borne elements through gaps and breaks in the intima which is known to accompany the transformation process.[2,13] The number of circular smooth-muscle layers continues to increase for approximately six months, whereas the degree of subintimal proliferation of longitudinal smooth-muscle cells tends to regress between 8 and 26 weeks following the initial stimulus.

After six months of wall remodeling, the coronary collateral appears to resemble an arteriole. The transformed vessel is almost normal. However, there are segments of the vessel with focal patches of subintimal proliferation consisting of longitudinal smooth-muscle cells. Also, the density of endothelial cells is still increased, resulting in persistent luminal infolding. Perhaps even these abnormalities would disappear with time. But Takahashi et al.[14] have identified persistent areas of subintimal proliferation containing fibroblasts and extracellular components such as collagen and ground substance at one year after coronary occlusion in dogs, and Schaper and her colleagues[10] have never observed a completely smooth and normal inner endothelial surface after similar periods of coronary occlusion and collateral development. It is possible that the collateral histology can never be completely normal. Small defects in the internal elastic lamina probably account for the observed tortuosity of coronary collateral vessels. As a result of this transformation process, the thickness of the vascular wall increases from $2-3\mu m$ to 27 μm, while the total volume of the vascular wall increases by a factor of 173 (Figure 5-1 [colorplates]). The diameter of the collateral vessel is increased by a factor of 10 within the first week following coronary occlusion and thereafter is 0.8 mm after six months and may exceed 1 mm after one year.

II. Changes in Collateral Flow Following Coronary Occlusion

This striking histologic tranformation is accompanied by equally remarkable changes in collateral flow following coronary occlusion. As early as 1939, Gregg, Thornton, and Mautz[15] chronically occluded the coronary artery of a dog by progressively tightening an encircling screw clamp during the course of three to six separate thoracotomies. They noted tremendous increases in both retrograde flow and peripheral coronary pressure. Whereas retrograde flow and peripheral coronary pressure shortly after abrupt coronary occlusion in their normal dogs were less than 1.5 ml/min and 36/22 mmHg, respectively, these investigators documented increases in flow to $6-105$ ml/min and average rises in distal pressure to 82/38 mmHg following chronic occlusion of the left anterior descending coronary artery. Hence, with time, coronary hemodynamics in the distal occluded vessel almost returned to normal. Several years later, Eckstein, Gregg, and Pritchard[16] observed that retrograde flow was already significantly increased as soon as 48 hours following coronary occlusion.

A. Coronary Autoregulation and Reactive Hyperemia

Since these early attempts to evaluate collateral flow following coronary occlusion, other techniques, as described in Chapter 4, have been developed

*The colorplates for this chapter appear on pp. 290–292.

for sequential monitoring of changes in flow in the same animal. However, before these adaptive changes can be appreciated, it is necessary to understand how the intact coronary circulation defends itself against encroaching stenoses. Coronary autoregulation is the first line of defense.[17,18] The arteriolar resistance vessels are responsible for establishing coronary tone. The degree of vasoconstriction is finely tuned to the metabolic state and demands of the heart. A coronary stenosis causing a fall of perfusion pressure would produce a transient fall in myocardial flow. In face of an unchanged cardiac metabolic state, the decreased flow would cause a reduction in myocardial oxygen tension which would result in an accumulation of metabolic byproducts and a net breakdown of the high-energy phosphate compounds, ATP and ADP. The enzyme 5′-nucleotidase located at the myocardial cell membranes and transverse tubules dephosphorylates AMP which is formed as a result of the hypoxic degradation of ATP.[19,20] Adenosine, a potent vasodilator,

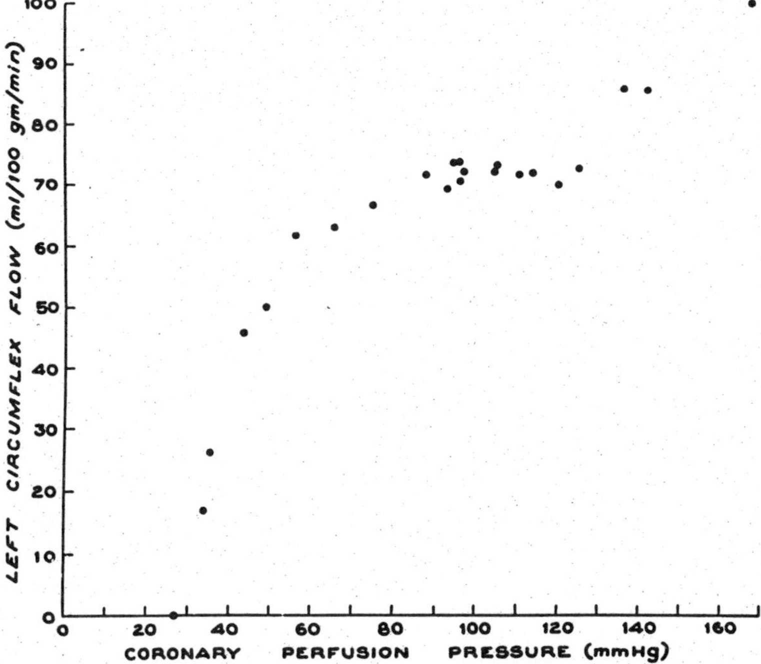

Figure 5-2   Steady-state coronary pressure-flow curve from a single experimental animal during constant cardiac function. Coronary flow is essentially constant over the pressure range of 70–130 mmHg. Despite changes in perfusion pressure in this range, flow is maintained by adjustment of the vascular tone of the arteriolar resistance vessels. At a pressure of 70 mmHg the vessels are maximally dilated. Any further diminution of perfusion pressure results in a striking linear decrease in flow. Conversely, the arterioles are maximally constricted at 130 mmHg. Thus, any additional increase in pressure is accompanied by a rise in flow. (Reprinted with permission of the American Heart Association from Mosher et al.[17])

is the product of this dephosphorylation. It diffuses into the interstitial space and causes relaxation of the coronary arterioles, thus diminishing vascular resistance and returning flow to the original level. This process of autoregulation occurs over a wide range of perfusion pressures (Figure 5-2) and aims to maintain a normal resting flow. Only after a fall in perfusion pressure has elicited maximal compensatory vasodilatation of the coronary arterioles, will further reductions of perfusion pressure result in actual declines in coronary flow. Further evidence of this autoregulatory response is noted when a coronary artery is transiently occluded and then released. With total cessation of antegrade flow during vessel occlusion, the accumulation of vasodilatory compounds including adenosine results in complete relaxation and hence maximal dilatation of the coronary arterioles. Following release of the occlusion, flow through these dilated vessels is greatly increased[21,22] (Figures 2-8 and 5-3). As the vasodilatory compounds are either washed away or metabolized, coronary tone is gradually reestablished and flow returns to baseline levels. The increased flow or reactive hyperemia almost always exceeds the flow debt incurred during the occlusion period, probably because of the actual time necessary to remove or to inactivate the metabolites.[23,24] If the coronary artery is first stenosed prior to complete occlusion, the initial autoregulation following narrowing results in a partially dilated arterial bed. Additional dilatation during subsequent occlusion is therefore attenuated, and less than that occurring in the normal artery without any narrowing. Therefore, maximal flow on release of the occlusion is less (Figure 5-3) and the reactive hyperemic response is diminshed. The magnitude of the reactive hyperemic response begins to diminish when the coronary artery diameter narrowing exceeds 50%, although resting flow will not be affected until the vessel is narrowed by more than 85–90%[25] (Figure 5-4). Such critical narrowing initiates the first phase of collateral transformation, the next defense of normal myocardial perfusion. Eckstein[26] and Gregg and his co-workers[27–30] have documented significant increases in collateral indices and flow even before complete vessel occlusion when a chronic stenosis had attenuated the reactive hyperemic response. In one group of experimental animals, critical coronary stenosis initiated collateral development, which resulted ultimately in an average collateral flow during test occlusions of the critically stenosed vessel of 58% (range, 40–70%) of the antegrade coronary flow.[29]

B. Left Ventricular Transmural Flow Distribution

Normal resting myocardial blood flow is approximately 1 ml/min/g. However, there is a broad normal range which may extend from 0.5 to 1.5 ml/min/g. This flow is fairly homogeneous in all left ventricular coronary distributions. The transmural flow distribution deserves special attention. The endocardial/epicardial or inner/outer left ventricular wall flow ratio normally

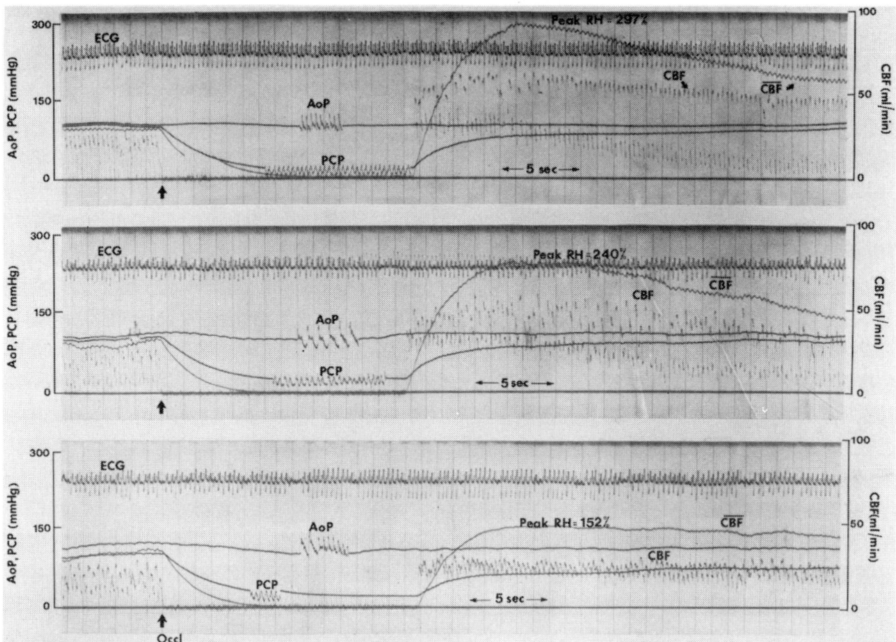

Figure 5-3   Aortic pressure (AoP), peripheral left circumflex coronary pressure (PCP), and phasic (CBF) and mean ($\overline{\mathrm{CBF}}$) left circumflex blood flow in a dog with a normal left circumflex artery (top panel) and then with mild (middle panel) and moderately severe (bottom panel) left circumflex stenoses. A balloon occluder encircling the left circumflex artery was inflated at the points indicated by the vertical arrows in the three panels. Total occlusion of the vessel was verified by prompt decline of flow to zero and decrease in PCP to 20–25 mmHg. After 15 secs the balloon was deflated, thus permitting flow to resume. In the top panel where the left circumflex was normal (aortic–left circumflex pressure gradient ~ 2 mmHg), a striking hyperemic response was apparent with a maximal threefold increase in flow over the preocclusion level. This reactive hyperemia (RH) is caused by vasodilatory metabolites produced during the previous ischemic interval. In the middle panel the left circumflex artery was made stenotic with a ligature. Although resting flow was unaffected, the aortic–left circumflex pressure gradient increased to 8 mmHg. In order to maintain normal flow in face of this stenosis, the distal coronary vasculature was forced to dilate. The smaller peak reactive hyperemic response of 240% documents that coronary reserve was diminished. The more severe stenosis in the bottom panel increased the aortic–left circumflex gradient to 18 mmHg. Significant vasodilatation was required to keep the resting flow normal. Because of this decrease in vascular tone at rest, the vessels were unable to dilate much more following release of the transient coronary occlusion. Consequently, the peak reactive hyperemic response was only 152% of the baseline flow.

exceeds 1.0. This homogeneity is either the result of regional autoregulation in the subendocardium[31] and/or increased subendocardial vascularity.[32,33] Approximately 10 to 20% of coronary flow normally occurs during the systolic phase of the cardiac cycle.[34–36] During systole there is an intramyocardial pressure gradient.[37,38] The pressure or wall stress in the subendocardium

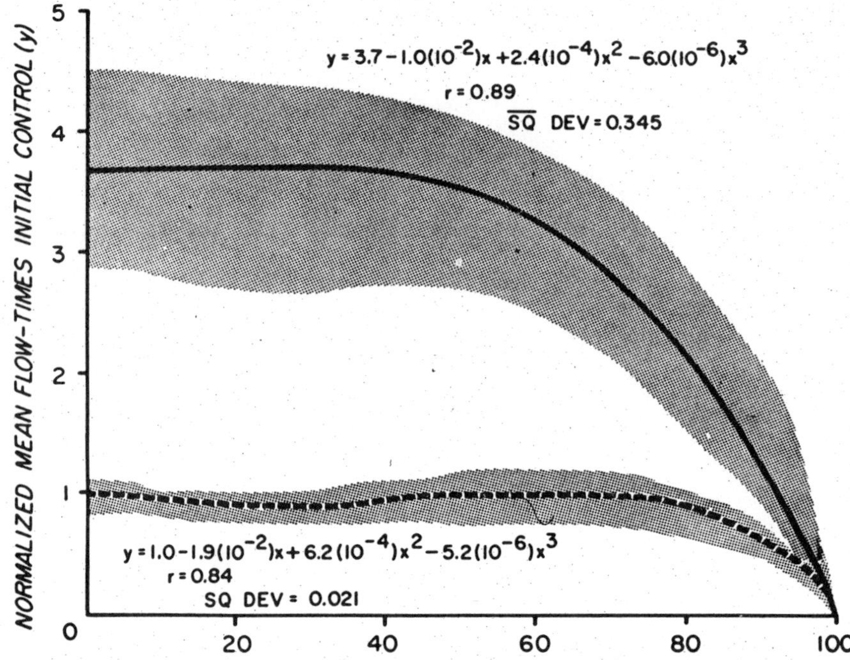

Figure 5-4   Relationship between stenosis of the left circumflex coronary artery of dogs and resting coronary flow (dotted line) and the hyperemic response following intracoronary injection of angiographic contrast medium (Hypaque-M) (solid line). The hyperemia after injection of contrast medium is comparable to that following release of a transient coronary occlusion. Hyperemic flows (ordinate) have been normalized for the control resting mean values at the beginning of each experiment. The reactive hyperemic response begins to diminish when the stenosis reduces the artery's diameter by more than 50%, whereas resting flow does not decrease until 85% of the vessel's diameter is compromised. The dotted and solid lines in the diagram are the best fits to the experimental data, while the shaded areas indicate the limits of the relations plotted for individual dogs. (Reprinted with permission of Dun-Donnelly Publishing Corp. from Gould et al.[25])

actually exceeds intraventricular and therefore intracoronary pressure, while that in the subepicardium is less than the pressure generated within the chamber. The augmented endocardial wall stress results in increased oxygen demands. But the greater endocardial compressive forces restrict flow in the inner half of the left ventricular wall.[39-44] Consequently, autoregulation would result in relative dilatation of the subendocardial vessels and hence increased flow during diastole when intramyocardial forces are minimal, thus making up for the systolic flow deficit. The price for this resting transmural flow homogeneity (averaged over a complete cardiac cycle), however, is partial diminution of the endocardial vascular reserve. This postulated mechanism of regional autoregulation is felt by many advocates to be strengthened by the observation that subendocardial vessels, already assumed to be partially dilated under resting conditions, are unable to dilate and increase flow as much as subepicardial arterioles after maximal pharmacologic vasodilatation with adenosine.[45]

Despite the obvious appeal of this explanation, Downey et al.[46] have presented additional data suggesting that endocardial autoregulation cannot fully explain the uniformity of transmural perfusion. When Cobb et al.[45] infused adenosine into conscious dogs, they noted a reversal of the normal relationship between endocardial and epicardial flows, and concluded that the diminished responsiveness of the endocardial vasculature proved the latter was partially dilated before adenosine administration. However, their results may have been influenced by choice of a conscious animal model. Because of maximal vasodilatation and abolition of any possible autoregulation, the transmural flow distribution might have been adversely affected by changes in extravascular coronary resistance (increase in heart rate and fall in blood pressure) accompanying administration of adenosine. Consequently, Downey et al.[46] studied the effect of maximal coronary vasodilation with adenosine on fibrillating dog hearts supported by a donor dog, thus avoiding the possible complicating effects of changing hemodynamics. In the absence of systolic vascular compression, adenosine increased endocardial flow to 9.8 ml/min/g and epicardial flow to 7.2 ml/min/g. Thus, the endo/epi flow ratio averaged approximately 1.37. Wüsten[33] performed similar experiments in empty, supported dog hearts, but he arrested the hearts with procainamide. Maximal adenosine vasodilatation produced significant increases in transmural flow and an endo/epi flow ratio of 1.62. Therefore, in the absence of any myocardial compression and under experimental conditions where extravascular coronary resistance is minimal and unvarying, the increase in endocardial flow during maximal vasodilatation exceeded that to the epicardium. Autoregulation cannot explain these results. A plausible alternate explanation is the presence of a gradient of vascularity increasing toward the endocardium. Winbury and Weiss[32] have indeed demonstrated a small gradient in small vessel vascular volume favoring the endocardium (endo/epi ratio = 1.05:1) in canine hearts during asphyxia. Wüsten[33] also measured intramural coronary vascularity in his arrested, supported dog hearts with maximally dilated coronary arteries by infusing a barium-gelatin mixture containing radioactive microspheres into a cannulated coronary vessel. After counting the radioactivity in myocardial samples, he was able to determine the sample's content of barium sulphate which was used as an index of vascular capacity. When portions of the left ventricle were cut into eight transmural layers, the lowest coronary artery volume was found in the most superficial slice. The vascular capacity increased gradually toward the endocardium and peaked in the sixth layer and then fell slightly in the two remaining subendocardial layers. These data suggest that there is an increased subendocardial vascularity in the dog, and hence a lower minimal subendocardial vascular resistance, which helps to compensate for the effects of extravascular compression during normal cardiac contraction. Curiously, Gerdes et al.[47] have reported that the rat epicardium has 38% more capillaries than the endocardial region, although neither Rakušan and colleagues[48] nor Wright and Hudlická[49] has been able to confirm this increased epicardial vascularity.

C. Time Course of Changes in Coronary Flow Following Coronary Occlusion

Following acute coronary occlusion in the dog, myocardial blood flow generally falls to 10–30% of the preocclusion flow.[50–59] However, there is a wide range of flows possible which is undoubtedly related to the magnitude and state of development of the native collateral circulation which in turn is genetically determined. In individual dogs the collateral circulation may be so well developed that there is little or no evidence of a flow deficit when antegrade flow is abolished.[56,58,60,61] Following coronary occlusion, transmural flow is typically inhomogeneous with inner/outer left ventricular wall flow ratios of 0.3–0.7.[51–53,55,56,58] It is possible that the diminished diastolic perfusion pressure is insufficient to open all of the endocardial vessels compressed during the residual systolic contraction of the ischemic myocardium. Furthermore, any element of diminished endocardial vascular reserve prior to coronary occlusion would be expressed as a more marked decline in endocardial flow following the occlusion.

Although it is accepted that collateral flow increases following coronary occlusion, the precise time course of the changes is not entirely clear. Confusion stems from the use of multiple methodologies and the nonuniform method of sampling the ischemic myocardium. Earlier studies employed either ^{133}Xe or [85]Kr clearance to monitor changes in ischemic myocardial flow.[62–68] Aside from the difficulty of having to measure flow in multiple compartments, as previously described, this technique monitors flow only in large myocardial areas. Therefore, changes in flow in some areas might be obscured by simultaneously occurring and possibly directionally opposite changes in other regions. Furthermore, these clearance studies yield no information about possible transmural flow alterations. Thermocouples inserted into the myocardium to measure thermal conductivity directly and hence indirectly to evaluate blood flow can monitor changes in flow to only very small, discrete myocardial areas.[69–71] In such situations it is not logical to assume that these small areas are representative of the entire ischemic myocardial region. More recently, radioactive microspheres have been employed to measure changes in perfusion of ischemic myocardium.[8,9,51–53,55,57,59,61,72–77] With this method it is possible to evaluate flows to multiple areas of interest as well as the epicardium and endocardium, although the animal must be sacrificed and the heart sectioned. In spite of the use of radioactive microspheres for quantitation of myocardial flow in most recent studies, the technique used to select tissue for analysis may greatly influence the results. Whereas some investigators define vascular perfusion territories with either Evans blue or other dye[59,72,73,75] or postmortem angiography,[55,61] others prefer to select the myocardium to be sampled visually on the basis of surface distribution of the branches of the occluded vessel.[51-53,57,76] In some studies the ischemic tissue is divided into infarcting and noninfarcting portions, whereas other investigators appear not to make this distinction. Thus, discrepancies in data from the various studies can often be related to methodological differences.

1. 0—30 Minutes

Following the abrupt decrease in tissue perfusion which occurs within the first 30 seconds beyond an acutely obstructed coronary artery in the dog, those studies that have measured collateral flow again at five minutes have documented significant flow increases.[51,55] Marcus et al.[51] measured 120% increases in flow to severely hypoperfused myocardium (from approximately 0.10 to 0.22 ml/min/g) while Jugdutt and colleagues[55] measured 150% increases. Thus, the histologic dilatation and stretching of the collateral channels described above have physiologic and functional correlates. Davenport et al.[59] measured blood flow to the vascular territory of the occluded vessel at five and again at 20 minutes after cessation of antegrade flow. Although flows increased throughout the area at risk, the increases were substantially smaller in the muscle destined to infarct. Thus, in the infarcting myocardium average flow rose from 2.2 to 4.3 ml/min/100g, whereas the change in the normal-appearing myocardium immediately adjacent to the necrotic zone was from 8.5 to 13.2 ml/min/100g. The collateral flow increases present at 20 minutes are also evident at 30 minutes after coronary occlusion.[63,64,67]

2. 1—6 Hours

Despite evidence of increasing collateral flow during the initial 30 minutes following coronary occlusion, further increases are not assured over the ensuing five-hour period. Marcus's group[51] measured a further increase in collateral flow from approximately 0.22 ml/min/g at five minutes to 0.27 ml/min/g one hour following occlusion in dogs. Jugdutt et al.[61] also reported increased collateral flow 60 minutes after coronary obstruction, but the data at one hour were compared to flows determined only immediately following coronary occlusion and, therefore, did not account for the increase acknowledged to occur 5 to 15 minutes after cessation of antegrade perfusion. Other investigators reporting early increases in collateral flow in dogs have reported no additional change[55] or even absolute decreases[63,64,67] in flow at one hour. Schaper and Pasyk[9] were also unable to detect increased flow at one hour.

These confusing results are not clarified by additional studies measuring flows at later intervals. In their studies Rees and Redding[63,64] noted that collateral flow decreased within minutes following coronary occlusion to approximately 25% of control levels but then gradually increased to 45% of control over the next 30 to 120 minutes. However, at one to two hours in most animals flow began to decrease, and by the third hour of the experiment mean ^{133}Xe clearance from the ischemic myocardium was usually less than that measured at five minutes. Further gradual declines were noted up to six hours following occlusion. Comparable changes were noted by Weisse et al.[67] who documented decreases in collateral flow from a peak of 0.39 ml/min/g at 30 minutes following occlusion to 0.18 ml/min/g at two to three hours. Grayson and colleagues[69-71] also measured a gradual and progressive decrease in collateral flow following coronary occlusion. In their earlier canine study[69] and their investigations in primates,[71] collateral flow was nearly zero at four to five hours after coronary obstruction, while the later study in dogs[70] demonstrated flow at six hours had decreased from 54% of control immediately after coronary ligation to 10%. In contrast, Marshall and Parratt[68] noted no change in collateral flow in dogs for the duration of the four-hour observation period following the initial decrease to 20% of control levels. These earlier studies used either ^{133}Xe or [85]Kr clearance techniques or implanted thermocouples to measure thermal conductivity. More recent investigations have used radioactive microspheres, but there is still no unanimity of results in this canine model. Significant increases in collateral flow to the central ischemic region from 0.11 ml/min/g at 15 minutes to 0.20 ml/min/g two hours following coronary ligation were observed by Smith et al.[74] Rivas and colleagues[53] also documented increases in collateral flow from 0.25 ml/min/g 45 seconds after occlusion to 0.39 ml/min/g at two hours. However, their protocol did not permit evaluation of the flow increase occurring at 5−15 minutes, and therefore it is not possible to determine whether the increase occurred soon after coronary ligation or was delayed. These same investigators[53] noted no change in flow from two to six hours. Davenport and colleagues[59] who documented increased perfusion of the ischemic myocardium from 5 to 20 minutes following coronary occlusion also observed additional increases at four hours in both infarcting (4.3 to 8.8 ml/min/ 100g) and adjacent (13.2 to 24.0 ml/min/100g) myocardium. Bishop et al.[52] and Schaper and Pasyk[9] found no change in collateral flow at two hours, and Bishop[52] also found no change at six hours.

Thus, between one and six hours following coronary ligation it is difficult to predict the changes in collateral flow. Some of the variation in results may be related to use of different methodologies. However, other possibilities have been suggested. Grayson believed the decrease in collateral flow was related to vasospasm of adjacent normal coronary arteries supplying the collateral channels.[69-71] To prove his hypothesis he demonstrated not only abolition of the decline but also a significant increase in collateral flow in those animals with either intramyocardial procaine infiltration along the course of the ligated artery or administration of bretylium or bethanidine, agents known to block adrenergic neurons, prior to ligation.[69,70] However, Redding and Rees[64] attempted to duplicate Grayson's results, and were unable to reverse the fall in collateral flow observed at two to six hours following coronary ligation with either sympathectomy, procaine infiltration, or administration of agents (bethanidine, phenoxybenzamine, propranolol) believed to have direct effects on ganglionic transmission. Furthermore, numerous investigations of the effect of coronary artery ligation on flow in adjacent normal vessels have never documented falls in flow, but often have shown rises[52,78-82] presumably related to the increased work and oxygen consumption of the muscle adjacent to the akinetic or dyskinetic zone.[80] Hence, it is unlikely that the fall in collateral flow seen several hours following coronary occlusion is related to generalized vasospasm of the adjacent normal vessels.

The "no reflow" phenomenon[83-86] provides an alternative explanation for the decrease in collateral flow often observed between one and six hours following coronary occlusion. This phenomenon refers to compression of the microvasculature by swollen myocardial cells, and was clearly demonstrated by the dye injection studies of Krug[83] and Kloner.[84] After variable periods of coronary occlusion lasting from 30 to 120 minutes, the myocardium was reperfused by removing the ligature. Immediately prior to animal sacrifice, either acridine orange[83] or thioflavin S[84] fluorescent dye was injected intravenously. Myocardium perfused without interruption showed normal fluorescence, whereas the distribution of fluorescence was inhomogeneous in the reperfused areas, and the inhomogeneity increased with increasing duration of the coronary occlusion prior to its release. Thus, reflow following a 40-minute coronary occlusion usually produced homogeneous distribution of fluorescence in the examined posterior papillary muscle, while after 90 minutes portions of the subendocardium and sometimes inner midmyocardium of the papillary muscle contained areas of nonfluorescence.[84] An occlusion of 120 minutes followed by reflow was associated with fluorescence in only the peripheral portions of the ischemic region.[83] Histologic studies have confirmed the presence of myocardial and capillary endothelial cell swelling producing obstruction of the microvasculature from within as well as from without. These qualitative observations are further supported by quantitative measurements. Three minutes of reflow following release of a 120-minute coronary occlusion does not result in restoration of normal flow to the previously nonperfused area. The reperfused tissue has diminished blood flow and a significant increase in regional coronary vascular resistance.[85]

3. 24 Hours

Progressive myocardial edema in the ischemic region may result in diminishing collateral flow. Diminution of collateral flow to the most ischemic areas destined to become necrotic represents the heart's second line of defense against the consequences of diminished or absent antegrade perfusion. Collateral flow to necrotic areas has little purpose, and therefore redistribution of this flow to somewhat less ischemic areas would perhaps insure the ultimate viability of these latter myocardial regions. This redistribution of collateral flow is most apparent when one examines the changes in transmural flow during the initial hours following coronary occlusion. As previously discussed, the endocardial/epicardial flow ratio decreases in acutely ischemic myocardium. Although some investigators have observed proportional increases in flow to the ischemic subendocardial and subepicardial myocardium during the first 24 hours following coronary occlusion in the dog,[51,53,76] most have documented a dramatic and progressive increase in flow to the subepicardium at the expense of flow to the subendocardium.[8,9,52,72,73,75] Hirzel et al.[75] showed that average flow to the necrotic subendocardium fell from 0.11 ml/min/g ten minutes following coronary occlusion to 0.05 ml/min/g at 24 hours, while flow to the normal appearing subepicardium rose over the same period from 0.24 to 0.39 ml/min/g. Thus, while total transmural flow increased from 0.12 to 0.18 ml/min/g, there was evidence of significant flow redistribution. Schaper and Pasyk[9] also showed that at two to four hours after coronary occlusion, subendocardial flow fell to nearly zero, while subepicardial flow was increasing. In similar experiments by Cox et al.[73] average endocardial flow following coronary occlusion initially fell to 0.10 ml/min/g and epicardial flow to 0.28 ml/min/g. Over the course of the next 24 hours there was no significant change in endocardial flow, but epicardial flow increased to 82% of the control level. Because of the more marked initial decline in endocardial flow following coronary occlusion, the subendocardium becomes more ischemic, accounting for quicker and more obvious disruption of cellular processes and production of tissue edema. The latter produces "no-reflow," and endocardial flow becomes even more limited. This chain of events perhaps explains the increased frequency of the subendocardial location of nontransmural infarcts and the greater endocardial extent of transmural infarcts. Furthermore, the simultaneous occurrence of "no-reflow" resulting in both decreasing flow and redistribution and the first phase of collateral transformation or stretching leading to increasing flow may account for the different patterns of collateral flow described by investigators during the initial 6-hour period following a coronary occlusion.

Whereas collateral flow in dogs is not clearly increased by six hours following coronary occlusion, most studies have documented significant flow increases by 24 hours.[9,52,57,61,66,72,73,75,76,87] Cox et al[72,73] measured an increase in transmural flow from approximately 20% of the preocclusion level immediately after coronary ligation to 57% at 24 hours. It must be reemphasized, however, that this early increase was accounted for solely by a change in subepicardial flow. In Bishop's studies,[52] average endocardial flow was increased from 26 to 39% of normal by 24 hours, while epicardial flow had increased from 47 to 67%. In the studies by Murdock and Cobb,[57] two- to threefold increases in ischemic zone flow were observed between 15 minutes and 24 hours following coronary occlusion in those regions where blood flows were initially less than 0.5 ml/min/g. Curiously, the greatest increases were noted in the most ischemic tissue (0.042 ± 0.004 to 0.172 ± 0.045 ml/min/g, $p < 0.01$).

In monkeys, left anterior descending coronary artery occlusion resulted in striking falls in flow in the jeopardized myocardium.[88] In the central ischemic area flows at five minutes after occlusion were only approximately 2% of their normal levels. There was virtually no change at 24 hours (0.02 to 0.04 ml/min/g in the endocardium and 0.04 to 0.07 ml/min/g in the epicardium, $p = NS$).

4. 4 Days to 3 Months

Beyond 24 hours following coronary occlusion in the dog collateral flow appears to increase quickly. It is at this time that the second phase of collateral transformation is initiated. Bishop et al.[52] showed that ischemic endocardial flow increased to 49% of normal four days after occlusion, while epicardial flow rose to 74% of normal. Although Rees and Redding[62] did not observe an increase in collateral flow in the first four days following coronary occlusion, ischemic myocardial blood flow was noted to rise to normal between the fourth and tenth days. In his review Schimmler[87] noted significantly increased collateral flow by 12 hours following coronary occlusion, a doubling by two days, and an increase to 40–100% of normal within three to four weeks.

Several days after coronary occlusion the third phase of collateral transformation is begun. However, long before transformation of the thin-walled conduit into an arteriole is complete, resting flow to the myocardium beyond the coronary occlusion is normal.[58,62,89–98] Thus, Rees and Redding[62] recorded normal flows in the previously ischemic areas as early as ten days after occlusion, and Schaper and colleagues[91,92] made similar observations four weeks after implantation of ameroid constrictors around a coronary artery, or approximately two weeks after completion of vessel occlusion. Perhaps a more sensitive indicator of the adequacy of collateral development than total flow itself is the transmural distribution. Following coronary occlusion, the endo/epi ratio falls from approximately 1.0–1.2 to 0.3–0.7.[51–53,55,56,58] Collateral development also restores this ratio to normal,[58,90–101] sometimes in as few as two to three weeks.[99,100]

In one recent study,[58] the homogeneity of collateral blood flow beyond a chronic coronary occlusion was graphically demonstrated by constructing flow histograms. In this study beagles were chronically instrumented with catheters and a flow probe and balloon occluder around the proximal left circumflex coronary artery. In addition, the left circumflex artery was constricted by encircling and snugly tying a ligature around it and an interposed 18 gauge needle which was then withdrawn. The stenosis resulted in approximately a 75–85% narrowing of the vessel's diameter. After recovery from surgery, collateral flow was measured with radioactive microspheres during a one-minute balloon inflation and left circumflex artery occlusion while the dog was resting quietly. Subsequently all animals were observed for three months. During this interval the coronary artery became occluded in six dogs. The time of occlusion was not known because of malfunction of all implanted flow probes within approximately four to five weeks of the initial surgery. Coronary angiography after three months demonstrated the coronary occlusion, and the occlusions were later confirmed by direct examination. Prior to animal sacrifice collateral flow was again measured while the animals were resting quietly. Three to five milliliters of a concentrated aqueous solution of Evans blue dye were injected into the distal LCf to outline the perfusion territory. The heart was removed, frozen, and serially sectioned from apex to base into 0.5-cm-thick slices. The rings of left ventricular tissue

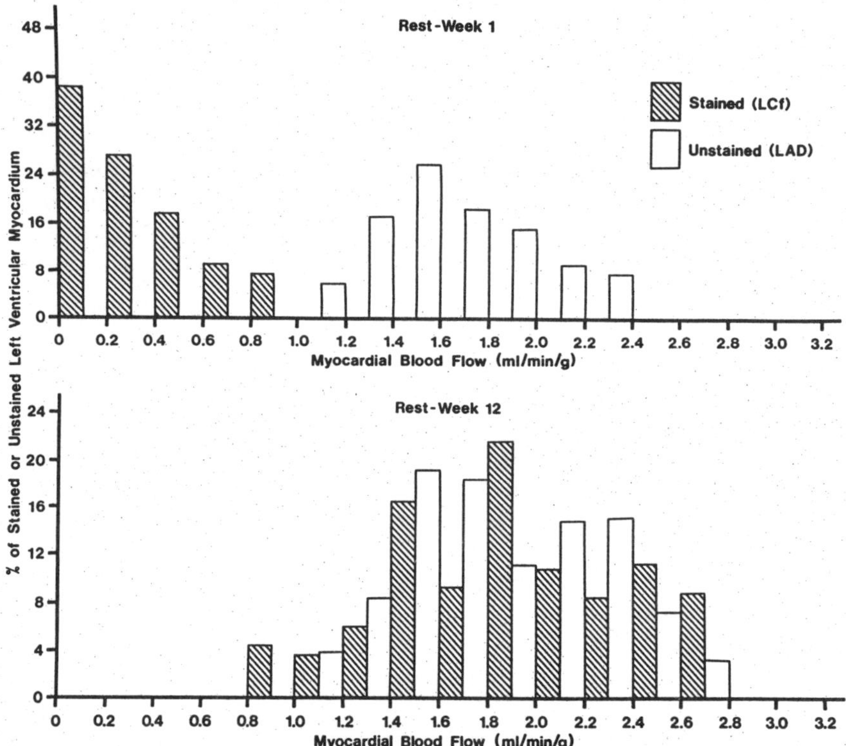

Figure 5-5   Histograms of myocardial blood flow at rest in the same dog during transient occlusion of the left circumflex coronary artery (LCf) during first week of protocol (top) and again 12 weeks later after chronic LCf occlusion (bottom). Hatched bars represent stained (Evans blue injected into distal LCf at time of animal sacrifice) or ischemic myocardium distal to LCf occlusion, whereas blank bars represent normal, unstained, or left anterior descending (LAD) myocardium. The abscissa is not a continuous function of blood flow, but is divided into discrete increments of 0.2 ml/min/g. During week one there was no overlap of flows to stained and unstained myocardial regions, and average flows were 0.35 and 1.66 ml/min/g, respectively. In contrast, there was complete overlap of flows to stained and unstained myocardium at week 12 following chronic coronary occlusion and collateral transformation and development, and flows to LCf and LAD myocardium were 1.90 and 1.86 ml/min/g, respectively. (Modified and reprinted with permission of the American Physiological Society from Cohen et al.[58])

were subdivided into stained (ischemic, left circumflex) and unstained (normal, left anterior descending) pieces by carefully following the serpiginous border separating the two. These large pieces were cut into wedges weighing 0.4−0.8 g , which were further subdivided into inner and outer halves. Isotope activities were determined and flows calculated. Whereas the average ratio of ischemic to normal blood flow was 0.37 in week one at the time of the first study, it averaged 1.03 after three months. Also, the average left ventricular endo/epi flow ratio increased from 0.57 to 1.11 over the same three-month period. A flow histogram from one representative dog is shown in Figure 5-5. The hatched bars represent stained or ischemic myocardium, whereas blank bars represent unstained or normal tissue. The abscissa is not a continuous function of blood flow, but is divided into discrete increments of 0.2 ml/min/g. Average ischemic and normal flows during week one were 0.35 and 1.66 ml/min/g, respectively. During the initial study there was no overlap of flows to these two myocardial regions, and it is not difficult to select two distinct populations of flows corresponding to the two regions. During week 12 resting flows to the normal and stained myocardial regions averaged 1.86 and 1.90 ml/min/g, respectively. The histogram shows there is now complete overlap of the flows, and examination of the bar graph does not allow one to distinguish stained from unstained tissue.

It is not coincidence that the dynamic process of histologic transformation of the collateral is paralleled by changing flows. Enlargement and remodeling of the collateral vessel make it more suitable for transport of the flows necessary to support normal myocardial function. Scheel et al.[102] examined collateral conductance in beagles at various time intervals following coronary occlusion. They observed that conductance increased rapidly during the first month after cessation of antegrade flow, also the time of greatest histologic change. During the second month collateral conductance increased further, but at a slower rate. Scheel[102] observed that after several weeks collateral conductance seemed to be high enough to supply enough blood to satisfy the resting requirements of the myocardium in the distribution of the occluded vessel.

III. Coronary Collateral Vascular Reserve

A. Vasodilators

Although collaterals may restore myocardial flow to normal under resting conditions, this observation should not be interpreted to imply that collaterals are a perfect substitute for the obstructed coronary artery. Schaper[92,103,104] and Scheel[105,106] have attempted to determine the minimal vascular resistance of the collateral bed following chronic coronary occlusion. Both have used isolated, supported canine heart preparations in which either adenosine[103,106] or dipyridamole[104] has been added to the perfusate to insure maximal coronary vasodilatation. The minimal vascular resistance of the normal coronary bed is 0.16 mmHg/ml/min/100g (or 0.16 resistance unit or 0.16 RU), and rises to 3.54 RU following acute coronary occlusion.[103] Four weeks following ameroid implantation around a coronary artery or approximately two weeks after vessel occlusion, the resistance of the collateral-dependent area has fallen dramatically to 0.58 RU in the subepicardium and 0.69 RU in the subendocardium. Further small decreases in epicardial and endocardial resistance occur at six (0.49 RU and 0.48 RU, respectively) and 16 (0.38 RU and 0.48 RU, respectively) weeks after occlusion. Thus, this study suggests collaterals are able to compensate for only 33% of the normal coronary conductance. Scheel[105,106] also has concluded that the coronary reserve of an occluded bed after three to five months is only 34−50% of the reserve of an unoccluded vessel. However, the isolated empty beating heart is not a physiologic preparation, and extrapolation to the intact organism may not be justified. Three determinations of minimal vascular resistance or conductance in open-chest, anesthetized canine preparations have been made.[92,104,107] Although collaterals appear to supply only 38 to 47% of the conductance of a normal bed, two of the studies[92,104] were completed at approximately two and four weeks following coronary occlusion—barely enough time for the third phase of collateral transformation to be initiated. Thus, these results are inconclusive. The third study by Walter et al[107] in dogs with coronary occlusions of four to five weeks reported the minimal collateral resistance to be 0.27 RU, a more promising result.

Although the minimal vascular resistance of well-developed collaterals in the intact heart is not yet known, several assessments of vascular reserve of the canine collateral bed have been made. Vasodilators such as lifoflazine[100] and dipyridamole[91,92,104,107,108] increase collateral flow but to a lesser degree than the observed rise in flow to normal beds. The magnitude of the flow deficit is dependent on the duration of the occlusion and extent of collateral transformation. Dipyridamole was able to double collateral flow two weeks after coronary occlusion, while flow to normal myocardium increased three- to fourfold.[108] After five months of occlusion dipyridamole increased normal epicardial and endocardial flows to 5.17 and 5.46 ml/min/g, respectively, still significantly higher than the flows of 3.72 and 2.50 ml/min/g in the collateral-dependent epicardium and endocardium.[108] Although maximal dilating doses of vasodilators usually depress the endo/epi ratio in normal myocardium,[45] submaximal vasodilatation results in significant increases in the endo/epi ratio.[109] Nonetheless, the redistribution away from the endocardium is exaggerated in the collateralized areas with all doses of vasodilators.[91,108] Again, the effect is less significant as the duration of occlusion increases. Thus, in two-week occlusions all doses of dipyridamole result in inhomogeneity of transmural flow, whereas transmural flow remains homogeneous in collateralized areas 22 weeks after coronary occlusion until dipyridamole causes total flow to exceed 2 ml/min/g.[91] Higher doses of the vasodilator will further raise the level of collateral flow, but the endo/epi flow ratio significantly decreases. All flow deficits observed during vasodilation can be abolished if antegrade coronary flow through the occluded vessel is resumed.[107]

B. Norepinephrine

By increasing myocardial oxygen consumption, norepinephrine causes secondary increases in coronary flow. In normal canine coronary beds, endocardial and epicardial flows increase linearly with norepinephrine-generated increases in pressure-rate product.[92,95,104] The response of the collateralized epicardium is somewhat blunted, whereas the endocardial response is nearly absent. However, these studies were conducted approximately two to four weeks after coronary occlusions, and, therefore, abnormal responses in the collateralized tissue are not unexpected. Only a study by Pass et al.[90] evaluated the response of collateral blood flow to norepinephrine infusion three months after implantation of ameroid constrictors. This inotropic agent increased normal subendocardial flow by 192%, while the increase in the collateralized endocardial layer was limited to 99%. Reestablishment of antegrade coronary flow beyond the obstruction restored normal coronary reactivity in all studies.[90,92,95,104]

C. Atrial Pacing

The tachycardia induced by atrial or ventricular pacing abbreviates diastole and therefore the time during which most of coronary flow occurs. Three to four days following occlusion of the proximal left circumflex and mid-left anterior descending coronary arteries in dogs, Patterson et al.[110] noted that subendocardial and mid-myocardial ischemic layers contained infarcted tissue and had low collateral flows and conductances which became even lower with right ventricular pacing at average rates of 222 beats/min. In the overlying subepicardial layer, which was usually free of necrosis, resting vascular conductance was normal, although it did not change during pacing (1.17 to 1.21 ml · min^{-1} · g^{-1}/100 mmHg). In contrast, conductance in normal zone subepicardium increased 35% during pacing from 1.24 to 1.69 ml · min^{-1} · g^{-1}/100 mmHg ($p < 0.03$). Therefore, collateral blood flow in the surviving myocardium within the initial zone of ischemia was normal at rest by three to four days after coronary occlusion. But there was no reserve capacity to increase collateral conductance during the stress of pacing.

Eight to nine weeks following coronary occlusion, pacing stress causes rises in ischemic subepicardial blood flow and either an inadequate or no increase in ischemic subendocardial flow resulting in transmural inhomogeneity.[97] One study documented an absolute decrease in flow to the collateralized area during atrial pacing which was abolished after revascularization of the area.[90] At atrial rates of 200 bpm, Neill and Oxendine[96] found few regional or transmural flow abnormalities in dogs with five-week occlusions.

But when the pacing rate was increased to 250 beats/min, the ischemic/normal myocardial blood flow ratio decreased significantly to 0.90, and the average endo/epi flow ratio in the myocardium beyond the ameroid occluder fell to 0.82.

Many of these studies have demonstrated that collaterals may deliver normal amounts of properly distributed blood at rest, but an inadequate flow of inhomogeneously distributed blood during administration of vasodilators or inotropic agents or induction of tachycardia. However, some of these investigations were conducted long before the transformation process had a chance to shape the changing collateral into a form even remotely resembling the final arteriolelike vessel. Others have employed unphysiologic techniques to examine collateral resistance. It is perhaps the minimal resistance (or maximal conductance) of the well-developed collateralized bed during physiologic stress that is most meaningful. This latter determination should yield the best estimate of functional value of coronary collaterals. It must be emphasized that the histologic studies revealing persistent abnormalities of collateral structure as long as six months to a year after coronary occlusion[8,10,14] suggest that collateral function may never be absolutely normal. It is, therefore, not completely surprising that maximal collateral conductance measured in the isolated, supported canine heart is only 40−50% of that of a normal coronary bed.[103,105,106]

D. Exercise

Exercise combines inotropic stimulation of the heart, direct and indirect stimuli of coronary flow, and tachycardia, and therefore represents a potent physiologic stress. Several investigators have examined the effectiveness of collaterals in exercising animals. In a recent study, quantitative ^{201}Tl scintigraphy has been employed to follow collateral development after coronary ligation, and exercise has been used to demonstrate the limitations and/or adequacy of collateral flow.[111] Briefly, ^{201}Tl is a radioisotope that is handled much like K^+ or Rb^+. It is a flow-limited tracer that is taken up by the myocardium in proportion to the flow to the tissue, and mixed in the intracellular pool. With time the isotope leaks from the cell back into the circulation. The isotope's presence within the myocardium is detected with an externally positioned gamma scintillation camera. Thallium perfusion scans will, therefore, detect the relative amounts of radioisotope in normal and poorly perfused regions. To magnify the differences between the two areas, exercise stress is commonly used. While flow to normal myocardium will increase severalfold, the increased flow to ischemic regions will be limited because of absent or nearly exhausted coronary reserve. Therefore, in the present study a ^{201}Tl scan was performed in a dog shortly after completion of treadmill running at a speed and incline adjusted so that the animal's heart rate was approximately 210−230 beats/min. While the dog was running, 1.5 mCi of ^{201}Tl was injected and exercise was continued for one minute. The dog was then anesthetized and scanning commenced ten minutes after injection. A baseline scan was performed prior to coronary occlusion, three days following surgical ligation of the left circumflex coronary artery, and at two, four, and six weeks thereafter.

The method employed for quantitative analysis is a modification of the circumferential profile method described by Burow et al.[112] The left ventricle is manually outlined. The computer then finds the centroid of this irregular region for the generation of profiles or radii radiating from this centroid to each pixel or point in the circumference (Figure 5-6). The computer then analyzes the number of radioactive counts at each of these points on the circumference. With the basal half of the major axis as 0° and proceeding in a clockwise fashion, the computer constructs 24 15° radials. The myocardium supplied by the left circumflex coronary artery extends from 30° to 150°, while the left anterior descending perfusion territory encompasses the circumfer-

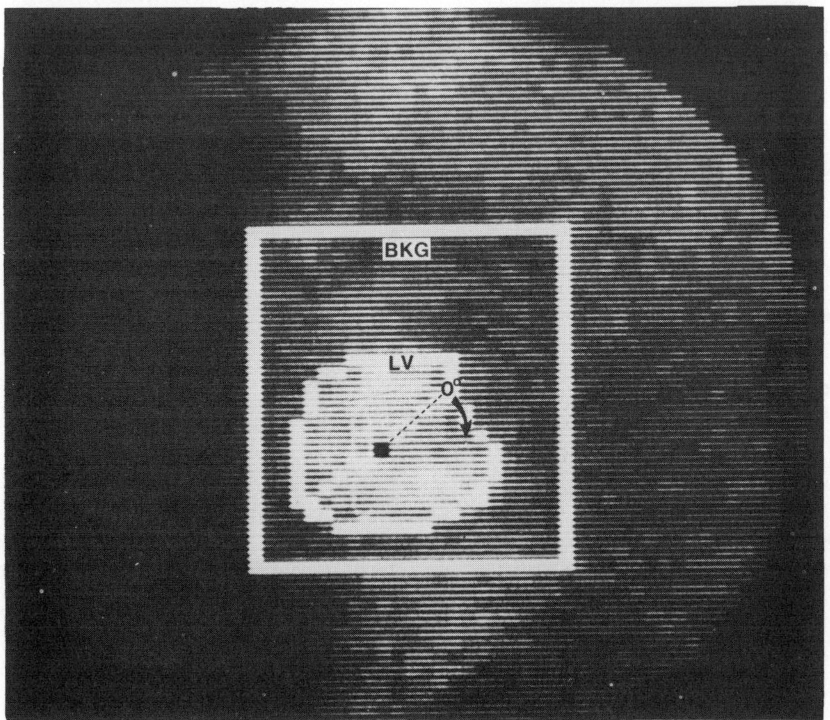

Figure 5-6　　Frame from ^{201}Tl perfusion scan with outline of region of interest (left ventricle—LV) and surrounding background (BKG) area. Computer techniques are employed to locate the center or centroid of the left ventricle (black dot). The 0° reference axis or radial is indicated, and the circumference of the chamber is then divided clockwise into 24 15° segments. In this projection the myocardium supplied by the left circumflex coronary artery extends from 30° to 150°, while the left anterior descending perfusion territory encompasses the circumference from 195° to 255°.

ence from 195° to 255°. The radial count data were expressed as a percentage of the highest radial activity in that frame.

The circumferential profiles from the exercising dogs at each of the scanning intervals were grouped and averaged. The group profiles are presented in Figures 5-7 and 5-8. The abscissa represents the left ventricular circumference where each 15° arc represents a radial, and the ordinate represents the averaged normalized radial count rates for the first five-minute frame of the scan. The solid line represents the preocclusion profile and the dashed line the profile at three days following occlusion of the left circumflex artery. The dotted line in Figure 5-7 is the averaged circumferential profile at four weeks following occlusion, while in Figure 5-8 the dotted line represents the six-week profile. The shaded area is the defect in the left circumflex area count rate noted in the initial postocclusion exercise study. The ischemic myocardium takes up less ^{201}Tl than normally perfused tissue. An important cause of the initially poor exercise performance of these animals was the development of significant left ventricular dysfunction, with left atrial pressures increasing to more than 20 mmHg and cardiac outputs rising inadequately. Presumably this dysfunction was related to exercise-

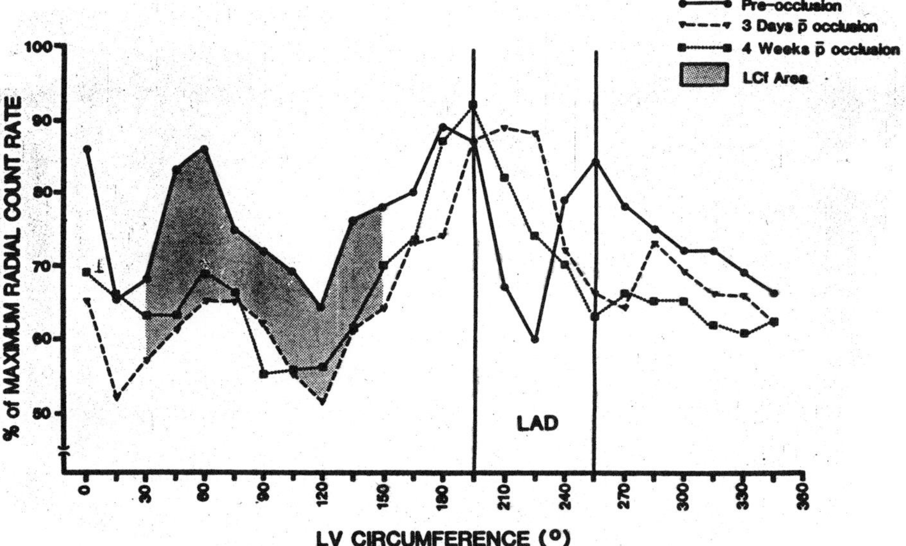

Figure 5-7   Circumferential profiles averaged from the five minute frames of exercise ^{201}Tl perfusion scans obtained in a group of dogs before (solid line) and three days (dashed line) and again four weeks (dotted line) following ligation of the left circumflex coronary artery. The abscissa represents the left ventricular circumference with radials extending every 15° from the chamber's centroid to its circumference. The ordinate represents the radioactive count data along the radials normalized for the highest radial activity appearing in that frame. The shaded area is the defect in the left circumflex area count rate noted in the initial postocclusion exercise study. Ischemic myocardium takes up less ^{201}Tl than normally perfused tissue. At four weeks after occlusion there was a tendency for the defect to be smaller.

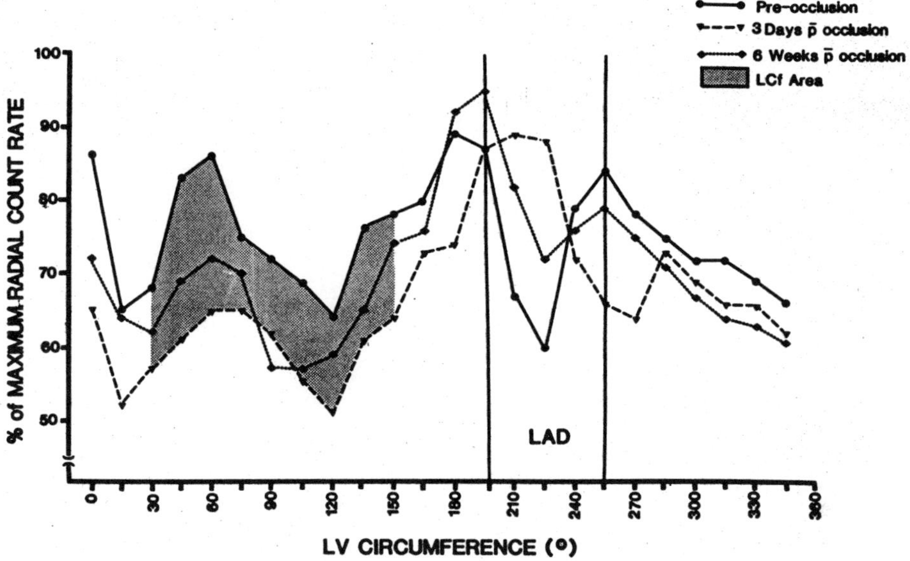

Figure 5-8   Circumferential profiles averaged from the five minute frames of exercise ^{201}Tl perfusion scans obtained in a group of dogs (same as in Figure 5-7) before (solid line) and three days (dashed line) and again six weeks (dotted line) following ligation of the left circumflex coronary artery. The shaded area is the defect in the left circumflex area count rate noted in the initial postocclusion exercise study. At six weeks after occlusion the defect is clearly smaller, and perfusion to portions of the left circumflex myocardium has normalized.

induced ischemia. Consequently, the heart rate-pressure double product was lower than that in the control period. Therefore, if anything, the magnitude of the defect is underestimated. In subsequent studies the double products were back to control levels. Exercise hemodynamics had improved, probably because collateral development resulted in attenuation of left ventricular ischemia. At four weeks (Figure 5-7) there was a tendency for the defect to be smaller, while at six weeks (Figure 5-8), the defect is clearly smaller and perfusion to portions of the left circumflex myocardium has normalized. In some dogs in which scans were done at longer intervals after the coronary occlusion, the process of flow normalization was observed to continue. The effect of collateral development on ^{201}Tl uptake by the myocardium in the distribution of the occluded left circumflex artery is perhaps best illustrated by Figure 5-9. In *A*, the scintigram and selective coronary angiogram were obtained three and two days, respectively, after coronary occlusion. A large scintigraphic defect in the left circumflex region is apparent. Furthermore, neither collaterals nor opacification of the distal artery is evident. In *B*, however, the scintigram and angiogram done four weeks later in the same animal demonstrate nearly normal uptake of the radioactive tracer and extensive collateralization of the distal left circumflex artery. Hence, col-

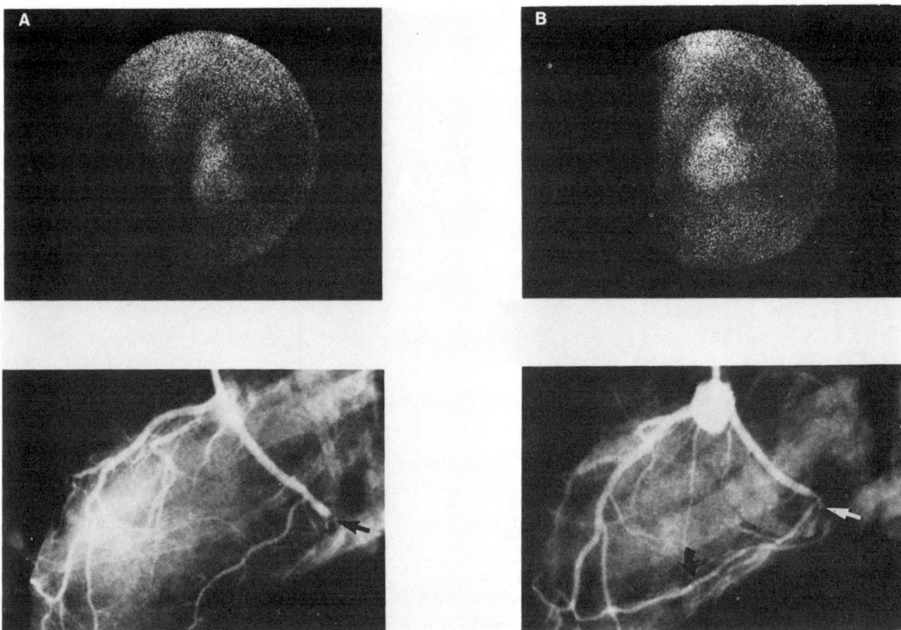

Figure 5-9   **A:** Unretouched Polaroid picture of a 201-thallium scintigram taken ten minutes after cessation of exercise performed three days following coronary occlusion. A frame from a coronary angiogram completed one day earlier appears beneath the scintigram. A large scintigraphic defect is apparent in the distribution of the left circumflex (LCf) coronary artery. The arrow in the angiographic frame indicates the site of LCf ligation. The radiopaque contrast agent injected into the ostium of the left coronary artery flowed only to the point of arterial obstruction. There were no visualized collateral channels, and no contrast agent was ever observed in the distal LCf. **B:** Scintigraphic and angiographic frames from studies performed four weeks following those presented in A. Only a small scintigraphic defect remains. The level of the LCf ligation is again indicated by the straight arrow, but now the entire distal LCf artery (curved arrow) is normally opacified by numerous intra- and inter-coronary collateral channels. Runoff from the distal LCf was only slightly slower than that from normal vessels. (Reprinted with permission of the American Heart Association from Cohen and Steingart.[111])

lateral development parallels and probably accounts for the improvement in the ^{201}Tl scintigrams observed in the weeks following coronary occlusion.

Coronary collaterals can, therefore, reestablish nearly normal myocardial flow even during the stress of exercise. The ^{201}Tl technique outlined above permits evaluation of myocardial perfusion over an extended period during both the early and the late phases of myocardial infarction, and hence complements investigations using radioactive microspheres. Several studies using microspheres generally confirm and in part extend the conclusions of the ^{201}Tl experiments. Hill et al.[113] implanted ameroid constrictors around the left circumflex arteries of dogs that then ran on a treadmill approximately two days after coronary occlusion (three weeks following ameroid implantation). At the time of study, resting flows in the collateralized myocardium were nearly normal with endo/epi ratios averaging 0.91. During exercise, blood flow to the subepicardium increased normally by 150%, but endocardial flow did not change. Consequently, the endo/epi ratio fell sharply to 0.36. Thus, at this point in the development of coronary collaterals, the defect in vascular reserve was clearly apparent during stress. Hess and Bache[114] measured collateral flow in dogs during submaximal treadmill exercise two weeks following occlusion of the left circumflex coronary artery. In collateralized myocardium containing minimal (1−25%) necrotic tissue, collateral flow increased during exercise to 80% of the level in normal regions. On the other hand, exercise flow in myocardium containing significant amounts of infarcted tissue was only 11% of normal flow. Thus, after only two weeks of coronary occlusion, collateral reserve is improved but is obviously not normal.

One study in dogs approximately seven weeks following coronary occlusion with an ameroid constrictor found that mild exercise that raised average normal myocardial flow to 1.83 ml/min/g increased flow to the collateralized tissue to only 1.49 ml/min/g.[94] However, most exercising dogs studied eight to nine weeks following coronary occlusion have had normal perfusion of the myocardium distal to the occluder (2.38 and 2.50 ml/min/g in normal and collateralized myocardium, respectively) and normal transmural distribution.[97]

In a study described previously,[58] coronary flow was measured during transient balloon occlusion of a previously constricted left circumflex coronary artery while dogs were resting quietly and again three months later. Coronary flow was also evaluated at the same times while the dogs were running at 4 mph and 12% grade (stage V of the Tipton test protocol[115]). After a stable exercise heart rate had been achieved, the balloon occluder was inflated and microspheres injected. Sometime between the two studies the constricted artery became totally occluded. During the initial study when the left circumflex was transiently occluded during running, average blood flow to normal myocardium was 2.78 ml/min/g, or double the resting level, while the endo/epi flow ratio was 1.05. Flow increases to normal tissue were actually limited by the development of cardiac failure during the coronary occlusion with a 28% decrease in cardiac output and increases in left atrial pressure to 21 mmHg. There was only a minor increase in ischemic flow from 0.53 at rest to 0.66 ml/min/g during exercise, and the transmural flow ratio was 0.53. At the time of the three-month study, after chronic coronary occlusion, exercise increased blood flow to the collateralized myocardium to 3.93 ml/min/g while the average endo/epi flow ratio was 0.97. These values were not different from those measured in normally perfused tissue. Flow histograms (Figure 5-10) of the exercise flows to the normal unstained and ischemic stained myocardium were constructed as detailed above. The resting and exercise flow histograms of Figures 5-5 and 5-10, respectively, are from the same animal. During the initial treadmill experiment the separation of flow to ischemic and normal myocardium following acute transient coronary occlusion is obvious.

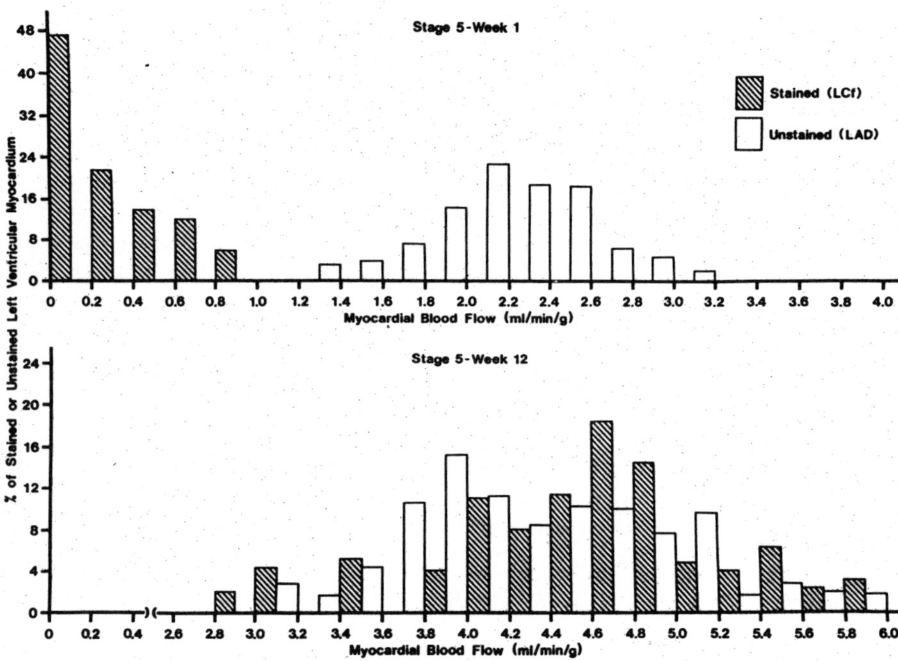

Figure 5-10   Histograms of myocardial blood flow measured at stage V of the Tipton exercise test (4 mph and 12% grade) during transient occlusion of the left circumflex coronary artery (LCf) during the first week of protocol (top) and again 12 weeks later after chronic LCf occlusion (bottom) in the same dog whose data are presented in Figure 5-5. Hatched bars represent stained (Evans blue injected into distal LCf at time of animal sacrifice) or ischemic myocardium distal to LCf occlusion, whereas blank bars represent normal, unstained, or left anterior descending (LAD) myocardium. The abscissa is not a continuous function of blood flow, but is divided into discrete increments of 0.2 ml/min/g. During week one there was no overlap of flows to stained and unstained myocardial regions, and average flows were 0.30 and 2.20 ml/min/g, respectively. In contrast, there was complete overlap of flows to stained and unstained myocardium at week 12 following chronic coronary occlusion and collateral transformation and development, and flows to LCf and LAD myocardium were 4.54 and 4.35 ml/min/g, respectively. (Modified and reprinted with permission of the American Physiological Society from Cohen et al.[58])

However, at 12 weeks there is complete overlap, and even careful scrutiny does not allow one to distinguish stained from unstained tissue.

Finally, a study completed 6.5 months following coronary occlusion demonstrated that running at approximately 6 mph and 8% grade in mongrel dogs increased normal coronary flows by 212% to 2.99 ml/min/g, while flow to the collateralized myocardium increased by 232% to 3.25 ml/min/g.[93] Transmural distribution was homogeneous in both normally perfused and collateralized regions.

Bache[116] studied dogs during light (heart rate 185 beats/min) and heavy (heart rate 230 beats/min) treadmill exercise one month after gradual coronary occlusion. Blood flow was measured with microspheres and coronary sinus blood was sampled for lactate and adenosine metabolites. In one group endocardial flow did not increase normally and even declined, resulting in a sharp drop in the endo/epi flow ratio. These animals had production of abnormal metabolites. In another group, however, heavy exercise increased collateralized endocardial and epicardial flows to 3.48 and 2.92 ml/min/g, respectively, without appearance of abnormal metabolites. The flow response was not different from that in normally perfused myocardium. Thus, as in Cohen's study,[58] collateral flow more than tripled without the appearance of regional or transmural flow inhomogeneities.

Schaper[117] studied dogs 100 days after coronary occlusion produced by ameroid constrictors. During exercise both collateral and normal myocardial flows rose equally to approximately 3 ml/min/g (W. Schaper, personal communication). Therefore, exercise was unable to elicit any abnormal responses. These same hearts were then excised and perfused with blood from a support dog. Adenosine was added to the perfusate to elicit maximal vasodilatation. In these hearts in which the physiologic stress of moderate to heavy exercise had been unable to exhaust the vascular reserve of the collateral bed, maximal collateral conductance was only 40% of that of the normal coronary arteries.

The exercise studies demonstrate that collaterals do have the ability to restore normal myocardial flow to collateralized regions during physiologic stress. Obviously, the vascular reserve of the collateral bed will increase over the first few months following coronary occlusion as the collaterals themselves undergo the transformation process, and, therefore, the exercise response is unlikely to be normal early after antegrade flow is blocked. It would be instructive to measure maximal collateral conductance of a collateral bed 6 to 12 months after coronary occlusion when the histologic transformation is known to be essentially complete. But regardless of these measurements, the exercise studies clearly point out that the typical physiologic stresses are not enough to exhaust the collateral bed's admittedly limited dilatory reserve.

IV. Myocardial Border Zones Following Coronary Occlusion

A. Transmural

The increase in collateral flow that occurs over the weeks and months after coronary occlusion in the dog is clearly a dynamic process that parallels a dramatic structural transformation. It must be reemphasized, however, that the described changes in collateral flow are not necessarily uniform throughout the region of tissue at risk or perfusion territory of the obstructed vessel. Although collateral flow after several months of collateral development is homogeneously distributed throughout the once-ischemic area, perfusion of the acutely ischemic myocardium is uneven. Gradients of flow can and do develop that profoundly affect ultimate infarct development and potential for modification of the necrotic process.

Immediately following coronary occlusion in the dog, residual collateral flow is inhomogeneously distributed across the left ventricular wall. The lower subendocardial and higher subepicardial flows result in a transmural flow gradient. This transmural flow gradient correlates well with the development of a transmural gradient of metabolites and metabolic byproducts.[118–120] Glycogen and high-energy phosphate compounds are more depleted while lactate accumulates more rapidly in the subendocardial myocardium. Whereas the more ischemic subendocardium must rely mainly on anaerobic metabolism, the higher blood flow and therefore greater oxygen and substrate availability in the subepicardium permit more efficient energy production with preservation of many aerobic reactions and maintained washout and clearance of inhibitory byproducts. The significance of the transmural flow gradient is further emphasized by the studies of Banka et al.[121] and Jennings et al.[122] who identified rapid appearance of ultrastructural ischemic changes in the endocardium with progression to loss of mitochondrial cristae, vacuolization, appearance of amorphous mitochondrial densities, and I bands by three to four hours following coronary ligation. These morphologic changes were associated with a reversal of the endocardial K^+/Na^+ ratio.[121] In contrast, however, structural and ionic alterations in the epicardium were minimal. Reimer and his colleagues[123,124] have also shown that cell death does not occur uniformly in an ischemic zone, but rather in a wave from subendocardium to subepicardium, and Hirzel et al.[125] have reported greater creatine kinase loss from the endocardium than from the epicardium following coronary ligation. The epicardium following coronary occlusion is, therefore, myocardium with levels of flow and metabolism intermediate between those of normal myocardium and the central ischemic zone (endocardium) with resultant delayed appearance of often mild morphologic and structural alterations. Thus, the epicardium in the dog is a true border zone. The concept of a border zone has important implications when one considers the possibility that an intervention might result in salvage of ischemic myocardium (see Chapter 7).

In the pig, coronary collaterals are poorly developed, and therefore, endocardial and epicardial flows are equally severely depressed following coronary occlusion. Hence, in this animal model transmural gradients are virtually absent.[126] It is interesting to note that even in the pig there is a transmural damage gradient at 40 minutes after coronary occlusion.[127] At this time there is significantly more cellular disruption in the inner than outer third of the left ventricular wall. But by 120 minutes a gradient is no longer apparent and necrosis is equally severe in all layers.

B. Radial

The traditional view of the existence of a simultaneous radial flow gradient and border zone shortly following coronary occlusion with the lowest flows in the center of the ischemic area and progressively higher flows toward the periphery has recently been challenged. The discrete nature of coronary arterial beds has been well documented.[128,129] However, despite the absence of significant overlap of branches of adjacent vascular territories and improbable occurrence of a dual vascular supply of normal myocardium, the collateral network does serve to interconnect otherwise distinct and separate myocardial perfusion areas. It had been reasoned that the anatomic center of the perfusion territory of an occluded artery would be farthest from the adjacent normal vessels giving rise to the collaterals. According to Poiseuille's law, the longer length of the collateral conduits to the center would increase vascular resistance and hence diminish flow. Early investigations by Linder[130] using intramyocardial depots of ^{85}Kr in the dog paradoxically suggested that there was a very steep gradient between normal and ischemic myocardium. Just within the ischemic border, flows fell to 10% of normal, with a further small decline to 5% at the center of the abnormally perfused area. On the other hand, microsphere studies by Becker and colleagues[131] purported to demonstrate multiple concentric rings of increasing flow surrounding the central core of an ischemic region. Ischemic border flows were reported to be ten times greater than the flows in the center. But methodologic difficulties, including lack of identification of the perfusion area at risk and therefore the impossibility of excluding inadvertent sampling of adjacent normal tissue and contamination of the alleged border zone, diminish the significance of the results. Marcus[60] claimed there was no distinct geometric border zone in dogs following coronary occlusion since he noted that severely ischemic myocardium was equally likely to be adjacent to tissue with normal or depressed flows. However, this latter study again did not attempt to identify a region at risk, and sampling of very large myocardial pieces certainly could have resulted in obfuscation of a border zone even if one were present.

It is now obvious that the peripheral border of ischemic myocardium is truly a mixture of normal and abnormal myocardial cells. When the perfusion territory of an occluded vessel is outlined by injecting Evans blue dye into the vessel distal to the obstruction, it is apparent that the boundary between the stained ischemic and unstained normal myocardium is serpiginous and impossible to follow with a scalpel blade. Therefore, inclusion of some normal tissue when the ischemic myocardium is excised is unavoidable, resulting in the creation of a spurious border zone composed of a combination of normal and abnormal tissue. Histologic examination of this peripheral ischemic area also emphasizes that there are prominent and deep invaginations or peninsulas of normal myocardium extending into the abnormal tissue[132] Therefore, measurements of flow in these peripheral zones would typically overestimate the true ischemic area flow. Techniques have been developed to account for this contamination of the ischemic region by adjacent normal tissue,[54,133,134] and Kirk and his colleagues[133,134] have concluded that there is no radial border zone. They contend that flow is uniform throughout the ischemic region, and further support this observation with studies that CPK depletion[125,134] and histologic evidence of necrosis[129] at 24 hours following coronary occlusion are also uniform with sharp transitions between ischemic and normal tissues. Others have confirmed the absence of radial flow gradients in dogs,[135] pigs,[125] and nonhuman primates[88] following coronary occlusion.

However, these overly pessimistic results are in part balanced by the later studies of Becker and colleagues[55,61] who have identified ischemic, noninfarcted tissue well within the borders of the perfusion territory at risk with flows two to three times higher than the ischemic core and border zones with flows two-thirds of normal. Furthermore, other studies have demonstrated that the infarct developing after coronary occlusion is smaller than the perfusion territory at risk with sparing of the lateral borders.[59,124,136,137] Thus, the issue of a radial flow gradient is still controversial. It is quite possible that all of these studies are correct and that a radial border zone is evident during only one phase of the evolution of infarcting myocardium. To this end it is instructive to note that 40 minutes following coronary occlusion in the pig there is a transmural ischemic damage gradient with the inner third of the left ventricular wall displaying significantly more evidence of cellular disruption than the outer third.[127] However, by 120 minutes there is no longer any gradient, and necrosis is equally severe in all transmural layers. Therefore, consideration of the time interval following coronary occlusion may be crucial. An early gradient may be obscured at a later time. In addition, Koyanagi et al.[135] demonstrated radial flow gradients between frankly ischemic and normal myocardium extending over only 3–5 mm in the endocardium or mid-myocardium. However, in the epicardium the flow transition could extend over a distance up to 33 mm. Thus, a radial flow gradient may exist in some layers but not in others.

Multiple correlative studies have been completed either to support or to refute the concept of a radial border zone, and many of these results have recently been reviewed by Hearse and Yellon.[138] Most investigations suggesting that there is a border zone of intermediate values for metabolites including glycogen and high-energy phosphate compounds,[139–141] ST-segment changes,[142] and segmental contraction and systolic thickening[143,144] have not been able to exclude the possibility that the intermediate values are the result of sampling artifacts, i.e., a mixed population of ischemic and normal cells. As already indicated, this cell mixture toward the periphery of the ischemic zone is virtually unavoidable.

Studies concluding that there is not a discrete metabolic border zone are instructive. Chance and his associates[145–149] have used epicardial NADH fluorescence photography to demonstrate that there is a very narrow border between anoxic (NADH enzyme predominating) and normoxic (NAD enzyme predominating) tissue, and by inference, a very sharp oxygen gradient. This metabolic change may occur within the width of several cells, and implies that a mitochondrion has either complete oxidative metabolism or none at all without any intermediate state. However, because tissue flow may decrease substantially before cellular oxygen tension falls below the critical level, which results in a metabolic shift toward the reduced NADH moiety, this technique cannot establish the absence of a radial flow gradient. Furthermore, this technique limits conclusions about mitochondrial function to only the epicardial surface. Janse et al[150] have detected glycogen-depleted cells adjacent to normal ones without evidence of significant numbers of cells with intermediate glycogen levels. Although this evidence suggests that a true border zone is not present, these investigators realized that it was possible that some of the glycogen-depleted cells were only reversibly damaged. However, they also noted that electrically unresponsive cells were in close proximity to cells with normal transmembrane action potentials. Using a specially designed tool that was able to cut multiple adjacent 2-mm-diameter biopsies, Yellon et al[151] have recently shown that the transition from normal to ischemic levels of ATP, CP, and lactate in a dog with an occluded coronary artery must occur in a band of myocardium narrower than 4 mm. However, the biopsies sampled only the superficial 10% of the left ventricular wall. Therefore, conclusions about the absence of a metabolic border zone would have to be restricted to only the most superficial myocardial layers.

Perhaps the most provocative evidence for lateral heterogeneity within the ischemic zone is derived from numerous histologic and histochemical studies. Thus, for 18 to 24 hours following coronary ligation in the dog, Cox et al[152] showed that there were different concentric myocardial zones with differing rates of enzyme depletion, and that mitochondrial swelling and accumulation of neutral fat droplets occurred in myocardium with preserved architecture. Fishbein and colleagues[153] have shown in the rat with a coronary ligation that a central myocardial area of combined glycogen and enzyme loss is surrounded by myocardium with glycogen depletion but only mild enzyme loss. This latter zone was itself surrounded by lipid-containing myocardium. These radial zones were evident for only 9 to 12 hours. Deloche et al[154] have also demonstrated myocardial zones with different enzyme-staining characteristics within the ischemic region, while others have noted architecturally normal myocardial cells with either glycogen depletion,[155] abnormal sarcomere relaxation and vacuole formation,[156] or mild degrees of cellular disorganization.[157] Buja et al[157] also demonstrated mitochondrial calcifications in only the peripheral necrotic zones, implying differences in residual blood supply to the central and peripheral areas. It is of interest that after a variable period of time in most of these studies (up to 48 hours) the multiple zones disappeared, leaving only a residual uniform necrotic area. Finally, Lie et al[158] have measured decreased K^+/Na^+ and Mg^{++}/Ca^{++} ionic ratios in histologically normal tissue adjacent to infarcted myocardium. Of course, all of these results may be influenced by artifactual admixture of normal and ischemic cells.

The foregoing histologic studies strongly suggest that ischemic and even infarcting myocardium following coronary occlusion is not homogeneous. Lateral zones, although possibly small, probably do exist, but one cannot justifiably claim that a radial flow gradient accounts for the inhomogeneity. Fujiwara and his colleagues[127] have observed transient transmural gradients of ischemic cellular damage following coronary occlusion in pigs in the absence of any identified flow gradient. It is possible that other unknown factors may be responsible. Because of the physiologic and clinical importance of the concept of a lateral border zone, additional investigations must be undertaken. Questions of the existence of a discrete anatomic border zone as well as the possible influence of duration of the ischemic interval must continue to be addressed.

V. Collateral Regression—Fact or Fancy?

The transformation of a thin-walled collateral conduit into a thick-walled arteriole occurs following occlusion of a coronary artery. The collateral vessel in effect revascularizes the ischemic myocardium. The fate of these collaterals should they no longer be necessary has intrigued several investigators. Revascularization of ischemic myocardium by anastomosis of a saphenous vein graft between the aorta and coronary artery distal to the obstruction restores antegrade blood flow to the affected region. Thus, the perfusion pressure of this coronary arterial bed will once again approximate aortic pressure and will abolish the pressure gradient that had previously stimulated collateral growth. In the absence of a pressure gradient across the collateral vessel, collateral blood flow will cease. Schaper[5,13] has provided evidence that remodeling and involution of collaterals during the transformation process can occur, but it is not known whether the now unused collateral that has already been transformed will undergo similar changes.

Several studies have evaluated collateral indices and reactive hyperemia responses following release of hydraulic occluders and relief of coronary obstruction.[159–161] The coronaries were occluded either abruptly[159–161] or gradually over 3 to 12 days.[159] One to six days following the occlusion, antegrade flow was restored. Immediately after release of the occlusion the reactive hyperemic response to a brief reocclusion of the vessel was blunted.[159,161] This observation implies that significant blood flow from other sources, presumably collaterals, was perfusing the distal arterial bed and attenuating myocardial ischemia during the reocclusion. Within minutes[159] to days,[161] the reactive hyperemic response returned to normal, suggesting rapid suppression of the collateral circulation and its functional effects. Collateral flow measured by the ^{133}Xe clearance technique and the traditional collateral indices of peripheral coronary pressure and retrograde flow also returned to low preocclusion levels during the hours following reestablishment of antegrade flow.[159-161] But subsequent vessel reocclusion two days to two months following restoration of patency resulted in rapid (30–60 minutes) increases in collateral function.[159-161] Thus, in less than one hour after reocclusion, peripheral coronary pressure, retrograde flow, and ^{133}Xe clearance from the ischemic region were at levels not reached for at least 24 hours following the initial occlusion of the vessel. Furthermore, reocclusion produced no electrocardiographic abnormalities.[159] Hence, coronary channels become nonfunctional when the need for them is removed, but they remain ready to supply the affected myocardium within a very short time when a subsequent reocclusion occurs up to at least two months later. However, in each of these investigations the initial stimulus for collateral development was shortlived, and the results may have been influenced by the incomplete vascular transformation.

Oldham and his colleagues[162] attached a venous graft between the aorta and left circumflex artery approximately six weeks after occlusion of the coronary vessel by an ameroid constrictor. Initial graft flow was 16 ml/min, whereas a graft inserted into an acutely occluded, otherwise normal left circumflex artery typically had flows of 65 ml/min. Presumably, the volume of collateral flow was enough to limit graft inflow. The meager graft flow remained constant for two and a half hours, suggesting absence of a tendency for collateral involution. Observations were not made beyond two and a half hours.

Cibulski et al.[163] studied the effects of anastomosis of an internal mammary artery to the left circumflex coronary artery occluded by an ameroid constrictor implanted 8 to 12 weeks before revascularization. Peripheral coronary pressure and retrograde flow were measured at the time of the anastomosis and again one day to 12 weeks later with an angiographic catheter wedged into the grafted internal mammary artery. Angiography revealed collaterals from the left anterior descending and right coronary arteries to the left circumflex artery before and one day after grafting, but no collaterals were seen 4 and 12 weeks later. The ratio of peripheral coronary pressure to aortic pressure was 0.85 just before revascularization and unchanged one day later. But after two weeks the ratio had fallen to 0.125. Similarly, retrograde flows in two dogs fell dramatically from 140 and 77 ml/min at the time of revascularization to 11.0 and 8.5 ml/min 12 weeks later. This evidence of diminished collateral function was confirmed by the electrocardiographic results of transient graft occlusion. Whereas occlusion one day after graft anastomosis in two dogs had no effect, occlusion at 12 weeks produced ST-segment elevation and ventricular fibrillation. Thus, the effects of even well-developed collateral vessels are lost within weeks following resumption of antegrade flow. There is little reason to expect that the collateral vessels involute, but reocclusion studies in animals with well-developed collaterals are necessary. Most likely, reestablishment of a pressure gradient across the already transformed vessel would result in stretching of the unused vessel's walls and rapid resumption of near-maximal collateral flow.

VI. Coronary-Luminal Communications

The previous discussion has dealt exclusively with the anatomic and functional development of inter- and intracoronary collateral vessels. However, as noted in Chapter 1, physiologists have been intrigued by the possibility of direct connections between the heart's chambers and the coronary arteries for almost as long as they've known about the existence of coronary collaterals. Interest and curiosity have prompted many studies to prove both the existence of these direct connections, Thebesian vessels and arterioluminal channels, and their functional significance. Vieussen's original demonstration[164] of plugs of carmine and glue protuding into the right and left ventricular cavities from the myocardium after injection into the coronary arteries and Thebesius's later observations of air injected into the coronary sinus bubbling from endocardial "pores" into fluid-filled ventricular chambers (see Roberts[165]) initiated the search for direct vascular-luminal communications. Careful inspection of the endocardial lining of the right and left ventricular chambers reveals multiple openings ranging from pinpoint size to nearly 1 mm in diameter. As previously described (see Chapter 1), Wearn's injection and microscopic studies[166] demonstrated direct vascular connections between the coronary arterial system and the ventricular lumen (arterioluminal channels) as well as myocardial sinusoids, which then communicated with the cavities. Using a combination of Schlesinger injection mass (barium sulphate–gelatin) and microscopic examination, others[167,168] have confirmed the presence of canine intramyocardial sinusoids that communicate with the ventricular lumen (Figure 5-11 [colorplate]). But Truex and Angulo[167] identified these sinusoids only after injection of the coronary sinus, and rarely after injection of the Schlesinger mass into the aortic root. Young and Fell[169] also were unable to document the presence of direct arterial-luminal connections. They injected an india ink-formalin solution into the right ventricle of excised rat hearts and observed india ink particles fill the entire cardiac vasculature. Microscopic examination revealed numerous channels (designated Thebesian veins) connecting coronary veins with the ventricular chambers but absence of connections with the arterial vasculature. Earlier studies by Pratt[170] with celloidin casts of the coronary vasculature had also demonstrated large connections between the Thebesian vessels and coronary veins but only small capillaries connecting the Thebesian channels and coronary arteries. After injecting the coronary vessels of either sheep, dog, or human hearts with celloidin or dilute chrome yellow gelatin, Grant and Viko[171] observed the injectate to leak from endocardial orifices in the walls of both ventricles. They then introduced into the endocardial foramina of other hearts fine glass cannulae through which the celloidin or gelatin was delivered. After further preparation of the specimen and partial clearing of the myocardium, the Thebesian vessels could be traced into the myocardium. The Thebesian vessels were frequently observed either to divide into a "tree" or to give off anastomoses to veins and other Thebesian channels. However, there were no large arterioluminal channels as described by Wearn.[166] Only fine capillary vessels were observed to anastomose with arterial branches. It appears clear from these descriptive studies that there are vascular channels that pass from endocardial openings in both ventricles into the myocardium. But most, if not all, are Thebesian veins, although it is still possible that arterioluminal channels also exist (Figure 5-11).

Under experimental conditions it can be readily demonstrated that flow occurs through these endomural channels. Net flow may be either toward the ventricular lumen or from the ventricular cavity into the coronary vascular system. Perfusion of the coronary arteries of excised hearts of either dogs, rabbits, or sheep with saline or defibrinated blood,[170] gelatin,[171] or synthetic resins[172] reveals pooling of the injectate in both the right and left ventricles. Lendrum et al.[173] quantitated the amount of direct ventricular drainage in isolated dog hearts by sealing the right and left atrioventricular orifices with special umbrellalike occlusive devices and perfusing the coronary system from the aorta with a mixture of serum and saline at 150 mmHg. A cannula was inserted into the coronary sinus to collect the effluent, and the remainder of right atrial drainage represented flow mainly from anterior cardiac veins. The effluent pooling in either ventricle was believed to have passed through arterioluminal channels. Of total coronary flow drainage, 36.4 ± 11.8% (SD) was collected in the coronary sinus, 24.5 ± 6.5% in the right atrium, and 30.8 ± 5.4% in the right ventricle. Left ventricular flow was 7.0 ± 3.3% of the total coronary effluent, and 1.4 ± 1.7% was recovered from the left atrium. Therefore, ventricular endomural channels were felt to be significant vascular components, at least in the right ventricle.

Skepticism concerning the applicability of these results to in-situ working hearts prompted others to study the possible direct transport of markers from the coronary circulation to the left ventricular cavity in intact animal models. Both Roberts et al.[174,175] and Watanabe[172] injected dyes into cannulated coronary arteries of dogs and sampled blood from the root of the aorta. The dye appeared in the aortic root within a few seconds, and its appearance often preceded that in the pulmonary artery. This early appearance was evident even after pulmonary artery blood was diverted to exclude any possibility of recirculation.[174] Thus, shunting of the dye appeared to occur between the coronary arterial system and lumen of the left heart. Moir and colleagues[176] attempted to further localize the site of this left-sided shunt by cannulating the left coronary artery or one of its major branches in the dog and perfusing it from a systemic artery. Then ^{131}I-albumin was injected into the coronary perfusion line, blood was sampled from the aortic root, and early appearance or shunting of the isotope was sought. In contrast to Watanabe's results,[172] the seven dogs with cannulation of the left anterior descending coronary artery never had any evidence of shunting. Only one of ten dogs with cannulation of the first septal artery showed any evidence of direct drainage of this vessel into the left heart, which is not surprising since previous reports by these same investigators[177] had demonstrated that as much as 80% of first septal flow (13% of total left coronary flow) entered the right ventricle directly. However, shunting was detected in every animal with cannulation of either the main left coronary or left circumflex artery, and Moir et al.[176] calculated that 6% of the isotope injected into the left circumflex coronary artery appeared early in the aortic root. Further studies revealed that the major shunt was through the left anterior atrial artery in the left atrium. Cannulation of the left circumflex artery below the origin of this branch decreased the amount of isotope shunted through the left cardiac chambers to less than 2%.

Perhaps the potentially more clinically important route would be chamber cavity to myocardium or coronary artery. Bohning et al.[178] cannulated the coronary arteries of a canine heart-lung preparation and perfused them from an isolated reservoir at a pressure of 60−100 mmHg while left ventricular pressure was 10−60 mmHg. Following intravenous injection of bismuth oxychloride suspension, histologic evidence of bismuth deposition in the coronary sinus, myocardial sinusoids, and intramural coronary veins and arteries was found in two-thirds of the specimens. Similar experiments with suspensions of killed bacteria confirmed the results. In these studies coronary perfusion pressure actually exceeded left ventricular pressure. However, other investigators were able to demonstrate transport from either the right or left ventricular lumen into the myocardium only when coronary pressure was lower than ventricular pressure. Eckstein[179] in Wearn's laboratory showed that Berlin blue or india ink injected into a sealed right ventricle of a beating heart produced complete capillary injection of the right and parts of the left ventricles only when right ventricular pressure exceeded that in the left ventricle. India ink in the right ventricle of excised rat hearts in which the coronary vasculature was empty has also been noted to fill the heart's vasculature.[169] Transport of dye from the left ventricular lumen into the arteries and veins of the myocardium after elimination of all other possible routes of entry has also been observed.[175,180,181] But, as noted above for the right ventricle, net flow into the myocardium was documented only when there was a pressure gradient from left ventricular cavity to coronary artery.

Stella[182] attempted to prove that there was no flow through Thebesian vessels by decreasing coronary perfusion pressure to nearly zero while maintaining left ventricular pressure at 30−150 mmHg. He never observed any coronary backflow. Gregg, Thornton, and Mautz[15] were more successful. In dogs with chronic occlusion of either the left anterior descending or left circumflex coronary artery, they measured retrograde flow from the chronically obstructed vessel after occluding the right and remaining patent left coronary artery. Despite occlusions of all coronary vessels, they were still able to collect retrograde flow. Many years later Hammond et al.[183] performed similar experiments. Retrograde flow following left circumflex cannulation averaged 5.4 ml/min, and fell by only 70% to 1.7 ml/min after acute occlusion of both the right and left coronary arteries. Although these investigators felt this continued blood flow represented squeezing of residual blood from the myocardium, it is quite possible that flow through Thebesian vessels was occurring. In the heart-lung preparation of Katz et al.[184] the volume of coronary sinus outflow was compared to that of coronary artery inflow. They observed that the venous outflow consistently exceeded total arterial inflow when the mean pressure in the heart cavities was high relative to coronary perfusion pressure. This effect was more pronounced for the right side of the heart. These experiments imply that a second source of coronary venous blood existed. Because of the experimental conditions, it could only have come from the ventricular cavities.

The aforementioned experiments strongly suggest that, at least under certain conditions (even if somewhat artificial), flow did occur through endomural channels. Of course, these demonstrations that flow does exist do not imply that it has any functional significance. In 1898 Pratt[170] cannulated the right ventricle of freshly excised, nonbeating cat hearts and then sealed the chamber's inflow and outflow tracts. Warm, defibrinated, oxygenated blood injected into the right ventricle led to resumption of cardiac contraction. As the blood in the chamber became venous in nature, the heart slowed. Replacement with oxygenated blood produced resumption of contractions. If the cannula was placed instead in the left ventricle, contractions of that chamber were similarly sustained. Ringer's solution instead of blood led to cessation of cardiac function, implying that more than mere mechanical stimulation of the endocardium was responsible for resumption of contractions. Wiggers[185] also tried to show the significance of arterioluminal vessels by cannulating and perfusing the coronary arteries of an isolated cat heart with Tyrode's solution. Drugs such as ephedrine, ouabain, epinephrine, and potassium chloride introduced into a sealed right ventricle had the same stimulating or depressant effects on the left ventricle that would ordinarily be seen after their injection into the aortic root or directly into the coronary system. Numerous histologic studies following experimental coronary artery ligation have demonstrated extensive endocardial infarction with relatively less epicardial involvement. Despite the significant endocardial involvement, the frequent occurrence of a rim of viable subendocardial tissue bordering the left ventricular cavity[124] provides strong evidence for the participation of luminal blood flow in the nutrition of ventricular myocardium. Of course, it is not possible to separate the effects of simple diffusion from active blood delivery by arterioluminal vessels (see below).

Despite this evidence and even his own experiments demonstrating the effects of an endomural circulation, Wiggers[186] in 1952 was prompted to write that "the connections between the ventricular cavity and coronary arteries are compressed by myocardial contraction. It is therefore dynamically inconceivable that any material volume of blood could be transferred from the ventricular cavity even if communications of very large caliber were present." Several investigators have attempted to quantitate the amount of blood flowing directly between coronary artery and ventricular lumen under basal conditions as well as during specific perturbations of the coronary perfusion and ventricular luminal pressures. Most experiments have been done by isolating the coronary arterial circulation and perfusing the heart from either a donor dog or a blood reservoir. In this manner, either a radioisotope or dye injected systemically would be excluded from the coronary circulation following recirculation, and any myocardial concentration of radioactivity or coronary venous effluent containing dye would be evidence of direct passage from the ventricular lumen.

Moir[187,188] injected ^{131}I-albumin systemically while perfusing the coronaries with nonradioactive blood. After two to five minutes the heart was excised and the amount of labeled arterial blood in the left ventricular myocardium determined. With normal coronary perfusion and left ventricular pressures, an average of 0.40 ml/100g of arterial blood, or 7% of the total myocardial blood volume, had entered the myocardium from the left ventricular lumen. This amount did not change as coronary perfusion pressure was diminished and/or left ventricular pressure raised. However, following coronary occlusion and restoration of normal left ventricular pressure, the amount of blood entering the myocardium from the ventricular lumen increased to 0.92 ml/100g.

In additional experiments, Moir and DeBra[189] injected ^{86}Rb into the systemic circulation of dogs in which coronary artery perfusion was from an isolated reservoir. This radioisotope is a positively charged, nonlipid soluble moiety that is considerably smaller than the albumin molecule. Clearance of rubidium by the endocardial half of the left ventricular wall averaged 17 ml/min/100g, considerably greater than the clearance of albumin (0.3 ml/min/100g). Of note was the virtual absence of rubidium from the epicardium. Parallel studies by Myers and Honig[190] confirmed the appreciable clearance of ^{86}Rb by the left ventricular endocardium. These investigators injected both ^{51}Cr-labeled red blood cells and ^{86}Rb into the systemic circulation. The left coronary artery was perfused with nonradioactive blood from a reservoir, while the right coronary artery was supplied normally from the aorta. Because it was reasoned the ^{51}Cr label would remain in the myocardial vasculature, the ^{51}Cr content of a myocardial sample represented a measure of the amount of luminal blood that it contained. From determination of the blood content of a tissue sample and measurement of the arterial concentration of ^{86}Rb at the time of removal of the heart, the amount of ^{86}Rb in the channels communicating with the left ventricular lumen could be calculated. In addition, the difference between the total ^{86}Rb content of a myocardial sample and this intravascular component represented the amount of ^{86}Rb which diffused from the luminal channels and accumulated in the myocardium, i.e., extravascular [86]Rb. The transmural myocardial samples were cut into 150 μm-thick sections from inner to outer surfaces. Labeled blood was detected 5.5 mm from the left ventricular lumen or at approximately midwall, and the innermost millimeter contained from 1.5 to 16% luminal blood by weight. In the innermost millimeter ^{86}Rb uptake ranged from 30 to 120% of the maximum right ventricular uptake. Assuming right and left ventricular extraction rates are similar, this uptake is equivalent to flows of 30–90 ml/min/100g. The concentration of ^{86}Rb decreased rapidly with increasing distance from the lumen, and little was detected in the outermost sections. Autoradiographs revealed that the radioactive label was essentially confined to the 2—3-mm rim of tissue immediately beneath the endocardium. If the luminal transport of ^{86}Rb to the entire left ventricle is considered, total luminal flow represents approximately 4% of the average coronary blood flow. Myers and Honig[190] believed that the charged, lipid-insoluble ^{86}Rb ion would not diffuse readily into the myocardium, and studies by Page and Bernstein[191] support the likelihood of insignificant diffusion from the luminal surface. It was therefore reasoned that appearance of the isotope at midwall implied the existence of functional channels. Nonetheless, placement of ^{86}Rb in the cavity of an excised heart rapidly leads to appearance of significant quantities of the isotope in the subendocardial layer,[192] suggesting that diffusion from the lumen should not be discounted.

Cohen and Kirk (unpublished observations) examined the contribution of luminal flow to the perfusion of both normal and ischemic canine myocardium in the same heart. The main left coronary artery was cannulated and perfused from a reservoir at a flow rate previously demonstrated to preserve normal myocardial contraction. The right coronary artery was ligated to eliminate possible contribution of this vessel to left ventricular perfusion, and the left anterior descending coronary artery was ligated to produce an ischemic region. [42]K and ^{86}Rb were simultaneously injected into the pulmonary artery and coronary perfusion tubing, respectively. After isotope injection the cannulated coronary sinus drained into a reservoir. Thus, the coronary circulation and left ventricular lumen were each exposed to only one isotope. Excised myocardium was divided into five pieces from endo- to epicardium. The results in one representative animal are presented in Figure 5-12. In the normal myocardium, endocardial clearance of ^{86}Rb, 0.89 ml/min/g, exceeded epicardial clearance, and the endo/epi ratio was 1.39. On the other hand, clearance of this isotope by the innermost layer of ischemic myocardium following intracoronary injection was 0.014 ml/min/g, and the endo/epi ratio was 0.033. Clearance of the systemically injected [42]K by the subendocardial myocardium was approximately 0.04 ml/min/g in both the normal and ischemic regions. Thus, the luminal flow to the ischemic subendocardium in this animal actually exceeded the flow derived from the coronary vasculature, and this pattern was observed in each of the other five animals studied. Of course the luminal flow proved to be a negligible fraction of the perfusion of normal tissue. Of great interest was the virtually identical myocardial clearance of [42]K by the ischemic and normal myocardium. There was a precipitous decrease in isotope clearance as the distance from the endocardium increased with an unexplained rise in the epicardial layer.

Using right heart bypass[193,194] or isolated heart[195] preparations it has been possible to monitor luminal flow continuously by measuring coronary inflow and collecting coronary sinus effluent. With coronary pressure exceeding left ventricular systolic pressure by 80—110 mmHg, 5 to 6% of coronary flow passed directly into the left ventricular lumen, while a coronary pressure 50—60 mmHg less than ventricular pressure characteristically led to coronary sinus flow being 3 to 7.5% greater than coronary inflow.[193,194] Blood flow into the coronary vasculature from the left ventricular lumen appeared

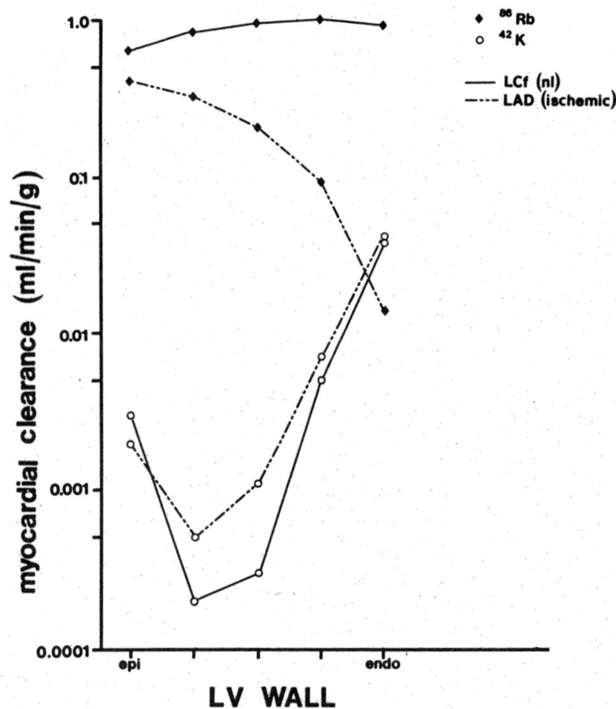

Figure 5-12 ^{86}Rb and ^{42}K clearance data from an experimental animal with a ligated left anterior descending coronary artery (LAD) in which the isotopes were injected into the coronary perfusion tubing and pulmonary artery, respectively, and prevented from mixing. Therefore, ^{86}Rb entered the myocardium from the coronary circulation, while ^{42}K was excluded from the coronary vasculature and contacted only the left ventricular endocardium. The left circumflex (LCf) myocardium represents normally perfused tissue. Uptake of ^{42}K by the left ventricular myocardium from the intravascular pool was highest in the endocardium, but was still negligible compared to normal levels of perfusion. A precipitous decrease in clearance in the inner layers is apparent. Of interest, the clearances of ^{42}K by ischemic and normal myocardium were virtually identical.

to commence when left ventricular and coronary perfusion pressures were equal.[193] Of course, these contributions represent blood flows to the full-thickness left ventricular myocardium. It is conceivable that the benefits to the subendocardium were significantly greater than those to the rest of the myocardium.

Most of these studies suggest that the luminal contribution to left ventricular perfusion is 5% or less of normal coronary flow. Brandfonbrener's results[196] confirm this impression. Only small amounts of Evans blue injected systemically were ever detected in the coronary sinus effluent of dogs with reservoir-perfused coronary arteries. The maximum shunt amounted to 0.041 ml/min/g. Studies with left atrial injections of microspheres while the coronary arteries were being perfused with nonradioactive blood have similarly demonstrated minor contributions of luminal flow to myocardial perfusion.[98,197,198] Maximal luminal flow was less than 0.006 ml/min/g, while total left ventricular perfusion from the lumen did not exceed 0.15 ml/min. However, larger contributions to subendocardial perfusion might have been found if thinner transmural sections had been studied.

Direct myocardial perfusion from the ventricular lumen probably does occur but it is hard to consider this an important source of oxygen and other nutrients. The immediate subendocardial tissue may benefit when antegrade coronary flow is significantly reduced, but it is doubtful that these endomural channels could account for significant epicardial or even midwall perfusion. Inter- and intracoronary collateral vessels must still be considered to be the most important pathway for delivery of blood to ischemic myocardium following coronary artery obstruction.

VII. Extracardiac Collateral Vessels

Frequently treated merely as anatomic curiosities, retrocardiac collateral vessels were universally observed by Omar[199] in excised canine hearts in which the coronary arteries had been injected with india ink solution. These collaterals are derived in part from the vasa vasorum of the great arteries and veins, and also develop around the lines of the pericardial reflection. They act as bridges connecting the atrial branches of the coronary arteries with bronchial and mediastinal arteries.

Battezzati,[200] Griffin,[201] and Glover[202–204] also demonstrated collateral connections between the internal mammary artery and coronary arterial system in dogs. When Evans blue was injected into the internal mammary artery at the level of the pericardiophrenic artery, dye was observed throughout the parietal pericardium, in the mediastinal pleura and fat, around the base of the aorta, pulmonary artery, and vena cavae, in the walls of the atria, in epicardial fat overlying the atrioventricular groove, and repeatedly in the small plexus of vessels underlying the epicardium.[202,203] In one dog the entire thickness of the left ventricular myocardium was stained with dye, even into the base of the papillary muscles. When ^{131}I was injected into the internal mammary artery, this isotope was routinely found in the left ventricular myocardium.[202,203]

Nomura[205] noted that the right subclavian artery supplied the sinoatrial node in the mouse heart. The heart of the rat has an obvious dual blood supply—coronary and extracoronary.[206] The right and left coronary arteries supply the ventricles and interventricular septum, and the right coronary artery supplies the interatrial septum. The extracoronary (or accessory) arteries to the rat heart are branches of the right and left cardiacomediastinal arteries which arise from the internal mammary artery and less frequently from the subclavian or common carotid arteries. The right cardiocomediastinal artery divides at the lower portion of the right superior vena cava into a deep mediastinal artery (to the right bronchus, trachea, esophagus, and posterior mediastinal structures) and a superficial cardiac branch. The cardiac branch gives rise to lateral, middle, and medial branches supplying the sinus node (node artery) and portions of the right and left atria and pulmonary veins. The left cardiacomediastinal artery divides at the middle of the left superior vena cava, also into a deep mediastinal artery and a superficial cardiac artery. The latter supplies portions of the left atrium, interatrial septum, pulmonary veins, and vasa vasorum to the coronary sinus. Thus, in the rat, the ventricles and small portions of each atrium are supplied by the coronary arteries, but the remaining atrial tissue is supplied by cardiac branches of the cardiacomediastinal arteries. Because the right coronary and accessory arteries supply the atria together, a potential anastomotic pathway between extracoronary and coronary arteries is established. These extracardiac arteries are homologous to similar arteries found in lower animal forms which disappeared during phylogenetic development. These accessory arteries are also anatomically reminiscent of the extracardiac coronary vessels in man.

Halpern[207] also studied the arterial supply of the sinoatrial node in the dog by clearing the heart after intracoronary injection with either latex, vinyl acetate, or nylon. In 90 of the 107 hearts examined, the major artery to the sinus node was the cristal artery, a branch of the dorsal right atrial artery which is itself a branch of the right coronary artery. In addition to forming an arterial ring around the superior vena cava with branches of the left atrial artery, the cristal artery sent twigs that became the vasa vasorum of the superior vena cava. Other small tributaries originating from the cristal artery anastomosed with pericardial arteries and branches of the pericardiophrenic artery.

The vasa vasorum of the canine aorta may arise directly from the lumen of the ascending aorta. Direct injection of these vessels with an india ink-gelatin mass and then clearing of the heart revealed extensive anastomoses including many with the coronary arteries.[208]

Hence, the dog and other mammals have extracardiac arteries that supply cardiac tissue and anastomose with the coronary arterial system. These vessels have clinical analogs, and in some cases may play important roles in the perfusion of the left ventricular myocardium.

References

1. Schaper W, and Vandesteene R: The rate of growth of interarterial anastomoses in chronic coronary artery occlusion. *Life Sci.* 6:1673–1680, 1967.
2. Schaper W, Schaper J, Xhonneux R, and Vandesteene R: The morphology of

intercoronary anastomoses in chronic coronary artery occlusion. *Cardiovasc. Res.* 3:315−323, 1969.

3. Schaper W, DeBrabander M, and Lewi P: DNA synthesis and mitoses in coronary collateral vessels of the dog. *Circ. Res.* 28:671−679, 1971.

4. DeBrabander M, and Schaper W: Quantitative histology of the canine coronary collateral circulation in localized myocardial ischemia. *Life Sci.* 10:857−868, 1971.

5. Schaper W: *The Collateral Circulation of the Heart.* North-Holland Publishing Co., Amsterdam, 1971.

6. Schaper J, Borgers M, and Schaper W: Ultrastructure of ischemia-induced changes in the precapillary anastomotic network of the heart. *Am. J. Cardiol.* 29:851−859, 1972.

7. Schaper W, Flameng W, and DeBrabander M: Comparative aspects of coronary collateral circulation. In *Comparative Pathophysiology of Circulatory Disturbances: Advances in Experimental Medicine and Biology,* Vol. 22 (ed CM Bloor). Plenum Press, New York, 1972, pp 267−276.

8. Schaper W, Schaper J, and Pasyk S: Development of a collateral circulation in chronic experimental coronary occlusion. In *Coronary Angiography and Angina Pectoris* (ed PR Lichtlen). Georg Thieme, Stuttgart, 1976, pp. 325−333.

9. Schaper W, and Pasyk S: Influence of collateral flow on the ischemic tolerance of the heart following acute and subacute coronary occlusion. *Circulation* 53 (Suppl. I):I-57−I-65, 1976.

10. Schaper J, König R, Franz D, and Schaper W: The endothelial surface of growing coronary collateral arteries. Intimal margination and diapedesis of monocytes: A combined SEM and TEM study. *Virchows Arch. (Path. Anat.)* 370:193−205, 1976.

11. Yabe Y, Takahashi T, Yoshimura S, et al: A study on cell proliferation kinetics of coronary collateral vessels and myocardial muscles in the ischemic heart in dog. (abstr) *Jpn. Circ. J.* 38:609, 1974.

12. Schaper W: Tangential wall stress as a molding force in the development of collateral vessels in the canine heart. *Experientia* 23:595−596, 1967.

13. Borgers M, Schaper J, and Schaper W: Acute vascular lesions in developing coronary collatals. *Virchows Arch. (Path. Anat.)* 351:1−11, 1970.

14. Takahashi T, Suzuki N, Ino-Oka E, et al: Morphological studies on coronary collateral vessels. (abstr) *Jpn. Circ. J.* 38:609, 1974.

15. Gregg DE, Thornton JJ, and Mautz FR: The magnitude, adequacy and source of the collateral blood flow and pressure in chronically occluded coronary arteries. *Am. J. Physiol.* 127:161−175, 1939.

16. Eckstein RW, Gregg DE, and Pritchard WH: The magnitude and time of development of the collateral circulation in occluded femoral, carotid and coronary arteries. *Am. J. Physiol.* 132:351−361, 1941.

17. Mosher P, Ross J Jr, McFate PA, and Shaw RF: Control of coronary blood flow by an autoregulatory mechanism. *Circ. Res.* 14:250−259, 1964.

18. Fam WM, and McGregor M: Pressure-flow relationships in the coronary circulation. *Circ. Res.* 25:293−301, 1969.

19. Rubio VR, Wiedmeier T, and Berne RM: Nucleoside phosphorylase: Localization and role in the myocardial distribution of purines. *Am. J. Physiol.* 222:550−555, 1972.

20. Berne RM, and Rubio R: Adenine nucleotide metabolism in the heart. *Circ. Res.* 35(Suppl. III):III-109−III-118, 1974.

21. Coffman JD, and Gregg DE: Reactive hyperemia characteristics of the myocardium. *Am. J. Physiol.* 199:1143−1149, 1960.

22. Olsson RA, and Gregg DE: Myocardial reactive hyperemia in the unanesthetized dog. *Am. J. Physiol.* 208:224−230, 1965.

23. Bache RJ, Cobb FR, and Greenfield JC Jr: Limitation of the coronary vascular response to ischemia in the awake dog. *Circ. Res.* 35:527−535, 1974.

24. Dunn RB, McDonough KM, and Griggs DM Jr: High energy phosphate stores and lactate levels in different layers of the canine left ventricle during reactive hyperemia. *Circ. Res.* 44:788−795, 1979.

25. Gould KL, Lipscomb K, and Hamilton GW: Physiologic basis for assessing critical coronary stenosis: Instantaneous flow response and regional distribution during coronary hyperemia as measures of coronary flow reserve. *Am. J. Cardiol.* 33:87−94, 1974.

26. Eckstein RW: Effect of exercise and coronary artery narrowing on coronary collateral circulation. *Circ. Res.* 5:230−235, 1957.

27. Elliot EC, Jones EL, Bloor CM, et al: Day-to-day changes in coronary hemodynamics secondary to constriction of circumflex branch of left coronary artery in conscious dogs. *Circ. Res.* 22:237−250, 1968.

28. Elliot EC, Bloor CM, Jones EL, et al: Effect of controlled coronary occlusion on collateral circulation in conscious dogs. *Am. J. Physiol.* 220:857−861, 1971.

29. Elliot EC: Hemodynamic evidence of the development of coronary collateral circulation in conscious dogs. In *Current Topics in Coronary Research: Advances in Experimental Medicine and Biology*, Vol. 39 (eds CM Bloor and RA Olsson). Plenum Press, New York, 1973, pp 173−190.

30. Gregg DE: The natural history of coronary collateral development. *Circ. Res.* 35:335−344, 1974.

31. Moir TW, and DeBra DW: Effect of left ventricular hypertension, ischemia and vasoactive drugs on the myocardial distribution of coronary flow. *Circ. Res.* 21:65−74, 1967.

32. Weiss HR, and Winbury MM: Nitroglycerin and chromonar on small-vessel blood content of the ventricular walls. *Am. J. Physiol.* 226:838−843, 1974.

33. Wüsten B: Biophysics of coronary artery narrowing. In *The Pathophysiology of Myocardial Perfusion* (ed W Schaper). North-Holland Biomedical Press, Amsterdam, 1979, pp 285−304.

34. Bache RJ, Cobb FR, and Greenfield JC Jr: Myocardial blood flow distribution during ischemia-induced coronary vasodilation in the unanesthetized dog. *J. Clin. Invest.* 54:1462−1472, 1974.

35. Hess DS, and Bache RJ: Transmural distribution of myocardial blood flow during systole in the awake dog. *Circ. Res.* 38:5−15, 1976.

36. Ball RM, and Bache RJ: Distribution of myocardial blood flow in the exercising dog with restricted coronary artery inflow. *Circ. Res.* 38:60−66, 1976.

37. Archie JP Jr: Intramyocardial pressure: Effect of preload on transmural distribution of systolic coronary blood flow. *Am. J. Cardiol.* 35:904−911, 1975.

38. Hoffman JIE: Determinants and prediction of transmural myocardial perfusion. *Circulation* 58:381−391, 1978.

39. Downey JM, and Kirk ES: Distribution of the coronary blood flow across the canine heart wall during systole. *Circ. Res.* 34:251−257, 1974.

40. Downey JM, Downey HF, and Kirk ES: Effects of myocardial strains on coronary blood flow. *Circ. Res.* 34:286−292, 1974.

41. Domenech RJ, and De La Prida JM: Mechanical effects of heart contraction on coronary flow. *Cardiovasc. Res.* 9:509−514, 1975.

42. Snyder R, Downey JM, and Kirk ES: The active and passive components of extravascular coronary resistance. *Cardiovasc. Res.* 9:161−166, 1975.

43. Downey JM, and Kirk ES: Inhibition of coronary blood flow by a vascular waterfall mechanism. *Circ. Res.* 36:753−760, 1975.

44. Downey J: Compression of the coronary arteries by the fibrillating canine heart. *Circ. Res.* 39:53−57, 1976.

45. Cobb FR, Bache RJ, and Greenfield JC Jr: Regional myocardial blood flow in awake dogs. *J. Clin. Invest.* 53:1618−1625, 1974.

46. Downey HF, Bashour FA, Boatwright RB, et al: Uniformity of transmural perfusion in anesthetized dogs with maximally dilated coronary circulations. *Circ. Res.* 37:111−117, 1975.

47. Gerdes AM, Callas G, and Kasten FH: Differences in regional capillary distribution and myocyte sizes in normal and hypertrophic rat hearts. *Am. J. Anat.* 156: 523−532, 1979.

48. Rakušan K, Moravec J, and Hatt P-Y: Regional capillary supply in the normal and hypertrophied rat heart. *Microvasc. Res.* 20:319−326, 1980.

49. Wright AJA, and Hudlická O: Capillary growth and changes in heart performance induced by chronic bradycardial pacing in the rabbit. *Circ. Res.* 49:469−478, 1981.

50. Wüsten B, Flameng W, and Schaper W: The distribution of myocardial flow. Part I: Effects of experimental coronary occlusion. *Basic Res. Cardiol.* 69:422−434, 1974.

51. Marcus ML, Kerber RE, Ehrhardt J, and Abboud FM: Effects of time on volume and distribution of coronary collateral flow. *Am. J. Physiol.* 230:279−285, 1976.

52. Bishop SP, White FC, and Bloor CM: Regional myocardial blood flow during acute myocardial infarction in the conscious dog. *Circ. Res.* 38:429−438, 1976.

53. Rivas F, Cobb FR, Bache RJ, and Greenfield JC Jr: Relationship between blood flow to ischemic regions and extent of myocardial infarction: Serial measurement of blood flow to ischemic regions in dogs. *Circ. Res.* 38:439−447, 1976.

54. Cohen MV: Quantitation of collateral and ischemic flows with microspheres and diffusible indicator. *Am. J. Physiol.* 234:H487−H495, 1978.

55. Jugdutt BI, Becker LC, and Hutchins GM: Early changes in collateral blood flow during myocardial infarction in conscious dogs. *Am. J. Physiol.* 237:H371−H380, 1979.

56. Cohen MV, and Yipintsoi T: Myocardial performance and collateral flow after transient coronary occlusion in exercising dogs. *Am. J. Physiol.* 237:H520−H527, 1979.

57. Murdock RH Jr, and Cobb FR: Effects of infarcted myocardium on regional blood flow measurements to ischemic regions in canine heart. *Circ. Res.* 47:701−709, 1980.

58. Cohen, MV, and Yipintsoi T: Restoration of cardiac function and myocardial flow by collateral development in dogs. *Am. J. Physiol.* 240:H811−H819, 1981.

59. Davenport N, Goldstein RE, Bolli R, and Epstein SE: Blood flow to infarct and surviving myocardium: Implications regarding the action of verapamil on the acutely ischemic dog heart. *J. Am. Coll. Cardiol.* 3:956−965, 1984.

60. Marcus ML, Kerber RE, Ehrhardt J, and Abboud FM: Three dimensional geometry of acutely ischemic myocardium. *Circulation* 52:254−263, 1975.

61. Jugdutt BI, Hutchins GM, Bulkley BH, and Becker LC: Myocardial infarction in the conscious dog: Three-dimensional mapping of infarct, collateral flow and region at risk. *Circulation* 60:1141−1150, 1979.

62. Rees JR, and Redding VJ: Anastomotic blood flow in experimental myocardial infarction: A new method, using [133]Xenon clearance, for repeated measurements during recovery. *Cardiovasc. Res.* 1:169−178, 1967.

63. Rees JR, and Redding VJ: Experimental myocardial infarction by a wedge method: Early changes in collateral flow. *Cardiovasc. Res.* 2:43−53, 1968.

64. Redding VJ, and Rees JR: Early changes in collateral flow following coronary artery ligation: The role of the sympathetic nervous system. *Cardiovasc. Res.* 2:219−225, 1968.

65. Haft JI, and Damato AN: Measurement of collateral blood flow after myocardial infarction in the closed-chest dog. *Am. Heart J.* 77:641−648, 1969.

66. Pasyk S, Bloor CM, Khouri EM, and Gregg DE: Systemic and coronary effects of coronary artery occlusion in the unanesthetized dog. *Am. J. Physiol.* 220:646−654, 1971.

67. Weisse AB, Senft A, Khan MI, and Regan TJ: Effect of nitrate infusions on the systemic and coronary circulations following acute experimental myocardial infarction in the intact dog. *Am. J. Cardiol.* 30:362−370, 1972.

68. Marshall RJ, Parratt JR, and Ledingham IM: Changes in blood flow and oxygen

consumption in normal and ischaemic regions of the myocardium following acute coronary artery ligation. *Cardiovasc. Res.* 8:204−215, 1974.

69. Grayson J, and Lapin BA: Observations on the mechanisms of infarction in the dog after experimental occlusion of the coronary artery. *Lancet* 1:1284−1288, 1966.

70. Grayson J, Irvine M, Parratt JR, and Cunningham J: Vasospastic elements in myocardial infarction following coronary occlusion in the dog. *Cardiovasc. Res.* 2:54−62, 1968.

71. Grayson J, and Irvine M: Myocardial infarction in the monkey: Studies on the collateral circulation after acute coronary occlusion. *Cardiovasc. Res.* 2:170−178, 1968.

72. Cox JL, Pass HI, Wechsler AS, et al: Evolution and transmural distribution of collateral blood flow in acute myocardial infarction. *Surg. Forum* 24:154−156, 1973.

73. Cox JL, Pass HI, Wechsler AS, et al: Coronary collateral blood flow in acute myocardial infarction. *J. Thorac. Cardiovasc. Surg.* 69:117−125, 1975.

74. Smith HJ, Singh BN, Norris RM, et al: Changes in myocardial blood flow and S-T segment elevation following coronary artery occlusion in dogs. *Circ. Res.* 36:697−705, 1975.

75. Hirzel HO, Nelson GR, Sonnenblick EH, and Kirk ES: Redistribution of collateral blood flow from necrotic to surviving myocardium following coronary occlusion in the dog. *Circ. Res.* 39:214−222, 1976.

76. Henry PD, Shuchleib R, Borda LJ, et al: Effects of nifedipine on myocardial perfusion and ischemic injury in dogs. *Circ. Res.* 43:372−380, 1978.

77. White FC, Sanders M, and Bloor CM: Regional redistribution of myocardial blood flow after coronary occlusion and reperfusion in the conscious dog. *Am. J. Cardiol.* 42:234−243, 1978.

78. Levy MN, and Cutarelli R: Effect of acute coronary artery ligation upon blood flow to the normal myocardium. *Am. J. Cardiol.* 13:48−50, 1964.

79. Herzberg RM, Rubio R, and Berne RM: Coronary occlusion and embolization: Effect on blood flow in adjacent arteries. *Am. J. Physiol.* 210:169−175, 1966.

80. Driscol TE, and Eckstein RW: Coronary inflow and outflow responses to coronary artery occlusion. *Circ. Res.* 20:485−495, 1967.

81. Joyce EE, and Gregg DE: Coronary artery occlusion in the intact unanesthetized dog: Intercoronary reflexes. *Am. J. Physiol.* 213:64−70, 1967.

82. Domenech RJ: Total and regional coronary blood flow during acute coronary occlusion in anaesthetized and conscious dogs. *Cardiovasc. Res.* 8:415−422, 1974.

83. Krug A, du Mesnil de Rochemont W, and Korb G: Blood supply of the myocardium after temporary coronary occlusion. *Circ. Res.* 19:57−62, 1966.

84. Kloner RA, Ganote CE, and Jennings RB: The "no-reflow" phenomenon after temporary coronary occlusion in the dog. *J. Clin. Invest.* 54:1496−1508, 1974.

85. Willerson JT, Watson JT, Hutton I, et al: Reduced myocardial reflow and increased coronary vascular resistance following prolonged myocardial ischemia in the dog. *Circ. Res.* 36:771−781, 1975.

86. Frame LH, and Powell WJ Jr: Progressive perfusion impairment during prolonged low flow myocardial ischemia in dogs. *Circ. Res.* 39:269−276, 1976.

87. Schimmler W: Interarterielle Anastomosen im Koronarkreislauf: Und ihre prophylaktische Bedeutung. *München. Med. Wschr.* 107:1748−1750, 1965.

88. Lavallee M, and Vatner SF: Regional myocardial blood flow and necrosis in primates following coronary occlusion. *Am. J. Physiol.* 246:H635−H639, 1984.

89. Shaw DJ, Pitt A, and Friesinger GC: Autoradiographic study of the [133]xenon disappearance method for measurement of myocardial blood flow. *Cardiovasc. Res.* 6:268−276, 1971.

90. Pass HI, Cox JL, Wechsler AS, et al: Response of coronary collateral circulation to

increased myocardial demands. (abstr) *Circulation* 48(Suppl. IV):IV-92, 1973.

91. Schaper W, Wüsten B, Flameng W, et al: Local dilatory reserve in chronic experimental coronary occlusion without infarction. Quantitation of collateral development. *Basic Res. Cardiol.* 70:159−173, 1975.

92. Schwarz F, Flameng W, Mack B, et al: Vascular and cardiac contractile reserve in the dog heart with chronic multiple coronary occlusions. *Am. Heart J.* 92:600−608, 1976.

93. Lambert PR, Hess DS, and Bache RJ: Effect of exercise on perfusion of collateral-dependent myocardium in dogs with chronic coronary artery occlusion. *J. Clin. Invest.* 59:1−7, 1977.

94. Heaton WH, Marr KC, Capurro NL, et al: Beneficial effect of physical training on blood flow to myocardium perfused by chronic collaterals in the exercising dog. *Circulation* 57:575−581, 1978.

95. Flameng W, Schwarz F, Schaper W, and Hehrlein F: Functional significance of coronary collaterals. In *Coronary Heart Disease: 3rd International Symposium Frankfurt* (eds M Kaltenbach, P Lichtlen, R Balcon, and W-D Bussmann). Georg Thieme, Stuttgart, 1978, pp 67−72.

96. Neill WA, and Oxendine JM: Exercise can promote coronary collateral development without improving perfusion of ischemic myocardium. *Circulation* 60:1513−1519, 1979.

97. Fedor JM, Rembert JC, McIntosh DM, and Greenfield JC Jr: Effects of exercise- and pacing-induced tachycardia on coronary collateral flow in the awake dog. *Circ. Res.* 46:214−220, 1980.

98. Crystal GJ, Downey HF, and Bashour FA: Evaluation of noncoronary sources of left ventricular perfusion to intercoronary collateral-dependent myocardium due to chronic major vessel occlusion: Absent contribution of luminal and extracardiac channels. *Am. Heart J.* 102:841−845, 1981.

99. Becker LC, and Pitt B: Collateral blood flow in conscious dogs with chronic coronary artery occlusion. *Am. J. Physiol.* 221:1507−1510, 1971.

100. Schaper W, Lewi P, Flameng W, and Gijpen L: Myocardial steal produced by coronary vasodilation in chronic coronary artery occlusion. *Basic Res. Cardiol.* 68:3−20, 1973.

101. Schaper W, Flameng W, Wüsten B, and Palmowski J: The distribution of coronary and of coronary collateral flow in normal hearts and after chronic coronary occlusion. In *Current Topics in Coronary Research: Advances in Experimental Medicine and Biology,* Vol. 39 (eds. CM Bloor and RA Olsson). Plenum Press, New York, 1973, pp 151−160.

102. Scheel KW, Banet M, Ott C, and Lehan PH: A quantitative approach to collateral and antegrade flows after coronary occlusion. *Am. J. Physiol.* 222:687−694, 1972.

103. Schaper W, Flameng W, Winkler B, et al: Quantification of collateral resistance in acute and chronic experimental coronary occlusion in the dog. *Circ. Res.* 39:371−377, 1976.

104. Flameng W, Schwarz F, and Schaper W: Coronary collaterals in the canine heart: Development and functional significance. *Am. Heart J.* 97:70−77, 1979.

105. Scheel KW, Galindez TA, Cook B, et al: Changes in coronary and collateral flows and adequacy of perfusion in the dog following one and three months of circumflex occlusion. *Circ. Res.* 39:654−658, 1976.

106. Scheel KW, Ingram LA, and Wilson JL: Effects of exercise on the coronary and collateral vasculature of beagles with and without coronary occlusion. *Circ. Res.* 48:523−530, 1981.

107. Walter P, Flameng W, Görlach G, and Hehrlein FW: Restoration of coronary reserve by bypass grafting in relation to the collateral circulation. In *Coronary Heart Disease: 3rd International Symposium Frankfurt* (eds. M Kaltenbach, P Lichtlen, R Balcon, and W-D Bussmann). Georg Thieme, Stuttgart, 1978, pp 27−33.

108. Flameng W, Wüsten B, Winkler B, et al: Influence of perfusion pressure and heart rate on local myocardial flow in the collateralized heart with chronic coronary occlusion. *Am. Heart J.* 89:51−59, 1975.

109. Rembert JC, Boyd LM, Watkinson WP, and Greenfield JC Jr: Effect of adenosine on transmural myocardial blood flow distribution in the awake dog. *Am. J. Physiol.* 239:H7−H13, 1980.

110. Patterson RE, Jones-Collins BA, and Aamodt R: Impaired collateral blood flow reserve early after nontransmural myocardial infarction in conscious dogs. *Am. J. Cardiol.* 50:1133−1140, 1982.

111. Cohen MV, and Steingart RM: Exercise 201-thallium scintigraphy in dogs: Effects of chronic coronary occlusion and collateral development on early and late scintigraphic images. *Circulation* (in press).

112. Burow RD, Pond M, Schafer AW, and Becker L: "Circumferential profiles": A new method for computer analysis of thallium-201 myocardial perfusion images. *J. Nucl. Med.* 20:771−777, 1979.

113. Hill RC, Kleinman LH, Tiller WH Jr, et al: Myocardial blood flow and function during gradual coronary occlusion in awake dog. *Am. J. Physiol.* 244:H60−H67, 1983.

114. Hess DS, and Bache RJ: Regional myocardial blood flow during graded treadmill exercise following circumflex coronary artery occlusion in the dog. *Circ. Res.* 47:59−68, 1980.

115. Tipton CM, Carey RA, Eastin WC, and Erickson HH: A submaximal test for dogs: Evaluation of effects of training, detraining, and cage confinement. *J. Appl. Physiol.* 37:271−275, 1974.

116. Bache RJ: Effects of exercise on blood flow to collateral-dependent myocardium in the dog. (abstr) *Circulation* 64(Suppl. IV):IV-117, 1981.

117. Schaper W: Influence of physical exercise on coronary collateral blood flow in chronic experimental two-vessel occlusion. *Circulation* 65:905−912, 1982.

118. Griggs DM Jr, Tchokoev VV, and Chen CC: Transmural differences in ventricular tissue substrate levels due to coronary constriction. *Am. J. Physiol.* 222:705−709, 1972.

119. Dunn RB, and Griggs DM Jr: Transmural gradients in ventricular tissue metabolites produced by stopping coronary blood flow in the dog. *Circ. Res.* 37:438−445, 1975.

120. Allison TB, Ramey CA, and Holsinger JW Jr: Transmural gradients of left ventricular tissue metabolites after circumflex artery ligation in dogs. *J. Mol. Cell. Cardiol.* 9:837−852, 1977.

121. Banka VS, Bodenheimer MM, Ramanathan KB, et al: Progressive transmural electrographic, myocardial potassium ion/sodium ion ratio and ultrastructural changes as a function of time after acute coronary occlusion. *Am. J. Cardiol.* 42:429−443, 1978.

122. Jennings RB, Ganote CE, and Reimer KA: Ischemic tissue injury. *Am. J. Pathol.* 81:179−198, 1975.

123. Reimer KA, Lowe JE, Rasmussen MM, and Jennings RB: The wavefront phenomenon of ischemic cell death. I. Myocardial infarct size vs. duration of coronary occlusion in dogs. *Circulation* 56:786−794, 1977.

124. Reimer K, and Jennings RB: The "wavefront phenomenon" of myocardial ischemic cell death. II. Transmural progression of necrosis within the framework of ischemic bed size (myocardium at risk) and collateral flow. *Lab. Invest.* 40:633−644, 1979.

125. Hirzel HO, Sonnenblick EH, and Kirk ES: Absence of a lateral border zone of intermediate creatine phosphokinase depletion surrounding a central infarct 24 hours after acute coronary occlusion in the dog. *Circ. Res.* 41:673−683, 1977.

126. Sjoquist P-O, Duker G, and Almgren O: Distribution of the collateral blood flow at the lateral border of the ischemic myocardium after acute coronary occlusion in the pig and the dog. *Basic Res. Cardiol.* 79:164−175, 1984.

127. Fujiwara H, Ashraf M, Sato S, and Millard RW: Transmural cellular damage and blood flow distribution in early ischemia in pig hearts. *Circ. Res.* 51:683–693, 1982.

128. Fulton WFM: *The Coronary Arteries: Arteriography, Microanatomy, and Pathogenesis of Obliterative Coronary Artery Disease.* Charles C. Thomas, Springfield, IL, 1965.

129. Factor SM, Okun EM, and Kirk ES: The histological lateral border of acute canine myocardial infarction: A function of microcirculation. *Circ. Res.* 48:640–649, 1981.

130. Linder E: Measurements of normal and collateral coronary blood flow by close-arterial and intramyocardial injection of krypton[85] and xenon[133]. *Acta Physiol. Scand.* 68(Suppl. 272):5–31, 1966.

131. Becker LC, Ferreira R, and Thomas M: Mapping of left ventricular blood flow with radioactive microspheres in experimental coronary artery occlusion. *Cardiovasc. Res.* 7:391–400, 1973.

132. Factor SM, Sonnenblick EH, and Kirk ES: The histologic border zone of acute myocardial infarction—Islands or peninsulas? *Am. J. Pathol.* 92:111–124, 1978.

133. Fischl SJ, Sonnenblick EH, and Kirk ES: Collateral blood flow in the border zone following acute coronary occlusion. (abstr) *Am. J. Cardiol.* 35:136, 1975.

134. Kirk ES, and Hirzel HO: Critical role of coronary collateral blood flow in the pathophysiology of myocardial infarction. In *Coronary Heart Disease: 3rd International Symposium Frankfurt* (eds M Kaltenbach, P Lichtlen, R Balcon, and W-D Bussmann). George Thieme, Stuttgart, 1978, pp 11–20.

135. Koyanagi S, Eastham CL, Harrison DG, and Marcus ML: Transmural variation in the relationship between myocardial infarct size and risk area. *Am. J. Physiol.* 242:H867–H874, 1982.

136. Wüsten B, Winkler B, and Schaper W: Influence of collateral circulation on infarct size in acute myocardial infarction. In *The First 24 Hours in Myocardial Infarction* (eds F Kaindl, O Pachinger, and P Probst). Verlag Gerhard Witzstrock, Baden-Baden, 1977, pp 140–142.

137. Jugdutt BI, Hutchins GM, Bulkley BH, and Becker LC: Similar relation between size of infarct and occluded bed in dog and man: Evidence for collateral protection. (abstr) *Clin. Res.* 29:212A, 1981.

138. Hearse DJ, and Yellon DM: The "border zone" in evolving myocardial infarction: Controversy or confusion? *Am. J. Cardiol.* 47:1321–1334, 1981.

139. Opie LH: Effects of regional ischemia on metabolism of glucose and fatty acids: Relative rates of aerobic and anaerobic energy production during myocardial infarction and comparison with effects of anoxia. *Circ. Res.* 38(Suppl. I):I-52-I-68, 1976.

140. Opie LH, and Owen P: Effect of glucose-insulin-potassium infusions on arteriovenous differences of glucose and of free fatty acids and on tissue metabolic changes in dogs with developing myocardial infarction. *Am. J. Cardiol.* 38:310–321, 1976.

141. Hearse DJ, Opie LH, Katzeff IE, et al: Characterization of the "border zone" in acute regional ischemia in the dog. *Am. J. Cardiol.* 40:716–726, 1977.

142. Kléber AG, Janse MJ, van Capelle FJL, and Durrer D: Mechanism and time course of S-T and T-Q segment changes during acute regional myocardial ischemia in the pig heart determined by extracellular and intracellular recordings. *Circ. Res.* 42:603–613, 1978.

143. Theroux P, Franklin D, Ross J Jr, and Kemper WS: Regional myocardial function during acute coronary artery occlusion and its modification by pharmacologic agents in the dog. *Circ. Res.* 35:896–908, 1974.

144. Ross J Jr, and Franklin D: Analysis of regional myocardial function, dimensions, and wall thickness in the characterization of myocardial ischemia and infarction. *Circulation* 53(Suppl. I):I-88–I-92, 1976.

145. Chance B: Discussion of effects of regional ischemia on metabolism of glucose and fatty acids. *Circ. Res.* 38(Suppl. I):I-69—I-71, 1976.
146. Barlow CH, and Chance B: Ischemic areas in perfused rat hearts: Measurement by NADH fluorescence photography. *Science* 193:909—910, 1976.
147. Steenbergen C, Deleeuw G, Barlow C, et al: Heterogeneity of the hypoxic state in perfused rat heart. *Circ. Res.* 41:606—615, 1977.
148. Harken AH, Barlow CH, Harden WR III, and Chance B: Two and three dimensional display of myocardial ischemic "border zone" in dogs. *Am. J. Cardiol.* 42:954—959, 1978.
149. Simson MB, Harden W, Barlow C, and Harken AH: Visualization of the distance between perfusion and anoxia along an ischemic border. *Circulation* 60: 1151—1155, 1979.
150. Janse MJ, Cinca J, Moréna H, et al: The "border zone" in myocardial ischemia: An electrophysiological, metabolic, and histochemical correlation in the pig heart. *Circ. Res.* 44:576—588, 1979.
151. Yellon DM, Hearse DJ, Crome R, et al: Characterization of the lateral interface between normal and ischemic tissue in the canine heart during evolving myocardial infarction. *Am. J. Cardiol.* 47:1233—1239, 1981.
152. Cox JL, McLaughlin VW, Flowers NC, and Horan LG: The ischemic zone surrounding acute myocardial infarction. Its morphology as detected by dehydrogenase staining. *Am. Heart J.* 76:650—659, 1968.
153. Fishbein MC, Hare CA, Gissen SA, et al: Identification and quantification of histochemical border zones during the evolution of myocardial infarction in the rat. *Cardiovasc. Res.* 14:41—49, 1980.
154. Deloche A, Fabiani JN, Camilleri JP, et al: The effect of coronary artery reperfusion on the extent of myocardial infarction. *Am. Heart J.* 93:358—366, 1977.
155. Shnitka TK, and Nachlas MM: Histochemical alterations in ischemic heart muscle and early myocardial infarction. *Am. J. Pathol.* 42:507—527, 1963.
156. Page E, and Polimeni PI: Ultrastructural changes in the ischemic zone bordering experimental infarcts in rat left ventricles. *Am. J. Pathol.* 87:81—104, 1977.
157. Buja LM, Parkey RW, Stokely EM, et al: Pathophysiology of technetium-99m stannous pyrophosphate and thallium-201 scintigraphy of acute anterior myocardial infarcts in dogs. *J. Clin. Invest.* 57:1508—1522, 1976.
158. Lie JT, Pairolero PC, Holley KE, et al: Time course and zonal variations of ischemia-induced myocardial cationic electrolyte derangements. *Circulation* 51:860—866, 1975.
159. Khouri EM, Gregg DE, and McGranahan GM Jr: Regression and reappearance of coronary collaterals. *Am. J. Physiol.* 220:655—661, 1971.
160. Elliot EC, Khouri EM, Snow JA, and Gregg DE: Direct measurement of coronary collateral blood flow in conscious dogs by an electromagnetic flowmeter. *Circ. Res.* 34:374—383, 1974.
161. Pasyk S, Wüsten B, Flameng W, and Schaper W: Behaviour of the coronary collateral circulation after release acute left circumflex coronary artery occlusion in the presence of the massive myocardial infarction. *Verh. Dtsch. Ges. Kreislaufforsch.* 40:334—337, 1974.
162. Oldham HN Jr, Kakos GS, Dixon SH Jr, et al: The effect of coronary collateral circulation on experimental aorto-coronary bypass. *J. Surg. Res.* 12:87—92, 1972.
163. Cibulski AA, Lehan PH, Timmis HH, and Hellems HK: Regression of intercoronary collateral vessels in mongrel dogs after coronary bypass grafting. *Am. J. Cardiol.* 31:480—483, 1973.
164. Vieussens R: *Nouvelles Découvertes sur le Coeur, Expliquées dans une Lettre écrite á Monsieur Boudin, Conseiller d'Etat, premier Medecin de Monseigneur.* Laurent d'Houry, Paris, 1706.
165. Roberts JT: Arteries, veins, and lymphatic vessels of the heart. In *Cardiology: An Encyclopedia of the Cardiovascular System* (ed AA Luisada). McGraw-Hill, New York, 1959, p I-93.

166. Wearn JT, Mettier SR, Klumpp TG, and Zschiesche LJ: The nature of the vascular communications between the coronary arteries and the chambers of the heart. *Am. Heart J.* 9:143−164, 1933.

167. Truex RC, and Angulo AW: Comparative study of the arterial and venous systems of the ventricular myocardium with special reference to the coronary sinus. *Anat. Rec.* 113:467−491, 1952.

168. Vineberg A: Experimental background of myocardial revascularization by internal mammary artery implantation and supplementary technics, with its clinical application in 125 patients: A review and critical appraisal. *Ann. Surg.* 159:185−207, 1964.

169. Young DAB, and Fell BF: Vascular connections between the coronary circulation and the ventricles of the rat heart. *Anat. Rec.* 144:149−153, 1962.

170. Pratt FH: The nutrition of the heart through the vessels of Thebesius and the coronary veins. *Am. J. Physiol.* 1:86−103, 1898.

171. Grant RT, and Viko LE: Observations on the anatomy of the Thebesian vessels of the heart. *Heart* 15:103−123, 1929.

172. Watanabe Y: An experimental study on the coronary-luminal communicating channels in coronary circulation. *Jpn. Circ. J.* 24:11−26, 1960.

173. Lendrum B, Kondo B, and Katz LN: The role of Thebesian drainage in the dynamics of coronary flow. *Am. J. Physiol.* 143:243−246, 1945.

174. Roberts JT, Spencer FD Jr, and Browne RS: Drainage of myocardium by cardial lumenal (Thebesian) vessels of the left ventricle. (abstr) *Fed. Proc.* 2:90−91, 1943.

175. Roberts JT, and Spencer FD Jr: The role of the Thebesian or arterio-luminal vessels in nourishment and drainage of the myocardium, especially in the left ventricle. (abstr) *Anat. Rec.* 94:547, 1946.

176. Moir TW, Driscol TE, and Eckstein RW: Thebesian drainage in the left heart of the dog. *Circ. Res.* 14:245−249, 1964.

177. Moir TW, Eckstein RW, and Driscol TE: Thebesian drainage of the septal artery. *Circ. Res.* 12:212−219, 1963.

178. Bohning A, Jochim K, and Katz LN: The Thebesian vessels as a source of nourishment for the myocardium. *Am. J. Physiol.* 106:183−200, 1933.

179. Eckstein RW, Roberts JT, Gregg DE, and Wearn JT: Observations on the role of the Thebesian veins and luminal vessels in the right ventricle. *Am. J. Physiol.* 132:648−653, 1941.

180. Roberts JT: Experimental studies on the nourishment of the left ventricle by the lumenal (Thebesial) vessels. (abstr) *Fed. Proc.* 2:90, 1943.

181. Roberts JT, and Spencer FD Jr: The accessory mechanism for drainage and nourishment of the myocardium by the Thebesian or arterio-luminal vessels, especially in the left ventricle. (abstr) *Proc. Am. Fed. Clin. Res.* 3:101, 1947.

182. Stella G: The part played by the Thebesian vessels in the blood supply to the heart. *J. Physiol.* 73:36−44, 1931.

183. Hammond GL, Juca ER, and Austen WG: The nature of intercoronary arterial flow in the normal heart. *Am. Heart J.* 78:559−568, 1969.

184. Katz LN, Jochim K, and Bohning A: The effect of the extravascular support of the ventricles on the flow in the coronary vessels. *Am. J. Physiol.* 122:236−251, 1939.

185. Wiggers CJ: The absorption of drugs from the right ventricular cavity. *J. Pharmacol. Exp. Ther.* 39:209−219, 1930.

186. Wiggers CJ: The functional importance of coronary collaterals. *Circulation* 5:609−615, 1952.

187. Moir TW: Luminal (Thebesian) coronary blood flow in the left ventricle. (abstr) *J. Lab. Clin. Med.* 70:868, 1967.

188. Moir TW: Study of luminal coronary collateral circulation in the beating canine heart. *Circ. Res.* 24:735−744, 1969.

189. Moir TW, and Debra DW: Measurement of the endocardial distribution of left ventricular coronary blood flow by Rb[86] chloride. *Am. Heart J.* 69:795−800, 1965.

190. Myers WW, and Honig CR: Amount and distribution of Rb[86] transported into myocardium from ventricular lumen. *Am. J. Physiol.* 211:739−745, 1966.

191. Page E, and Bernstein RS: Cat heart muscle in vitro. V. Diffusion through a sheet of right ventricle. *J. Gen. Physiol.* 47:1129−1140, 1964.

192. Gillespie WJ, and Love WD: Gradients in the regional rates of myocardial rubidium-86 clearance in tranquilized dogs. *Circ. Res.* 20:606−615, 1967.

193. Hammond GL, and Moggio RA: Function of microvascular pathways in coronary circulation. *Am. J. Physiol.* 220:1463−1467, 1971.

194. Moggio RA, Kabemba JM, and Hammond GL: Coronary-ventricular lumen blood exchange demonstrated by ^{51}Cr-labeled erythrocytes. *Am. J. Physiol.* 221:955−960, 1971.

195. Hammond GL, and Austen WG: Drainage patterns of coronary arterial flow as determined from the isolated heart. *Am. J. Physiol.* 212:1435−1440, 1967.

196. Brandfonbrener M: Left ventricular blood supply from sources other than left coronary artery. *J. Appl. Physiol.* 27:313−315, 1969.

197. Fixler DE, Wheeler M, and Huffines D: Extent of myocardial flow from luminal collateral circulation. *J. Appl. Physiol.* 37:282−285, 1974.

198. Brazier J, Hottenrott C, and Buckberg G: Noncoronary collateral myocardial blood flow. *Ann. Thorac. Surg.* 19:426−435, 1975.

199. Omar BK: Retrocardiac collateral circulation of heart: An anatomical study. *Indian Heart J* 20:177−180, 1968.

200. Battezzati M, Tagliaferro A, and DeMarchi G: La legatura delle due arterie mammarie interne nei disturbi di vascolarizzazione del miocardio: Nota preventiva relativa ai primi dati sperimentali e clinici. *Minerva Med.* 46:1178−1188, 1955.

201. Griffin JC Jr, Hardy JD, and Turner MD: Does internal mammary ligation increase arterial flow to the myocardium? *Surg. Forum* 8:325−327, 1957.

202. Glover RP, Davila JC, Kyle RH, et al: Ligation of the internal mammary arteries as a means of increasing blood supply to the myocardium. *J. Thorac. Surg.* 34:661−678, 1957.

203. Glover RP, Kitchell JR, Kyle RH, et al: Experiences with myocardial revascularization by division of the internal mammary arteries. *Dis. Chest* 33:637−657, 1958.

204. Glover RP, Kitchell JR, Davila JC, and Barkley HT Jr: Clinical and experimental study of bilateral internal mammary artery ligation (Bimal) for the relief of angina pectoris. (abstr) *Circulation* 20:701−702, 1959.

205. Nomura S: On the structure, distribution and innervation of the special heart muscle systems of the mouse. *Cytol. Neurol. Studies* 10:211−256, 1952.

206. Halpern MH: The dual blood supply of the rat heart. *Am. J. Anat.* 101:1−16, 1957.

207. Halpern MH: Arterial supply to the nodal tissue in the dog heart. *Circulation* 9:547−554, 1954.

208. Woodruff CE: Studies on the vasa vasorum. *Am. J. Pathol.* 2:567−569, 1926.

Functional Significance of Coronary Collaterals in Experimental Animals

I. Introduction

Coronary collateral vessels are present in normal hearts. Following coronary occlusion, collaterals undergo a striking transformation that results in reshaping of a 40 µm capillarylike channel into an arteriole with an internal diameter of up to 1 mm. Large collaterals have also been observed in other conditions associated with hypoxia where the major coronary arteries have been normal. Although it is logical to assume that this transformation process as well as the collaterals themselves should benefit the heart as well as the organism by providing an alternate source of blood supply to myocardial tissue, this assumption has been challenged often. Morphology does not provide reliable estimates of function, and the presence of collaterals that can enlarge is not sufficient to prove their importance. In 1900, Porter[1] wrote:

> The objection that one of the coronary arteries can be injected from another, and that therefore they are not terminal, is based on the incorrect premise that terminal arteries cannot be thus injected, and has no weight against the positive evidence of the complete failure of nutrition following closure. The passage of a fine injection-mass from one vascular area to another proves nothing concerning the possibility of the one area receiving its blood-supply from the other. Such supply is impossible if the resistance in the communicating vessels is greater than the blood-pressure in the smallest branches of the artery through which the supply must come. It is the fact of this high resistance, due to the small size of the communicating branches, which makes the artery "terminal". This condition of high resistance is really present during life, or infarction could not take place.

In spite of Porter's arguments, numerous investigators have determined that flow to acutely ischemic myocardium following coronary occlusion in dogs is not absent, but averages 10 to 30% of normal levels,[2–9] and intravenous injections of either fluorescein[10,11] or ^{32}P-erythrocytes[10] or intracoronary injection of Evans blue dye into patent vessels[12] demonstrate obvious staining or radioactivity in distal myocardial areas deprived of antegrade flow. Wiggers,[13–15] however, another proponent of the lack of importance of coronary collateral vessels, believed that this blood flowing through the ischemic area was too sluggish to serve a useful purpose. This conclusion was in part based on the early work of Tennant and Wiggers[16] with myocardiographs or superficial strain gauges sewn to the epicardium. These gauges were stitched parallel to the superficial fibers and recorded the force of the contractile effort of the fibers stretching between the feet of the gauges. Following coronary ligation, evidence of decreasing systolic contraction was observed with appearance of bulging of the cyanotic area as early as 14 seconds after ligation in some dogs. By one minute there was absence of active contraction, and within 40 to 60 minutes, marked expansion was noted during the period of isometric contraction. These results with superficial strain gauges have been confirmed by many.[17–22] Puri[23] developed a two-pronged miniature-length gauge attached to the end of an intravascular catheter. The catheter could be positioned in either the right or left ventricle and advanced to embed the prongs in the ventricular wall to evaluate changes in endocardial segment length. He observed complete loss of fiber shortening followed by paradoxical passive systolic lengthening within one minute of coronary occlusion. More recently, pairs of ultrasonic crystals have been implanted within the myocardial wall. One crystal is a transmitter and the other a receiver of emitted sound waves. Because the speed of sound transmission through myocardium is known, measurement of the time interval between emission and reception may be converted into instantaneous determination of the distance separating the crystals. Normally, the intercrystal distance shortens during systole as myocardial fibers shorten, and lengthens during diastolic relaxation. The myocardial response to acute coronary occlusion is similar in dogs,[24–27] pigs,[28,29] and baboons.[30] There is an abrupt decrease in percent shortening of the myocardial segments and an increase in end-diastolic segment length. Paradoxical increases in segment length during systole, or bulging, are also frequently observed.

To explain the rapid and marked deterioration of regional myocardial function following coronary occlusion, Saÿen and co-workers[31] measured the myocardial oxygen tension in the center of an ischemic area of a canine heart and noted that it dropped quickly to near zero after coronary ligation. Administration of 100% oxygen to the animal did not alter the oxygen tension in the central area although the PO_2 increased significantly in border zones and remote normal areas. These results also helped to explain the decreased ventricular fibrillation threshold known to occur in the ischemic area.[32]

These myocardial contraction abnormalities and difficulties with oxygen delivery must occur because of ineffective myocardial perfusion, and to this extent Wiggers[13–15] was correct. However, although coronary collaterals may be inadequate immediately following coronary occlusion, this observation does not disprove some functional significance either at the time of occlusion or subsequently. Many investigators have obtained data to support the conclusion that coronary collateral vessels play an important role in attenuating or even abolishing myocardial ischemia. Evidence that collaterals improve survival, preserve function, and diminish necrosis following coronary occlusion supports the impetus to learn to control or at least modify the collateral circulation to effect an increase in its salutary role in ischemic heart disease.

II. Animal Survival Following Abrupt Coronary Ligation

Survival of animals following coronary ligation has been successfully correlated with the extent of collateral development. Abrupt coronary ligation in pigs, which normally have very poor natural coronary collaterals,[33] is nearly always fatal with close to a 100% immediate mortality.[34-38] On the other hand, 56 to 71% of dogs, with their relative abundance of coronary collateral vessels,[33] survive acute coronary occlusion for at least eight hours.[39] Support of the conclusion that the adequacy of the collateral circulation, and not other species differences, accounts for the changing survival rates in pigs and dogs was obtained by further analysis of those animals that died and those surviving after coronary occlusion. Several studies designed to evaluate factors influencing mortality in the initial hours following coronary ligation have used postmortem angiography to assess the adequacy of the collateral circulation.[39-43] Injection of the patent coronary arteries with a barium-sulphate-gelatin mass 24 hours after the animal's death or sacrifice results in retrograde filling of the occluded vessel. The magnitude of this retrograde opacification in the ischemic area has been equated with the adequacy of the coronary collateral circulation. Thus, left circumflex occlusion in all 19 and left anterior descending obstruction in five of nine dogs without collaterals produced fibrillation in less than 30 minutes.[43] Conversely, all animals with left anterior descending ligation and good collaterals lived for 30 minutes, while 27 of 28 dogs with good collaterals and left circumflex occlusion survived. Identical results were apparent when the observation interval was prolonged to eight[39] and twelve[41,42] hours.

As noted, the meager coronary collateral circulation of the domestic pig puts this animal at great risk for sudden death following coronary occlusion. Blumgart and his associates[34-37] studied the effects of initial narrowing of a coronary artery in the pig before total occlusion. By tying a ligature around the coronary vessel and an interposed wire or 0.8-mm probe and then removing the latter, the coronary artery was effectively narrowed by 75 to 85%. Whereas abrupt occlusion or vessel narrowing in excess of 87% produced predictable ventricular fibrillation or standstill, 5 of 12 pigs with occlusion after more than 12 days of narrowing survived. The collateral circulation was studied by selectively injecting lead-agar mass into the coronary arteries.

Only 3 of 161 normal pigs had some form of visible collateralization, and in two of these only fine twigs were observed. Pigs that survived less than two days had no further evidence of collateralization, but 77% of pigs sacrificed between 2 and 29 days had collaterals. Of the 12 pigs that survived for more than 12 days with a narrowed coronary vessel, nine had a rich collateral network. Five of these nine survived sudden superimposed total occlusion of the stenotic vessel.

Lumb et al.[38] studied pigs with either acute right coronary artery ligation or gradual occlusion with an ameroid constrictor. They again noted that there were no survivors in the former group. But some of the pigs with slow occlusion did survive, and the survival rate increased as the occlusion was more gradual. Presumably, the longer interval to total obstruction permitted increased collateral development. Thus, these results extend those of Blumgart and colleagues.[34–37]

Robertson,[44] and later Hahn and Beck,[45] attempted to ligate proximally the three major coronary arteries of dogs. The ligations were performed in stages. There were some survivors even after all three vessels were ligated. Although not demonstrated by the investigators, it may be presumed that collaterals from the first septal branch and extracoronary vascular anastomoses through adhesions permitted continued myocardial function. Nonetheless, the inescapable conclusion is that collaterals were responsible for survival in these animals.

III. Ventricular Fibrillation Following Coronary Ligation

It would appear, then, that there is a definite relationship between survival following coronary occlusion and the extent of prior coronary collateral development. Because ventricular fibrillation is usually the direct cause of death in animals after coronary obstruction, the relationship between ventricular fibrillation threshold and presence of coronary collaterals has also been examined. Current delivered during early diastole through an electrode inserted into normal myocardium can induce ventricular fibrillation. If the myocardium is ischemic, it is well known that the minimal current required to produce ventricular fibrillation is less.[32] The lowered fibrillation threshold implies that ischemic myocardium is easier to fibrillate than normal tissue. In dogs with ligation of either the left circumflex[46] or left anterior descending[43] coronary artery, the fall in fibrillation threshold was observed to be directly dependent on the degree of collateralization. Thus, in dogs with minimal evidence of coronary collaterals evaluated by retrograde filling of the occluded coronary vessel during postmortem angiography, ligation of the left circumflex artery lowered the threshold from 28 to 4.3 mA, whereas in those animals with prominent collaterals, the fall was only from 24.8 to 14.1 mA, significantly higher ($p < 0.001$) than in the first group. Meesmann and colleagues[47−49] examined the time course of change in the ventricular fibrillation threshold in these animals. They documented decreases in the threshold at approximately four to eight minutes after ligation. After several additional minutes the threshold gradually increased and was near normal by 30 minutes. However, the threshold fell more in dogs with no or poor collaterals (from 16.5 to 5.0 mA in dogs with poor collaterals and from 18.0 to 13.5 mA in those with good collaterals, $p < 0.01$). Furthermore, the nadir of the decrease in the threshold occurred later in those animals with good collateral vessels. Garza et al.[50] also documented a fall in ventricular fibrillation threshold following coronary artery occlusion in dogs, and noted that the magnitude of the decrease was inversely proportional to the anastomotic index, a determination using collateral counts from histologic sections (see Chapter 4). However, these investigators did not observe return of the ventricular fibrillation threshold to normal until two to four weeks later after substantial increases in the anastomotic index.

IV. Myocardial Infarct Size and Region at Risk

Coronary occlusion results in cessation of antegrade flow through the obstructed vessel. But as already described for survival rates and ventricular fibrillation threshold, the consequences of the occlusion to the myocardium and the organism are favorably modified by the collateral circulation. Myocardial infarction occurs when the cell's chemical reactions and transport mechanisms are no longer able to maintain cellular integrity. This happens when oxygen delivery is inadequate and supply of high-energy phosphate compounds is insufficient. However, myocardial infarction is not a necessary outcome of coronary occlusion. Studies have demonstrated that even abrupt coronary obstruction may result in no myocardial damage or only a small scar,[26,51,52] although many more reports have made a distinction between abrupt coronary ligation and progressive obstruction with either an ameroid constrictor or mechanical occlusive device.[35,52−68] While acute ligation may produce a large infarct, slower occlusion is often not accompanied by myocardial necrosis. The effect of delayed occlusion on infarct size is readily appreciated in dogs,[52−55,59−68] but the results are more dramatic in pigs, which, as described above, have initially poor coronary collateral circulations[33] and very high mortality rates following acute coronary ligation.[34−38] Although progression of stenosis of a porcine coronary artery to total occlusion over six to seven days results in myocardial infarction in all animals that survive more than two days,[57] the coronary collateral circulation shows evidence of significant development over the initial two to three weeks. If the coronary artery is first narrowed by 75 to 85% for at least 12 days prior to complete occlusion, then no infarct is produced and postmortem radiographic study demonstrates an abundant collateral circulation.[35] Ramo et al.[58] compared the effects of gradual occlusion of the left anterior descending and right coronary arteries in pigs. Right coronary artery occlusion produced faster and more extensive collateral development. Although all pigs had evidence of myocardial necrosis, only 42% of those with right coronary artery obstruction had transmural infarcts, whereas all infarcts in the group with left anterior decending artery occlusion extended from endo- to epicardium. Schaper et al.[56] compared the infarcts of collateral-rich dogs and collateral-poor pigs caused by gradual coronary occlusion. Only 21% of the dogs had evidence of necrosis, and the infarcts were small and nontransmural, whereas 44% of the surviving pigs had large infarcts that were transmural.

Wilson and Scheel[68] quantitated the volume of infarcted myocardium after either abrupt circumflex ligation or gradual occlusion with an ameroid constrictor in dogs. In both groups of dogs the occlusions were proximal to all circumflex branches. Sudden ligation of the coronary vessel produced infarcts averaging 15.6% of the left ventricular volume, and all dogs had evidence of myocardial necrosis. In contrast, only 2 to 3% of the left ventricle was infarcted in dogs with gradual occlusion of the circumflex artery ($p < 0.001$), and 24% of the animals had no histologic evidence of infarction.

Although the above studies were done with external compression of the coronary arteries, similar conclusions have been made for endogenous obstruction. Thus, the narrowing of coronary arteries induced by feeding cholesterol to rabbits was also associated with development of increased myocardial vascularity, presumably collaterals, and minimal scarring.[69]

The protection from a delayed occlusion may be seen with as little as a five- to ten-hour interval between stenosis and occlusion. Cohen and Eldh[63] studied a series of dogs after embolizing hollow or solid plugs down the left anterior descending coronary artery in a closed-chest preparation. The solid plugs created immediate total occlusion of the vessel, whereas the hollow plugs created a narrowing of the vessel lumen that became progressively more severe as thrombus filled the plug. Complete occlusion in these latter animals occurred within five to ten hours of embolization. Two to four weeks after the occlusion survivors were sacrificed and the extent of infarction measured from photographs of several transverse sections. Hollow plugs produced average infarct sizes of only 4% of the left ventricular cross-sectional area with half of the animals having no grossly detectable necrosis, while solid plugs caused infarction of 20% of the left ventricle. The only apparent difference between the groups was the initial period during which the hollow plugs were slowly becoming occluded, an interval permitting collateral stretching and delivery of maximal blood supply to the ischemic tissue prior to complete cessation of antegrade flow.

Schaper and his co-workers[70] produced chronic stenosis of the left circumflex coronary artery in dogs by implanting a Teflon ring around the vessel which reduced the peak reactive hyperemic flow response following a transient occlusion by 50%. Six weeks following this operation a branch of the stenotic vessel within the risk region and a second branch beyond the perfusion territory of the narrowed vessel were occluded. The ensuing infarct six hours after occlusion was considerably smaller in the distribution of the stenotic vessel (19% versus 52% of risk region). Therefore, the presence of a critical stenosis and delay before coronary occlusion result in myocardial salvage. Again, it is postulated that collateral development accounts for the effect on infarct size. In a subsequent study using a similar protocol, Schaper[71] ligated the left circumflex artery of 17 dogs after five weeks of stenosis. Eleven dogs had large infarcts averaging 44.1% of the left circumflex risk area. In each of these dogs collateral flow prior to coronary stenosis was poor and there was no increase during the five-week period of stenosis (from 0.12 to 0.15 ml/min/g). In contrast, the other six dogs had no evidence of infarction. Collateral flow increased from 0.22 to 1.02 ml/min/g ($p < 0.05$) after five weeks of left circumflex stenosis. The significant collateral development, thus, prevented infarction.

The dependence of the extent of necrosis on collateral flow is further demonstrated by investigations of Koke and Bittar.[72] They created ischemia in a canine model by either conventional coronary ligation or ligating a diagonal branch and then virtually severing a transmural piece of myocardium in its distribution to eliminate possible collateral flow and then suturing it back into place. Collateral flow and ultrastructural evidence of myocardial damage in the two groups of dogs were evaluated in the distribution of the ligated vessel and the isolated segment. In the isolated segment where virtually no collateral flow was evident, uniform glycogen depletion, prominent intracellular edema, and severe morphologic abnormalities of the mitochondria were apparent. These changes were much less evident in the animals with conventional ischemic areas caused by simple coronary ligation where collateral flows were 20 to 40 times greater.

Coronary occlusion deprives myocardium of antegrade perfusion and jeopardizes the structural integrity of the tissue. By supplying an alternate source of blood, the coronary collateral circulation may modify the extent and severity of the potential infarction. The ability of collaterals to modify or attenuate infarction is perhaps underscored by the observation that the infarct developing after coronary occlusion is generally far smaller than the perfusion territory of the involved vessel. The vascular distribution of a vessel should represent the area of potentially jeopardized myocardium following obstruction of that vessel. This risk region should therefore also represent the largest possible infarct size, although as noted in Chapter 5, some investigators have attempted to show that reflex vasoconstriction of adjacent vessels following coronary ligation results in infarcts larger than the primary risk region.[73–79] Hirsch and Spalteholz[80] first reported a discrepancy between infarct size and apparent risk region, and their observation has been confirmed many times. Prinzmetal also noted that the area of cyanosis[10] or bulging myocardium[20] following abrupt coronary ligation was typically smaller than the vessel's perfusion area.

These visual or qualitative estimates of the disproportion between areas of ischemia or infarction and vascular perfusion territory have been supported by quantitative measurements. Schaper et al.[81] ligated the proximal left anterior descending coronary artery of mongrel dogs and sacrificed the animals 16 hours later. The hearts of 45 dogs were serially sectioned from apex to base, and the slices incubated in 2,3,5-triphenyl tetrazolium chloride (TTC). TTC interacts with dehydrogenase enzymes of viable myocardium producing a formazan pigment which stains normal tissue dark red. The ischemic or infarcted myocardium remains pale. After this incubation the slices were put in formaldehyde solution, and then the ischemic area was excised and weighed. The ischemic tissue averaged 11.2 ± 4.1% of the heart's fresh weight. In an additional 46 hearts the occluded vessel was cannulated at the site of the ligature and perfused with formaldehyde solution while the remaining coronary arteries were perfused with Ringer's solution containing a blue dye. The hardened, unstained tissue representing the risk region was excised and weighed, and averaged 20.1 ± 5.3% of the heart's fresh weight. Thus, in these dogs approximately 55% of the area at risk was infarcted.

It is easy to object to Schaper's study[81] because the coronary risk region and infarct size were not determined in the same hearts. Various protocols have since been designed to relate the area or volume of ischemic and/or infarcted myocardium to the risk region in the same animal. The vascular perfusion territory has usually been defined by either intravascular injection of Evans blue with staining of the perfused tissue or postmortem angiography, and the ischemic area identified by either histologic techniques or staining with nitroblue tetrazolium chloride (similar to TTC). Large coronary artery occlusions in the dog thus result in ischemia and/or infarction of from 23 to 79% of the defined region at risk[5,7,82−91] with an average of approximately 47% and a median of 36.6−44.3%. Ligation of smaller branches produces infarction of as little as 14% of the vessel's perfusion territory.[83] Jugdutt et al.[7,85,88] determined that dogs with sudden left circumflex artery occlusion had no infarction if the left ventricular risk region area was less than 20 g. They also reported that there was a strong correlation between the mass of infarcted myocardium and the size of the risk region[85,88] (Figure 6−1), an observation previously recorded by Lowe et al.[92] If, however, the extent of infarcted tissue was expressed as a percentage of the risk region (Figure 6−2), then it became apparent that in these animals the maximal size of infarction could not exceed 53% of the total risk region.[85] In other words, there was always at least 47% natural salvage of the risk region following coronary occlusion. Vokonas and colleagues[93] ligated a branch of the left circumflex coronary artery, and injected ^{14}C-antipyrine intravenously 24 hours later. After one minute the animals were sacrificed, and the hearts excised and sliced. Macroradioautograms were prepared and the myocardial isotope concentration determined by scanning the film with a densitometer and comparing the results to those obtained with known standards. Thus, the coronary risk region was determined as the total region with decreased isotope uptake, while the extent of abnormal myocardium was quantified histologically. After making several geometric assumptions, these authors concluded that the volume of infarcted myocardium was 40.9% of the entire risk region.

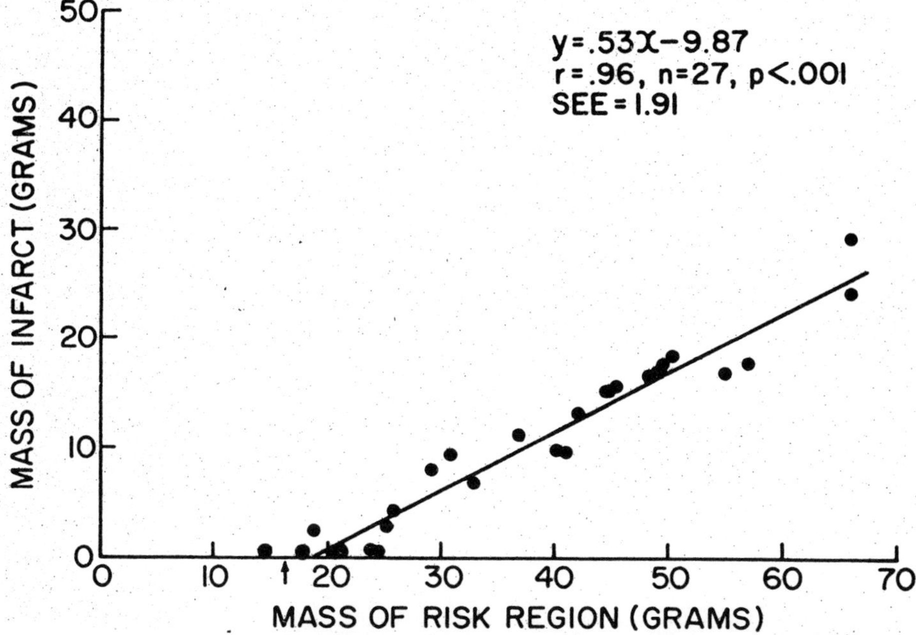

Figure 6–1   Relationship of infarct size to the myocardial mass at risk following ligation of the left circumflex coronary artery in dogs. The risk region is equivalent to the perfusion territory of the occluded vessel. Infarct size was linearly related to the size of the region at risk. The horizontal axis intercept at approximately 18 g suggests no infarct occurs when the nonperfused mass of myocardium beyond the occlusion is smaller than this critical size. The slope of the linear regression equation is less than 1.0, implying that a significant amount of the risk region does not undergo infarction following coronary occlusion. (Reprinted with permission of the American Heart Association from Jugdutt et al.[85])

Schaper and his colleagues[82,84,94] have made additional interesting observations regarding the relationship of the mass of ischemic tissue to the coronary risk region. The left anterior descending coronary artery of dogs was proximally ligated. In some animals the vessel was reperfused after varying periods of time up to six hours. The dogs were then sacrificed after 48 hours. In those animals with reperfusion after 45 minutes, 20% of the risk region was infarcted. Involvement of the risk region increased to 60% if reperfusion was delayed to 90 minutes following coronary ligation. Reperfusion had no effect if delayed for more than four hours, and permanent ligation produced infarction of approximately 75% of the risk region. Identical results have been obtained by Reimer et al.[86] who reperfused the left circumflex bed of dogs after occlusions lasting from 40 minutes to 6 hours.

The discrepancy between size of the myocardial region at risk and ultimate extent of damaged tissue must in some way be related to differential perfusion of various portions of the jeopardized tissue. Bobb et al.[95] attempted to establish the effect of collaterals on infarct size by cauterizing the edges of the distribution area of the left anterior descending coronary artery.

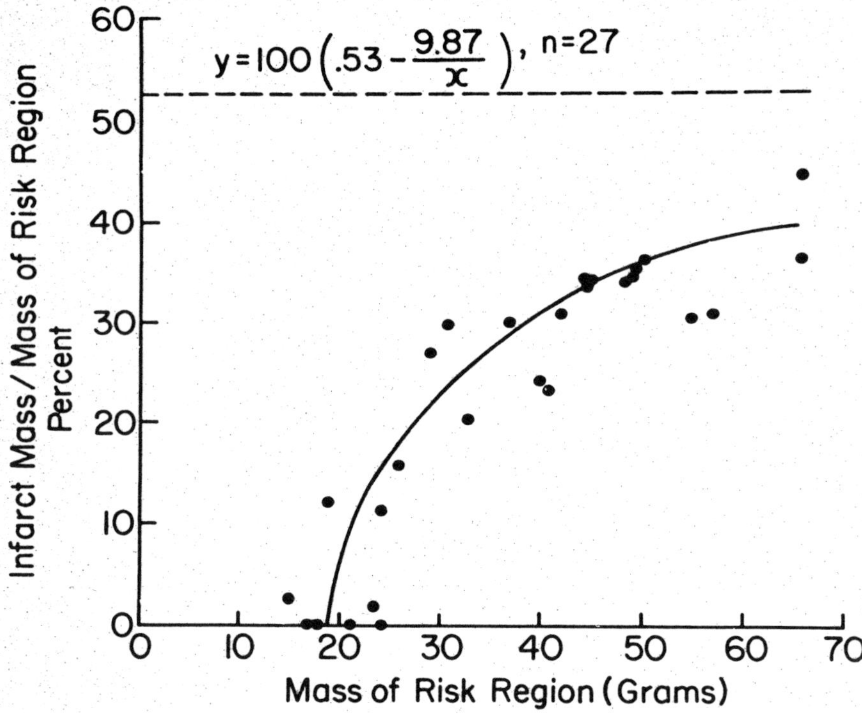

Figure 6–2   Hyperbolic relationship between size of left ventricular region at risk (perfusion territory of occluded vessel) and infarct size normalized for the mass of the risk region. The same experimental data used in Figure 6–1 were replotted to derive this relationship. The equation relating the two variables appears at the top of the figure. The upper limb of the negative hyperbola is asymptotic with a horizontal line through an infarct/risk region value of 53%. Thus, these data suggest that under natural conditions the maximum size of an infarct is 53% of the total risk region. (Reprinted with permission of the American Heart Association from Jugdutt et al.[85])

The epicardial burns were 3–5 mm wide and less than 1 mm deep, and never caused any central infarction in dogs with patent coronary arteries. All dogs surviving the cauterization and associated ligation of the left anterior descending artery for 24 hours developed transmural infarctions extending to the cauterized boundaries. In contrast, of eight dogs with coronary ligation and no cauterization, two had no infarction, four had infarcts significantly smaller than the risk region, and only two had large areas of necrosis. Differences in extent of necrosis between the two groups with coronary ligation prompted the authors to suggest that epicardial collaterals were an important determinant of infarct size. Although logical, this assumption that epicardial collaterals were the important factor in minimizing the consequences of coronary occlusion was never directly proven.

More recent investigations have clearly demonstrated an inverse correlation between collateral blood flow and infarct size following coronary occlusion. In one study,[96] the left anterior descending coronary artery of closed-chest dogs was embolized with fluoroscopically placed plugs.[63] Vessel occlusion in the middle third was confirmed by coronary angiography. Myocardial blood flow immediately following occlusion was measured with radioactive microspheres. The animals were permitted to recover and were sacrificed one week later. The hearts were removed and sectioned from apex to base, and the size of the visible infarct measured by planimetry from photographs of the fresh specimens. Blood flows were determined in normal and infarcted endocardial and epicardial halves, and ratios of abnormal to normal endocardial and epicardial perfusion rates calculated. Infarct size ranged from 0 to 32% of the left ventricular cross-sectional area. Myocardial necrosis was observed only when endocardial blood flow was reduced below approximately 50%. Below this flow level there was a significant reciprocal linear relationship ($r = 0.80$) between total infarct size normalized for left ventricular mass and normalized endocardial flow distal to the plug measured immediately after occlusion (Figure 6−3). A significant reciprocal relationship ($r = 0.86$) between infarct size and normalized epicardial flow was also apparent (Figure 6−4). The conclusion that collateral blood flow at the time of coronary obstruction directly affected the extent of myocardial infarction, and hence the degree of myocardial salvage, seemed evident.

Additional detailed studies have confirmed these results. Inverse linear relationships exist between collateral blood flow to the ischemic and/or infarcted tissue and infarct size whether expressed as a fraction of the total left ventricular mass[4,7,97] or of the myocardial region at risk.[5,7,90] Investigators have also measured collateral blood flow and quantitated the extent of necrosis by histologic techniques in the same transmural wedge of myocardium excised from the risk region.[27,29,85,86,98] Excellent inverse correlations between blood flow and extent of necrosis were again confirmed. Some studies have found better correlations between collateral blood flow and extent of infarction when only endocardial[4,90] or epicardial [86] collateral flow had been analyzed, although Jugdutt[85] and Cohen[96] found significant correlations in both endocardial and epicardial layers. These studies prove that collateral flows measured less than 20[5,7,27,29,85,86,97,98] and even less than five[5,27,85,97] minutes following coronary occlusion are predictive of the amount of eventual necrosis. Flows determined as late as 24 to 96 hours after cessation of antegrade perfusion are also highly correlated with the amount of myocardial necrosis and can predict the subsequent outcome.[4,5,27,29,85,90] The inverse relationship is still apparent after reperfusion of the occluded vessel.[97,99]

These data inversely correlating residual collateral flow and infarct size are consistent with the results reported by Koyanagi[89] on the relationship between size of infarction and different risk areas in the same heart. He and his colleagues reported that the ratio of infarct size to risk area for the entire left ventricle following left circumflex occlusion in dogs was 36.6%. But within the heart there were identifiable areas at greater or lesser risk. Thus, the average ratio for the endocardium was 50.7%, whereas only 18.8% of the

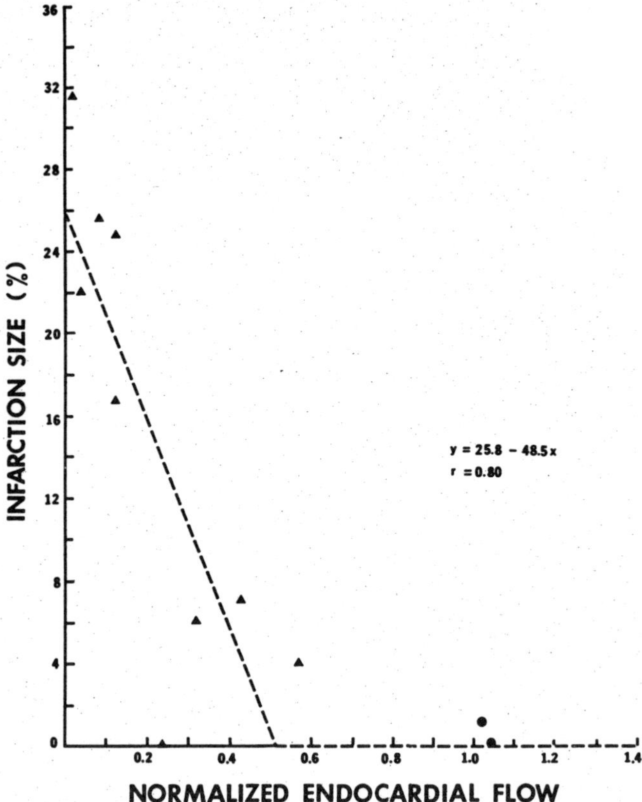

Figure 6–3   Graph of infarct size normalized for left ventricular mass as a function of endocardial flow in the ischemic and/or infarcted tissue measured immediately after occlusion of the left anterior descending coronary artery in dogs. The ischemic endocardial flows have been normalized for simultaneously measured flows in normal tissue. Infarction occurred only when the endocardial flow fell to less than 50% of normal values. Below this critical level there was a linear reciprocal relationship between infarct size and endocardial flow in these animals ($r = 0.80$).

epicardium at risk infarcted. Schaper and his colleagues[82,84] have reported very similar observations. As noted in Chapter 5, endocardial flows following coronary occlusion are typically much less than epicardial flows. It is not surprising that more jeopardized endocardium will infarct than epicardium. Papillary muscles with their single central artery generally have very poor collateral circulation and hence low flow after cessation of normal antegrade flow. For papillary muscles the infarct size/risk area ratio averaged 74.0%.[89]

In Koyanagi's dogs[89] myocardial perfusion five minutes after coronary occlusion fell by an average of 86% in those areas going on to infarct, while the decrease was only 34% in that portion of the area at risk in which infarction

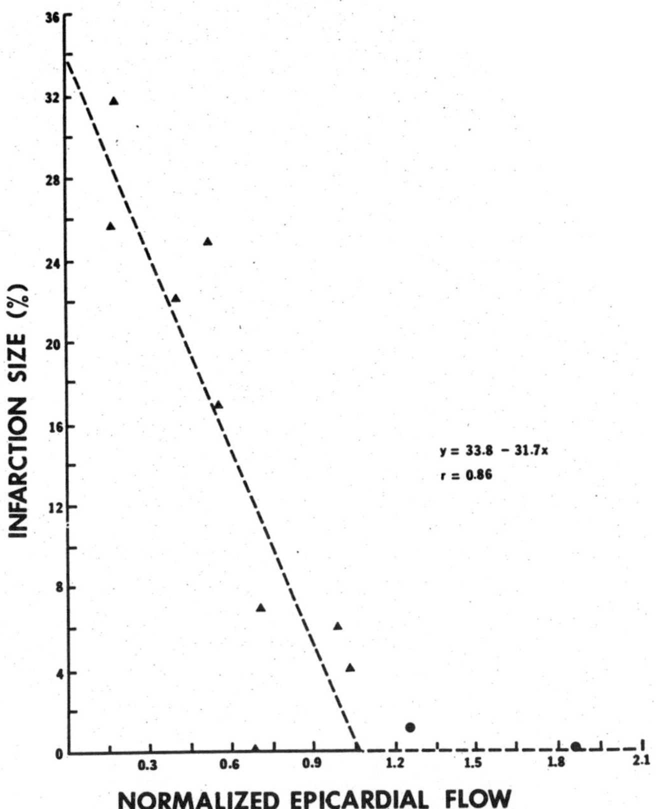

Figure 6−4   Graph of infarct size normalized for left ventricular mass as a function of epicardial flow in the ischemic and/or infarcted tissue measured immediately after occlusion of the left anterior descending coronary artery in dogs. The ischemic epicardial flows have been normalized for simultaneously measured flows in normal tissue. There is a linear reciprocal relationship between infarct size and epicardial flow ($r = 0.86$). However, because changes in epicardial flow usually lag behind changes in endocardial flow in ischemic tissue, the relationship between endocardial flow and infarct size depicted in Figure 6−3 probably has greater physiologic significance (see text).

did not occur. This study[89] as well as that of Jugdutt et al.[7] and the preliminary investigation of Glogar et al.[87] have identified critical levels of collateral or coronary flow in dogs which result in total sparing of myocardium after coronary occlusion. Thus, early collateral flow in areas eventually demonstrating infarction was always less than 0.3−0.4 ml/min/g. Conversely, spared regions always had flows exceeding 0.5 ml/min/g. These absolute flow levels are comparable to the critical 50% endocardial flow reduction necessary for infarction noted previously by Cohen et al. (Figure 6−3).[96] Of interest was Cohen's observation that infarction was apparent with any reduction in epicardial flow (Figure 6−4). Coronary stenosis causes endocardial flow to fall before epicardial flow, and infarction begins to appear when endocardial perfusion declines to 50% of normal. When epicardial flow starts to decrease, endocardial flow is already at or near critical levels. The amount of infarcted myocardium that results is therefore more a reflection of the endocardial rather than the epicardial flow deficit.

Kirk and his co-workers[100,101] have used creatine phosphokinase (CPK), an enzyme contained in myocardial cells, as a marker of tissue damage. CPK leaks out of damaged cells with leaky membranes, and therefore enzyme depletion is a measure of the extent of loss of myocardial cellular integrity. There was an inverse correlation between the collateral blood flow in the central ischemic area measured at ten minutes and the degree of CPK depletion at 24 hours ($r = 0.90$).

It is apparent that the extent of collateral circulation existing at the time of coronary occlusion is a major determinant of the size of the ensuing infarct. This evidence serves to document the functional importance of the collateral circulation and gives direction to those who seek to develop techniques and/or pharmacologic agents to limit the extent of myocardial necrosis in the clinical arena. It must be emphasized, however, that these studies demonstrate the benefits and functional significance of only the collateral circulation existent at the time of coronary occlusion. One may not extrapolate from these observations and assume that collaterals undergoing the expected histologic transformation following chronic coronary occlusion have increased functional value. Perhaps they are only biological markers of the coronary occlusive process.

V. Electrocardiographic Changes Following Coronary Occlusion

Mortality, ventricular fibrillation, and myocardial infarction are dramatic end-points of the ischemic process initiated by coronary obstruction. Although coronary collaterals appear to decrease mortality, limit the fall in ventricular fibrillation threshold, and minimize the extent of myocardial infarction, their effect is also evident in the earliest stages of myocardial ischemia. ST-segment shifts and changes in QRS morphology appear within minutes, and sometimes within seconds, of coronary occlusion. These changes are easily recorded from standard limb and precordial leads in closed-chest animals, and from the epicardial surface in those animals with exposed hearts. These electrocardiographic abnormalities reflect changes in ionic currents and are initially reversible if coronary perfusion is resumed shortly after its interruption. Meesmann and his colleagues[46,102−108] have documented that dogs with good coronary collaterals have less ST-segment elevation than those animals with poor or minimal coronary collateral development. In these investigations the coronary collateral circulation was evaluated with postmortem coronary angiography, and the degree of retrograde opacification of the occluded vessel considered to be an index of collateral flow. In addition to the lesser degree of ST-segment elevation following left circumflex coronary artery ligation in dogs with well-developed collaterals, there were also fewer QRS abnormalities.[103] Thus, in more than 50% of dogs with good collaterals, the QRS remained normal, while in the remainder the changes were minimal and appeared late. The ratio of ST-segment elevation to R-wave amplitude was also significantly less in those animals with prominent collaterals.[102] The ratio of QRS duration before and after coronary ligation was 2.33 in animals with minimal evidence of collaterals and 1.15 in those with a prominent collateral circulation.[102] Furthermore, in 15 of the 28 dogs with good collaterals, left circumflex ligation resulted in no QRS prolongation (ratio 1.0).[102]

Epicardial ST-segment mapping has been used to quantitate the magnitude of ischemia in experimental animals. Various interventions have been employed to affect myocardial ischemia by altering myocardial oxygen consumption and therefore the relationship between myocardial oxygen supply and demand. Right atrial pacing directly increases oxygen consumption of the heart and limits the time available for diastolic perfusion of the coronary vessels, while vagal stimulation has opposite effects. Practolol, a negative inotropic agent, depresses the rate of rise of left ventricular pressure during isovolumic contraction (dP/dt), and thus reduces myocardial oxygen consumption. Although these interventions had qualitatively similar effects on dogs with either good or poor collaterals following ligation of the left anterior descending coronary artery, i.e., increased ischemia and ST-segment elevation during pacing and decreased ischemia and ST-elevation during practolol infusion, ST-segment elevation at any given level of myocardial oxygen consumption was greater in those animals with a poorly developed collateral circulation.[104−108] Thus, despite conditions requiring the same oxygen demand and utilization in dogs with good and poor collaterals, the greater substrate availability in the animals with prominent collaterals minimized the resulting myocardial ischemia. Alternatively, myocardial ischemia was comparable in the two groups of dogs only when oxygen demand was higher in the dogs with good collaterals.

Eckstein[109] compared the electrocardiographic changes in pigs and dogs following coronary artery ligation. As discussed in Chapter 4, the collateral circulation in pigs is much more meager than that in dogs. Eckstein quantitated retrograde flow in pigs as 0.3 − 0.6 ml/min, whereas the range was 0.4 − 17.1 ml/min in dogs.[109] Eight of nine pigs with acute coronary ligation had marked ST-segment abnormalities. There was no evidence in these animals of passage into other coronary territories of a barium sulphate suspension injected into the left anterior descending coronary artery at a pressure of 100 mmHg. In contrast, 11 of 25 dogs with similar abrupt coronary occlusion had minimal or no electrocardiographic changes, and the barium suspension appeared in adjacent left circumflex branches.

Janse and Wilms-Schopman[110] have recently reported similar observations. They studied isolated, perfused dog and pig hearts with coronary occlusions by recording extracellular electrograms from the left ventricular epicardium. The effects of changing perfusion pressure to the nonoccluded arteries on the electrophysiologic border where the TQ-segment potentials became negative were observed. In dogs with abundant epicardial collaterals, the border shifted outward (more abnormal myocardium) when the perfusion pressure was decreased and inward (less abnormal myocardium) when the pressure was increased. On the other hand, pigs with sparse collaterals had no change in the electrophysiologic border as perfusion pressure was varied. Thus, changes in perfusion pressure could enlarge or reduce the area of ischemic myocardium only in animals with collateral flow that could be altered. Increased perfusion pressure was unable to spare myocardium in the pig with negligible preexisting collaterals.

In a further attempt to document the salutary effect of collaterals on ischemic electrocardiographic manifestations, Eckstein[111] bled dogs until the hemoglobin concentration was 15 to 30% of normal, and maintained this level of anemia in the dogs for four weeks. At the end of this period, he acutely transfused the animals to restore the normal hemoglobin level. These animals had an average retrograde flow of 9.6 ml/min, nearly triple the rate of control animals. After clamping the left circumflex artery, only 23% of the experimental group developed severe electrocardiographic abnormalities, in contrast to 70% of the control group.

Katada et al.[112] recorded intramyocardial electrograms three to twelve weeks after implantation of ameroid constrictors around the left anterior descending coronary artery in dogs. There was no evidence of ST-segment shifts at rest. During right atrial pacing, 6 of the 15 animals studied demonstrated ST-segment elevation. However, the remaining nine dogs had normal electrograms. These latter animals developed ST-segment elevation during atrial pacing only after the left circumflex artery had also been narrowed by 50 to 85%. The group of nine dogs with ST-segment elevation only during combined right atrial pacing and left circumflex stenosis had higher retrograde flows from the distal left anterior descending artery ($p < 0.02$), and higher ratios of peripheral coronary pressure to aortic pressure ($p < 0.02$) than the other group of six dogs. Thus, coronary collaterals attenuated the electrographic evidence of myocardial ischemia.

VI. Reactive Hyperemia during Coronary Stenosis and Occlusion

Reactive hyperemia, or increased blood flow to ischemic myocardium following release of a temporary coronary occlusion, is normally considered a measure of coronary reserve. For the few seconds after release when the flow is greatest, the arterioles are maximally dilated. In the presence of a coronary stenosis the distal vasculature dilates to compensate for the pressure drop across the vessel narrowing, and the reactive hypermic response during a superimposed arterial occlusion declines.[113] As the stenosis nears total occlusion, the coronary resistance vessels become maximally dilated. Temporary occlusion of the stenotic vessel cannot therefore induce additional dilatation. Consequently there is no increase in flow when the occlusion is released, and reactive hyperemia is abolished. Thus, abolition of reactive hyperemia is related to the presence of myocardial ischemia. Under certain conditions, however, the absence of reactive hyperemia may signify lack of ischemia. Reperfusion or restoration of antegrade flow following an interval of coronary occlusion might not be associated with a hyperemic response if the myocardium was not formerly ischemic, but was instead adequately perfused by collaterals. Absence or attenuation of ischemia in spite of the coronary occlusion would not necessitate maximal compensatory dilatation of the resistance vessels. Consequently, the hyperemic response following resumption of normal antegrade flow would also be less than maximal, and in fact might be negligible.

Khouri et al.[61] gradually occluded the left circumflex artery of dogs over three to twelve days, and then released the occlusion after a period ranging from one to six days. Following resumption of antegrade perfusion, the left circumflex coronary flow quickly increased to normal levels and there was no reactive hyperemia. The reactive hyperemic response to transient coronary reocclusion slowly returned over a two-minute interval following resumption of antegrade flow, implying gradually less dependence on collateral flow from the left anterior descending artery. Despite the short time allowed for collateral development during vessel occlusion, there was sufficient collateral flow under resting conditions immediately after deflation of the occluding balloon to minimize myocardial ischemia and the reactive hyperemic response. Oldham and colleagues[114] used ameroid constrictors to occlude the left circumflex artery of dogs, and six weeks later attached a venous graft between the aorta and coronary artery distal to the obstruction. Graft flow in these animals with well-formed collateral vessels was only 16 ml/min compared to a flow of 65 ml/min when grafts were anastomosed distal to acute occlusions in control animals. Furthermore, in nine of ten dogs with chronic left circumflex obstruction, release of a transient occlusion of the venous graft was not associated with any reactive hyperemic response. As in Khouri's experiments,[61] these observations suggest the collateral circulation was able to supply the myocardium adequately.

The experiments of Tomoike et al.[115] in chronically instrumented animals further emphasize this latter point. Ameroid constrictors on the left circumflex artery gradually occluded the vessel over a two- to three-week period. The reactive hyperemic response during this period of progressing stenosis was sequentially examined by transiently inflating a hydraulic occluder and totally occluding the left circumflex vessel for one minute. On the fourth day after implantation of the constrictor the reactive hyperemic response was 300 ± 12%. The flow response diminished to 201 ± 44% on the eighth day and 88 ± 37% on the 15th day. By the 22d day the one-minute inflation and then deflation of the hydraulic occluder produced no reactive hyperemic response. Before these changes are simply attributed to collateral development, it must be pointed out that in these experiments, in contrast to those of Khouri[61] and Oldham,[114] the reactive hyperemic response of an increasingly stenotic vessel was being determined. Therefore, disappearance of the reactive hyperemia could in part have been related to gradual dilatation of the resistance arterioles as compensation for the ischemia-generating proximal stenosis,[113] and collateral development may not have been involved. But the progressive lessening of deterioration of regional myocardial function during test coronary occlusions over the same three-week period confirms the initial impression that collateral development was occurring during this time interval. Hence, absence of reactive hyperemia in all of these experiments and therefore of metabolically induced vasodilatation of the coronary arterioles implies that ischemia was not present when the coronary artery was occluded or made stenotic, and that the collateral circulation played a functionally important role.

VII. Myocardial Fiber Shortening and Regional Left Ventricular Function Following Coronary Occlusion

Perhaps the most direct consequence of myocardial perfusion is contraction of muscle fibers. In the early investigations of the effects of coronary collaterals, Tennant and Wiggers[16] and Wiggers and Green[17] emphasized that contraction of myocardium was the best index of collateral flow. They advocated the use of myocardial strain gauges sewn directly to the epicardium for accurate and reliable assessment of collateral capacity and adequacy. More recent studies using epicardial length gauges or intramyocardial ultrasonic crystals have clearly demonstrated a direct relationship between coronary blood flow and regional myocardial function in both dogs[27,116,117] and pigs.[28] Therefore, elimination of antegrade flow would be expected to depress segmental function severely. Preservation of function or later improvement would then be a direct consequence of myocardial perfusion through coronary collaterals. Global cardiac function in the resting animal is not usually affected until regional blood flow is severely depressed,[28] and therefore cannot often be used to evaluate the adequacy of myocardial perfusion. However, global left ventricular function of the exercising animal has proved to be an adequate index of coronary collateral flow.[8,9] The significant increases in metabolic demand and myocardial oxygen consumption accompanying the exercise state result in a need for increased coronary flow and therefore tax the circulation with already limited reserve. Stress-induced exhaustion of coronary reserve may result in inadequate increases in flow, and thus the effects of even small deficiencies in resting myocardial flow will be magnified. If the involved myocardial area is sufficiently large, the altered contractile state induced by the limited perfusion will in turn affect the pumping qualities of the entire left ventricle.

Abrupt coronary occlusion results in cyanosis, paradoxical bulging, and thinning of the myocardium in the distribution of the obstructed vessel.[14,16-23,26-30,116-118] Despite this weight of evidence, several studies have documented persistence of effective, albeit diminished, regional contraction following coronary occlusion,[27,119,120] thereby establishing the effectiveness of collateral function at even this early time. Furthermore, any abnormal contraction pattern appearing after acute coronary occlusion does not persist. Numerous studies in experimental animals (dogs and pigs) with gradual coronary occlusions created by either ameroid constrictors, screw clamps, or plugs embolized into selected coronary arteries have demonstrated return of regional contraction and even complete normalization of the contractile pattern of the myocardium previously perfused by the occluded vessel.[19,20,22,26,54,115,121-128] Tomoike et al.[115] instrumented dogs with ameroid constrictors, hydraulic occluders, and myocardial ultrasonic crystals to evaluate segmental contractile function during superimposed abrupt transient occlusion of the left circumflex coronary artery as it was becoming critically narrowed and then permanently occluded by swelling of the hygroscopic material. Systolic shortening of myocardial fibers in the left circumflex distribution was only $9 \pm 6\%$ of control when the vessel was occluded on the fourth day after ameroid implantation. However, function was improved by the eighth day when shortening was $24 \pm 11\%$ of control during balloon inflation. The improvement was progressive and systolic shortening was $45 \pm 16\%$ of control by day 15. On the 22d day following implantation, inflation of the hydraulic occluder elicited no change in systolic function. Thus, at this time complete loss of antegrade coronary flow had no effect on myocardial contractile function, which was presumably preserved by collateral development occurring during the slowly progressive vessel obstruction. The nearly identical protocol of Hill et al.[127] produced very similar conclusions. During the three-week period of gradual occlusion of the left circumflex artery by the ameroid constrictor, transient inflation of a pneumatic snare produced diminishing deterioration of systolic function of the circumflex perfusion territory as the interval between implantation and testing lengthened. Finally after total arterial occlusion by the ameroid constrictor, there was no discernible defect in resting regional myocardial function. Serial measurements of collateral blood flow at the same intervals as determination of regional myocardial shortening during balloon inflation also revealed diminishing flow deficit and increasing transmural flow homogeneity as the time following implantation increased. Therefore, the direct beneficial effect of collateral blood flow on regional myocardial function was apparent. Similar experiments by Franklin et al.[128] demonstrated normal myocardial fiber systolic shortening after gradual coronary occlusion with an ameroid constrictor. Quantitated collateral blood flow was equivalent to normal tissue perfusion at the time of these functional measurements.

In other experiments, Theroux et al.[26] acutely occluded the left circumflex artery of conscious instrumented dogs and followed segmental myocardial function. Paradoxical bulging was initially observed in all animals. In those dogs without myocardial infarction, resting segmental function recovered completely. However, in the animals with gross infarction, end-diastolic lengths were decreased four weeks after coronary occlusion and shortening was still depressed. There was a positive correlation between the amount of scarring and the persistent abnormalities in this group of dogs. Although Nakhjavan and his colleagues[22] also demonstrated that myocardium distal to critically narrowed or occluded coronary vessels resumed contraction after the development of collateral vessels, characteristics of the systolic function were not entirely normal. The myocardial length-active tension curve for the collateralized region had a flat slope or even a descending limb, while the instantaneous rate of tension development was mildly depressed, implying a diminished contractile state.

Nakamura et al.[123] used serial left ventriculograms to study contraction abnormalities in dogs with coronary occlusions. These investigators constricted the left circumflex artery until the diameter ranged from 1 to 2 mm. Over the course of three to four weeks the stenoses progressed to total occlusions. Despite progression of the coronary lesion wall motion of the posteroinferior wall which was depressed following initial vessel narrowing demonstrated significant improvement.

Hood and colleagues[129] fortuitously documented that coronary collaterals help to preserve left ventricular function. They inflated balloon occluders around either the left anterior descending or left circumflex coronary artery to occlude the vessel. Damage to the balloon tubing in two dogs necessitated release of the occlusion after six days. In these two dogs, subsequent inflation of the occluder around the remaining previously normal major coronary artery produced either no or minimal electrocardiographic or hemodynamic alterations, including measurements of left ventricular pressure and dP/dt. Thus, the collaterals that had already developed during the initial coronary occlusion helped to preserve function of the myocardium perfused by that vessel from which the collaterals had originated. Therefore, blood was able to flow in either direction along the collaterals, and the only important determinant of direction of flow was the pressure gradient itself.

The effect of coronary collaterals on myocardial contraction following abrupt coronary occlusion was examined in dogs that had had a left circumflex ameroid constrictor implanted four to five weeks earlier.[130] In these animals with left circumflex stenosis, acute occlusion of the left anterior descending artery resulted in a 57.6 ± 11.1% decrease in myocardial contractile force measured with epicardial strain gauges in the ischemic region. Deterioration of myocardial function was considerably more marked in control animals without prior left circumflex stenosis and subsequent collateral development. In these dogs, contractile force fell by 93.2 ± 17.2%. Increasing perfusion pressure and flow to the distal left circumflex artery produced with a mechanical pump markedly improved myocardial function in the perfusion territory of the occluded vessel in those animals with additional chronic left circumflex stenosis and collateral development. There was no effect in the control dogs. Postmortem angiography documented few collaterals in the latter dogs and many in the others. Therefore, coronary collaterals were again able partially to preserve myocardial function following cessation of normal antegrade perfusion.

This improvement of myocardial function in the resting animal weeks to months following coronary occlusion is the result of collateral development. Collateral flow shortly after coronary occlusion is often as low as 10 to 30% of flow to normally perfused myocardium. However, several weeks following interruption of antegrade flow, resting myocardial perfusion of the previously ischemic region is again normal.[9,64,66,123,131−146] Measurement of myocardial blood flow with radioactive microspheres during acute coronary occlusion at the time of implantation of an ameroid constrictor in dogs and again six weeks later following chronic occlusion of the vessel permitted Walter et al.[65] to determine minimal collateral resistance before and during the transformation process. Prior to the stimulus for development, collateral resistance after dipyridamole infusion was 6.17 ± 1.28 mmHg/(ml/min)/100g. Six weeks later, after chronic coronary artery occlusion, resistance in the same vascular bed in dogs without evidence of gross infarction had decreased to 0.27 ± 0.04 mmHg/(ml/min)/100g. This marked fall in resistance attests to the magnitude of the histologic transformation of the coronary collaterals, and accounts for restoration of tissue flow. As previously discussed, resting perfusion following chronic occlusion is homogeneous[9] (see Figure 5−5), and it is often not possible to distinguish myocardium perfused by normal coronary arteries from that perfused by collaterals. Furthermore, the endocardial/epicardial flow ratio after chronic coronary artery obstruction is also normal.[9,64,66,131,133,135,137−147] Hence, collateral development results in restoration of blood flow to ischemic myocardium. The renewed source of oxygen and metabolites in turn restores myocardial contractile function. Millard[125] constricted a coronary artery in pigs. The stenosis progressed to become critical as the animals grew from 10 to 30 kg. Hemodynamics and blood flow were measured after eight weeks. At this time collateral flow had increased manyfold from less than 0.05 ml/min/g in acutely ischemic endocardium and epicardium to 0.49 ± 0.05 ml/min/g in the endocardium and 0.85 ± 0.07 ml/min/g in the epicardium. Although not quite back to normal, this remarkable increase in myocardial perfusion was accompanied by normalization of systolic shortening of the myocardial fibers in the distribution of the narrowed vessel.

VIII. Left Ventricular Function during Stress Following Coronary Occlusion

Although collaterals may be responsible for eventual normalization of myocardial flow and function at rest, their functional reserve capacity cannot be inferred from the above observations. Stresses such as exercise and positive inotropic agents increase myocardial oxygen consumption and therefore the need for enhanced myocardial perfusion, vasodilators decrease aortic pressure and therefore the coronary and collateral perfusion pressures, and tachycardia abbreviates diastole and therefore the time available for collateral perfusion. Is collateral development sufficient to maintain normal function and perfusion of collateral-dependent regions under such conditions?

A. Changes in Left Ventricular Volume and Pressure

Volume overloading[122] and increased afterload[122,125] have been observed to produce deterioration of cardiac function in animals with prior coronary occlusions. On the other hand, peak isovolumetric pressure and left ventricular dP/dt following cross-clamping of the aorta before and during norepinephrine infusion were not different in control dogs and those with four-week occlusions of the right and left circumflex coronary arteries.[139] However, measurement of global ventricular function may obscure dysfunction of ischemic myocardium because of compensatory hyperfunction of normal regions. Cohen et al.[121] noted that a modest decrease in coronary perfusion pressure that had little effect on normal muscle significantly diminished regional function of myocardium in the perfusion territory of occluded vessels. It should be noted, however, that in those studies the coronary artery had been occluded for only two and a half to four weeks, and therefore, collateral development was in an early stage.

B. Pacing-Induced Tachycardia

Atrial or ventricular pacing may produce deterioration of regional or segmental function of collateralized myocardium even when resting function is normal.[26,122,126,128] However, the amount of dysfunction is related to the interval between coronary occlusion and subsequent testing. Thus, prompt deterioration of segmental function with holosystolic expansion of the ischemic myocardium is evident when pacing is attempted several hours after coronary occlusion, but one week later the response of the same segments to the induced tachycardia is normal.[26] In the experiments of Kumada et al.[126] ameroid constrictors were placed around the left circumflex artery and ultrasonic crystals were embedded in the myocardium for analysis of segmental contraction. By the 21st postoperative day when the coronary artery was totally occluded, resting function of all segments was normal. Ventricular pacing to rates of appproximately 250 beats/min resulted in deterioration of function of the segments in the left circumflex distribution with decreases in shortening of 42% and wall thickening of 63%. However, by the 29th postoperative day pacing to the same heart rates produced no significant functional alteration. Although myocardial flows were not quantitated, it is reasonable to assume that sufficient collateral development had occurred by the time of the follow-up studies to ensure enough blood flow to maintain normal regional function during the stress of pacing. Franklin's parallel studies[128] demonstrated deterioration of myocardial function during pacing three weeks after implantation of ameroid constrictors, but function was unaffected when pacing was performed more than one month after surgery. Whereas resting blood flow was normal, pacing flows at three weeks revealed abnormal endocardial perfusion with reversal of the left ventricular endo/epi flow ratio. But the normal functional response during pacing beyond one month was accompanied by normal increases in endocardial flow.

Franklin's data[128] suggest a definite relationship between collateral flow and the functional significance of these developing vessels, and a strong influence of the time interval between coronary occlusion and testing. Other investigators have also evaluated the effects of an elevated heart rate on blood flow to ischemic myocardium. In animals with critical coronary stenoses and exhausted coronary reserve, atrial pacing results in smaller increases in flow to the affected myocardium than to normally perfused tissue as well as a fall in the average endocardial/epicardial flow ratio to 0.67 in the abnormal regions.[148] Collateral blood flow is known to be inhibited by myocardial compression occurring during systolic contraction.[149] Because coronary reserve is abolished following coronary occlusion and the proportion of the cardiac cycle occupied by systole increases with increasing heart rate, it is reasonable to expect significant abnormalities of regional and transmural flow during pacing in animals with recent coronary occlusion. Three to four days following proximal left circumflex and mid-left anterior descending coronary occlusions right ventricular pacing which increased heart rate from 110 to 222 beats/min caused subendocardial collateral vascular conductance, which was already abnormal, to diminish further.[90] Vascular conductance to the surviving subepicardium of the ischemic zone was normal at rest and did not change during pacing, an abnormal response. Thus, pacing caused transmural flow to become significantly more heterogeneous. Fedor et al.[143] studied the effects of right ventricular pacing in dogs 11 to 12 weeks after implantation of ameroid constrictors around right and left circumflex coronary arteries. The effects of pacing on blood flow to the collateralized region were dependent on the quality of the collateral response to the stimulus of coronary occlusion. In those animals with deficient collateral formation, total flow to the collateralized area increased normally but the increase was almost entirely in the epicardium. The change in endocardial flow was minimal, accounting for the fall in the endocardial/epicardial flow ratio to 0.56. In the animals with more complete collateral revascularization, endocardial flow in the collateralized myocardium rose during pacing, although the increase was not as great as that in the epicardium. Thus, in these latter animals there was minimal maldistribution of blood flow in the collateralized region. Other studies by Flameng et al.[135] and Pass and colleagues[134] performed approximately two to three months after implantation of ameroid constrictors have yielded inconsistent results. In one study atrial pacing resulted in an absolute decrease in blood flow to the collateralized myocardium,[134] while in the other, blood flow rose and was homogeneously distributed.[135] The ultimate blood flow response depends on the extent of collateral development following coronary occlusion, and it is unreasonable to believe that the collaterals of all dogs have the same ability to develop and transform. Rather, the important lesson must be that function of the postocclusion myocardium must be correlated with the actual flow response in order to determine the true role of the coronary collateral.

C. Exercise

Exercise is a powerful stress of the cardiovascular system and its reserve because of greatly increased metabolic requirements of the organism and marked hemodynamic alterations, including tachycardia. Because of the increased cardiac work, coronary flow normally increases two- to fourfold. Therefore, even subtle defects in vasodilatory reserve would rapidly become evident. Several studies have reported the effects of exercise on segmental function,[115,124,126,127,150] and each has documented appearance of exercise-induced contraction abnormalities in the myocardium beyond the occluded vessel, even when the resting contraction pattern was normal. Kumada and his colleagues[126] demonstrated that exercise uncovered defects in fiber shortening and transmural thickening of the left ventricular wall in those animals in which regional function had been normal during and after pacing. Thus, myocardial flow and reserve in the "ischemic" region were adequate for pacing but not for exercise. Hill[127] also demonstrated that exercise produced marked deterioration of shortening and rate of shortening of ischemic myocardium, as well as striking flow redistribution away from the inner myocardial layers several days after coronary occlusion by implanted ameroid constrictors, even though resting function and flow had been normal or near normal. However, all of these studies[115,124,126,127,150] were performed in animals in which ameroid constrictors had recently produced complete coronary occlusions. Therefore, collaterals were not well developed, and could not have been expected to respond normally to the metabolic stimuli of an exercising heart. But after as few as two weeks of collateral development following coronary occlusion, the flow response to exercise in the ischemic tissue can be much improved.[151] Hess and Bache[151] showed that after two weeks of coronary occlusion exercise blood flow in myocardium containing minimal necrotic tissue was 80% of that in normally perfused regions. It therefore seemed important to evaluate the functional effects of exercise in animals likely to have better collateral development and consequently less abnormal flow responses.

Other studies have indeed documented beneficial effects of well-developed or transformed collaterals on global left ventricular function in exercising animals.[8,9,140] While studying the effects of transient left circumflex coronary occlusion in dogs running on a treadmill, Cohen and Yipintsoi[8] noted that the degree of hemodynamic deterioration from left ventricular failure appeared to be related to the magnitude of collateral blood flow to the left circumflex myocardium. Beagles had previously been instrumented with left circumflex flow probes and balloon occluders and catheters to measure pressures and cardiac output and sample arterial blood. Controlled constrictions of the left circumflex artery had also been produced. After surgery, hemodynamics were measured while the dogs were resting quietly. Left circumflex collateral flow was quantitated by injecting 15-μm radioactive microspheres into the left atrium during a one-minute balloon occlusion of the vessel. Decline of the flow probe signal to zero confirmed the adequacy of the occlusion. Hemodynamics were again measured after the dogs began to run on the treadmill, and as the speed and incline were increased to 4 mph and 12% (stage V of the Tipton test[152]). During steady-state exercise the left circumflex was again transiently occluded for one minute. Immediately after onset of the occlusion, microspheres were injected into the left atrium to quantitate collateral flow during exercise. Repeat hemodynamic measurements were made, and then the occlusion was released. After completion of other protocols the left circumflex region was demarcated by intracoronary injection of Evans blue. The animals were sacrificed and the hearts excised, and the myocardium divided into multiple slices and pieces for gamma spectrometry. There was a wide spectrum of hemodynamic results in the animals studied. However, two distinct patterns emerged when the animals were segregated into groups based on the ratio of resting collateral to normal myocardial blood flow. When the normalized collateral blood flow was less than 50% of normal perfusion levels, the exercising animals developed significant left ventricular failure during left circumflex occlusion. Prior to occlusion heart rate averaged 220 beats/min, cardiac output 4.5 l/min, and left atrial pressure 10.4 mmHg. Following occlusion cardiac output fell by more than 40% to 2.6 l/min ($p < 0.001$). Because there was little change in heart rate, this decrease was entirely related to a fall in stroke volume from 20.2 to 12.5 ml/beat ($p < 0.001$). Left atrial pressure tripled to 30 mmHg ($p < 0.001$). In contrast, hemodynamic abnormalities were minimal in the animals in which resting normalized collateral flow exceeded 50% of expected normal perfusion. In these latter exercising dogs left atrial pressure rose slightly following coronary occlusion from 13.0 to 18.0 mmHg ($p < 0.05$). Although cardiac output declined from 6.9 to 5.5 l/min ($p < 0.05$), this fall was solely related to the modest decrease in heart rate. Stroke volume (30.8 to 28.0 ml/beat) was unchanged. Thus, those dogs with high collateral flows seemed to be protected and had minimal hemodynamic deterioration when the coronary artery was occluded during exercise.

The above study[8] adequately documented a beneficial effect of collaterals on the stressed canine left ventricle. However, the collaterals studied were those present in previously normal hearts, and the protocol design required comparison of different groups of dogs. Because it was not possible to exclude completely the effects of uncontrolled genetic or physiologic factors on the group results, a second study was undertaken in which the same dogs were examined at two different times, and hence served as their own controls.[9] By examining markers of collateral function at two different times and at two different levels of collateral development in individual dogs, it was possible to determine the specific beneficial effects of collateral vessels. Genetic variability or potential differences of the individual animal's tissue responsiveness to a physiologic perturbation would no longer require specific reservations.

The revised protocol[9] included study of the beagles at one week and reexamination of the same dogs after twelve weeks. The initial measurements were identical to those outlined above, and similar hemodynamic and blood flow studies were completed at three months. In these animals, an initial stenosis of 80–90% of the lumen's diameter progressed to complete occlusion at some unknown time during the three-month period. Thus, the first study was performed while the left circumflex was narrowed but still patent and the collaterals were those already present in the normal heart, whereas at the time of the second study the vessel was totally occluded and the collateral vessels had begun their transformation. In the initial week one study, exercise doubled blood flow to the normal myocardium from 1.39 to 2.78 ml/min/g, whereas collateral blood flow to the left circumflex myocardium increased negligibly from 0.53 to 0.66 ml/min/g. Thus, the ratio of ischemic to normal blood flow declined from 0.37 to 0.22. There was no change in transmural distribution in either region. Left ventricular failure was again observed during transient left circumflex coronary occlusion in the running dogs during this first week. Average cardiac output declined from 5.4 to 3.9 l/min ($p < 0.001$), while left atrial pressure increased from 9.2 to 20.9 mmHg ($p < 0.001$). The situation was quite different three months later. Blood flow to normally perfused myocardium again increased significantly during running from 1.52 to 3.78 ml/min/g. This time, however, collateral blood flow, which had risen to normal in the animals at rest, also increased normally during exercise from 1.54 to 3.93 ml/min/g and was homogeneously distributed. The ischemic/normal blood flow ratio was 1.03 at rest and 1.04 during exercise. That the exercise flows to normal and collateralized myocardium were equivalent can be seen from a representative flow histogram (Figure 5–10) where there is complete overlap of flows to the two regions in contrast to the exercise flow distribution in week one when no overlap was evident. After chronic coronary occlusion, running at the same speed and incline as in the first week produced a cardiac output of 6.5 l/min and left atrial pressure of 12.1 mmHg, both of which were unaffected by inflation of the balloon around the left circumflex artery. This latter hemodynamic profile was similar to that observed in the dogs with constricted but patent coronary arteries while running on the treadmill during the initial week one studies. Thus, collateral development definitely affected global left ventricular performance during the stress of exercise by virtually eliminating the disastrous hemodynamic consequences previously recorded during coronary occlusion.

Lambert et al.[140] implanted ameroid constrictors around the left circumflex artery of mongrel dogs and then restudied the animals 6.5 months later. Global left ventricular performance was studied while the dogs were running at 6 mph and 8% grade. The average heart rate during this period of moderate exertion was 228 beats/min. Blood pressure increased normally in these animals, and the left atrial pressure of 4.6 mmHg during exercise was unchanged from the resting level of 3.3 mmHg. These results in animals with mature, histologically transformed coronary collateral vessels parallel those described in beagles with occlusions of less than three months,[9] as well as those in dogs with well-developed but naturally occurring collaterals.[8]

Other exercise studies in dogs with chronic coronary occlusion have also confirmed that collateral flow may be normal during the stress of exercise.[140,141,143,144,153] After sufficient time for development, coronary collaterals can triple blood flow to collateralized myocardium during strenuous treadmill exercise.[140,143,144,153] The flow increases to the myocardium distal to the coronary occlusion are comparable and sometimes greater than the flow increments to normally perfused myocardium. Furthermore, the endocardial/epicardial flow ratio, a sensitive index of myocardial ischemia, remains normal in the collateralized region during running. Therefore, 12 to 26 weeks after implantation of ameroid constrictors there is no evidence of regional or transmural flow inhomogeneity either at rest or during strenuous exercise.

D. Vasodilators

Vasodilators increase blood flow to normal myocardium by relaxing the arteriolar resistance vessels. Because the tunica media of developing collaterals is incompletely formed, collateral vessels do not display similar responsiveness to these agents. Since collateral flow is in large part dependent on perfusion pressure in the source vessel, the slight drop in pressure in the coronary tree noted during vasodilatation of the distal arteriolar beds may affect perfusion of collateralized myocardium. Thus, while the potent vasodilator adenosine may double or triple flow to normal myocardium, flow to ischemic regions in the same dogs 7 to 14 days after coronary ligation may actually decrease.[154] This absolute decrease in ischemic flow, or coronary steal, is typical of the earliest stages of collateral development. Lidoflazine administered three to six weeks after implantation of ameroid constrictors, somewhat later than in the above study,[154] actually results in increases in total blood flow to the collateralized myocardium, but the increases are less than those to normal tissue.[146,147] However, there may still be an absolute decrease in flow to the endocardium.[146,147] The increase in collateral flow induced by carbochromen 8 to 12 weeks following ameroid implantation and coronary occlusion, and therefore after additional collateral transformation, is again less than normal, but there is now no endocardial steal until an external stress such as atrial pacing is superimposed.[135,147] The effects of dipyridamole, another potent vasodilator, have been documented both early and late following coronary occlusion, and differences reflect the changing capacity of the collateral circulation. As already noted, minimal collateral resistance after dipyridamole infusion decreases from 6.17 ± 1.28 mmHg/

(ml/min)/100g immediately after acute coronary occlusion to 0.27 ± 0.04 mmHg/(ml/min)/100g six weeks following ameroid constrictor implantation (or approximately three to four weeks following coronary occlusion).[65] Studies comparing maximal collateral flows following dipyridamole infusion at 4 and 20 to 28 weeks after ameroid implantation have documented significantly higher flows at the later time.[64,137] Furthermore, at four weeks, dipyridamole was much more likely to produce inhomogeneous flow across the left ventricular wall.[137] Only minimal increases in collateral flow induced by dipyridamole resulted in redistribution of flow away from the endocardium at four weeks, whereas redistribution was not observed at 24 to 28 weeks until dipyridamole had increased collateral flow above 2 ml/min/g.[137] Hence, vasodilators produce abnormal flow patterns in collateralized myocardium, but these inhomogeneities again become less obvious as the interval between coronary occlusion and drug administration lengthens. (See Chapter 7 for reservations about flow measurements in ischemic tissue following administration of vasodilators.)

E. *Norepinephrine*

Infusion of a positive inotropic agent such as norepinephrine may also uncover collateral deficiencies. Four weeks after ameroid implantation (or one to two weeks following total coronary occlusion) norepinephrine-mediated increases in endocardial and epicardial flows in the collateralized myocardium are significantly less than those in normally perfused tissue.[139] In studies in which the coronary occlusion was more remote, norepinephrine increased epicardial flows normally, but endocardial flows were still unable to increase to normal levels, resulting in a decline in the left ventricular wall endocardial/epicardial flow ratio.[66,134] The pattern of greatest flow deficit soon after coronary occlusion and more subtle abnormalities in hearts with more remote occlusions is similar to that noted with vasodilators.

IX. Coronary Collateral Reserve

Regional performance of collateralized myocardium and global function of a heart with occluded coronary arteries during stresses as atrial pacing, dynamic exercise, and pharmacologic interventions are dependent on the adequacy of collateral vessels. The amount of collateral blood flow is, in turn, largely dependent on the interval between coronary occlusion and subsequent study. In general terms, longer intervals imply increased development and therefore greater collateral capacity and flow.

Poorly developed collaterals are not able to respond fully to the demands of imposed stresses, and flow in myocardium supplied by collateral channels cannot increase appropriately and is inhomogeneously distributed. But collaterals permitted to develop for longer periods can fully restore blood flow to collateral-dependent myocardium even during strenuous exercise. If the increase in collateral blood flow in response to an intervention can match the changes in perfusion of normal areas, then function will remain normal. The above studies demonstrate that in the canine model this is a realistic expectation. On the other hand, less than normal increases may be expected to result in regional myocardial, and possibly global ventricular, dysfunction.

It is unlikely that many physiologic stresses would impose demands on the heart's vasculature exceeding those of strenuous exercise and revealing significant maldistribution of flow. Therefore, as described above, collaterals in the experimental canine model are capable of complete functional revascularization. It should be noted, however, that collateral capacity or conductance is not normal in these animals. As already indicated, several attempts have been made to measure maximal collateral conductance. One study examined collateral responsiveness to norepinephrine and reactive hyperemia in in-situ hearts and concluded that collateral conductance was 38% of normal vessel conductance.[139] However, the dogs in this study had had ameroid constrictors implanted just four weeks earlier, and therefore it is surprising that the collateral conductance was as high as it was. Other measurements by Scheel[155,156] and Schaper[153,157] have been made in dogs with occlusions of approximately 9 to 20 weeks. To ensure maximal vasodilatation of coronary and collateral vessels the hearts were excised and perfused with blood from support dogs to which adenosine had been added. Collateral conductance ranged from 33 to 50% of that of normal coronary vessels. In one study Schaper[153] measured the collateral conductance of trained and sedentary dogs three to four months after implantation of ameroid constrictors around the right and left circumflex coronary arteries. Prior to the final study, the dogs exercised strenuously and collateral flows were approximately 3 ml/min/g without any evidence of flow inhomogeneity (W. Schaper, personal communication). After excision of the hearts and addition of adenosine to the blood perfusing the coronary vasculature, flows to myocardium perfused by normal coronary arteries approached 8 ml/min/g, but obvious deficiencies of collateral perfusion were evident. Schaper concluded that collateral conductance was only 40% of normal.

The available studies of collateral reserve have all been done after coronary occlusions of less than six months, and in most the interval has been less than three to four months.[139,153,155−157] Since the collateral transformation process is still known to be active at these times, perhaps it would be better to determine maximal collateral conductance at a longer interval, perhaps one year, after coronary occlusion. Because the luminal diameter of even well-developed coronary collaterals will be smaller than the occluded vessels they are replacing and because the collaterals will be tortuous, minimal collateral resistance (or maximal conductance) can never be expected to be the same as that of the native circulation. Nonetheless, collateral development is capable of producing total functional revascularization during physiologic stresses. Only unphysiologic interventions that are capable of raising normal myocardial flows to more than 4−5 ml/min/g would be expected to uncover evidence of regional or transmural flow heterogeneity in collateral-dependent tissue.

X. Correlation between Coronary Collateral Flow and Global and Regional Left Ventricular Function

The studies already quoted have documented that regional and global left ventricular function significantly deteriorates shortly after coronary occlusion, but is less disturbed and possibly normal as the time of occlusion becomes more remote. Other investigations have demonstrated that blood flow to collateral-dependent myocardium is depressed and inhomogeneous early after coronary occlusion, but with further collateral development eventually becomes normal to all regions and transmural layers even during exercise stress. This concordance between flow and functional data is not coincidence, but rather is cause and effect. As collaterals develop in the interval following coronary occlusion, flow that can be delivered increases, and functional capacity of the myocardium is enhanced. This association between collateral flow and myocardial function is central to the position that coronary collaterals are beneficial. It should be noted, however, that this association is based on observations at only two times—early and late after coronary occlusion. Furthermore, the described investigations have generally examined either only function or only flow, and there has been little effort to correlate the two directly. Studies able to demonstrate a direct correlation between collateral flow and myocardial function would prove the contention that collaterals are not merely markers of disease but have salutary functional effects.

In one such study,[8] already briefly described, hemodynamics and myocardial blood flow were evaluated in chronically instrumented beagles. The animals were initially divided into two groups on the basis of the ratio of resting collateral to normal myocardial blood flow. Those animals with ratios less than 0.5 had marked evidence of left ventricular failure when the coronary artery was occluded during treadmill running. Left atrial pressure tripled to 30 mmHg and cardiac output and stroke volume declined by 40%. However, in those animals with flow ratios exceeding 0.5, coronary occlusion elicited only minor hemodynamic changes. Stroke volume did not change, and left atrial pressure increased from 13 to only 18 mmHg. Although these data seemed to define a definite correlation between collateral flow and myocardial function in beagles with naturally occurring collateral channels, it was realized that the separation of the animals into two groups was somewhat arbitrary. Therefore, the absolute changes in left atrial pressure (mmHg) and stroke volume (ml) following coronary occlusion for all dogs were plotted as functions of the ratio of collateral to normal blood flow measured at rest. The relationship for left atrial pressure is presented in Figure 6-5. In the resting animals there was no correlation between normalized collateral flow and the response of the left atrial pressure to left circumflex occlusion. However, when the coronary artery was occluded during running, an inverse relationship ($y = 3.78\ x^{-1.08}$, $r = -0.84$) between the change in left atrial pressure and resting normalized collateral flow was observed. Thus, as collateral flow increased in these dogs, there was less tendency for the left ventricle to fail and left atrial pressure to rise when the left circumflex was occluded during running. Coronary collaterals had a protective effect. A similar relationship was observed for the changes in stroke volume (Figure 6-6). At rest left circumflex occlusion produced a

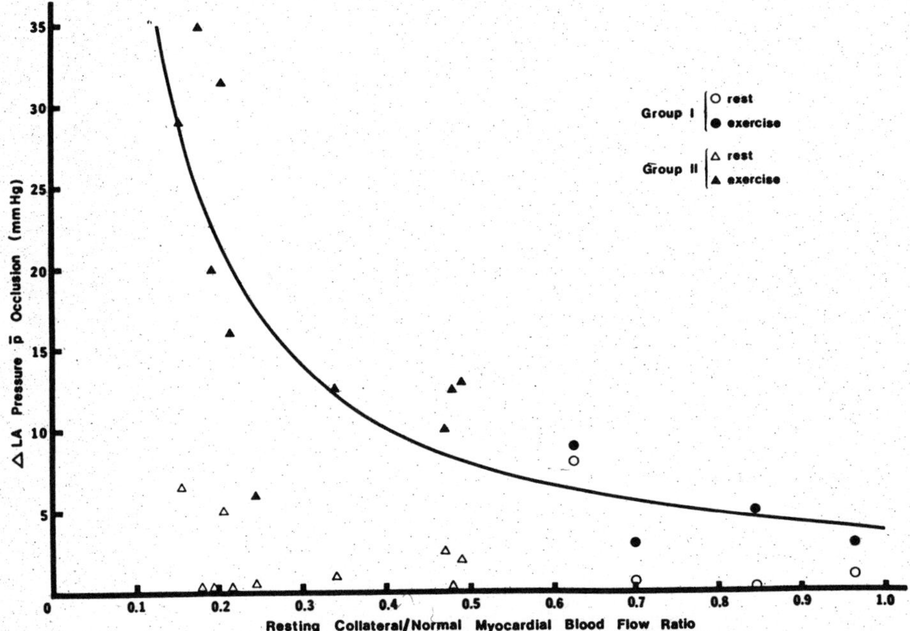

Figure 6-5 Graphic presentation of the change in left atrial (ΔLA) pressure after acute occlusion of the left circumflex coronary artery in dogs as a function of normalized collateral blood flow measured under resting conditions. Open symbols represent hemodynamic changes at rest in group I (O) (collateral/normal myocardial blood flow ratio > 0.5) and group II (Δ) (ratio ≤ 0.5). Closed symbols represent left atrial pressure changes during running in group I (●) and group II (▲). At rest, left atrial pressure response to coronary occlusion is minimal and does not appear to be correlated with amount of collateral flow, probably because metabolic demand of the myocardium does not greatly exceed the ability of the beleaguered supply to deliver oxygen and metabolites. However, during running, demand greatly exceeds supply, and now an obvious inverse relationship between collateral blood flow and change in left atrial pressure following coronary occlusion is evident. Dogs with higher collateral flows had smaller rises in left atrial pressure and therefore less deterioration of cardiac function. (Reprinted with permission of the American Physiological Society from Cohen and Yipintsoi.[8])

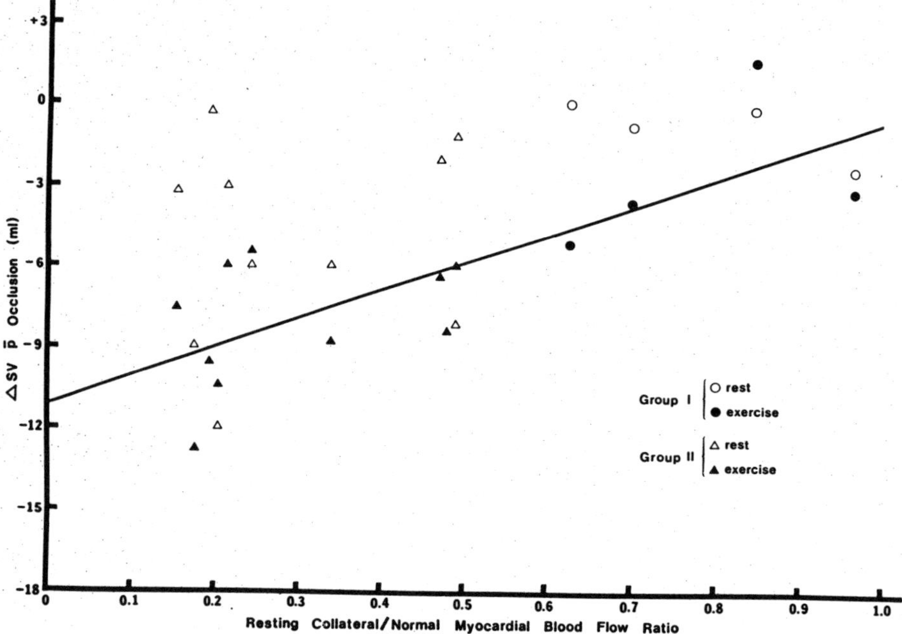

Figure 6–6   Graphic presentation of the change in stroke volume (ΔSV) after acute occlusion of the left circumflex coronary artery as a function of normalized collateral blood flow measured under resting conditions. Symbols are identical to those used in Figure 6–5. At rest there is a weak linear relationship ($r = 0.49$) between changes in stroke volume following coronary occlusion and collateral blood flow. However, the fall in stroke volume is magnified when the coronary artery of the running dog is occluded, and the linear relationship between stroke volume change and collateral flow is better ($r = 0.78$). This relationship between collateral flow and change in stroke volume emphasizes the significant effect of collateral flow on myocardial function. (Reprinted with permission of the American Physiological Society from Cohen and Yipintsoi.[8])

small decrease in stroke volume, but this appeared to be largely independent of the normalized collateral flow ($r = 0.49$). During running, the decreases in stroke volume following left circumflex occlusion were magnified, and the relationship of the two variables could be approximated by a straight line ($y = -11.11 + 10.44x, r = 0.78$). Again, there was less tendency for left ventricular failure and for stroke volume to fall in the animals with higher collateral flows. This relationship between collateral flow and change in stroke volume again emphasizes the significant effect of collateral flow on myocardial function. It is obvious that there is a continuous relationship between collateral flow and function of ischemic myocardium. This realization goes far toward convincingly documenting the primary beneficial effect of collaterals on cardiac performance.

For further proof of this relationship, the effect of collateral development on both flow to ischemic myocardium and global left ventricular function was examined by measuring collateral flow and evaluating exercise hemodynamics in the same beagles at two times.[9] Thus, the animals were instrumented as previously detailed and the described blood flow and hemodynamic measurements were made at rest and during exercise with and without left circumflex occlusion approximately two weeks following recovery from surgery. For the purposes of a separate protocol the animals were then divided into two groups. One group was subjected to daily exercise training consisting of sprint and endurance running, while the other served as sedentary controls. Ater 10 to 12 weeks, hemodynamic and blood flow measurements at rest and during exercise were repeated in all dogs. Fifteen dogs completed the study protocol. Of the total, seven were runners and eight were sedentary. By the end of the 10- to 12-week program, none of the coronary flow probes implanted around the left circumflex artery three to four months earlier was functional. Coronary angiography was performed in all animals to determine left circumflex patency and reliable functioning of the balloon occluders. In nine dogs (five controls and four runners, Group I) the left circumflex was patent, whereas in the other six animals (three controls and three runners, Group II), it was occluded at the site of either the flow probe or balloon occluder. However, late vessel patency was not felt to be important for the purposes of the study because it was the coronary collateral independent of its developmental stimulus that was being evaluated.

The dogs in Group I with patent left circumflex coronary arteries at weeks one and twelve developed significant left ventricular failure when the left circumflex artery was transiently occluded during treadmill running. Although there was a modest increase in resting collateral flow in these animals over the three-month observation period from 0.58 to 0.96 ml/min/g, the average ischemic/normal blood flow ratio rose from 0.48 to only 0.66. The increase in collateral flow was not sufficient to eliminate the adverse response to coronary occlusion during exercise. On the other hand, collateral flow in the dogs with left circumflex vessels that became occluded increased from 0.53 ml/min/g in week one to 1.54 ml/min/g in week twelve. Thus, the ischemic/normal blood flow ratio rose from 0.37 to 1.03. As already described, this increase in collateral flow was accompanied by the notable absence of significant hemodynamic abnormalities when the balloon occluder was inflated in the running animals. These data again suggest a cause-and-effect relationship between collateral flow and preservation of left ventricular function. It should be pointed out, however, that the average group changes in hemodynamics and myocardial blood flows with and without left circumflex occlusion from the first to the second study partially obscure their dependent relationship, especially in Group I. The data in individual dogs are presented graphically in Figures 6−7 and 6−8. The changes in left atrial pressure (Figure 6−7) and stroke volume (Figure 6−8) after transient left circumflex occlusion during treadmill running for both the initial and final studies are plotted as functions of the ratio of resting collateral flow to normal myocardial flow. Data points in individual dogs are connected, making it possible to view each dog as its own control and to compare hemodynamics

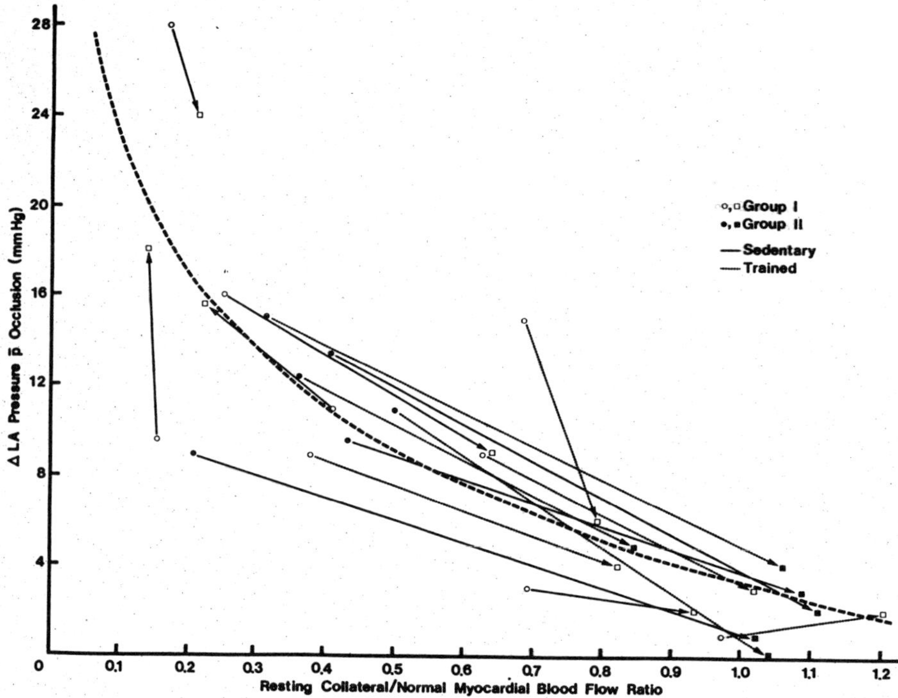

Figure 6–7   Change in left atrial (ΔLA) pressure after transient left circumflex (LCf) occlusion in exercising dogs as a function of collateral/normal myocardial blood flow ratio measured at rest. Measurements were made twice in all dogs, weeks one (○,●) and twelve (□, ■) of the study protocol, and the data points from the initial and final studies in individual dogs are connected. The arrowhead indicates data from the second study. In Group I dogs (○, □) the LCf was stenotic but patent just prior to transient balloon occlusion during the two studies. In Group II dogs (●, ■) the LCf became permanently occluded sometime between weeks one and twelve of the protocol, and, therefore, these animals had the greatest collateral development. In 13 of the 15 dogs collateral flow increased from week one to twelve, and in all 13 left atrial pressure rose less when the encircling balloon occluder was inflated during running (4 mph and 12% grade) in week twelve. The two animals with less collateral flow in week twelve, possibly related to platelet emboli and occlusion of collateral vessels, had significant increases in the left atrial pressure rise when the LCf was occluded during running. The curve (long dashes) represents the best-fit line for all data points ($r = -0.83$), and clearly demonstrates the significant effect of collateral flow on left ventricular function during the stress of exercise. During the twelve-week protocol some dogs were sedentary whereas others were trained. This division is indicated by either solid (sedentary) or short dashed (trained) connecting lines. (Reprinted with permission of the American Physiological Society from Cohen and Yipintsoi.[9])

and myocardial blood flows at two points while other unspecified variables remain unchanged.

As noted in Figures 6–7 and 6–8, changes in the hemodynamic response to transient coronary occlusion may be directly related to observed differences in collateral flow. In 13 of the 15 dogs in Groups I and II, the

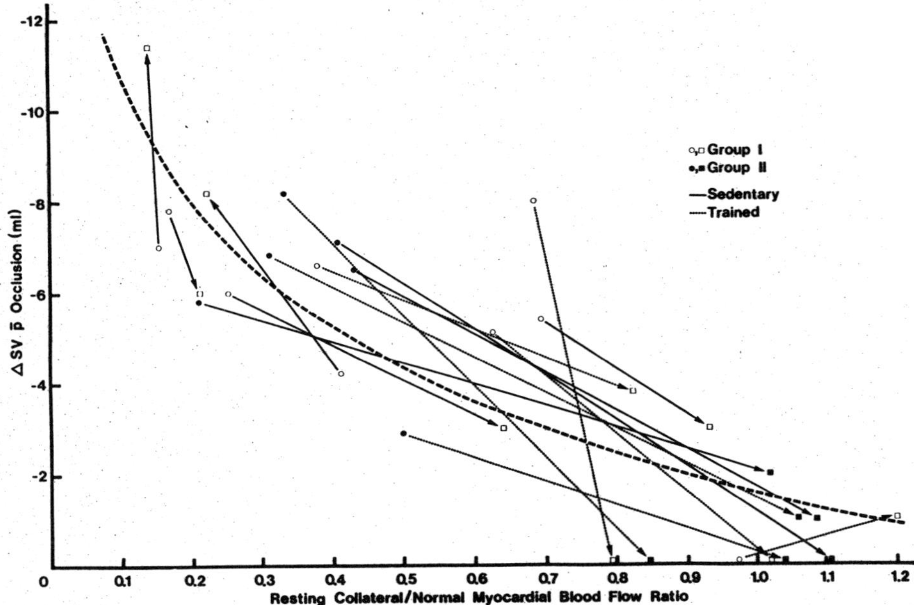

Figure 6–8   Change in stroke volume (ΔSV) after transient left circumflex (LCf) occlusion in exercising dogs as a function of collateral/normal myocardial blood flow ratio measured at rest. Symbols as in Figure 6–7. Again, the 13 dogs with increasing collateral flow from week one to week twelve had smaller drops in stroke volume when the coronary artery was transiently occluded during treadmill running in week twelve. In contrast, the two animals with decreased collateral flow in week twelve had more marked falls in stroke volume. The best-fit curve (r = 0.84) also demonstrates the dependence of left ventricular function on collateral flow. (Reprinted with permission of the American Physiological Society from Cohen and Yipintsoi.[9])

collateral flow ratio increased from the initial to the final study, and in 12 of these 13 dogs the rise in left atrial pressure and fall in stroke volume during stage V exercise and transient left circumflex occlusion were significantly less at week twelve than at week one. In the 13th dog, the one with the highest collateral flows, the changes in stroke volume (1 ml/beat) and left atrial pressure (1 mmHg) responses from week one to twelve were negligible. In these 12 dogs running at 4 mph and 12% grade (stage V), the average left atrial pressure increase after inflation of the coronary balloon occluder declined from 11.7 ± 1.8 mmHg at week one to 5.0 ± 1.7 mmHg at week twelve (p < 0.001), while the decrement in stroke volume diminished from 5.9 ± 0.6 to 1.6 ± 0.5 ml/beat (p < 0.005). In the two animals in which the measured collateral/normal blood flow ratio actually declined from week one to twelve, the average rise in left atrial pressure after transient left circumflex occlusion increased from 10.2 to 16.8 mmHg (Figure 6–7), while the fall in stroke volume was further exaggerated (5.6 ml/beat at week one to 9.9 ml/beat at week twelve) (Figure 6–8). Logarithmic curves were fitted to all the data points (r = −0.83 for left atrial pressure and r = 0.84 for stroke volume).

Although the abscissa in Figures 6–7 and 6–8 was the resting collateral/normal blood flow ratio, alternate use of the exercise flow ratio produced little change in the relationship between the ratio and changes in left atrial pressure or stroke volume during transient left circumflex occlusion. The resting and exercise flow ratios were linearly related with a correlation coefficient of 0.94.

This second study[9] thus supports the conclusions based on the initial observations in groups of collateral-poor and collateral-rich dogs.[8] Collateral development was stimulated by a combination of intentional coronary constriction, unplanned slowly progressive coronary occlusion, and possible chronic endurance exercise training (see Chapter 7). Left ventricular function in running dogs during a standardized stress induced by transient coronary occlusion was closely linked to the level of resting collateral flow and development (Figures 6–7 and 6–8). When all data are considered, the same inverse relationships between resting normalized collateral flow and rise in left atrial pressure (compare Figures 6–5 and 6–7) or fall in stroke volume (compare Figures 6–6 and 6–8) are evident. But more convincing, perhaps, is the effect of changing collateral flow on left ventricular function in each individual animal. In the 13 dogs in which collateral flow increased after three months, cardiac failure as assessed by changes in left atrial pressure and stroke volume either improved during the second coronary occlusion (12 of 13 dogs) or did not change significantly (1 of 13) when compared to the response during the initial occlusion. In the two dogs in which collateral flow decreased, perhaps related to small platelet emboli occluding some of the collateral channels, cardiac hemodynamics during the second coronary occlusion deteriorated further. Thus, the collateral/normal blood flow ratio accurately predicted the extent of dysfunction of the stressed left ventricle. The excellent correlation between collateral flow and myocardial function over a wide range of flows in both groups of animals as well as individual dogs supports the central importance of collateral perfusion. Coronary collaterals are beneficial and do limit the adverse hemodynamic effects of coronary occlusion.

Whereas the experiments by Cohen and Yipintsoi[8,9] measured collateral flow and its effect on global left ventricular function, at least two attempts have been made to document similar effects of collateral vessels on regional segmental function.[27,127] Roan et al.[27] implanted ultrasonic crystals in the myocardium in the distribution of the left anterior descending artery and correlated abnormalities of net systolic wall thickening following balloon occlusion of the vessel with the amount of collateral perfusion to the affected myocardium. On the basis of postocclusion segmental thickening they were able to divide the experimental animals into three groups. Those with minimal abnormalities of thickening also had no perfusion abnormalities. Those dogs with moderate defects in systolic thickening also had moderate decreases in blood flow. Finally, the animals with paradoxical thinning of the myocardium following coronary occlusion had the most marked perfusion defects, especially of the endocardium. There was a significant nonlinear correlation between regional segmental function and myocardial blood flow.

Thus, the general expectation of preservation of myocardial function by coronary collaterals is again supported by Roan's results.

Hill et al.[127] implanted ameroid constrictors and pneumatic occluders around the left circumflex artery of dogs. After approximately 19 days the vessel was occluded. Regional myocardial function was evaluated with miniature ultrasonic crystals embedded in the myocardium. Systolic function was evaluated under control conditions and during transient coronary occlusion produced by the encircling balloon 7 and 14 days after surgery, and collateral flow was measured with radioactive microspheres during coronary occlusion at the same times. Approximately two days after permanent coronary occlusion (21 days after surgery), regional myocardial function and collateral blood flow were measured again. During the study on day seven collateral flows to the ischemic endocardium and epicardium were 0.10 and 0.27 ml/min/g, respectively, and systolic function of the ischemic myocardium deteriorated markedly during transient coronary occlusion. At 14 days the endocardial and epicardial flows were 0.42 and 0.70 ml/min/g, and systolic function deteriorated less when the balloon was inflated. Finally, at 21 days both systolic shortening and rate of shortening were normal despite permanent coronary occlusion, and collateral flows and transmural distribution were nearly normal. The relationship between collateral development and maintenance of function is again apparent.

These observations and experimental data document the ability of coronary collaterals to modify and even prevent sequelae of coronary obstruction and ischemic heart disease. Coronary collaterals account for improved survival following coronary occlusion, higher ventricular fibrillation thresholds, less myocardial ischemia and necrosis, restoration of blood flow to ischemic regions, and, finally, preservation of function of myocardium in the distribution of the occluded vessel. The magnitude of the beneficial effect is proportional to the degree of collateral development or the success with which the collaterals revascularize the ischemic region. Demonstration of the salutary effect of collaterals in both pig and dog provides hope that these channels will have similar effects in humans. Presumably, the lingering question of the usefulness of the coronary collateral circulation in the clinical area is a function only of the less exacting and precise investigational tools available. The impressive data supporting the beneficial role of coronary collaterals in animal models provide enough justification to warrant further investigation to uncover pharmacologic agents or physiologic maneuvers that can stimulate collateral growth and development and thereby flow even before coronary occlusion occurs.

References

1. Porter WT: The nutrition of the heart. In *An American Text-Book of Physiology*, Vol. 1, 2nd ed. (ed WH Howell). W.B. Saunders and Co., Philadelphia, 1900, p 180.

2. Wüsten B, Flameng W, and Schaper W: The distribution of myocardial flow. Part I: Effects of experimental coronary occlusion. *Basic Res. Cardiol.* 69:442–443, 1974.

3. Marcus ML, Kerber RE, Ehrhardt J, and Abboud FM: Effects of time on volume and distribution of coronary collateral flow. *Am. J. Physiol.* 230:279–285, 1976.

4. Bishop SP, White FC, and Bloor CM: Regional myocardial blood flow during acute myocardial infarction in the conscious dog. *Circ. Res.* 38:429–438, 1976.

5. Rivas F, Cobb FR, Bache RJ, and Greenfield JC Jr: Relationship between blood flow to ischemic regions and extent of myocardial infarction: Serial measurement of blood flow to ischemic regions in dogs. *Circ. Res.* 38:439–447, 1976.

6. Cohen, MV: Quantitation of collateral and ischemic flows with microspheres and diffusible indicator. *Am. J. Physiol.* 234:H487–H495, 1978.

7. Jugdutt BI, Becker LC, and Hutchins GM: Early changes in collateral blood flow during myocardial infarction in conscious dogs. *Am. J. Physiol.* 237:H371–H380, 1979.

8. Cohen MV, and Yipintsoi T: Myocardial performance and collateral flow after transient coronary occlusion in exercising dogs. *Am. J. Physiol.* 237:H520–H527, 1979.

9. Cohen MV, and Yipintsoi T: Restoration of cardiac function and myocardial flow by collateral development in dogs. *Am. J. Physiol.* 240:H811–H819, 1981.

10. Prinzmetal M, Bergman HC, Kruger HE, et al: Studies on the coronary circulation. III. Collateral circulation of beating human and dog hearts with coronary occlusion. *Am. Heart J.* 35:689–717, 1948.

11. Cohn PF, Kirk ES, Downey JM, et al: Autoradiographic evaluation of myocardial collateral circulation in the canine heart. *Cardiovasc. Res.* 7:181–185, 1973.

12. Hammond GL, Juca ER, and Austen WG: The nature of intercoronary arterial flow in the normal heart. *Am. Heart J.* 78:559–568, 1969.

13. Wiggers CJ: The inadequacy of the normal collateral coronary circulation and the dynamic factors concerned in its development during slow coronary occlusion. *Am. Heart J.* 11:641–647, 1936.

14. Wiggers CJ: The problem of functional coronary collaterals. *Exp. Med. Surg.* 8:402–421, 1950.

15. Wiggers CJ: The functional importance of coronary collaterals. *Circulation* 5:609–615, 1952.

16. Tennant R, and Wiggers CJ: The effect of coronary occlusion on myocardial contraction. *Am. J. Physiol.* 112:351–361, 1935.

17. Wiggers CJ, and Green HD: The ineffectiveness of drugs upon collateral flow after experimental coronary occlusion in dogs. *Am. Heart J.* 11:527–541, 1936.

18. Gregg DE, and Dewald D: The immediate effects of the occlusion of the coronary veins on collateral blood flow in the coronary arteries. *Am. J. Physiol.* 124:435–443, 1938.

19. Gregg DE, Thornton JJ, and Mautz FR: The magnitude, adequacy and source of the collateral blood flow and pressure in chronically occluded coronary arteries. *Am. J. Physiol.* 127:161–175, 1939.

20. Prinzmetal M, Schwartz LL, Corday E, et al: Studies on the coronary circulation. VI. Loss of myocardial contractility after coronary artery occlusion. *Ann. Intern. Med.* 31:429–449, 1949.

21. Goldman A, Shaw C, Corday E, et al: Experimental methods for detection of changes of blood supply to the heart. *J. Thorac. Surg.* 24:105–115, 1952.

22. Nakhjavan FK, Son R, and Goldberg H: Myocardial contractility in areas with chronic ischaemia: Studies on isometric tension. *Cardiovasc. Res.* 2:226–233, 1968.

23. Puri PS, and Bing RJ: Effect of drugs on myocardial contractility in the intact dog and in experimental myocardial infarction: Basis for their use in cardiogenic shock. *Am. J. Cardiol.* 21:886–893, 1968.

24. Theroux P, Franklin D, Ross J Jr, and Kemper WS: Regional myocardial function

during acute coronary artery occlusion and its modification by pharmacologic agents in the dog. *Circ. Res.* 35:896−908, 1974.

25. Heyndrickx GR, Millard RW, McRitchie RJ, et al: Regional myocardial functional and electrophysiological alterations after brief coronary artery occlusion in conscious dogs. *J. Clin. Invest.* 56:978−985, 1975.

26. Theroux P, Ross J Jr, Franklin D, et al: Regional myocardial function and dimensions early and late after myocardial infarction in the unanesthetized dog. *Circ. Res.* 40:158−165, 1977.

27. Roan PG, Buja LM, Izquierdo C, et al: Interrelationships between regional left ventricular function, coronary blood flow, and myocellular necrosis during the initial 24 hours and 1 week after experimental coronary occlusion in awake, unsedated dogs. *Circ. Res.* 49:31−40, 1981.

28. Stowe DF, Mathey DG, Moores WY, et al: Segment stroke work and metabolism depend on coronary blood flow in the pig. *Am. J. Physiol.* 234:H597−H607, 1978.

29. Savage RM, Guth B, White FC, et al: Correlation of regional myocardial blood flow and function with myocardial infarct size during acute myocardial ischemia in the conscious pig. *Circulation* 64:699−707, 1981.

30. Crozatier B, Ross J Jr, Franklin D, et al: Myocardial infarction in the baboon: Regional function and the collateral circulation. *Am. J. Physiol.* 235:H413−H421, 1978.

31. Saÿen JJ, Sheldon WF, Horwitz O, et al: Studies of coronary disease in the experimental animal. II. Polarographic determinations of local oxygen availability in the dog's left ventricle during coronary occlusion and pure oxygen breathing. *J. Clin. Invest.* 30:932−940, 1951.

32. Wiggers CJ, Wégria R, and Piñera B: The effects of myocardial ischemia on the fibrillation threshold—The mechanism of spontaneous ventricular fibrillation following coronary occlusion. *Am. J. Physiol.* 131:309−316, 1940.

33. Bellman S, and Frank HA: Intercoronary collaterals in normal hearts. *J. Thorac. Surg.* 36:584−603, 1958.

34. Blumgart HL, Gilligan DR, Zoll PM, et al: Studies of experimentally produced intercoronary collateral circulation. *Trans. Assoc. Am. Phys.* 57:152−156, 1942.

35. Blumgart HL, Zoll PM, Freedberg AS, and Gilligan DR: The experimental production of intercoronary arterial anastomoses and their functional significance. *Circulation* 1:10−27, 1950.

36. Zoll PM, and Norman LR: The effects of vasomotor drugs and of anemia upon interarterial coronary anastomoses. *Circulation* 6:832−842, 1952.

37. Paul MH, Norman LR, Zoll PM, and Blumgart HL: Stimulation of interarterial coronary anastomoses by experimental acute coronary occlusion. *Circulation* 16:608−614, 1957.

38. Lumb G, Singletary HP, and Hardy LB: Collateral circulation following experimental gradual narrowing of the coronary arteries. *Angiology* 13:463−465, 1962.

39. Meesmann W, Schulz F-W, Schley G, and Adolphsen P: Überlebensquote nach akutem experimentellem Coronarverschluss in Abhängigkeit von Spontankollateralen des Herzens. *Z. Ges. Exp. Med.* 153:246−264, 1970.

40. Amann L, Meesmann W, Schley G, et al: Der Einfluss gesteigerten Laufbandtrainings auf die Entwicklung von Koronarkollateralen und die Mortalität nach akuter Koronarligatur bei Hunden. (abstr) *Pflügers Arch. Ges. Physiol.* 332:R80, 1972.

41. Schley G, Meesmann W, and Schulz FW: Die Bedeutung von Spontankollateralen des Herzens für die frühen elektrokardiographischen Veränderungen nach akutem experimentellem Koronarverschluss. *Med. Welt.* 23:1373−1374, 1972.

42. Schulz FW, Meesmann W, and Schley G: Der Einfluss von Spontankollateralen auf akute experimentelle Myokardinfarkte. *Med. Welt.* 23:1375−1376, 1972.

43. Meesmann W, Stephan K, Gülker H, et al: Arrhythmias, vulnerability, and focal blocks in the early phase of experimental myocardial infarction in relation to

coronary collateral vessels. In *Coronary Heart Disease: 3rd International Symposium Frankfurt* (eds M. Kaltenbach, P Lichtlen, R Balcon, and W-D Bussmann). Georg Thieme, Stuttgart, 1978, pp 55−60.

44. Robertson HF: The reestablishment of cardiac circulation during progressive coronary occlusion: An experimental study on dogs. *Am. Heart J.* 10:533−541, 1935.

45. Hahn RS, and Beck CS: Revascularization of the heart: A study of mortality and infarcts following multiple coronary artery ligation. *Circulation* 5:801−809, 1952.

46. Schley G, Meesmann W, Wild U, and Wild A: Der Einfluss von Infarktgrösse und Spontankollateralen auf die Flimmerschwelle des Herzens nach akutem experimentellem Koronarverschluss. *Verh. Dtsch. Ges. Kreislaufforsch.* 39:203−207, 1973.

47. Meesmann W, Gülker H, Krämer B, and Stephan K: Time course of changes in ventricular fibrillation threshold in myocardial infarction: Characteristics of acute and slow occlusion with respect to the collateral vessels of the heart. *Cardiovasc. Res.* 10:466−473, 1976.

48. Krämer B, and Meesmann W: Akuter oder protrahierter Koronarverschluss. *ZFA* (Stuttgart) 54:9−14, 1978.

49. Meesmann W: Early arrhythmias and primary ventricular fibrillation after acute myocardial ischaemia in relation to preexisting coronary collaterals. In *Early Arrhythmias Resulting from Myocardial Ischaemia: Mechanisms and Prevention by Drugs* (ed JR Parratt). Oxford University Press, New York, 1982, pp 93−112.

50. Garza DA, White FC, Hall RE, and Bloor CM: Effect of coronary collateral development on ventricular fibrillation threshold. *Basic Res. Cardiol.* 69:371−378, 1974

51. Smith FM: The ligation of coronary arteries with electrocardiographic study. *Arch. Intern. Med.* 22:8−27, 1918.

52. Burchell HB: Adjustments in coronary circulation after experimental coronary occlusion: With particular reference to vascularization of pericardial adhesions. *Arch. Intern. Med.* 65:240−262, 1940.

53. Blum L, Schauer G, and Calef B: Gradual occlusion of a coronary artery: An experimental study. *Am. Heart J.* 16:159−164, 1938.

54. Gregg DE, and Mautz FR: Dynamics of collateral circulation following chronic occlusion of coronary arteries. (abstr) *Am. J. Physiol.* 123:84, 1938.

55. Kattus AA, and Gregg DE: Some determinants of coronary collateral blood flow in the open-chest dog. *Circ. Res.* 7:628−642, 1959.

56. Schaper W, Jageneau A, and Xhonneux R: The development of collateral circulation in the pig and dog heart. *Cardiologia* 51:321−335, 1967.

57. McIntosh HD, Zeft HJ, Hackel DB, and Kong Y: The time-course of the development of collateral circulation following gradual coronary occlusion in the pig. *Trans. Am. Clin. Climatol. Assoc.* 79:124−131, 1968.

58. Ramo BW, Peter RH, Ratliff N, et al: The natural history of right coronary arterial occlusion in the pig: Comparison with left anterior descending arterial occlusion. *Am. J. Cardiol.* 26:156−161, 1970.

59. Elliot EC, Bloor CM, Jones EL, et al: Effect of controlled coronary occlusion on collateral circulation in conscious dogs. *Am. J. Physiol.* 220:857−861, 1971.

60. Schaper W, Flameng W, Snoeckx L, and Jageneau A: Der Einfluss körperlichen Trainings auf den Kollateralkreislauf des Herzens. *Verh. Dtsch. Ges. Kreislaufforsch.* 37:112−121, 1971.

61. Khouri EM, Gregg DE, and McGranahan GM Jr: Regression and reappearance of coronary collaterals. *Am. J. Physiol.* 220:655−661, 1971.

62. Schaper W: Collateral circulation. In *Quantitation in Cardiology: Proceedings of the Boerhaave Courses* (eds HA Snellen, HC Hemker, PG Hugenholtz, and JH van Bemmel). Leiden University Press, Leiden, 1971, pp 55−58.

63. Cohen MV, and Eldh P: Experimental myocardial infarction in the closed-chest

dog: Controlled production of large or small areas of necrosis. *Am. Heart J.* 86: 798−804, 1973.

64. Flameng W, Wüsten B, Winkler B, et al: Influence of perfusion pressure and heart rate on local myocardial flow in the collateralized heart with chronic coronary occlusion. *Am. Heart J.* 89:51−59, 1975.

65. Walter P, Flameng W, Görlach G, and Hehrlein FW: Restoration of coronary reserve by bypass grafting in relation to the collateral circulation. In *Coronary Heart Disease: 3rd International Symposium Frankfurt* (eds M Kaltenbach, P Lichtlen, R Balcon, and W-D Bussmann). Georg Thieme, Stuttgart, 1978, pp 27−33.

66. Flameng W, Schwarz F, Schaper W, and Hehrlein F: Functional significance of coronary collaterals. In *Coronary Heart Disease: 3rd International Symposium Frankfurt* (eds M Kaltenbach, P Lichtlen, R Balcon, and W-D Bussmann). Georg Thieme, Stuttgart, 1978, pp 67−72.

67. Flameng W, Schwarz F, and Schaper W: Coronary collaterals in the canine heart: Development and functional significance. *Am. Heart J.* 97:70−77, 1979.

68. Wilson JL, and Scheel KW: Myocardial infarction in dogs with acute and gradual occlusion of the circumflex or right coronary arteries. *Anat. Rec.* 204:113−122, 1982.

69. Ullrich H, Bötticher H, and Guski H: Experimentelle Koronarsklerose und ischämische Herzkrankheit. II. Mitteilung: Morphometrische Untersuchungen zum Nachweis von Anpassungsvorgängen an den Koronararterien und am Myokard. *Zentralbl. Allg. Pathol.* 124:15−19, 1980.

70. Schaper W, Nienaber C, and Gottwik M: The importance of the collateral circulation for myocardial survival. *Acta Med. Scand. Suppl.* 651:29−34, 1981.

71. Schwarz F, Wagner HO, Sesto M, et al: Native collaterals in the development of collateral circulation after chronic coronary stenosis in mongrel dogs. *Circulation* 66:303−308, 1982.

72. Koke JR, and Bittar N: Functional role of collateral flow in the ischaemic dog heart. *Cardiovasc. Res.* 12:309−315, 1978.

73. Manning GW, McEachern CG, and Hall GE: Reflex coronary artery spasm following sudden occlusion of other coronary branches. *Arch. Intern. Med.* 64:661−674, 1939.

74. McEachern CG, Manning GW, and Hall GE: Sudden occlusion of coronary arteries following removal of cardiosensory pathways: An experimental study. *Arch. Intern. Med.* 65:661−670, 1940.

75. LeRoy GV, Fenn GK, and Gilbert NC: The influence of xanthine drugs and atropine on the mortality rate after experimental occlusion of a coronary artery. *Am. Heart J.* 23:637−643, 1942.

76. Guzman SV, Swenson E, and Jones M: Intercoronary reflex: Demonstration by coronary angiography. *Circ. Res.* 10:739−745, 1962.

77. Moschos CB, Lehan PH, Oldewurtel HA, et al: Coronary vascular reactivity following arterial versus arteriolar obstruction. (abstr) *Clin. Res.* 12:190, 1964.

78. Grayson J, and Lapin BA: Observations on the mechanisms of infarction in the dog after experimental occlusion of the coronary artery. *Lancet* 1:1284−1288, 1966.

79. Grayson J, Irvine M, Parratt JR, and Cunningham J: Vasospastic elements in myocardial infarction following coronary occlusion in the dog. *Cardiovasc. Res.* 2:54−62, 1968.

80. Hirsch C, and Spalteholz W: Coronararterien und Herzmuskel: Anatomische und experimentelle Untersuchungen. *Dtsch. Med. Wochenschr.* 33:790−795, 1907.

81. Schaper W, Remijsen P, and Xhonneux R: The size of myocardial infarction after experimental coronary artery ligation. *Z. Kreislaufforsch.* 58:904−909, 1969.

82. Wüsten B, Winkler B, and Schaper W: Influence of collateral circulation on infarct

size in acute myocardial infarction. In *The First 24 Hours in Myocardial Infarction* (eds F Kaindl, O Pachinger, and P Probst). Verlag Gerhard Witzstrock, Baden-Baden, 1977, pp 140−142.

83. Schaper W: Experimental coronary artery occlusion. III. The determinants of collateral blood flow in acute coronary occlusion. *Basic Res. Cardiol.* 73:584−594, 1978.

84. Schaper W, Frenzel H, Hort W, and Winkler B: Experimental coronary artery occlusion. II. Spatial and temporal evolution of infarcts in the dog heart. *Basic Res. Cardiol.* 74:233−239, 1979.

85. Jugdutt BI, Hutchins GM, Bulkley BH, and Becker LC: Myocardial infarction in the conscious dog: Three-dimensional mapping of infarct, collateral flow and region at risk. *Circulation* 60:1141−1150, 1979.

86. Reimer K, and Jennings RB: The "wavefront phenomenon" of myocardial ischemic cell death. II. Transmural progression of necrosis within the framework of ischemic bed size (myocardium at risk) and collateral flow. *Lab. Invest.* 40: 633−644, 1979.

87. Glogar D, Ertl G, Kloner RA, et al: Coronary collateral flow in relationship to coronary bed-size. (abstr) *Clin. Res.* 28:174A, 1980.

88. Jugdutt BI, Becker LC, Hutchins GM, et al: Effect of intravenous nitroglycerin on collateral blood flow and infarct size in the conscious dog. *Circulation* 63:17−28, 1981.

89. Koyanagi S, Eastham CL, Harrison DG, and Marcus ML: Transmural variation in the relationship between myocardial infarct size and risk area. *Am. J. Physiol.* 242:H867−H874, 1982.

90. Patterson RE, Jones-Collins BA, and Aamodt R: Impaired collateral blood flow reserve early after nontransmural myocardial infarction in conscious dogs. *Am. J. Cardiol.* 50:1133−1140, 1982.

91. Davenport N, Goldstein RE, Bolli R, and Epstein SE: Blood flow to infarct and surviving myocardium: Implications regarding the action of verapamil on the acutely ischemic dog heart. *J. Am. Coll. Cardiol.* 3:956−965, 1984.

92. Lowe JE, Reimer KA, and Jennings RB: Experimental infarct size as a function of the amount of myocardium at risk. *Am. J. Pathol.* 90:363−380, 1978.

93. Vokonas PS, Malsky PM, Paul SJ, et al: Radioautographic studies in experimental myocardial infarction: Profiles of ischemic blood flow and quantification of infarct size in relation to magnitude of ischemic zone. *Am. J. Cardiol.* 42:67−75, 1978.

94. Schaper W, Hofmann M, Müller K-D, et al: Experimental occlusion of two small coronary arteries in the same heart. A new validation method for infarct size manipulation. *Basic Res. Cardiol.* 74:224−229, 1979.

95. Bobb JRR, Kunze DC, McCall W Jr, and Green HD: Location of communications between cognate bed of descending ramus of left coronary and adjacent collateral vascular beds. *Proc. Soc. Exp. Biol. Med.* 69:115−117, 1948.

96. Cohen MV, Holman BL, and Kirk ES: Coronary collaterals: Determinant of infarct size. (abstr) *Clin. Res.* 22:678A, 1974.

97. White FC, Sanders M, and Bloor CM: Regional redistribution of myocardial blood flow after coronary occlusion and reperfusion in the conscious dog. *Am. J. Cardiol.* 42:234−243, 1978.

98. Irvin RG, and Cobb FR: Relationship between epicardial ST-segment elevation, regional myocardial blood flow, and extent of myocardial infarction in awake dogs. *Circulation* 55:825−832, 1977.

99. Tanabe M, Fujiwara S, Ohta N, et al: Pathophysiological significance of coronary collaterals for preservation of the myocardium during coronary occlusion and reperfusion in anaesthetized dogs. *Cardiovasc. Res.* 14:288−294, 1980.

100. Hirzel HO, Sonnenblick EH, and Kirk ES: Absence of a lateral border zone of

intermediate creatine phosphokinase depletion surrounding a central infarct 24 hours after acute coronary occlusion in the dog. *Circ. Res.* 41:673−683, 1977.

101. Kirk ES, and Hirzel HO: Critical role of coronary collateral blood flow in the pathophysiology of myocardial infarction. In *Coronary Heart Disease: 3rd International Symposium Frankfurt* (eds M. Kaltenbach, P Lichtlen, R Balcon, and W-D Bussmann). Georg Thieme, Stuttgart, 1978, pp 11−20.

102. Schley G, Meesmann W, Schulz FW, et al: Der Einfluss von Spontankollateralen des Herzens auf die frühen elektrokardiographischen Veränderungen nach akutem experimentellem Coronarverschluss. *Verh. Dtsch. Ges. Inn. Med.* 77: 869−872, 1971.

103. Schley G, Meesmann W, Schulz F-W, and Adolphsen P: Das Elektrokardiogramm nach akutem experimentellem Koronarverschluss in Abhängigkeit von Spontankollateralen des Herzens. *Z. Kreislaufforsch.* 60:405−420, 1971.

104. Sadony V, Stephan K, and Meesmann W: Das Ausmass der Myokardischämie nach experimentellem Koronarverschluss in Abhängigkeit vom Sauerstoffbedarf und Spontankollateralenstatus des Herzens. *Thoraxchirurgie* 22:320−324, 1974.

105. Stephan K, Sadony V, and Meesmann W: Das epikardiale Elektrokardiogramm nach experimentellem Koronarverschluss in Abhängigkeit vom Sauerstoffbedarf und dem Kollateralenstatus des Herzens. *Verh. Dtsch. Ges. Inn. Med.* 80:1154− 1156, 1974.

106. Stephan K, Meesmann W, and Sadony V: Oxygen demand and collateral vessels of the heart: Factors influencing the severity of myocardial ischaemic injury after experimental coronary artery occlusion. *Cardiovasc. Res.* 9:640−648, 1975.

107. Sadony V, Stephan K, and Meesmann W: Die Ischämieveränderungen im epikardialen Elektrokardiogramm nach experimentellem Koronarverschluss in Abhängigkeit vom Sauerstoffbedarf und Kollateralenstatus des Herzens. *Langenbecks Arch. Chir. Suppl.:* 15−18, 1974.

108. Stephan K, Sadony V, and Meesmann W: Einfluss der Spontankollateralen und assistierten Zirkulation auf das Ischämieausmass im EKG nach experimentellem Koronarverschluss. *Med. Welt.* 26:1310−1312, 1975.

109. Eckstein RW: Coronary interarterial anastomoses in young pigs and mongrel dogs. *Circ. Res.* 2:460−465, 1954.

110. Janse MJ, and Wilms-Schopman F: Effect of changes in perfusion pressure on the position of the electrophysiologic border zone in acute regional ischemia in isolated perfused dog and pig hearts. *Am. J. Cardiol.* 50:74−82, 1982.

111. Eckstein RW: Development of interarterial coronary anastomoses by chronic anemia. Disappearance following correction of anemia. *Circ. Res.* 3:306−310, 1955.

112. Katada Y, Mizutani T, Maekawa K, et al: An electrographic study on the functional capacity of the coronary collateral circulation in dogs with chronic coronary occlusion. *Jpn. Circ. J.* 44:294−302, 1980.

113. Gould KL, Lipscomb K, and Hamilton GW: Physiologic basis for assessing critical coronary stenosis: Instantaneous flow response and regional distribution during coronary hyperemia as measures of coronary flow reserve. *Am. J. Cardiol.* 33:87−94, 1974.

114. Oldham HN Jr, Kakos GS, Dixon SH Jr, et al: The effect of coronary collateral circulation on experimental aorto-coronary bypass. *J. Surg. Res.* 12:87−92, 1972.

115. Tomoike H, Franklin D, Kemper WS, et al: Functional evaluation of coronary collateral development in conscious dogs. *Am. J. Physiol.* 241:H519−H524, 1981.

116. Wyatt HL, Forrester JS, Tyberg JV, et al: Effect of graded reductions in regional coronary perfusion on regional and total cardiac function. *Am. J. Cardiol.* 36:185−192, 1975.

117. Gallagher KP, Kumada T, Koziol JA, et al: Significance of regional wall thickening abnormalities relative to transmural myocardial perfusion in anesthetized dogs. *Circulation* 62:1266−1274, 1980.

118. Selmonosky CA, King GE, and Ellison RG: Synchronous diastolic coronary perfusion in experimental acute coronary ischemia. *Ann. Thorac. Surg.* 11:409–416, 1971.

119. Jones CE, Thomas JX, Parker JC, and Parker RE: Acute changes in high energy phosphates, nucleotide derivatives, and contractile force in ischaemic and nonischaemic canine myocardium following coronary occlusion. *Cardiovasc. Res.* 10:275–282, 1976.

120. Yoran C, Sonnenblick EH, and Kirk ES: Contractile reserve and left ventricular function in regional myocardial ischemia in the dog. *Circulation* 66:121–128, 1982.

121. Cohen MV, Downey JM, Sonnenblick EH, and Kirk ES: The effects of nitroglycerin on coronary collaterals and myocardial contractility. *J. Clin. Invest.* 52:2836–2847, 1973.

122. Marlon AM, Adams MH, Wexler L, and Harrison DC: Angiographic demonstration of collateral development in experimental coronary artery occlusion with ameroid constrictors. *Invest. Radiol.* 8:131–137, 1973.

123. Nakamura M, Mitsutake A, Matsuguchi H, et al: Effects of collateral circulation on regional myocardial blood flow and left ventricular wall motion (A preliminary note). *Basic Res. Cardiol.* 72:492–504, 1977.

124. Kumada T, Gallagher KP, Shirato K, et al: Reduction of exercise-induced regional myocardial dysfunction by propranolol: Studies in a canine model of chronic coronary artery stenosis. *Circ. Res.* 46:190–200, 1980.

125. Millard RW: Induction of functional coronary collaterals in the swine heart. *Basic Res. Cardiol.* 76:468–473, 1981.

126. Kumada T, Gallagher KP, Battler A, et al: Comparison of postpacing and exercise-induced myocardial dysfunction during collateral development in conscious dogs. *Circulation* 65:1178–1185, 1982.

127. Hill RC, Kleinman LH, Tiller WH Jr, et al: Myocardial blood flow and function during gradual coronary occlusion in awake dog. *Am. J. Physiol.* 244:H60–H67, 1983.

128. Franklin D, Millard RW, and Nagao T: Responses of coronary collateral flow and dependent myocardial mechanical function to the calcium antagonist, diltiazem. *Chest* 78(Suppl):200–204, 1980.

129. Hood WB Jr, Kumar R, Joison J, and Norman JC: Experimental myocardial infarction. V. Reaction to impaired circumflex flow in the presence of established anterior myocardial infarction in intact conscious dogs. *Am. J. Cardiol.* 26:355–364, 1970.

130. Yokoyama M, Mizutani T, Fujiwara K, et al: An experimental study on the role of coronary collateral development in preservation and improvement of contractile force in the ischemic myocardium. *Jpn. Circ. J.* 42:1249–1256, 1978.

131. Becker LC, and Pitt B: Collateral blood flow in conscious dogs with chronic coronary artery occlusion. *Am. J. Physiol.* 221:1507–1510, 1971.

132. Shaw DJ, Pitt A, and Friesinger GC: Autoradiographic study of the [133]xenon disappearance method for measurement of myocardial blood flow. *Cardiovasc. Res.* 6:268–276, 1971.

133. Cibulski AA, Lehan PH, and Hellems HK: Myocardial collateral flow measurements in mongrel dogs. *Am. J. Physiol.* 225:559–565, 1973.

134. Pass HI, Cox JL, Wechsler AS, et al: Response of coronary collateral circulation to increased myocardial demands. (abstr) *Circulation* 48(Suppl. IV):IV-92, 1973.

135. Flameng W, Schaper W, and Lewi P: Multiple experimental coronary occlusion without infarction: Effects of heart rate and vasodilation. *Am. Heart J.* 85:767–776, 1973.

136. Scheel KW, Banet M, Ott C, and Lehan PH: A quantitative approach to collateral and antegrade flows after coronary occlusion. *Am. J. Physiol.* 222:687–694, 1972.

137. Schaper W, Wüsten B, Flameng W, et al: Local dilatory reserve in chronic experimental coronary occlusion without infarction. Quantitation of collateral development. *Basic Res. Cardiol.* 70:159−173, 1975.

138. Brazier J, Hottenrott C, and Buckberg G: Noncoronary collateral myocardial blood flow. *Ann. Thorac. Surg.* 19:426−435, 1975.

139. Schwarz F, Flameng W, Mack B, et al: Vascular and cardiac contractile reserve in the dog heart with chronic multiple coronary occlusions. *Am. Heart J.* 92:600−608, 1976.

140. Lambert PR, Hess DS, and Bache RJ: Effect of exercise on perfusion of collateral-dependent myocardium in dogs with chronic coronary artery occlusion. *J. Clin. Invest.* 59:1−7, 1977.

141. Heaton WH, Marr KC, Capurro NL, et al: Beneficial effect of physical training on blood flow to myocardium perfused by chronic collaterals in the exercising dog. *Circulation* 57:575−581, 1978.

142. Neill WA, and Oxendine JM: Exercise can promote coronary collateral development without improving perfusion of ischemic myocardium. *Circulation* 60:1513−1519, 1979.

143. Fedor JM, Rembert JC, McIntosh DM, and Greenfield JC Jr: Effects of exercise- and pacing-induced tachycardia on coronary collateral flow in the awake dog. *Circ. Res.* 46:214−220, 1980.

144. Bache RJ: Effects of exercise on blood flow to collateral-dependent myocardium in the dog. (abstr) *Circulation* 64(Suppl. IV):IV-117, 1981.

145. Crystal GJ, Downey HF, and Bashour FA: Evaluation of noncoronary sources of left ventricular perfusion to intercoronary collateral-dependent myocardium due to chronic major vessel occlusion: Absent contribution of luminal and extracardiac channels. *Am. Heart J.* 102:841−845, 1981.

146. Schaper W, Lewi P, Flameng W, and Gijpen L: Myocardial steal produced by coronary vasodilation in chronic coronary artery occlusion. *Basic Res. Cardiol.* 68:3−20, 1973.

147. Schaper W, Flameng W, Wüsten B, and Palmowski J: The distribution of coronary and of coronary collateral flow in normal hearts and after chronic coronary occlusion. In *Current Topics in Coronary Research: Advances in Experimental Medicine and Biology*, Vol. 39 (eds CM Bloor and RA Olsson). Plenum Press, New York, 1973 pp 151−160.

148. Neill WA, Oxendine J, Phelps N, and Anderson RP: Subendocardial ischemia provoked by tachycardia in conscious dogs with coronary stenosis. *Am. J. Cardiol.* 35:30−36, 1975.

149. Russell RE, Chagrasulis RW, and Downey JM: Inhibitory effect of cardiac contraction on coronary collateral blood flow. *Am. J. Physiol.* 233:H541−H546, 1977.

150. Franklin D, Tomoike H, Shirato K, et al: Functional evaluation of coronary collaterals during ameroid coronary constriction in the conscious dog. (abstr) *Circulation* 56(Suppl. III):III-9, 1977.

151. Hess DS, and Bache RJ: Regional myocardial blood flow during graded treadmill exercise following circumflex coronary artery occlusion in the dog. *Circ. Res.* 47:59−68, 1980.

152. Tipton CM, Carey RA, Eastin WC, and Erickson HH: A submaximal test for dogs: Evaluation of effects of training, detraining, and cage confinement. *J. Appl. Physiol.* 37:271−275, 1974.

153. Schaper W: Influence of physical exercise on coronary collateral blood flow in chronic experimental two-vessel occlusion. *Circulation* 65:905−912, 1982.

154. Cohen MV: Coronary steal in awake dogs: A real phenomenon. *Cardiovasc. Res.* 16:339−349, 1982.

155. Scheel KW, Galindez TA, Cook B, et al: Changes in coronary and collateral flows and adequacy of perfusion in the dog following one and three months of circumflex occlusion. *Circ. Res.* 39:654−658, 1976.

156. Scheel KW, Ingram LA, and Wilson JL: Effects of exercise on the coronary and collateral vasculature of beagles with and without coronary occlusion. *Circ. Res.* 48:523−530, 1981.
157. Schaper W, Flameng W, Winkler B, et al: Quantification of collateral resistance in acute and chronic experimental coronary occlusion in the dog. *Circ. Res.* 39:371−377, 1976.

CHAPTER SEVEN

Modification of Collateral Flow and Stimulation of Collateral Development in Experimental Animals with Pharmacologic, Metabolic, and Mechanical Agents

I. Modification of Collateral Flow

Coronary collaterals are alternative vascular channels that become functional when antegrade perfusion through the major coronary arteries is either impeded or blocked. Because coronary collaterals and the flow they supply preserve the structural integrity and functional capacity of ischemic myocardium, mechanical interventions or pharmacologic agents have been used in attempts to maximize collateral flow. Following the onset of myocardial ischemia, even small increases in collateral flow would be expected to spare jeopardized myocardium. However, in this acute period when collaterals already present in the myocardium are nearly devoid of vasomotor activity and are overstretched, many vasoactive agents might be expected to be deleterious or at best inactive. Because hypoxia and myocardial ischemia are the only well-known stimuli of collateral development and transformation, attempts to promote growth of the collateral circulation prior to critical coronary stenosis or occlusion without affecting the well-being of the animal have not been very successful. Although it is not yet possible to claim that collateral flow can be successfully manipulated, past investigations have uncovered the determinants of collateral flow and promising areas for future research.

389

A. Vasodilators

1. Technical and Conceptual Difficulties Encountered in Available Studies

Because of the ability of known coronary vasodilators to dilate normal coronary arteries and hence increase myocardial perfusion, many of these same agents have been examined for possible effects on collateral vessels and flow. It is not possible to review the results of the scores of reported studies. Instead, the effects of several prototype pharmacologic agents will be described. Before these experimental results are presented, however, it is necessary to appreciate the difficulties inherent in interpretation of studies of vasodilators. In fact, many reports concluding that vasodilators increase collateral flow are misleading and possibly inaccurate.

Most recent protocols seeking to document the effect of vasodilators on coronary collaterals have employed the radioactive microsphere technique. Following coronary occlusion, differently labeled microspheres are injected into the left atrium, first before and then after administration of the vasoactive agent. Radioactivity of a sample of ischemic myocardium is then measured and flows calculated. An increase in flow to the ischemic myocardium following infusion of the vasodilator is then interpreted as an effect of the drug on collateral channels. Obviously, this conclusion can be accepted only if the increase in flow in the sampled ischemic region is related solely to an increase in collateral flow. But evidence from several reports[1,2] suggests that the expected increase in flow to the surrounding normal muscle and contamination of the sample of ischemic myocardium by normal tissue may be responsible for the apparent increase in flow to the ischemic region. This would imply that the observed increase in ischemic flow following administration of a vasodilator drug may be an artifact of the experimental design.

Cohen,[1] using a technique originally described by Eckstein et al.[3] and adapted to the coronary circulation by Kirk and his co-workers,[4-6] demonstrated that myocardium perfused by one major coronary artery could seemingly be perfused by the adjacent coronary system as well. By using the experimental preparation shown in Figure 7-1, the cannulated left anterior descending artery could be perfused either directly from a systemic artery or through a specially designed reservoir. By appropriate adjustment of the clamps, blood from the systemic artery could enter the balloon within the reservoir. The expanding balloon would then express blood from the surrounding reservoir into the perfusion tubing at normal flow rate and phasic perfusion pressure, resulting in preservation of normal perfusion of the left anterior descending myocardium. Radioactive microspheres injected into the left atrium during reservoir perfusion of the left anterior descending coronary artery would then lodge directly in the left circumflex myocardium. Microspheres that ordinarily would have entered the left anterior descending circulation would be trapped within the balloon. Therefore, any micro-

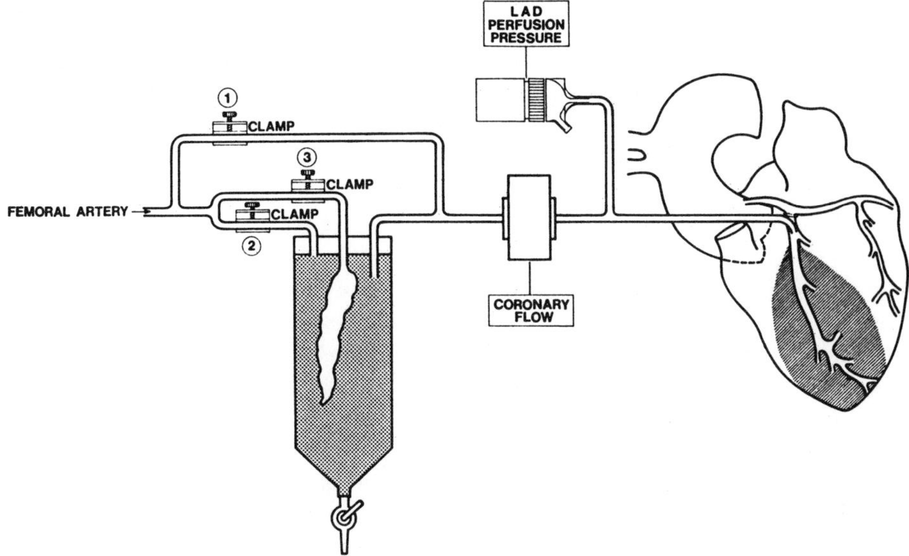

Figure 7-1   Experimental preparation allowing separate perfusion of the left anterior descending (LAD) coronary artery from either the femoral artery (removal of clamp 1) or from the reservoir (closing clamp 1 and opening either clamp 2 or 3). If clamp 2 is open, blood passes through the reservoir directly into the perfusion tubing to the LAD. But if clamp 2 is closed and clamp 3 is open, incoming blood enters the balloon, which expands and expresses reservoir blood into the LAD perfusion tubing. Thus, the LAD myocardium can be segregated and perfused with isotope-free reservoir blood while the other coronary arteries are perfused normally from the aorta with blood containing a radioactive marker. (Reprinted with permission of the American Physiological Society from Cohen.[1])

spheres found in the left anterior descending myocardium must have arrived from the left circumflex circulation through noncollateral channels while the left anterior descending artery was being perfused normally. This flow component, or overlap flow, would be determined only by left circumflex perfusion, and would be unaffected by changes in left anterior descending flow or pressure. Overlap flow would continue to be evident following occlusion of the left anterior descending artery. Therefore, quantitated flow to ischemic myocardium would be a function of both true collateral flow and the contaminating, noncollateral overlap flow component, and routine microsphere measurements of residual flow to myocardium following coronary occlusion would characteristically overestimate collateral flow. Cohen[1] found that overlap flow was present in all animals studied, but varied widely from 14 to 80% of total ischemic flow, and averaged 49.4%. Therefore, the average routine measurement of ischemic flow in mongrel dogs would overestimate true collateral flow by 100%. The histologic studies of Factor et al.[7] provide an anatomic basis for this overlap flow component. These authors observed peninsulas of myocardium supplied by the left circumflex artery jutting deep into left anterior descending territory. Thus, samples of left anterior descending myocardium would unavoidably include some myocardium supplied by the left circumflex vessel. The practical importance of these observations seems obvious. If a vasodilator increases flow to the normal left circumflex myocardium surrounding ischemic left anterior descending tissue, then overlap flow or left circumflex flow to these peninsulas will likewise increase, giving the false impression of an increase in collateral flow to the ischemic tissue even if collateral flow itself is unaffected. The effect of this contamination would be greater for lower baseline collateral flows.

Patterson and Kirk[2] have quantitated the effect of this overlap flow on measurements of ischemic flow during infusion of the vasodilator adenosine. Although adenosine is a potent vasodilator and increases flow to normal coronary beds, it can reduce collateral flow by diminishing systemic blood pressure and therefore coronary perfusion pressure as well as by causing an internal flow redistribution or coronary steal (see below). Patterson and Kirk infused adenosine intravenously into dogs and blood pressure fell by 20−35 mmHg. Blood flow to normal myocardium increased by 362%. However, true collateral flow calculated by discounting the quantitated total ischemic flow for the overlap component actually declined. This decrease in collateral perfusion was confirmed by significant declines in peripheral coronary pressure and retrograde flow. The observed fall in collateral flow was documented only when contamination of the ischemic tissue by the interdigitating peninsulas of normal tissue was accounted for. If as little as 4% of the ischemic myocardial sample was not actual ischemic muscle but instead contaminating normal zone tissue, then the decline in collateral flow would have been obscured. Contamination of the ischemic sample by normal myocardium equivalent to 8% of the sample's mass would have resulted in an apparent significant drug-induced increase in collateral flow. Obviously, the magnitude of the increase would depend on the degree of contamination. Thus, the inclusion of even very small amounts of normal tissue in the sample of ischemic myocardium may obscure the direct effects of a vasodilator on the ischemic coronary and collateral vasculature. Gross et al.[8] have reported nearly identical results with the selective coronary vasodilator chromonar. Contamination of the ischemic tissue by normal myocardium making up as little as 6% of the sample's mass would have successfully obscured the true deleterious effect of chromonar on collateral flow. These observations reinforce the importance of careful separation of myocardial zones and attention to the precise definition of myocardial ischemia. It is not difficult to imagine that previous studies claiming to have documented vasodilator-mediated increases in collateral flow might be subject to these objections.

A second methodologic limitation of many studies attempting to define the effect of pharmacologic agents on immature coronary collaterals was recently reported by Brazzamano and co-workers.[9] These investigators partially constricted the left circumflex coronary artery of dogs, and studied the animals 14 days later. Collateral blood flow was measured during transient occlusion of the left circumflex artery on two occasions separated by a period of reperfusion. This type of protocol is frequently employed in the study of pharmacologic agents, and a selected drug might be administered before or during the second occlusion to determine its effect on perfusion of the ischemic myocardium. Brazzamano, however, showed that ischemic flow during the second occlusion was significantly greater than flow in the same area during the first occlusion despite absence of any intervention (0.37 ± 0.22 versus 0.28 ± 0.17 ml/min/g, $p < 0.01$). Hence, even a drug without any vascular activity but by chance administered at the time of the second occlusion would mistakenly be considered capable of improving flow to ischemic tissue. One must be certain of stable baseline flows before the superimposed effects of external agents can be accurately assessed.

2. Conductance and Resistance Vessels

All vasodilator drugs do not have similar effects on the heart's vasculature. In part, differences may be related to nonuniformity of the arterial tree. The coronary bed can be divided both functionally and anatomically into two major categories of vessels.[10-27] Larger conductance vessels are most visible on the epicardial surface, and smaller precapillary resistance vessels lie in closer proximity to the contracting myocardial fibers. Numerous experimental studies have documented a distinction between the larger capacitance arteries and smaller resistance vessels. Isolated helical strips of coronary arteries with either attached force transducers to monitor tension[10,13,14,18] or impaling microelectrodes to record action potentials,[19] isolated heart preparations,[17,18] or intact, anesthetized animals[11,12,15,16,21] in which proximal and distal coronary pressures are measured to allow calculation of regional vascular resistance, and direct measurements of coronary arterial diameter with ultrasonic dimension gauges in either anesthetized[22,23] or conscious[20,24-27] animals have demonstrated that proximal and distal arterial segments respond differently and independently to pharmacologic agents and metabolic stimuli and have distinct time courses of reactivity.

At normal perfusion pressures the resistance of the larger epicardial segments of the coronary tree constitutes less than 10% of the total coronary resistance,[11,12,15] and the conductance vessel resistance increases to only 12% of the total resistance at mean pressures of 56 mmHg.[15] Thus, significant changes in total coronary resistance primarily reflect alterations in vascular tone of the smaller vessels, and regulation of coronary blood flow becomes a function of these resistance vessels. During conditions of myocardial ischemia, however, when arteriolar resistance vessels are maximally dilated and their resistance correspondingly diminished, the resistance of the larger arterial segments becomes a more meaningful part of the total vascular resistance of that coronary bed. Under these circumstances, changes in vascular tone of the capacitance vessels may have important physiologic consequences. Resistance of the larger arterial segments may be altered by vasoactive agents, and their response frequently differs significantly from that of the smaller arteriolar vessels. These differences often have significant effects on the volume of collateral flow to ischemic myocardium. Because the large capacitance vessels are proximal to the origin of most collateral channels, dilatation of the former results in less pressure loss from the aorta to the mouths of the collaterals. Since flow in most collateral channels is pressure dependent, a higher pressure at the collateral source in turn produces higher flows. Furthermore, well-developed collateral channels and the large capacitance arteries are felt to respond similarly to external stimuli. Thus, agents that dilate the latter can also potentially dilate collateral channels with subsequent improvement of perfusion of collateral-dependent myocardium.

Any vasodilating agent that is not specific for the coronary vascular bed may dilate peripheral arteriolar resistance vessels, resulting in variable declines in systemic blood pressure and therefore coronary perfusion pressure. Because the autoregulatory capacity of developing collateral vessels is limited and collateral perfusion of ischemic myocardium is often directly dependent on the coronary perfusion pressure, any fall in the latter will also decrease the former. Those agents capable of dilating the smaller coronary resistance vessels may also directly produce flow redistribution with resultant diminution of collateral flow. This type of redistribution is termed coronary steal.

3. Coronary Steal—Adenosine

By definition, coronary steal refers to absolute decreases in flow to ischemic regions in the face of increases to normal myocardium. An agent believed to cause a primary coronary steal should do so by its direct action on the coronary vasculature, and not by its systemic hypotensive effect caused by peripheral vasodilatation. Theoretical considerations would suggest that an agent that could dilate the resistance vessels of the coronary bed and therefore substantially increase flow would result in a decline in distal coronary and hence collateral perfusion pressure. Such an agent would be expected to decrease collateral flow. Adenosine, a potent dilator of the small coronary resistance vessels, is perhaps the prototype of such agents. Essentially all investigations[13–15,17–19] have demonstrated that adenosine has an intense, prolonged vasodilatory effect on these resistance vessels, but no or at most a negligible effect on large coronary artery segments. Cohen and Kirk[15] have demonstrated, however, that a vasodilatory response of the capacitance vessels to infused adenosine can be uncovered if the agent is infused during conditions of decreased coronary perfusion pressure, which itself leads to autoregulatory dilatation of the resistance vessels and hence attenuation of their response to adenosine. Because of adenosine's marked effect on the small resistance vessels, one would expect it to produce a coronary steal.

To document this theoretical prediction of an adenosine-induced coronary steal, mongrel dogs were instrumented with a flow probe and balloon occluder around the proximal left circumflex artery and aortic and left atrial catheters.[28] A small branch of the left circumflex vessel originating just beyond the balloon occluder was isolated, ligated distally, and cannulated retrogradely with a small catheter for measurement of intracoronary pressure and delivery of adenosine directly into the coronary circulation at doses that do not have systemic effects (Figure 7-2). The left circumflex artery was constricted to reduce the peak hyperemic response to a transient 15-second occlusion by 33−50%. By testing the responsiveness of the circumflex bed to transient occlusions and intracoronary bolus injections of adenosine both before (Figure 7-3) and after (Figure 7-4) stenosis of the vessel, obvious decreases in left circumflex perfusion pressure during the period of increased flow became apparent with appearance of (Figure 7-3) or increase in (Figure 7-4) the aortic−distal left circumflex pressure gradient. In the experimental model of Figure 7-2 an ischemic myocardial area was created by ligating the left anterior descending coronary artery in its middle third. The

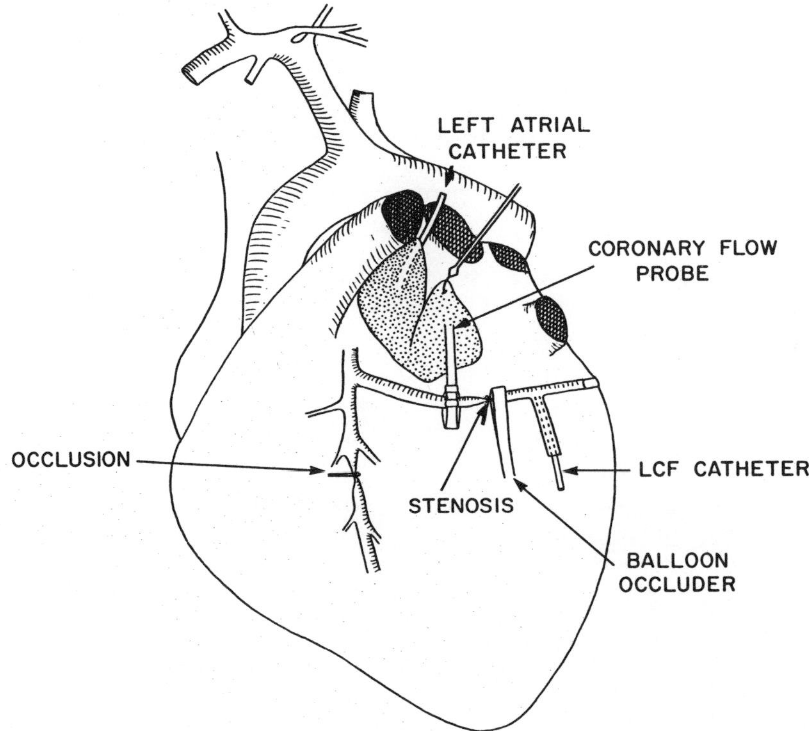

Figure 7-2   Experimental preparation with a left circumflex (LCf) coronary artery stenosis diminishing peak reactive hyperemia following release of a 15-sec LCf occlusion by 33−50% and ligation of the left anterior descending coronary artery in its middle third. A 16-gauge catheter was inserted into an LCf branch for pressure measurement and drug infusion. (Reprinted with permission of the British Medical Association from Cohen.[28])

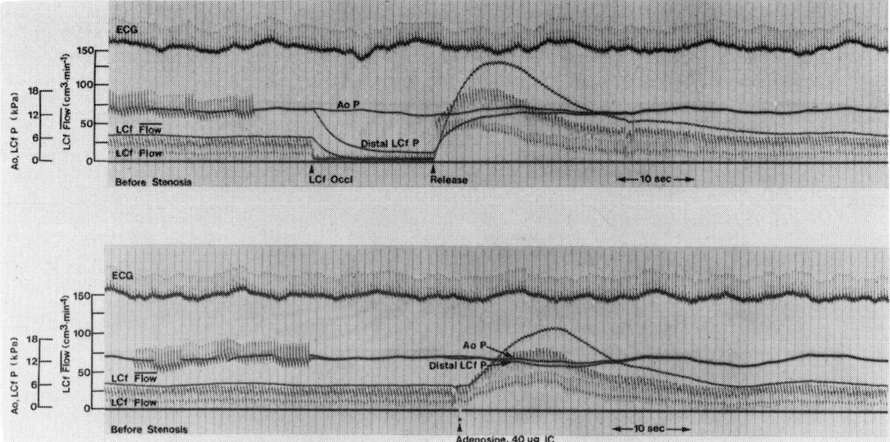

Figure 7-3   Records of aortic (AoP) and distal left circumflex artery (LCf) pressures and phasic and mean (flow) LCf flows prior to LCf stenosis in an experimental animal. The responses to both a 15-sec inflation of the encircling LCf balloon occluder and 40-μg bolus injection of adenosine into the LCf are depicted. Neither the transient vessel occlusion nor the intracoronary (IC) adenosine injection affected aortic pressure. No pressure gradient between aorta and distal LCf was initially present. However, following deflation of the balloon or pharmacologic vasodilatation, both of which increased LCf flow to nearly 400% of baseline, a small pressure gradient appeared. The gradient rapidly diminished and disappeared as the hyperemia waned. Conversion: 1 mmHg = 0.133 kPa. (Reprinted with permission of the British Medical Association from Cohen.[28])

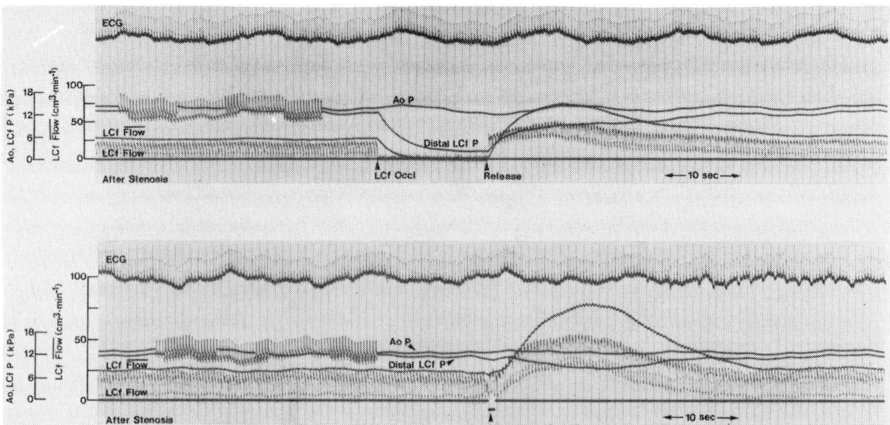

Figure 7-4   Records of aortic (AoP) and distal left circumflex artery (LCf) pressures and phasic and mean (flow) LCf flows following LCf stenosis from the same animal described in Figure 7-3. Following LCf narrowing, a fixed pressure gradient of 1.6 kPa across the stenosis developed, although baseline coronary flow was little affected. After release of a transient LCf occlusion or intracoronary (IC) injection of a 40-μg bolus of adenosine, LCf flow increased by approximately 233% and the gradient across the stenosis was magnified (note that the flow scale for the adenosine injection record has been changed). The gradient appeared to persist longer than in Figure 7-3, but also diminished as the hyperemic response disappeared. Conversion: 1 mmHg = 0.133 kPa. (Reprinted with permission of the British Medical Association from Cohen.[28])

animals were then permitted to recover and were studied in the conscious state 7 to 14 days later. While the animals were resting quietly, hemodynamics were measured and radioactive microspheres injected into the left atrium to quantitate collateral flow to the ischemic region. Thereafter an intracoronary adenosine infusion (280–320 μg/min) was begun. Hemodynamic measurements were repeated and microspheres labeled with a different isotope were injected into the left atrium.

When the hearts were excised, care was taken to delineate the three different perfusion areas. Evans blue dye was injected into the left anterior descending vessel beyond the ligature to identify the ischemic myocardium, and a colored silastic elastomere was injected through the indwelling left circumflex branch catheter to demarcate the tissue perfused with adenosine. The unstained myocardium supplied mainly by the proximal left anterior descending artery but also by the proximal left circumflex vessel was considered to represent normally perfused tissue. The demarcated myocardial areas were carefully excised, cut into wedges, and prepared for counting in the γ spectrometer. The effects of adenosine on flows to the three regions could thus be determined.

During adenosine infusion aortic pressure and other hemodynamic variables were unchanged, while pressure in the distal left circumflex artery declined from 86 to 55 mmHg, resulting in a dramatic increase in the pressure gradient across the arterial stenosis. The blood flow data are presented in Figure 7-5. In the control resting state average blood flows to the normal myocardium and left circumflex adenosine region beyond the left circumflex narrowing were similar (1.74 and 1.53 ml/min/g, respectively). Collaterals to the left anterior descending myocardium supplied approximately 60% of normal flow. Adenosine infusion resulted in doubling of the flow to the left circumflex adenosine myocardium, while flow to the normal region perfused by vessels not affected by the adenosine infusion was unchanged. It is important to note that blood flow to the collateral-dependent area beyond the left anterior descending ligation fell in each dog, and average flow decreased by 20% to 0.85 ml/min/g ($p < 0.005$). Thus, despite the maintenance of normal aortic pressure and absence of other systemic hemodynamic alterations, adenosine infusion produced a fall in blood flow to the collateral-dependent ischemic tissue while blood flow to the coronary bed giving rise to the collaterals doubled. Because increased flow across the stenosis resulted in a pressure drop, distal coronary pressure and therefore collateral perfusion pressure declined, resulting in a concomitant fall in collateral blood flow. Therefore, the increase in blood flow to the normal myocardium mediated by adenosine was at the expense of a fall in perfusion to the collateral-dependent region, a phenomenon aptly described by the term coronary steal.

To initiate this type of flow redistribution or steal, the pharmacologic agent must increase flow to the normal myocardium and decrease perfusion pressure responsible for regulating flow to the collateral-dependent ischemic area. Furthermore, the production of coronary steal is dependent on the presence of two parallel vascular pathways (in the above experiments

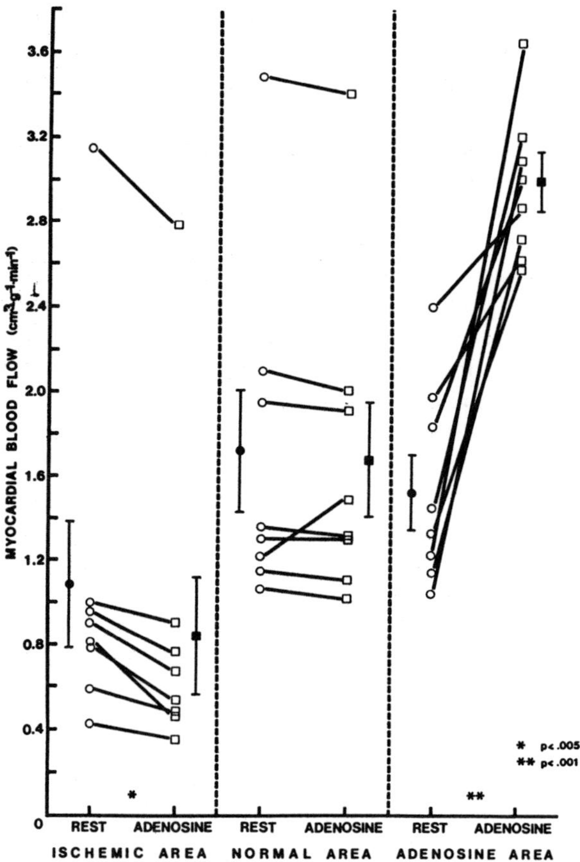

Figure 7-5   Myocardial blood flow data at rest (○) and during continuous intracoronary adenosine infusion (□), 280−320 µg/min, in eight dogs 7−14 days following recovery from surgical implantation of catheters and flow probes. The solid symbols (●, ■) denote group means, and the vertical bars indicate ± SE. The adenosine infusion had no detectable effects on systemic hemodynamics. While blood flow to the left circumflex myocardium directly affected by the intracoronary infusion of adenosine doubled, there was no change in blood flow to the proximal left anterior descending (LAD) myocardium perfused by adenosine-free blood directly from the aorta. In contrast, blood flow to the collateral-dependent ischemic area distal to the LAD ligation significantly diminished by 20% (p < 0.005). Because of the absence of change in systemic hemodynamics the decrease in flow to the ischemic region is related to an internal flow redistribution or coronary steal. Vasodilation of coronary arterioles in nonischemic myocardium results in a fall in intracoronary pressure and consequently a decrease in perfusion pressure at the origin of the collateral vessels. Hence, collateral flow falls. (Reprinted with permission of the British Medical Association from Cohen.[28])

the distal left circumflex arteriolar bed and the collaterals supplying the distal left anterior descending myocardium) with a proximal common segment. Each portion of the vascular system (large proximal precollateral vessels, collateral channels, and distal postcollateral nutritive vessels) has its own resistance. As demonstrated by Wichmann and colleagues,[29,30] the two factors governing the presence of a steal are the extent of pressure drop across the proximal large vessels (or ratio of precollateral to postcollateral resistance) and the dilating capacity of collaterals (or ratio of collateral to nutritive vessel resistance). Increase in these two resistance ratios as reflected by a more marked proximal coronary pressure fall and limited ability of the collaterals to dilate because of either already near-maximal dilation or impaired vasomotor tone in the face of dilation of resistance vessels set the stage for a coronary steal. In ischemic myocardium, autoregulation of resistance arterioles leads to near-maximal vasodilatation, and unresponsiveness to vasodilators. Nonetheless, vasodilators may dilate adjacent normal coronary beds, resulting in increased flow and fall in coronary pressure. Without effective dilatation of the proximal capacitance vessels, which would minimize the pressure drop, or of developed collaterals, or without a responsive ischemic arteriolar bed, which could dilate and increase flow, collateral perfusion pressure and thus flow decrease. Hence, drugs such as adenosine,[13–15,19] carbochromen (or chromonar),[8,12] and dipyridamole,[11,12,22,23] which mainly dilate arteriolar resistance vessels and have little or no effect on proximal large coronary artery segments do produce coronary steal[28,29,31–41] (see Figure 3-8). On the other hand, agents that principally dilate the large proximal coronary arteries, limiting the pressure drop in this precollateral segment, and/or collateral vessels would theoretically tend to increase collateral flow rather than cause a steal. Thus, the search for a coronary vasodilator with salutary effects should focus on this latter type of agent.

4. Nitroglycerin

Nitroglycerin briefly dilates small arteriolar resistance vessels, but has prolonged dilatory effects on the larger proximal capacitance arterial segments.[11,12,14,15,17–23,25] and possibly the collateral channels as well.[42] In general, the peak vasodilatory effect of nitroglycerin on the resistance vessels is observed approximately 20 seconds after intravenous infusion of the drug, while the peak effect on the larger capacitance vessels is delayed until approximately two minutes. Whereas baseline vascular tone of the smaller arterioles returns by two to three minutes, the more proximal segments remain dilated for approximately 12 minutes, and in some studies for considerably longer.[17,25] This striking effect of nitroglycerin on the large conductance arteries has been observed in both anesthetized[11,12,15,21–23] and conscious[20,25] experimental dog models as well as isolated heart preparations.[17] Thus, this agent is the prototype of the large artery dilators, and as such, would be expected to influence the coronary circulation and myocardial perfusion differently than adenosine.

Numerous experimental studies have attempted to define the effects of nitroglycerin and related nitrates on collateral blood flow. Unfortunately, most published protocols are plagued by significant design flaws that make the results difficult to interpret and possibly even misleading. When studying the effects of an agent such as nitroglycerin on coronary collateral vessels, it is imperative that only the drug's direct action on the vessels be examined.

Thus, small doses of the drug administered directly into the coronary circulation are required to maximize the drug's coronary effects and minimize unwanted peripheral actions. Nitrates, as well as most vasoactive agents, have multiple systemic effects capable of indirectly modifying collateral flow. As explained in more detail below, the frequently observed decline in perfusion pressure[43−46] and increase in heart rate[39,45] following administration of vasodilators diminish collateral flow, while the documented fall in left ventricular filling and therefore end-diastolic pressure[39,43] results in increases in perfusion of collateral-dependent myocardium. These systemic changes and therefore indirect effects on the collateral circulation are practically unavoidable if agents are infused intravenously. Attempts to counterbalance the systemic effects of vasodilators by simultaneous administration of α-agonists such as methoxamine are unsatisfying because of the potential complicating cardiac effects of the latter agents themselves.[20,47] Finally, as explained previously, small increases in blood flow to ischemic myocardium following vasodilator infusion may be artifactual. Unless adjustment of ischemic flow for the normal overlap component is made, the impossibility of perfect separation of ischemic from adjacent normal myocardium resulting in inadvertent contamination of collateral-dependent muscle by normal tissue with its vasodilator-mediated rise in coronary flow may make apparent drug-induced increases in ischemic flow meaningless. Thus, studies purporting to measure the response of collaterals to nitroglycerin and other vasodilators must be reviewed critically to ensure accurate interpretation of the results.

(a) Recent coronary occlusion

An additional theoretical drawback of most of the reports evaluating the effect of nitrates and other drugs on coronary collateral vessels has been the use of animal models with acute coronary occlusions. As described in Chapter 5, the coronary collateral immediately following coronary occlusion is a thin-walled, overstretched conduit virtually devoid of a smooth-muscle layer. Until development of medial smooth muscle these vessels are themselves incapable of responding to drugs. Therefore, it is not surprising that nitroglycerin in dogs with recent coronary obstructions has been unsuccessful in influencing either the angiographic appearance of coronary collaterals,[48] collateral indices of retrograde flow and/or peripheral coronary pressure,[42,49−53] xenon[51,54] and myocardial heat[55] clearance, or directly measured tissue flow.[9,56,57] The inability of nitroglycerin to diminish infarct size,[58,59] improve systolic wall thickening of ischemic myocardium,[60] or modify contractile force of ischemic tissue[42,61] shortly after coronary occlusion is further evidence of the inability of acute collaterals to respond to nitroglycerin. In the bulk of reports claiming that nitroglycerin either increases retrograde[45,62,63] or transmural ischemic[61,64−67] flow or causes flow redistribution from ischemic epicardium to endocardium,[58,59,68] nitroglycerin has been administered intravenously with resultant falls in left ventricular diastolic pressure and therefore diastolic wall tension and collateral vessel compression.[69] Thus, changes in collateral flow and function in these latter experiments may be the result of alterations in extravascular resistance and cannot be unequivocally ascribed to a direct vascular mechanism. In several studies methoxamine was administered to prevent changes in aortic and left atrial pressures during intravenous nitroglycerin infusion,[61,70] but direct effects of the α-agonist itself cannot be discounted.[20,47] Furthermore, the small increases in collateral flow observed in these studies following nitroglycerin administration could actually be related to contamination of the ischemic tissue by interdigitating normal myocardium despite attempts to select samples from only the center of the ischemic zone (see above), or to spontaneous flow increases observed shortly after coronary occlusion (see Chapter 5) or after repeated brief temporary coronary occlusions.[9]

Forman[67] used the balloon technique described above to account for possible contamination of ischemic myocardium by adjacent normal tissue, and documented a flow increase from 0.101 ± 0.019 to 0.149 ± 0.024 ml/min/g ($p < 0.001$) following intravenous nitroglycerin infusion when coronary perfusion pressure was not permitted to fall by use of a mechanical pump. Of course, other extravascular effects of nitroglycerin should not be discounted. One evaluation of intracoronary nitroglycerin in dogs with acute coronary occlusion has also demonstrated improvement in ischemic myocardial flow.[71] It is more likely that the nitrate in these situations was dilating large epicardial vessels rather than having any effect on the collaterals themselves. Decreased vascular tone of the large conductance vessels would be expected to diminish the pressure drop along this vascular segment and hence increase perfusion pressure at the source of the collaterals and in turn collateral flow. Thus, nitroglycerin is probably incapable of dilating coronary collaterals shortly after coronary occlusion, although a salutary effect is possible if the vascular resistance of the large epicardial vessels is reduced or if other hemodynamic variables are appropriately altered.

(b) Chronic coronary occlusion

In contrast to the data from animals with acute coronary occlusion, nitroglycerin and other nitrates do improve collateral function in dogs several weeks after coronary constriction has gradually progressed to total obstruction. As already described (see Chapter 5), collateral transformation in the first few weeks following coronary occlusion results in development of a demonstrable medial smooth-muscle layer and restoration of normal resting flows in the ischemic tissue. Nitrates dilate partially transformed coronary collaterals visualized angiographically,[48] and increase peripheral coronary pressure and retrograde flow in the vascular bed distal to the coronary occlusion.[37,42,50,53,72−74] These results have been confirmed by Schaper[57] who has studied the effects of nitroglycerin in canine hearts several weeks after occlusion of the right and left circumflex coronary arteries with ameroid constrictors. To eliminate all extravascular influence, isolated, supported, empty beating heart preparations were employed in which coronary perfusion pressure was maintained constant. Nitroglycerin injected into the perfusion line consistently raised peripheral coronary pressure in the collateralized beds. Because the experiments were designed to eliminate drug-mediated peripheral effects or changes in extravascular coronary resistance, the increase in peripheral coronary pressure can only be related to dilation of the coronary collateral vessels (and/or large epicardial channels). The time course of the effect of nitroglycerin on peripheral coronary pressure and retrograde flow in these animals with partially transformed collaterals is prolonged,[42, 53,72] and may persist for more than five minutes following an intracoronary bolus.[42] Because nitroglycerin transiently dilates coronary arteriolar vessels and increases coronary flow, a coronary steal is initially possible.[34,35,75, 76] However, this effect on the resistance vessels rapidly wanes, and the prolonged beneficial effect of coronary collateral dilatation then becomes obvious.

The salutary myocardial effects of nitrate-induced collateral dilatation were demonstrated by documenting the improved contractile response of the ischemic myocardium following intracoronary nitroglycerin injection.[42] Contractile force was studied in dogs by sewing isometric strain gauge arches onto the epicardium parallel to the superficial fibers two and a half to four weeks following gradual left anterior descending artery occlusion designed to produce minimal infarction. One gauge was sewn to the surface of the heart in the perfusion territory of the normal left circumflex artery, while a second monitored contraction in the collateralized myocardium distal to the occlusion. The strain gauge arch records contraction forces that are obviously dependent on local metabolic processes. Sequential falls in coronary flow are associated with progressive loss of amplitude of strain gauge arch deflections. Thus, the gauges permit assessment of the extent of myocardial ischemia. The increase in amplitude of the strain gauge arch recording with the resumption of a higher coronary flow indicates a flow-dependent state of the myocardium underlying the gauge and serves as an operational definition of ischemia. The main left coronary artery was cannulated to monitor coronary hemodynamics, administer intracoronary drugs, and maintain constant perfusion pressure. Because resting contractile force of the collateralized myocardium was normal, coronary perfusion pressure was lowered by an average of 40 mmHg. This fall in perfusion pressure had a differential effect on the two strain gauges. Whereas the left circumflex gauge measuring contractile force of a region with normal coronary reserve was depressed by only $4 \pm 1\%$, the left anterior descending gauge registering the response of collateral-dependent myocardium was depressed by $29 \pm 4\%$. Thus, the collateralized myocardium was ischemic. The response of one representative animal to the diminution of perfusion pressure and subsequent intracoronary injection of nitroglycerin is shown in Figure 4-6. In the control state, coronary perfusion pressure was 99 mmHg and the gradient between the main left coronary artery and distal left anterior descending artery beyond the occlusion was 45 mmHg. Before administration of nitroglycerin the perfusion pressure was decreased to 51 mmHg, leaving a gradient of 35 mmHg. At this level of perfusion the left anterior descending area clearly was ischemic, as shown by the marked fall in contractile force. In contrast, the contractile force in the nonischemic left circumflex area was essentially unchanged. Intracoronary administration of nitroglycerin (18 μg) increased coronary blood flow but had no effects on perfusion pressure, left atrial pressure, or other systemic hemodynamics. Peripheral coronary pressure in the distal left anterior descending vessel rose by 10 mmHg, and the pressure gradient across the occlusion decreased to 25 mmHg despite a constant coronary perfusion pressure. Concomitantly the contractile force in the ischemic collateralized myocardium increased markedly by 90% of the prenitroglycerin level while the strain gauge arch on normal myocardium was not affected. When the contractile force at the peak of nitroglycerin's effect is compared to the measurement at normal perfusion pressure, it is evident that nitroglycerin can transiently restore the contractile force in the ischemic myocardium to near-normal levels. The prolonged effect of the bolus nitroglycerin injection on coronary and collateral blood flow cannot be related to the drug's action on the autoregulating resistance vessels since the response of these vessels is quite transient.[11,12,15,20−23,25] Therefore, the increase in contractile force must be related to the augmented flow to the ischemic myocardium coursing through dilated collateral (and/or large epicardial) channels. The prolonged drug effect on peripheral coronary pressure is consistent with this impression. Thus, nitroglycerin can dilate well-developed collateral vessels. Presumably, it is that part of the collateral passing through normal tissue that is responsive to nitroglycerin, since the portion passing through ischemic tissue would already be maximally dilated because of autoregulation.

The observations that nitroglycerin can increase collateral flow, in contrast to agents such as adenosine, and can have beneficial functional effects on ischemic myocardium confirm the theoretical assertions that large and small vessel dilators should have different effects on collateral-dependent tissue. Thus, vasodilators should not be classified as a single group of agents. It is the large vessel dilating agents that hold promise as drugs capable of modifying collateral flow and function of ischemic myocardium in clinically desirable ways.

5. Other Pharmacologic Agents

An important consideration when the effects of pharmacologic agents on the coronary circulation are examined is their site of active vasodilatation. Dipyridamole, an agent that inhibits adenosine uptake by myocardial cells and erythrocytes and therefore decreases the rate of adenosine degradation, and that also decreases transport of the nucleoside across capillary endothelium into the venous circulation[77] would be expected to have the same effects on large and small coronary artery segments as adenosine itself. In fact, most studies[11,12,17,18,22,23] have demonstrated that dipyridamole has a prolonged vasodilatory action on the small resistance arterioles and has no effect on the large capacitance vessels. However, a recent study by Hintze and Vatner[27] in conscious dogs with ultrasonic dimension gauges around the proximal left circumflex coronary artery demonstrated that dipyridamole produced a 6.6% increase in mean coronary diameter. Furthermore, dipyridamole can relax helical strips of large coronary arteries.[18] Other drugs such as carbochromen, lidoflazine, and prenylamine which, like dipyridamole, markedly increase coronary blood flow almost exclusively dilate distal resistance vessels.[12,18] Papaverine was noted by Winbury[12] to be in this same class of small vessel dilators. However, Kamitani and colleagues[18] have documented that papaverine has significant dilatory actions on the large coronary arteries of the isolated canine heart preparation and can relax helical strips of these conductance vessels. Nitroprusside dilates both large and small coronary arteries.[21,25] In anesthetized dogs, the effect on large vessels appears to predominate,[21] while the reverse is true in conscious animals.[25] Calcium-channel entry blockers have recently been introduced as therapeutic agents in the treatment of various forms of heart disease. Both nifedipine[16,17,21] and verapamil[17,21] have been shown to have striking dilatory effects on small arterioles and no effect on large arterial segments. However, verapamil blocks calcium-dependent action potentials in isolated strips of both large and small coronary arteries,[19] and nifedipine inhibits potassium-induced contractions of large capacitance porcine coronary vessel strips.[78] Nifedipine can also increase proximal coronary artery diameter in conscious dogs.[26] In contrast, diltiazem dilates both large and small vessels, and the effect on the former appears to be of longer duration.[17] These observations again emphasize that various agents grouped together because of similar pharmacologic properties may not have identical effects on the coronary circulation.

(a) Recent coronary occlusion

Investigators have evaluated numerous vasoactive agents for their effects on collateral blood flow and resistance shortly following coronary occlusion, but the myriad studies cannot be cited here. As already noted, agents dilating the small coronary resistance vessels have generally been noted to cause deleterious flow redistribution. Thus, in studies in which hemodynamics have been closely monitored or even controlled, adenosine,[2,34−36,39,79] carbochromen,[8,29,31,32,34,35,38,40,41,80] and dipyridamole[29,33,35,38,81] have either resulted in flow shifts from ischemic regions to normal tissue or transmural redistribution from the more ischemic endocardium to the better perfused epicardium. Even the new calcium-channel blockers nifedipine[35] and lidoflazine[80] may cause a coronary steal. In other studies in which coronary perfusion pressure was either unaltered by drug administration or regulated, neither dipyridamole[61] nor verapamil[78,82] affected collateral flow. All of these investigations have used animal models with acute coronary occlusions. Because of the absence of vasomotor tone in acute collateral channels, the chances of detecting a deleterious repartitioning of flow after treatment with vasodilators are maximized. On the other hand, those studies in animals with acute coronary occlusions purporting to demonstrate vasodilator-mediated increases in collateral flow have in general either not excluded changes in peripheral hemodynamics as possible contributors to the observed flow increases or not considered the likelihood that the ischemic flow change is the result of sample contamination by adjacent normal tissue. Thus, most reported increases in flow and/or decreases in collateral resistance caused by carbochromen,[83] dipyridamole,[83-85] nifedipine,[86-89] and diltiazem[90] are probably not related to direct effects of the drugs on collateral vessels.

Even many studies claiming that vasodilators have no or deleterious effects on acute collaterals[53-55,63,91-93] are suspect because of the uncontrolled decreases in coronary perfusion pressure. Weintraub[93] used a balloon technique to correct blood flow measurements in ischemic regions for contamination by adjacent normally perfused myocardium. Nifedipine actually decreased collateral blood flow from 0.17 to 0.14 ml/min/g ($p < 0.05$). However, because coronary perfusion pressure also fell, the diminution in flow cannot be unequivocally attributed to a direct effect of the calcium-channel entry blocker on the coronary vasculature. In one study the effect of diltiazem on collateral blood flow was evaluated after the systemic effects of the drug had dissipated,[94] and in a second investigation nifedipine was administered to running dogs and blood flow measurements again delayed until hemodynamics had returned to normal.[95] Before and 30 minutes following infusion of these vasodilators, a coronary artery was acutely occluded and collateral flow measured with radioactive microspheres. Collateral flow was unaffected, but perhaps the drugs' effects on collateral vessels had also waned by this time.

The difficulty in evaluating these investigations of pharmacologic agents on collateral blood flow is exemplified by the simultaneous appearance of three preliminary reports of the effects of the vasodilator prostacyclin (PGI_2) on collateral flow. Whereas one report claimed that PGI_2 lowered aortic pressure and had no effect on collateral blood flow,[96] a second documented an increase in collateral flow,[97] while the third found directly measured collateral flow as well as retrograde flow to decrease.[98] Thus, before conclusions about the effects of vasodilators on collateral flow can be accepted, the experimental design and protocol must be carefully evaluated.

Hence, one must be skeptical of reports suggesting that acute collaterals can be dilated by drugs. Nonetheless, two studies claim that papaverine will increase retrograde flow[63,99] and peripheral coronary pressure,[99] especially when coronary perfusion pressure is controlled.[63] Perhaps this agent is having its effect on the proximal large epicardial arteries much like nitroglycerin rather than on the collateral vessels themselves. In dogs in which the hypotensive effect of both nifedipine and diltiazem has been eliminated by simultaneous infusion of phenylephrine, administration of the calcium-channel blockers is noted to increase flows to tissue made ischemic by acute coronary ligation.[100] Although this may be a true effect of the drugs, contamination of ischemic tissue by normal myocardium with subsequent obscuration of the agents' pharmacologic actions cannot be excluded. Using the balloon technique to account for contamination, Gross et al.[101] found no change in collateral flow during intravenous infusion of nifedipine. However, when the drug-induced fall in perfusion pressure was reversed by aortic constriction, epicardial and transmural flows in the ischemic zone significantly increased. Nitroprusside increased endocardial flow in the perfusion territory of an acutely occluded left anterior descending coronary artery despite significant falls in aortic pressure.[102] Perhaps the observed effect is related to the ability of nitroprusside to dilate large conductance vessels.[21,25] One recent report by Blumenthal and colleagues[103] has also claimed that dipyridamole may significantly increase epicardial flow in the ischemic region following coronary ligation and decrease the size of the infarct. In these experimental animals, dipyridamole's systemic hemodynamic effects were minimal and the flow increases in the adjacent normal tissue were small. Thus, it is not clear how dipyridamole produced the increase in flow and resultant salvage of ischemic myocardium. In light of the studies demonstrating dipyridamole's tendency to initiate a coronary steal,[29,33,35,38,81] the report by Blumenthal is certainly curious. However, Hintze's recent report[27] of large vessel dilatation by dipyridamole in conscious dogs affords one possible explanation.

(b) Chronic coronary occlusion

Whereas one would not expect acute collaterals to respond to vasodilator drugs, chronic or partially transformed collaterals may. Golenhofen et al.[104] studied the mechanical responses of helical strips of excised collateral vessels 1½ to 2½ months after coronary occlusion produced by implanted ameroid constrictors. They observed that the collateral vessels had spontaneous basal tone and dilatory β receptors. In addition, at least the stem part of the collateral channel had α receptors. In many respects the basal smooth-muscle tone of the collateral vessels was comparable to that of normal coronary arteries of similar size, and the responses of the two types of vessels to extrinsic agents were likewise comparable. Thus, transformed collaterals should respond directly to vasoactive agents. However, even though developed collaterals may have vasomotor tone, collateral flow is still very much dependent on perfusion pressure. Thus, coronary steal has been demonstrated with both adenosine[28] and dipyridamole.[37] Other reports claiming that drugs such as dipyridamole[105] and diltiazem[106] increase collateral flow are subject to the same criticisms leveled at the studies in animals with acute collaterals. Perfusion pressure must be controlled, changes in systemic hemodynamics must be minimized, and contamination of ischemic tissue by adjacent normal myocardium must be taken into account before the conclusions that the agents dilate collaterals can be accepted. Evidence has been presented that prostacyclin (PGI$_2$),[107] diltiazem,[53,100] and nifedipine[100] may indeed dilate collaterals. In the first report,[107] the hearts with well-developed collaterals were fibrillated, excised, and perfused from donor support dogs. Thus, perfusion pressure could be maintained constant during drug infusion and systemic hemodynamic alterations and possible drug-mediated changes in extravascular resistance were avoided. Both adenosine and prostacyclin increased total coronary blood flow and produced falls in peripheral coronary pressure, presumably the result of a coronary steal. Although ischemic endocardial flow was increased by the drugs, the increase may be artifactual since adjacent normal tissue blood flow was also substantially augmented. When the adenosine infusion was discontinued, blood flow and pressure alterations faded. In the animals treated with PGI$_2$, cessation of drug administration was also followed by the expected decrease in total coronary flow. But peripheral coronary pressure rose and increased to levels higher than control. This increase in peripheral coronary pressure must be the result of collateral (and/or large epicardial vessel) dilatation. The pattern of early coronary steal initially obscuring and then being replaced by longer-lasting coronary collateral dilatation is reminiscent of the previously described effects of nitroglycerin on ischemic myocardium. This pattern was also apparent after administration of diltiazem to dogs with chronic coronary occlusions,[53] although the agent was administered intravenously and therefore produced systemic effects that had to be discounted. Initially, there was a transient rise in total coronary blood flow accompanied by declines in aortic and peripheral coronary pressures. But as blood flow returned to its predrug baseline level, both retrograde flow and peripheral coronary pressure increased significantly above control values. Again, the effect of a vasoactive agent on collateral channels lasted longer than the dilatation of the coronary arterioles. When aortic pressure was supported by phenylephrine infusion, both nifedipine and diltiazem substantially increased collateral blood flow to the myocardium distal to a chronically occluded coronary artery.[100] Hence, several agents—nitroglycerin, prostacyclin, diltiazem, and nifedipine—appear to dilate coronary collateral vessels. In seeking clinically useful agents, nonselective vasodilators of the coronary vasculature are probably not helpful, since the tendency to produce deleterious flow redistribution will obscure the salutary effect of coronary collateral dilatation. Rather, an agent that specifically dilates large epicardial and collateral vessels or only transiently affects the coronary arterioles while having a prolonged effect on the collaterals would appear to be the ideal drug. Such agents deserve to be identified.

B. Changes in Coronary Perfusion Pressure: Aortic Counterpulsation

Although modification of smooth-muscle tone or vascular resistance of the coronary collateral channels with vasodilators is the most direct means of altering flow to the ischemic myocardium, collateral perfusion is also affected indirectly by changes in perfusion pressure and extravascular resistance. Alterations in both perfusion pressure and extravascular resistance may be caused by either mechanical or pharmacologic agents. Despite the lack of specificity of these agents, they may have important effects on the volume of flow to the collateral-dependent tissue. As suggested numerous times in the above discussion, unless these indirect effects on collateral perfusion are avoided in the design of an experimental protocol, it is often impossible to conclude that a change in ischemic flow is the result of an agent's direct effect on collateral vascular resistance.

Coronary perfusion pressure is the collateral driving pressure. Because of the small pressure drop across the large epicardial vessels at normal coronary flows, the pressure at the source of the collaterals is only slightly less than aortic pressure. Coronary collaterals in the early stages of transformation are passive tubes incapable of active modification of tone. Therefore, changes in perfusion pressure would be expected to have potentially great effects on flow. Both Anrep and Haüsler[108] and Brown et al.[44–46] have demonstrated positive relationships between retrograde flow from the distal segment of an acutely occluded coronary artery and perfusion pressure, while Johansson and colleagues[43] derived similar data using isotope clearance techniques to measure collateral flow. Brown[45,46] found that changes in aortic systolic pressure from 61 to 122 mmHg had virtually no effect on retrograde flow, whereas increases in mean aortic diastolic pressure over a similar range predictably increased retrograde flow. These workers derived a quadratic expression relating mean aortic diastolic pressure to retrograde flow.

Numerous other investigations have attempted to document the effect of intraaortic balloon counterpulsation on total coronary blood flow as well as collateral flow to acutely ischemic myocardium. Because diastolic expansion of the balloon partially empties the vascular reservoir, systolic pressure during the next cardiac cycle is lower, and the left ventricle is unloaded. Diminished left ventricular work reduces the obligatory myocardial oxygen consumption, and the result may be a secondary fall in coronary blood flow to normal, contracting tissue. The increased aortic diastolic pressure itself has little effect on flow to normal myocardium, since autoregulatory processes will result in arteriolar vasoconstriction and maintenance of a stable coronary flow. Hence, virtually all investigations measuring total coronary blood flow from normally perfused, normotensive hearts have documented either virtually no change or a small decrease in flow.[109–113] The major impact of balloon pumping on the determinants of collateral flow in acutely ischemic beds unable to autoregulate is elevation of diastolic perfusion pressure, although decreases in left ventricular end-diastolic pressure and systolic wall tension are also evident and may contribute to the effect of counterpulsation on collateral flow (see below). With rare exception,[114] aortic counterpulsation has been observed to augment ischemic myocardial flow significantly,[115–122] with often greater effects on endocardial than epicardial perfusion. In addition, aortic counterpulsation has been noted successfully to diminish ischemic ST-segment elevation, the size of infarcts, and mortality following acute coronary ligation.[123,124] Of course, in these latter studies the benefits of counterpulsation could be attributed to diminished cardiac work and hence oxygen demand as well as improvement of perfusion of ischemic myocardium. One interesting study of the effect of counterpulsation in pigs with subtotal coronary stenoses demonstrated decreases in flow to myocardium perfused by the compromised vessel.[125] However, because residual antegrade flow was still present, the specific effect of diastolic balloon inflation on collateral blood flow cannot be discerned.

It is now well accepted that perfusion pressure may significantly modify collateral perfusion. It is interesting to note, however, that all of the above studies were done in animals with acute coronary occlusions. To the extent that well-developed collaterals may be able to autoregulate, the dependence of collateral flow on perfusion pressure may be less apparent. There is only indirect evidence that collaterals are able to autoregulate. In the experiments described above, which documented the ability of intracoronary nitroglycerin to dilate coronary collaterals and improve contractile function of ischemic myocardium, the success of the drug depended on the collateral-dependent myocardium being selectively ischemic.[42] If nitroglycerin were administered before the perfusion pressure had been lowered to produce differential ischemia of the myocardium or if the perfusion pressure were lowered too much so that the entire heart became ischemic, nitroglycerin was ineffective. The results of the three parts of the experiment are diagrammatically depicted in Figure 7-6, and are easily explained by assuming the collateral vessel responds to metabolic stimuli and the segment of a collateral vessel in an ischemic area dilates maximally in response to the hypoxic stimulus. Thus, at a perfusion pressure where no portion of the myocardium is ischemic, intracoronary nitroglycerin dilates the collateral vessels but no myocardial effect is possible. With the collateral-dependent tissue selectively ischemic, the collateral segment passing through the hypoxic myocardium is already maximally dilated. Nitroglycerin dilates that portion of the collateral vessel passing through normal myocardium. The enhanced collateral flow improves the contractility of the depressed myocardium. With the initiation of global ischemia, all collateral and resistance vessels are maximally dilated, and now nitroglycerin can have no effect. This analysis of the experimental data is based on the premise that the coronary collateral is responsive to its metabolic milieu. Therefore, that portion of the collateral vessel in normal myocardium at the source has vascular tone that can be modified by nitroglycerin, and is not responsive to the needs of the distant ischemic area. When the myocardium surrounding the origin of the collateral becomes ischemic, then this section of the collateral also becomes maximally dilated, and its tone can no longer be affected by nitroglycerin. Further investigation must be performed to determine if well-developed collaterals indeed have

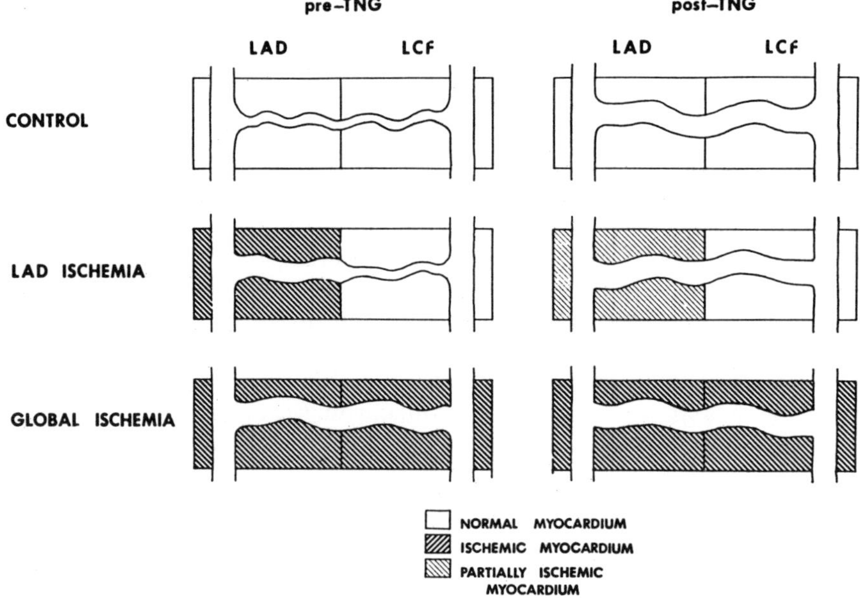

Figure 7-6   Model of collateral vascular bed before (pre-TNG) and after (post-TNG) intracoronary nitroglycerin administration under various conditions of myocardial perfusion. Changes in shading indicate changing myocardial ischemia. In the control state where no myocardium is ischemic, nitroglycerin is able to dilate the collateral vessel, but function of the already normally contracting myocardium cannot be improved. By modestly lowering coronary perfusion pressure the collateral-dependent left anterior descending (LAD) myocardium becomes ischemic, while the left circumflex (LCf) region continues to contract normally. That portion of the collateral in the ischemic muscle dilates (autoregulation), whereas the collateral in the nonischemic region retains its tone. Nitroglycerin dilates the collateral segement in the LCf territory, and thus increases collateral flow to the ischemic LAD tissue. As a result, this myocardium becomes less ischemic and contractile force is improved. If coronary perfusion pressure is lowered further, the LCf as well as the LAD myocardium becomes ischemic. Now both ends of the collateral vessel are surrounded by ischemic tissue, and the collateral is fully dilated. Nitroglycerin can have no effect on collateral tone, and therefore, cannot increase collateral flow or improve myocardial function. (Reprinted with permission of the American Society for Clinical Investigation from Cohen et al.[42])

acquired autoregulation, and whether this defense mechanism makes perfusion of the collateralized myocardium less pressure-dependent.

C. Changes in Extravascular Resistance

The effects of extravascular resistance on coronary and collateral perfusion were not well appreciated until Raff, Kosche, and Lochner published their carefully executed studies approximately 15 years ago.[126–129] They, as well as Gregg before them,[130,131] reasoned that the marked increase in left ventricular wall stress during systole would compress the coronary vasculature and impede flow. Therefore, factors accounting for increased wall stress such as enhanced contractility or a relative increase in the duration of systole as seen in tachycardia would be likely to increase systolic compression of the vasculature. Similarly, increasing end-diastolic pressure would increase diastolic wall tension and result in compression of vessels mainly in the subendocardium. Raff et al. investigated the effects of each of these three factors in preparations designed to permit significant changes of only one at a time. Thus, heart rate was changed by electrical pacing, contractility by administration of isoproterenol, and left ventricular end-diastolic pressure by intravenous infusion of barbiturates. In all experiments, aortic pressure was controlled and the coronary arteries were maximally dilated with adenosine to eliminate possible influence of changes in vascular tone. Under these conditions an increase in heart rate of 100 beats/min was found to raise extravascular resistance by 14%; an increase in left ventricular dP/dt of 1,000 mmHg/sec caused a 7.5% rise in extravascular resistance; and an elevation of left ventricular end-diastolic pressure of 10 mmHg resulted in an 11% increase in extravascular resistance. Of course, because extravascular resistance accounts for less than 15 to 20% of total coronary resistance when the coronary arteries are intrinsically normal, these increments would ordinarily have minor effects. But in animals with coronary occlusions intravascular collateral pressure is considerably lower than aortic perfusion pressure, and, therefore, it could be assumed that the collaterals would be more easily compressed and closed off by myocardial wall stresses.

In the isolated, empty, supported dog heart, wall stress and therefore extravascular resistance are eliminated. Under these conditions collateral flow to myocardium beyond a coronary occlusion is approximately 26 ml/min/100g and the left ventricular endocardial/epicardial flow ratio is 0.9.[132] When this is compared to the collateral flow of 6 ml/min/100g and endo/epi ratio of 0.5 in the in-situ beating heart, it is immediately obvious that consideration of extravascular resistance is imperative when the collateral circulation is under investigation.

Increasing heart rate causes a disproportionately greater diminution in the duration of diastole than systole. Therefore, as the heart beats faster, the time spent in systole during each minute rises while the diastolic time falls. Although Johansson et al.[43] used [85]Kr clearance techniques to measure collateral flow and observed no effect of a changing heart rate, Brown and colleagues[46] noted a small but definite decrease in retrograde flow as heart rate was raised. Schaper and Wüsten[39] have quantitated the effect of tachycardia in dogs with chronic coronary occlusion. Adenosine was used to induce maximal coronary vasodilatation so that changes in resistance could be attributed directly to the changing heart rate. In the collateralized epicardium total coronary resistance prior to induction of the tachycardia (heart rate 75–100 beats/min) was 0.3 mmHg/(ml/min)/100g, and increased negligibly to approximately 0.45 mmHg/(ml/min)/100g at 200 beats/min, a response similar to that seen in normally perfused myocardium. However, the resistance changed from 0.3 to 2.1 mmHg/(ml/min)/100g in the collateralized endocardium, a far steeper increase than that observed in normal endocardium. This increase in resistance is entirely related to a rise in the extravascular component and underscores the fact that tachycardia may have a profound effect on collateral flow and its distribution.

Left ventricular pressure and contractility also influence collateral flow by causing systolic compression of the vessels. In isolated, isovolumetrically beating, maximally vasodilated, supported dog hearts with chronic coronary occlusion, the effect of increasing left ventricular pressure was determined for normal and collateralized myocardium.[39] In both regions, total coronary resistance in the maximally dilated vascular beds correlated linearly with increasing left ventricular pressure, but the effect was more evident in the collateral-dependent region. For any given increase in left ventricular pressure the resistance in the collateralized bed increased 3.6 times more than that in normal tissues. Thus, the resistance in the collateral-dependent region increased from 0.20 in the unloaded ventricle to 0.63 mmHg/(ml/min)/100g when left ventricular pressure was 120 mmHg. As shown in Figure 7-7 increasing systolic wall stress also influences the transmural distribution of flow. Whereas the relationship between the left ventricular endo/epi flow ratio and left ventricular pressure is linear in normal areas, it is exponential in the collateralized region. With only modest increases in left ventricular pressure from 0 to 20 mmHg, the endo/epi ratio is little changed in the normal region but falls from 1.2 to 0.4 in the collateralized myocardium. Little additional change in the collateralized region is possible as left ventricular pressure is raised further because the endocardial vessels are already compressed.

In experiments in in-situ hearts with constant coronary perfusion pressure and acute coronary occlusion, Russell et al[133] also attempted to determine the inhibitory effect of cardiac contraction on collateral flow. They measured flow during resting conditions and again following cardiac arrest induced by vagal nerve stimulation. Whereas contraction had little effect on normal or collateralized epicardial flow, flows in the ischemic subendocardial layers were decreased by 50 to 71% during effective cardiac contraction, more than the 33 to 46% decrement seen in the normally perfused inner layers. These data again make apparent the adverse effects of increased extravascular resistance on coronary collateral flow.

Left ventricular end-diastolic pressure is a function of diastolic volume loading of the chamber. Although usually low, this pressure will be elevated during most forms of ventricular dysfunction, e.g., due to coronary occlusion. Normally the diastolic coronary perfusion pressure is considerably higher than this end-diastolic pressure, but following coronary occlusion the lowered intravascular peripheral coronary pressure often approaches the elevated extravascular diastolic filling pressure and hence diastolic myocardial pressure, resulting in compression of the subendocardial vasculature. Furthermore, the level of preload and end-diastolic pressure affects the distribu-

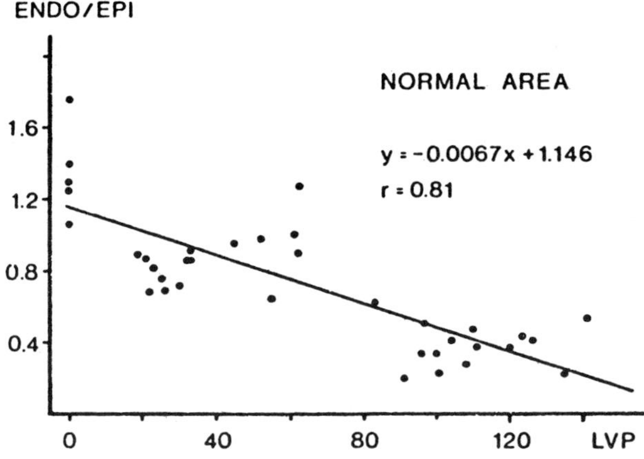

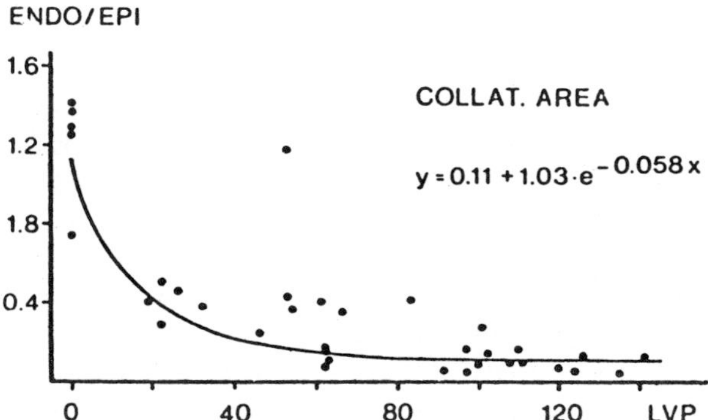

Figure 7-7   Graphs demonstrating the effect of left ventricular pressure on the left ventricular wall endocardial/epicardial flow ratio. Studies were performed in isolated, supported, isovolumetrically beating, maximally vasodilated dog hearts with chronic coronary occlusions. Thus, vascular resistance and hemodynamic variables affecting extravascular resistance could be controlled. Whereas in normally perfused myocardium there is an inverse linear relationship between the endo/epi ratio and left ventricular pressure, the endo/epi ratio changes rapidly at low values of left ventricular pressure in collateral-dependent areas and the relationship is an exponential function. Thus, the transmural flow distribution in myocardium perfused by collaterals is very much affected by intracavitary pressures and wall tension. (Reprinted with permission of Elsevier Biomedical Press from Schaper and Wüsten.[39])

tion of circumferential wall stress during the subsequent systole probably by influencing sarcomere lengths.[134] Thus, at end-diastolic pressures of 0 to 4 mmHg intramyocardial pressure is fairly uniform across the wall with higher values usually in the outer half of the ventricular wall. In contrast, when end-diastolic pressure exceeds 7 mmHg, there is a distinct transmural intramyocardial pressure gradient with the pressure in the subendocardium being substantially higher than that in the subepicardium. Kjekshus[69] acutely ligated a coronary branch and then measured the effect on collateral blood flow and distribution of a blood infusion which raised average left ventricular end-diastolic pressure from 5 to 18 mmHg. Although the infusion also increased left ventricular systolic pressure from 105 to 125 mmHg, increase in this range would be expected to have little effect on the left ventricular endo/epi flow ratio (Figure 7-7) and would account for only a 12% increase in extravascular resistance.[39] In these preparations, elevation of the end-diastolic pressure had no significant effect on ischemic epicardial flow while the endocardial flow in the collateral-dependent myocardium declined further by 30%. The endo/epi flow ratio decreased from 0.71 to 0.45.

Pharmacologic or mechanical agents that modify systemic hemodynamics and therefore extravascular coronary resistance may have little effect on perfusion of normal myocardium, but may be able to modify significantly blood flow to collateral-dependent cardiac muscle. Normal coronary arterioles are able to dilate actively to compensate for the increases in extravascular resistance that usually accompany increases in heart rate, contractility, and left ventricular systolic and end-diastolic pressures. But if the vessels are already maximally dilated and unable to decrease their vascular tone further, the increase in extravascular resistance is likely to have a significant effect. Collaterals in the early stages of transformation are unable to dilate actively, and even those collaterals with medial smooth muscle may not be able to autoregulate normally. Collateral vessels, therefore, may not be able to modify their tone when extravascular resistance increases, thus further jeopardizing the perfusion of already ischemic muscle.

D. Exercise

Exercise is a complex physiologic intervention that has been studied extensively in animals with coronary occlusions. During the exercise state there is a sympathetic drive that increases heart rate, cardiac output, and myocardial contractility. Blood pressure usually increases despite peripheral vasodilatation. The augmented heart rate and myocardial contractility increase myocardial oxygen consumption and therefore demand. The increased myocardial metabolism leads to production of vasoactive metabolites as adenosine which in turn produce coronary vasodilatation. In addition, circulating vasoactive metabolites may dilate coronary arterioles directly. The increased blood pressure also raises coronary and collateral perfusion pressures. On the other hand, catecholamines released from sympathetic nerve endings have direct vasoconstricting effects on the coronary arteries, while increased heart rate and contractility and higher left ventricular systolic and end-diastolic pressures increase extravascular coronary resistance. Because of the multiple positive and negative influences on the coronary and collateral circulation, it would be difficult to predict the net effect of exercise on collateral perfusion. Furthermore, acute and chronic collaterals would be expected to behave differently.

1. Recent Coronary Occlusion

The effect of exercise on collateral flow and myocardial function in running dogs whose left circumflex coronary artery is acutely occluded by inflation of a balloon occluder has been evaluated.[135] These studies provide a baseline and permit evaluation of the differences observed when animals with transformed collaterals are exercised. As described in Chapter 5, exercise in dogs with poorly developed collaterals at the time of balloon occlusion of the coronary artery has deleterious effects. In a group of ten dogs with average resting collateral flow of 0.33 ml/min/g, running at 4 mph and 12% grade produced a small increase in flow to 0.51 ml/min/g.[135] At the same time, flow in normal myocardium more than doubled. The increasing discrepancy between ischemic and normal myocardial blood flow during exercise in dogs with acute coronary occlusion is graphically depicted in week one flow histograms (Figures 5-5 and 5-10). Although there was a small but significant exercise-induced increase in collateral flow for this group of animals, it is noteworthy that flow during running actually declined in four dogs, and two of these four developed ventricular fibrillation after 53 and 55 seconds of the standard 60-second coronary occlusion. The precipitous rise in left atrial pressure to 30 mmHg and 40% fall in stroke volume during the one-minute coronary occlusion are satisfactory evidence that the small increase in collateral flow for the running dogs was insufficient to satisfy the increased metabolic demands of the exercise state. In Hill's evaluation of dogs approximately two days after final closure of the ameroid constrictor encircling the left circumflex artery, submaximal treadmill exercise produced an increased flow deficit and drastic deterioration of regional myocardial function.[136] Immediately following coronary occlusion the thin-walled collateral vessel is unable to respond actively to vasodilatory stimuli and, therefore, changes in collateral flow are governed by a competition between beneficial and adverse systemic hemodynamic alterations. The increased aortic and hence coronary perfusion pressure that occurs during exercise will increase collateral flow, while the increased extravascular resistance related to tachycardia and increased left ventricular systolic and diastolic wall stresses will impede perfusion of ischemic myocardium. The net result is either an absolute decrease or inadequate rise in collateral perfusion.

2. Chronic Coronary Occlusion

Collateral transformation with development of a smooth-muscle layer greatly changes the response of the collateral vasculature to the stress of exercise. Active vasodilatation in response to metabolic or pharmacologic stimulation allows the collateral channels to overcome the adverse effects of increasing extravascular resistance and to better satisfy the increased myocardial demands for oxygen and other metabolites. Six dogs studied during treadmill running one to two weeks after occlusion of the distal left anterior descending artery and mild stenosis of the left circumflex artery demonstrated two distinct responses.[28] Whereas collateral flow to the left anterior descending perfusion territory nearly doubled in three animals, there was no or only negligible change in the other three despite two- to threefold increases in flow to left circumflex myocardium. It is interesting to speculate that the limitation of flow in three of the animals was in part related to coronary steal caused by exercise-induced vasodilation of the left circumflex resistance vessels and increased pressure loss across the circumflex related to the higher flow with lower poststenosis collateral perfusion pressure. Alternatively, increases in extravascular resistance might have attenuated rises in collateral flow. In the other three animals, doubling of collateral flow was a distinct change from that seen in the animals with acute coronary occlusion, but the flow increase still lagged well behind that to the normal tissue.

Heaton et al.[137] also studied dogs two weeks following surgical implantation of an ameroid constrictor around the left anterior descending artery and stenosis of the left circumflex artery which resulted in a 60 to 90% decrease in the vessel's cross-sectional area. In these studies, the ameroid resulted in complete coronary occlusion within five days. Resting collateral and normal myocardial flows were comparable. During running at 3 mph and 5% incline, circumflex flow increased from 1.22 to 1.83 ml/min/g, while collateral flow rose from 1.16 to 1.49 ml/min/g. Although epicardial flows increased equally in the two regions, the increase in endocardial flow in the circumflex region (1.32 to 1.97 ml/min/g) was greater than that observed in the left anterior descending perfusion territory (1.10 to 1.36 ml/min/g). Thus, there appeared to be a relative endocardial hypoperfusion in the collateralized tissue accounting for a fall in the endo/epi flow ratio.

Hess and Bache[138] exercised dogs two weeks following left circumflex occlusion. Exercise collateral blood flow was 80% of normal if the amount of infarcted tissue in the samples did not exceed 25%. However, in myocardial samples in which necrotic tissue accounted for 75 to 100% of the sample's mass, exercise flow was only 11% of that in the normal muscle.

Bache and colleagues[95] measured exercise blood flows four weeks after implantation of ameroid constrictors around one of the two main branches of the left coronary artery. Whereas resting flow (1.08 ± 0.06 ml/min/g) and perfusion of the collateralized myocardium during mild exercise (heart rate 190 beats/min) were normal, the increment in flow during severe exercise (230 beats/min) was significantly less than that in normal tissue. Thus, flow was 3.16 ± 0.26 ml/min/g in normal myocardium and 2.22 ± 0.34 ml/min/g in the collateralized regions ($p < 0.05$). Furthermore, the endo/epi flow ratio in the myocardium beyond the occluded coronary artery declined sequentially from 1.12 at rest to 0.83 and 0.61 during the two levels of exercise. In contrast, transmural flow continued to be preferentially distributed to the normal endocardium at rest and during exercise. Thus, collateral vascular reserve was shown to be deficient only with moderately strenuous exercise. Sufficient collateral development had already occurred to meet the heart's needs adequately at rest and during low-level stress.

Endocardial hypoperfusion was also seen in some of the other dogs studied by Bache[139] approximately one month after occlusion of a coronary artery by an implanted ameroid constrictor. He measured myocardial flows and collected coronary sinus blood for detection of abnormal metabolites during light (average heart rate 185 beats/min) and heavy (average heart rate 230 beats/min) exercise. In four dogs epicardial flow in the collateralized myocardium increased normally from 0.91 ml/min/g at rest to 2.28 and 2.97 ml/min/g during light and heavy exercise, respectively. However, endocardial flow that was normal at rest (0.98 ml/min/g) actually declined during light exercise (0.65 ml/min/g) and fell further during heavy exercise (0.49 ml/min/g). This abnormal endocardial flow response was accompanied by production of abnormal myocardial metabolites. In a second group of five dogs, endocardial flows increased during exercise, although the increases were substantially less than those of the epicardial layers where flow increments were normal. The observation that the epicardium becomes fully collateralized before the endocardium is not surprising. Distribution of transmural wall stresses as well as the favored epicardial location of collateral vessels in the normal canine heart make the collateralization process easier in the outer myocardial layers.

In Bache's study[139] there was a third group of five dogs in which both endocardial and epicardial flows to collateral-dependent myocardium increased normally during exercise stress. Epicardial flows rose from an average resting value of 0.82 ml/min/g to 2.27 and 2.92 ml/min/g during the two stages of exercise studied. Resting endocardial flows averaged 1.11 ml/min/g with increases to 2.48 and 3.48 ml/min/g during light and heavy exercise, respectively. In these five dogs the endo/epi flow ratio exceeded 1.0 at rest, and there was no evidence of transmural redistribution during exercise. It is remarkable that in as few as four weeks following coronary occlusion the collaterals in these animals could have developed to such a degree that flows could increase normally to more than 3 ml/min/g. Although collateral development is the most likely explanation of these dramatic results, the lack of collateral flow measurements immediately following coronary occlusion leaves the nagging possibility that these five animals had excellent collateral flows even at the beginning of the protocol, and that little collateral development occurred in the subsequent four weeks. That this is not such a remote possibility is demonstrated by the observation in one dog studied by Cohen and Yipintsoi[140] of a collateral/normal blood flow ratio of 0.97 during sudden balloon occlusion of the left circumflex artery. Decline of the coronary flow probe signal to zero insured cessation of antegrade flow and proper functioning of the balloon occluder. It is unlikely that Bache studied five dogs like this, but the possibility must be entertained.

Others have also studied the effect of exercise on collateral flow in animals with well-developed collaterals. Schaper (personal communication) measured equal normal and collateral exercise blood flows of approximately 3 ml/min/g three months after implantation of ameroid constrictors and subsequent coronary occlusion. However, in other studies in dogs running at 10 km/hr and 16% incline,[39] he has noted myocardial flow to normal areas to increase to 6−8 ml/min/g, while flow to collateralized regions increased to only 2.5 ml/min/g. Fedor et al.[141] were able to distinguish two different flow responses to exercise 11 to 12 weeks after ameroid implantation. In one group normal myocardial flow increased to 3.18 ml/min/g and the endo/epi flow ratio remained greater than 1.0. The increase in total collateral flow to 2.65 ml/min/g in these same animals was significantly less than the increase to normal tissue, and the endo/epi flow ratio in the collateralized tissue fell to less than 1.0. This evidence of endocardial hypoperfusion resembles Bache's data.[95,139] Fedor and colleagues[141] also identified a second group of dogs with normal responses of the collateralized endocardium and epicardium to exercise. Lambert et al.[142] studied dogs during mild and moderate exercise six and a half months after implantation of ameroid constrictors. The increases in flow to the collateralized myocardium from average resting values of 0.97 ml/min/g to 2.14 and 3.25 ml/min/g during the two exercise levels exceeded the increments to the normal regions. Furthermore, the endo/epi flow ratios were normal. These authors were unable to discern any differences in regional or transmural blood flow between these exercising animals with chronically occluded vessels and a second group with all coronary arteries patent.[143]

Cohen and Yipintsoi[140] also studied six dogs with chronic left circumflex occlusions. Prior to the permanent obstruction, transient acute occlusion of the vessel proved the inadequacy of the existing collaterals. Average resting collateral flow was initially 0.53 ml/min/g or 37% of normal tissue flow. During running at 4 mph and 12% grade collateral flow increased to only 0.66 ml/min/g and the endocardial/epicardial flow ratio was 0.53. Following chronic coronary artery occlusion the effect of exercise on coronary collateral flow was again examined. This time, running increased collateral flow from 1.54 to 3.93 ml/min/g with an exercise endo/epi flow ratio of 0.97. These flow data and those from the normal left anterior descending myocardium were virtually identical. Flow histograms (Figures 5-5 and 5-10) demonstrate the equivalence of flows to the normal and collateralized tissue both at rest and during exercise.

Thus, in most of these experimental studies blood flow to chronically collateralized myocardium is normal at rest and increases normally during the stress of exercise. This evidence strongly suggests that transformed collaterals are able to dilate actively in response to the increased metabolic demands and augmented sympathetic drive of the exercise state. This vasomotor tone and the ability to change it accounts for the very different responses of acute and chronic collaterals. Of course, as already explained, a normal flow response to exercise should not imply that the collaterals have completely restored normal coronary reserve to the collateralized myocardium. Fedor et al.[141] have demonstrated relative endocardial hypoperfusion during right ventricular pacing at heart rates of approximately 200 beats/min in those dogs that had normal collateral flow responses to exercise, and Schaper[144] determined that collateral conductance was only 40% of normal vessel conductance in those dogs in which collateral flow increased normally during running.

Although the collateral flow response to a complex stimulus such as exercise can be normal, the degree of collateral transformation is obviously critical, as it was in the evaluation of drug effects on collateral perfusion. The response of the collateral circulation to any pharmacologic or mechanical agent or other stimulus must be interpreted in light of the degree of collateral development, and any complete investigation of the influence of an intervention must seek to establish its effects on collateral vessels appearing after both acute and chronic coronary occlusions.

E. Nonvasoactive Pharmacologic Agents

Clearly, the number of agents that can be evaluated is endless. This discussion has been concerned mainly with vasodilators, counterpulsation, and exercise. Drugs ordinarily not considered to have vasoactive properties should not be overlooked in future investigations. For example, aspirin has been reported to increase collateral flow after acute coronary occlusion, possibly because of its ability to block prostaglandin synthesis.[145] Mannitol was also thought to be effective in increasing acute collateral perfusion,[121,122,146,147] although a more recent investigation[148] has suggested the initial positive reports were inaccurate because of the failure to account for mannitol's effect on flow in adjacent normal myocardium and the contaminating overlap flow component. This latter observation underscores the necessity for careful evaluation of results when collateral flow is being measured. When flow to normal myocardium is increased, it is imperative that the investigator insure that simultaneously observed rises in collateral flow are independent of the possible artifactual contamination of ischemic samples by normal tissue. Investigators must also be aware of the agent's systemic hemodynamic effects, which may complicate interpretation of the results, and therefore should consider intracoronary application to determine direct effects on the collateral circulation.

II. Stimulation of Collateral Development

Only modification of collateral flow by a pharmacologic agent or other intervention at some finite point in time has been discussed. Identification of coronary collateral vasodilators and manipulations that can increase collateral flow has important clinical significance which justifies the continuing search. Another area that has intrigued physiologists and pharmacologists is the possible stimulation of collateral growth and development. Increased or more rapid growth of collaterals following coronary occlusion would minimize the duration of ischemic complications. A logical extrapolation of this reasoning would be the attempt to stimulate collateral growth even before the occurrence of coronary occlusion. If collateral development could be initiated in the animal with normal coronary arteries, then subsequent coronary obstruction would have minimal functional significance. This form of protection would clearly be highly desirable, and the clinical value of the agents offering such protection would be immeasurable.

A. Trigger of Collateral Development

It should be obvious from the multiple studies reviewed in the foregoing chapters that probably the most potent stimulus of coronary collateral development is coronary occlusion itself. It is, of course, self-evident that the goal is the ability to stimulate collateral development in the absence of coronary occlusion. Most of the interventions that have successfully influenced collateral growth cannot be used in the clinical arena. Nonetheless, even these latter interventions provide insight into the pathophysiology of collateral development.

It is widely assumed that myocardial hypoxia and/or creation of a pressure gradient across the collateral vessel somehow triggers collateral growth and development. However, the precise biophysical force or biochemical transmitter responsible for the initiation of collateral transformation is as yet unknown. Schaper[149-151] believes that increased tangential wall stress or tension is involved. According to the LaPlace relationship, wall tension (T) is proportional to the product of luminal pressure (P) and radius (r) and inversely proportional to wall thickness (h), or $T\alpha\,[(P\cdot r)/h]$. Schaper has theorized that dilatation of the thin-wall collateral from any cause will cause the r term of the expression to increase, resulting in a rise in wall tension. To restore tension to its equilibrium value, wall thickness, or h, will then increase until wall tension is again normal. Normalization of wall tension thus removes the stimulus for further increases in wall thickness, although the remodeling process is not necessarily terminated. Scheel's recent investigation[152] in dogs after four weeks of aortic banding perhaps lessens the significance of tangential wall stress as a stimulus of collateral transformation. In these animals with increased supravalvular pressures (average initial pressure gradient across the constriction = 46 mmHg), coronary perfusion pressures were chronically higher and tangential wall stress in the collateral channels would have logically increased. Yet there was no functional evidence of increased collateral development.

Humoral factors may play a significant role in the development of collateral vessels following occlusion of the native vessel. Cell hypoxia causes the release of products of anaerobic metabolism and intracellular constituents such as potassium from injured cells. These substances are themselves potent vasodilators. Cuttino et al.[153] presented evidence that a mitogenic factor was produced by ischemic renal tissue several weeks following renal artery stenosis. Additional evidence that implicates production by hypoxic tissue of a chemical substance that promotes cell division is found in the radioautographic studies of Schaper[154] and Ilich.[155] Schaper studied myocardium after coronary occlusion, while Ilich examined renal tissue following critical renal artery stenosis. Both investigators injected ^{3}H-thymidine to label dividing cells, and noted many mitoses in the collateral vessels themselves. However, Schaper also found evidence of cell division in vessels, fibroblasts and mesenchymal cells in the surrounding normal myocardium, and Ilich noted an increase in the labeling index of endothelial cells of the renal vein and periureteric vessels and epithelial cells of the ureters. These are areas and structures that are unlikely to experience biophysical forces, such as increased blood flow or tangential wall stress, which have been postulated to stimulate growth of collaterals to occluded arteries. A likely explanation for this evidence of mitotic activity at a distance would be local production of a circulating humoral factor.

B. Coronary Stenosis

The ability of a coronary constriction or stenosis to stimulate growth of coronary collaterals has been noted by several investigators.[39,132,156−167] Pigs which normally have very few coronary collaterals develop intercoronary anastomoses in as little as two days following narrowing of a major coronary artery with the aid of a 0.8-mm probe placed next to the vessel and then removed after secure ligation of an encircling suture.[156] In these same animals a rich network of collaterals which protected some from sudden death following total vessel occlusion was documented by postmortem coronary injection studies 12 days after creation of the stenosis.

Gregg and his colleagues[159−163] clearly demonstrated that coronary collateral indices in dogs improved during the period of progressive coronary constriction prior to total occlusion resulting from implantation of one of several occlusive devices. Implanted hydraulic or mercury-filled cuffs or ameroid constrictors occluded the coronary artery gradually over three to six days. During this interval peripheral coronary pressure, retrograde flow, and clearance of radioactive isotopes were measured during transient total occlusion of the vessel by a second occluder.[159−161,163] In one additional experimental protocol a flowmeter around the coronary vessel distal to the occluder permitted measurement of actual residual or collateral flow in the vessel following cessation of antegrade flow.[162] Significant increases in all collateral indices as well as directly measured collateral flow were observed during the process of vessel narrowing. Evidence of increasing collateral flow was apparent before antegrade flow had ceased. The greatest increase in collateral function was observed after the coronary stenosis had progressed to the point where release of the transient test coronary occlusion was unaccompanied by a reactive hyperemic response. Gregg[163] reported that stable constriction of the left circumflex artery which created a 10 mmHg gradient across the stenosis had no effect on left circumflex inflow but significantly diminished the vessel's reactive hyperemic response. After four to six days, peripheral coronary pressure following transient occlusion of the stenotic vessel had increased two- to fivefold and ^{133}Xe clearance from the ischemic myocardium had increased to equal that from the same myocardial area prior to critical coronary constriction. Gregg also noted that stenoses that produced higher gradients and were observed for longer intervals produced even greater evidence of collateral development.

Radioautographic studies support the physiologic evidence that coronary stenoses can stimulate collateral development. Pasyk and his co-workers[167] gradually constricted coronary arteries of dogs over periods of 36 hours to 5 days with previously implanted mercury-filled cuffs. Twenty-four hours after complete coronary occlusion the hearts were removed and the coronary arteries perfused with blood to which ^{3}H-thymidine had been added. Collaterals identified by coronary injection of micronized barium sulphate were excised and prepared for autoradiography. In general, the labeling index of dividing cells increased as the period of constriction prior to total occlusion lengthened. Thus, growth of collateral vessels began soon after initiation of coronary constriction, and progressed for the duration of the period of constriction.

Gregg's data[159–163] suggest that the process of collateral development is somehow dependent on the impairment of the reactive hyperemic response of the stenotic vessel. Because reactive hyperemia is a measure of a vessel's dilatory reserve, stressful situations would result in exhaustion of the already limited reserve of the vascular bed of the constricted vessel with subsequent production of myocardial ischemia. This chain of events might provide the stimulus for collateral development. Of course, because the stenoses usually did not significantly affect resting coronary arterial inflow, hypoxic episodes in these sedentary animals would not be expected to be frequent. In these situations, it is therefore possible that the always present pressure gradient across the collateral vessel rather than the myocardial hypoxia itself was the stimulus for collateral development.

Others have also noted that a critical coronary stenosis is necessary before collateral growth becomes apparent. Sewell[158] has written that the coronary lumen must be decreased to 4 to 10% of its normal size before collateral stimulation is observed. Millard[164] narrowed the coronary artery of 10-kg domestic pigs by approximately 50%. Over the ensuing six to eight weeks as the pigs grew to 30 kg, the relative severity of the fixed stenosis increased. At the end of the observation period the vessel was still patent. Endocardial and epicardial flows in the perfusion territory of the stenotic vessel following the vessel's occlusion were 0.49 and 0.85 ml/min/g, respectively. When compared to baseline collateral flows of less than 0.05 ml/min/g following acute coronary occlusion in the pig, the significance of the collateral development is apparent. Schaper[132] created stenoses of varying severity in dogs. "Mild" to "moderate" narrowings had no effect on collateral development, and subsequent total occlusion of these constricted vessels produced areas of infarction similar in size to those observed in animals with occlusion of previously normal vessels. On the other hand, prior stenosis of 80−90% did stimulate growth of collaterals, and subsequent total occlusion of the vessel produced only small areas of necrosis.

Schaper[165] narrowed the left circumflex artery of dogs with an implanted Teflon ring which diminished the peak reactive hyperemic response following release of a transient coronary occlusion by 50%. After six weeks a circumflex branch and a comparable branch of an adjacent artery were ligated. The size of the infarct related to occlusion of the circumflex branch was significantly smaller than that caused by ligation of the neighboring branch (19% versus 52% of the risk region). In further experiments[166] the stenotic vessel was occluded after five weeks. Eleven dogs developed large infarcts, whereas six did not. In the 11 with infarcts collateral flow was poor before stenosis and changed little over the ensuing five weeks (0.12 to 0.15 ml/min/g). In contrast, collateral flow increased markedly from 0.22 to 1.02 ml/min/g during the five-week period of coronary stenosis in the six dogs not developing infarcts after coronary occlusion. Therefore, stenosis stimulated collateral development and increased collateral perfusion.

Both Eckstein[157] and Schaper and Wüsten[39] have attempted to quantitate the influence of coronary stenosis on collateral development. Eckstein[157] narrowed the left circumflex coronary artery of dogs with the aid of probes with diameters varying from 0.75 to 1.3 mm. The probes were placed next to the vessel, tightly secured in an encircling ligature, and then removed. After six to eight weeks the left circumflex artery was cannulated distal to the ligature. Aortic pressure was adjusted to 100 mmHg and then timed antegrade flow through the stenosis was collected. This flow, which was inversely related to the degree of vessel narrowing, was used as a marker of the severity of the stenosis. Retrograde flow was employed as an index of collateral development. There was a reciprocal, nonlinear relationship between retrograde flow from the distal vessel and antegrade flow through the stenosis. A stenosis which approximately halved the 700−800 ml/min/100g flow through a normal left circumflex artery opened to atmospheric pressure was required before retrograde flow began to increase above the level measured in dogs with acute coronary occlusions. With more severe stenoses and further limitation of antegrade flow, retrograde flow rose rapidly.

Schaper and Wüsten[39] slightly modified Eckstein's approach. They placed Teflon rings with inner diameters of 1.5−2.0 mm around the left circumflex artery. This constriction resulted in diminution of the peak reactive hyperemic response following transient total occlusion of the circumflex vessel to 24−60% of the control level prior to stenosis. After ten weeks these hearts were removed and studied in an isolated, perfused, nonworking heart preparation. Maximal vasodilation was produced by adenosine infusion. Total blood flow through the stenosis was measured by an encircling flow probe while collateral blood flow to the myocardium beyond the constriction was assessed with radioactive microspheres injected during transient circumflex occlusion. As shown in Figure 7-8 an inverse relationship between stenosis flow and collateral blood flow is apparent. The conclusions are similar to those of Eckstein.[157] As the constriction becomes more severe, increasingly limiting blood flow through the stenosis, the development of the collateral circulation is accelerated and the conductive capacity of these vessels progressively enhanced. The best mathematical fit to the data points was an exponential function curve.

Thus, coronary constriction is a definite stimulus for the development and transformation of coronary collaterals. As the stenosis becomes more severe, the stimulus becomes more intense. Coronary occlusion merely represents one end of the spectrum. Of course these observations cannot

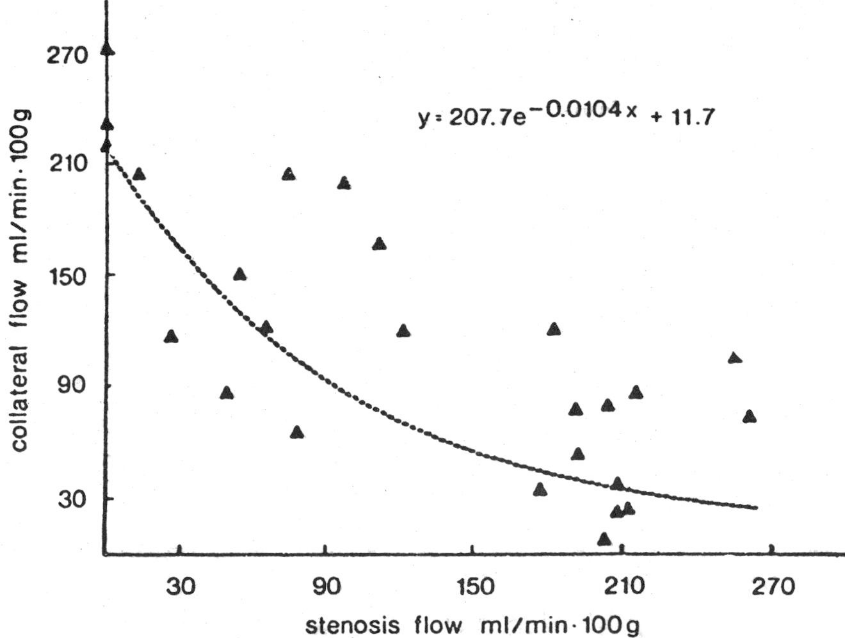

Figure 7-8   Relationship between collateral flow in dogs with chronic coronary artery stenoses and residual antegrade flow through the stenosed vessels. Teflon rings with internal diameters of 1.5 – 2.0 mm were implanted around the left circumflex arteries, and ten weeks later the hearts were removed and studied in an isolated, perfused, maximally vasodilated, nonworking heart preparation. Total antegrade blood flow through the stenosis was measured by an encircling external flow probe, while collateral flow was measured with radioactive microspheres during transient circumflex occlusion. A definite inverse relationship between stenosis flow and collateral flow is evident. Thus, as the constriction became more severe, resulting in increasing limitation of antegrade flow, the development of the collateral circulation was accelerated and the conductive capacity of these vessels progressively enhanced. (Reprinted with permission of Elsevier Biomedical Press from Schaper and Wüsten.[39])

prove the identity of the precise trigger. Collateral stimulation by less severe arterial narrowings may well be related to the development of a transcollateral pressure gradient. However, with more severe constrictions the ensuing myocardial ischemia and hypoxia are likely to play a role.

C. Hypoxemia

Hypoxia with resulting diminished myocardial oxygenation may itself be a primary trigger of coronary collateral development. However, like coronary constriction and occlusion, the willful production of hypoxia to stimulate collateral growth will not find ready clinical acceptance. But this approach does promote further understanding of the pathophysiology of collateral stimulation.

Day and colleagues[168,169] created a pulmonary artery−left atrial shunt in dogs with a 10−15-mm side-to-side anastomosis which diverted desaturated blood into the systemic circulation. Approximately 20% of the cardiac output passed through the shunt, resulting in an arterial oxygen saturation of 75 to 88%. After two to four weeks, closure of the shunt and ligation of the left circumflex artery resulted in 10% mortality within one hour, compared to 72% in a control series of experiments. These authors studied the collateral circulation in postmortem hearts by vinyl plastic coronary injections and then corrosion digestion. Whereas in control hearts their technique revealed no anastomoses between right and left coronary arteries and left-to-left collaterals in only 30% of specimens, 60% of animals with shunts had vascular connections between right and left coronary arteries and all had left-to-left collateral vessels. Furthermore, many of the casts from hypoxemic animals demonstrated retrograde filling of the distal ligated left circumflex artery and its branches from the directly injected left anterior descending artery. But MacLean et al.[170] were unable to document increased collateral blood flow measured with D_2O in empty, beating hearts six weeks to six months after creation of a pulmonary artery−left atrial shunt. Bishop and Bloor[171] adopted a similar approach to study the effects of chronic hypoxia on the heart. They surgically transposed the caudal vena cava of dogs to the left atrium, which successfully lowered the arterial oxygen saturation to 70%. Eighteen to thirty months after this initial surgery, balloon occluders were implanted around the left circumflex coronary artery of the animals. Normal dogs were treated similarly. Seven to fourteen days later coronary flow was measured in all animals with radioactive microspheres before, and 5 minutes, and 24 hours after inflation of the balloon and occlusion of the coronary artery. Gross infarct size as a percentage of the left ventricular mass averaged 17% in the normal dogs but only 6% in the hypoxemic animals. Prior to coronary occlusion, blood flow was homogeneously distributed to all parts of the left ventricle in both groups of dogs. Five minutes after coronary occlusion the ratio of flows in the infarcted to the noninfarcted epicardium of normal dogs was 0.31, whereas this ratio in the hypoxemic dogs was 0.80. The flow ratio of infarcted to noninfarcted endocardial tissue was 0.16 in normal and 0.56 in hypoxemic dogs. All flow ratios increased significantly by 24 hours. It is apparent that the collateral flows were significantly higher in the animals with surgically created shunts and resulting hypoxemia, and these higher flows accounted for the smaller infarcts. Hence, mild to moderate lowering of the arterial oxygen saturation for weeks to months can induce development of the coronary collateral circulation. Obviously, in these experiments there was never a pressure gradient across the collaterals until occlusion of a coronary artery in the final stage of the investigation. Myocardial hypoxia must therefore be able to trigger the transformation process.

D. Anemia

The effect of decreased oxygen-carrying capacity of the blood has also been studied by creating anemia in pigs[156] and dogs[172,173] by repeated venesection. Stable hematocrits of 15−30% have been produced, and in one protocol[173] average hemoglobin levels of 5.6 g/100ml were maintained for six weeks by feeding the dogs an iron-deficient diet. In the early studies of Zoll and Norman[156] coronary occlusion in the normal pig always had a disastrous outcome. However, anemia for as little as two weeks prior to coronary occlusion significantly increased the number of intercoronary anastomoses visualized in the postmortem heart injected with Schlesinger's lead-agar mass and improved survival after vessel ligation. These semiqualitative data were confirmed by Eckstein[172] in the dog. He measured retrograde flow in control and anemic animals after adjusting aortic pressure to 100 mmHg. Whereas retrograde flow was 3.8 ml/min in the control preparations, it averaged 17 ml/min in the anemic dogs. Furthermore, more anemic dogs had no or negligible electrocardiographic changes when the left circumflex artery was clamped. But Eckstein was concerned that the diminished blood viscosity might be contributing to the high retrograde flow in the dogs with anemia. Therefore, he acutely bled normal dogs and replaced the blood volume with saline. These animals with low hemoglobin concentrations and diminished blood viscosity had retrograde flows averaging 8.6 ml/min, considerably less than the 17 ml/min rate in the chronically anemic dogs with comparable hematocrits and similar blood viscosities. Finally, some of the chronically anemic animals were transfused with packed red blood cells to restore the hemoglobin level to normal. Retrograde flow in these transfused dogs averaged 9.6 ml/min, still significantly higher than in control dogs. Only 23% of the transfused dogs had significant electrocardiographic evidence of ischemia, in contrast to 70% of the control group which demonstrated marked changes.

More recently, Scheel et al.[173] reexamined the effect of anemia on coronary collateral development. After six weeks of a 15% hematocrit, the hearts of the experimental dogs were isolated and perfused with whole blood. Dipyridamole was added to the blood reservoir to produce maximal vasodilatation. Coronary flows were higher and resistances lower in the hearts from the anemic animals. A leftward shift of the coronary pressure-flow curve during maximal vasodilation suggested new vascular growth. Collateral flow was evaluated by measuring retrograde flow from all three major coronary arteries. The average retrograde flows for the left anterior descending, left circumflex, and right coronary arteries of hearts from anemic dogs were 31%, 28%, and 60%, respectively, higher than those from identically prepared control hearts. Despite the substantial differences, the changes were not significant because of the wide differences in collateralization among individual dogs.

E. Vasodilators

Hypoxemia and anemia appear to stimulate collateral growth. Although it is not known for certain, some investigators reasoned that these two stimuli cause inadequate oxygen delivery to the myocardium and therefore compensatory maximal vasodilatation of the coronary vasculature. It was further postulated that this chronic vascular dilatation could be the specific trigger of the resulting collateral transformation. Extrapolation of this reasoning suggested that chronic drug-induced vasodilatation might have similar effects. Because the administration of vasoactive agents is simple and could, if successful, be used clinically to promote collateral growth, great interest was aroused. Accordingly, the effects of chronic administration of several vasodilators and other promising drugs were evaluated in both pigs and dogs with normal coronary arteries, but without uniform success.

1. Dipyridamole

Perhaps the most frequently examined vasodilator has been dipyridamole. Autoradiographic[174,175] and morphometric[176] studies by Tornling and his co-workers have demonstrated that dipyridamole administered to rats for several weeks causes proliferation of capillary wall cells in the heart[174] and skeletal muscle,[175] and a 22% increase in skeletal muscle capillary density and 24% rise in capillary/muscle fiber ratio.[176] Thus, chronic vasodilatation does stimulate vascular growth, perhaps triggered by the increase in tangential wall stress resulting from the pharmacologically mediated increase in internal vascular dimensions.

Many of the older studies examining the effect of dipyridamole on coronary collateral development are somewhat unsatisfying because of the use of survival rates following coronary occlusion as the only measure of functional significance of drug administration and reliance on the qualitative angiographic analysis of the collateral circulation. Vineberg and his colleagues[177] began administration of dipyridamole to dogs two days before implantation of ameroid constrictors around both the left circumflex and left anterior descending coronary arteries and continued treatment until dogs died spontaneously or were sacrificed. The treated dogs, thus, received the drug during the three weeks of gradually progressing constriction of the vessels. Only 2 of 13 untreated dogs survived up to three months following surgery, whereas 6 of 12 dogs receiving dipyridamole survived for this interval. Postmortem angiograms done by the Schlesinger technique revealed much better retrograde opacification of the left coronary system following injection of the right coronary artery in the treated animals. Eleven control dogs died within 60 days of ameroid implantation. Seven of these animals had no evidence of right-to-left collaterals and only one had "good" collaterals (retrograde opacification of at least 50% of the major arteries but no filling of the smaller branches). Six treated dogs died from 12 to 27 days after surgery. Only one had no collaterals and four had "good" collaterals. The remaining two control animals were sacrificed at six and eight months after surgery and both had "good" collaterals. In contrast, the remaining six treated dogs either died or were sacrificed at four to nine months; one had "good" collaterals and the other five demonstrated "complete collateralization" (total retrograde opacification of major arteries and smaller branches of the left coronary system with reflux of angiographic mass through the left ostium).

Laustela[178] implanted ameroid constrictors around the left circumflex and left anterior descending coronary arteries of dogs and then, using a blinded protocol, treated one-half of the operated dogs with dipyridamole and the remaining dogs with a placebo. After ten to twelve weeks the left coronary artery of survivors was acutely ligated. Postmortem coronary injection studies revealed that dogs that received dipyridamole had better evidence of collaterals, and the duration of survival following coronary ligation was correlated with the degree of collateral formation.

Asada et al.[179] produced vessel narrowing by wrapping gelatin sponges containing dicetyl phosphate around the coronary artery. Fibrosis and granulation tissue produced constriction but, of course, it was not possible to know that the stenoses were equivalent in each animal. Dogs were started on dipyridamole during the period of gradual constriction. Collaterals were evaluated by postmortem injection studies. Treated dogs had more collaterals even when treated and untreated animals with similar degrees of coronary narrowing were compared. Treated dogs also had increased tolerance to hypoxia. When the oxygen content of the inspired gas was decreased, electrocardiographic changes of myocardial ischemia appeared at lower arterial oxygen contents in the dogs that had received dipyridamole.

Other investigators have pretreated pigs[180,181] and dogs[57,182–187] with dipyridamole for longer intervals before any manipulation of the coronary arteries. Ameroid constrictors were implanted in pigs following 13 to 16 months of dipyridamole administration.[180] All control animals died spontaneously, while 16 of 18 treated pigs lived for at least three months. Postmortem angiograms revealed that the treated pigs had numerous collaterals in contrast to the striking paucity in control animals. Halmagyi's investigations[181] in pigs were comparable. Similar conclusions were also made by Meesmann and Bachmann[183,184] who evaluated the treatment of dogs with dipyridamole for 7 to 36 weeks by doing postmortem angiography with a gelatin-barium sulphate mixture capable of filling arterioles but not capillaries. Injection into one coronary artery revealed no retrograde filling of the other coronary arteries in 7 of the 15 control hearts and only minimal cross-over in the other 8 hearts. On the other hand, all hearts from treated dogs demonstrated obvious retrograde filling of one vessel when a second coronary artery was injected antegradely. In this study, pretreatment for as few as seven weeks had the same effect on the collateral circulation as drug administration for longer intervals. In Suzuki's investigation,[186] the development of collaterals was monitored in each dog by performing serial coronary arteriography. Pretreated dogs had faster development of collaterals and less evidence of myocardial infarction after occlusion of the left anterior descending artery than control animals.

Attempts to quantitate collateral development in animals being treated with dipyridamole have involved measurement of collateral indices or collateral flow directly. Schmidt and Schmier[185] administered the drug to dogs for 3 to 23 weeks and then ligated a coronary artery. Arterial pressure was better maintained and there was less mortality from ventricular fibrillation in the treated group. Furthermore, retrograde flows in the treated animals were higher. These hemodynamic data were supported by corrosion casts which revealed a denser arterial network in the dogs that had received dipyridamole prior to coronary ligation. There were multiple arterio-arterial anastomoses in the perfusion territory of the ligated coronary artery in the treated animals which were not present in the controls. Schmier[188] subsequently pretreated dogs with dipyridamole for six weeks before ligating the left anterior descending coronary artery. Peripheral coronary artery pressure in these animals was 38.5 mmHg, whereas it was less than 10 mmHg in matched controls. The mortality was 91% in the control group and only 15.3% in the treated dogs. Again, Araldite corrosion casts in some dogs and barium sulphate injections in others revealed many larger collaterals in those animals that received dipyridamole. In the control animals, only 2% of coronary collaterals were as large as 200−300 μm, and there were none larger. In contrast, 7% of collaterals in treated dogs had diameters of 200−300 μm, and 5% exceeded this size. Fam et al.[182] confirmed the ability of long-term treatment of dogs with dipyridamole to promote collateral development. Retrograde flow in animals pretreated with the vasodilator for 10.5 to 23 weeks averaged 8.3 ml/min, whereas it was only 3.8 ml/min in control animals ($p < 0.025$).

Rees and Redding[187] measured ^{133}Xe clearance from myocardium beyond an acute left anterior descending coronary occlusion in control dogs and in dogs treated with dipyridamole for three months. Clearance of the isotope was 29% higher in the treated group, but the difference was not statistically significant ($p < 0.2$). However, the 50% increase in a proposed index of collateral capacity (^{133}Xe clearance/perfusion pressure) was significant ($p < 0.01$). Postmortem injection of a radiopaque solution also revealed more collateral vessels in the pretreated animals.

Despite all of the foregoing studies that have concluded that dipyridamole stimulates collateral development, Schaper's data [57] are not in agreement. His is the only study in which collateral flow was measured directly with radioactive microspheres. Although average collateral flow was higher in the animals pretreated with dipyridamole, the wide scatter of data points in the control and experimental groups made the difference statistically insignificant. Schaper's study is clearly outnumbered by those insisting dipyridamole can stimulate collaterals, but it is disturbing that the only investigation that has directly quantitated the action of the drug on collateral flow was unable to detect a significant effect. Even the ^{133}Xe clearance and flow data of Rees and Redding[187] did not reveal a difference between control and pretreated animals, although a derived index of collateral capacitance was successful at distinguishing one group from the other. More investigations such as Schaper's must be done. Additional careful studies of the functional and quantitative effects of chronic coronary vasodilatation with dipyridamole are necessary to provide data about this specific agent as well as information about the general applicability of chronic administration of vasodilators to coronary collateral stimulation.

2. Nitroglycerin, Nitrates, and Nitrites

As previously described, nitroglycerin and related nitrates dilate coronary collaterals in experimental animals with chronic coronary occlusions. However, few studies have been done with these agents to determine their ability to stimulate collateral growth in animals with normal coronary vessels. Zoll and Norman[156] treated pigs with sodium nitrite for two weeks and then studied the collateral circulation with postmortem injections of Schlesinger's lead-agar mass. Although they concluded that this vasodilator stimulated collateral growth, the evidence is tenuous. Only four pigs were in the treatment group and one had 2+ anastomoses. Because only 2 of the 132 animals in the control group had 1+ anastomoses, the difference between control and treated pigs was considered significant. However, the small number of experimental animals and the semiquantitative nature of the postmortem examination make one question the accuracy of the conclusions. Pentaerythritol tetranitrate was administered to pigs seven days before implantation of ameroid constrictors in one study[189] and to dogs two days prior to coronary embolization of steel cylinders in another investigation.[190] The only evidence that pretreatment had any effect was lower mortality rates in the animals receiving the nitrate before coronary occlusion[189,190] and less hemodynamic deterioration immediately following the occlusion.[190] Claims of decreased mortality in dogs pretreated with isosorbide dinitrate shortly before coronary occlusion have also been made.[191] Obviously, it is not possible to conclude whether there was any effect on coronary collaterals in these last three studies. These limited results reveal the level of our ignorance about the effects of drug pretreatment, and underscore the necessity of undertaking future investigations to demonstrate the possible utility of this approach.

3. Calcium-Channel Blocking Agents

Lidoflazine, a calcium-channel blocking agent, dilates coronary as well as systemic arteriolar resistance vessels. Schaper and colleagues[192] pretreated mongrel dogs for two weeks with this drug and continued treatment for four weeks after implantation of ameroid constrictors. After this treatment period peripheral coronary pressure distal to the coronary occlusion was measured in all experimental and control animals. Peripheral coronary pressure was significantly higher in the experimental group. The ratio of diastolic peripheral coronary pressure to diastolic arterial pressure was 0.23 in control dogs and 0.59 in dogs that received lidoflazine. In parallel studies done by Verheyen et al.[193] treatment of Labrador retrievers with lidoflazine was begun on the day of ameroid implantation and continued for four weeks or six months. Before animal sacrifice ^{3}H-thymidine was injected intravenously and epicardial collaterals excised. The number of mitoses in cells of the endothelium and subintimal layer of the collateral wall was increased in dogs treated with lidoflazine for four weeks. However, at six months there was no difference between the collaterals of control and treated animals. These data suggest that lidoflazine accelerated a naturally occurring phenomenon, and perhaps the higher peripheral coronary pressure in the treated animals in the initial weeks following coronary occlusion is a functional correlate. It should be pointed out, however, that the effect of lidoflazine on collateral resistance or flow is not known.

Nifedipine is another calcium-channel blocking agent currently being used extensively in the treatment of vasospastic and occlusive coronary artery disease. Schmier and his co-workers[194–197] administered this drug daily to dogs for periods of 6 to 20 weeks. The left anterior descending coronary artery was then ligated and dogs sacrificed 48 hours later. Detailed morphometric studies were done by making corrosion casts of the coronary system with either epoxy or acrylic resin. Superficial and intramyocardial anastomoses were counted with a microscope. This technique was able to identify 30 μm vessels. Seven of the 14 treated animals survived to 48 hours, whereas only 2 of 24 control dogs survived a similar interval. Treated dogs demonstrated obvious retrograde filling of the distal left anterior descending coronary artery and complete perfusion of its distal vasculature. In contrast, control animals had large nonperfused areas distal to the occlusion. There were approximately 30% more collaterals in treated dogs. In untreated animals the diameter of the collateral channels never exceeded 300 μm, while the narrowest collateral observed in 6.3% of the nifedipine group was 300 μm. Some of these latter animals had collaterals with diameters of 1 mm. Furthermore, the average diameter of collaterals in control animals was 95 μm, compared to 145 μm in the treated dogs. Thus, the cross-sectional area was three to four times higher in dogs pretreated with nifedipine. Therefore, chronic nifedipine therapy prior to coronary occlusion increased the size and number of collateral vessels. The results of collateral flows quantitated with radioactive microspheres were consistent with these morphometric data.[197] In control dogs endocardial and epicardial flows averaged 12.5 and 21.0 ml/min/100g, respectively, whereas flows were increased to 27.0 and 31.5 ml/min/100g in pretreated animals. These data are promising.

The morphometric data of Kanazawa[198] are similar to those of Schmier and colleagues.[194-197] In addition, Kanazawa quantitated myocardial flows by the hydrogen clearance technique. Whereas collateral flows were negligible in five of seven control dogs one week after ligation of the left anterior descending artery, flows in animals pretreated with nifedipine for four months averaged 80% of those measured in normally perfused regions. Unfortunately, these data may be incorrect since flows near the periphery of the ischemic area were quantitated where undoubtedly there was an intermingling of ischemic and normal tissue. However, other functional evidence also supported the efficacy of nifedipine pretreatment. The level of left coronary flow that elicited ST-segment elevation on epicardial electrograms recorded over the collateral-dependent left anterior descending perfusion territory tended to be lower in pretreated animals (161 versus 116 ml/min/100g). Finally, infarct size in the dogs that received nifedipine was half that of controls ($p < 0.05$).

Prenylamine[199] given to dogs for 12 weeks before coronary occlusion increased the number of collaterals visualized in corrosion casts. Although these results are encouraging, the absence of physiologic data or other objective measurements again diminishes the significance of the reported data.

F. Other Pharmacologic Agents

Other agents have been similarly tested. Papaverine[200] administered immediately following coronary occlusion improved survival and decreased infarct size. On the other hand, cortisone[201-203] started either before or shortly after coronary occlusion had no effect on retrograde flow, peripheral coronary pressure, mortality rate, or infarction size, although there was less perivascular inflammation evident in the wall of the developing collateral vessel. Future investigations with vasoactive agents will be necessary to define the role of prophylactic treatment further. Because of the ease of administration of such drugs, demonstrated success would have important clinical implications. However, current protocols should seek to quantitate coronary and collateral flows. Although casts and postmortem angiographic studies provide interesting insights, these techniques cannot furnish data that can be interpreted unequivocally.

G. Exercise

Much effort has been expended to determine the effects of exercise on collateral development. Although training programs have definite cardiovascular effects and increase fitness, their influence on the collateral circulation has been difficult to define. Exercise has widespread appeal because of the ease with which it can be prescribed for large populations. Thus if an obvious effect of this intervention on collateral channels could be proven, it would provide further justification for the clinical use of exercise programs.

Experiments in animals can generally be grouped into three distinct classifications based on the status of the coronary circulation: (1) normal coronary vessels, (2) coronary occlusion, and (3) critical coronary artery narrowing. The results of exercise training would be expected to be different in each of these three groups because of the differing degrees of compromise of the coronary vascular reserve. Both the dog and the pig have been used as experimental models and each has specific limitations, as already noted in Chapter 4. Many of the experimental protocols to be described have quantitated collateral blood flow with the radioactive microsphere technique, and, therefore, do not suffer from one of the major objections to the conclusions of the vasodilator studies. However, a deficiency of many of these investigations is the absence of flow data in the same dogs before and after the period of training or cage confinement. Use of each animal as its own control clearly eliminates other biological or statistical variations that might affect the results. In the absence of such internal comparisons conclusions can be based only on group data. Because of the natural wide variation in spontaneous collateral flow in animals such as the dog, group data tend to obscure the significance of all but major changes. These considerations may account for some of the negative results obtained in previous experiments.

1. Normal Coronary Arteries

Miniature swine[204,205] and dogs[206–211] with normal coronary arterial systems have been trained successfully to run on motorized treadmills or exercise tracks. Training effects of the repetitive exercise sessions frequently are apparent. Usually a lower heart rate for a given level of exercise after completion of the training program is sufficient to document that the training has had an effect on the cardiovascular system. The intensity of the daily exercise and duration of the training program vary with each protocol. Thus, the beagles in Scheel's study[210] ran at 3.6 mph and 25% incline for 45 minutes each day for six to eight weeks, while the dogs in the experiments of Burt and Jackson[206] were exercised for daily periods of 90 minutes at 10 mph for four to six weeks. The miniature pigs of Sanders et al.[204] trained for a ten-month period with daily hour endurance runs at 5 km/h. Cohen's studies[209,211] in beagles combined both sprint and endurance running for a three-month period. Despite the diversity of the training programs all of these studies have concluded that the collateral circulation is not affected by training in animals with normal coronary circulations.

Meesmann and his co-workers[207,208] examined the collateral circulation with postmortem coronary angiograms and found no difference in the occurrence of spontaneous collaterals in trained and sedentary dogs. Following acute ligation of the left circumflex coronary artery all trained and sedentary animals with abundant collateral circulations survived, while all with poorly visualized collaterals died. Eight of 46 control and 8 of 29 trained dogs had collateral networks intermediate between the two extremes. Curiously, all eight of the sedentary animals died in ventricular fibrillation following coronary ligation, while the eight trained animals survived. The difference in mortality is apparently not related to the collateral circulation. Burt and Jackson[206] measured retrograde flows in their sedentary and trained dogs. Although the average retrograde flow in the trained group (4.96 ml/min) exceeded that in the sedentary animals (4.10 ml/min), the difference was not statistically significant, and all dogs developed epicardial ST-segment changes during retrograde flow collection. Cohen et al.[209] quantitated collateral flow with radioactive microspheres following acute occlusion of the left anterior descending coronary artery in beagles after three months of training or cage confinement. Neither total collateral flow nor true collateral flow after subtraction of the overlap flow component was different in the two groups. Furthermore, subdivision of the transmural flow into endocardial and epicardial components did not reveal any differences. Finally, Scheel et al.[210] isolated the hearts of sedentary and trained beagles and perfused all major coronary arteries separately from a blood-filled reservoir at controlled perfusion pressures through individually inserted cannulae. Retrograde flow from each of the three major coronary arteries was measured during maximal dilatation of the other coronary arteries with adenosine. These authors calculated the resistance of the collaterals coursing between any two of the three major vessels. In sedentary dogs the resistance varied from a low of 17.2 mmHg/ (ml/min) for circumflex-to-anterior descending collaterals to a high of 187.2 mmHg/(ml/min) for anterior descending-to-right coronary anastomoses. There were no differences in the trained animals.

All of the above evaluations of collateral flow have been performed in either the isolated heart or the anesthetized, open-chest dog model. Cohen et al.[211] also evaluated the functional effect of collateral development in conscious beagles with normal coronary arteries. After a three-month training period, conditioned beagles as well as the sedentary control group underwent left thoracotomy for implantation of catheters and a snare around the left circumflex coronary artery immediately distal to the first large marginal branch. Three days after surgery the animals were able to run on a treadmill. Speed and incline were gradually increased until heart rates were approximately 200−220 beats/min, and 2 mCi of [201]TlCl were then injected into the right atrium. A thallium scintigram was then recorded in the anesthetized animal, and quantitative analysis performed as described in Chapter 5. Four days later the snare around the coronary artery was pulled to occlude the vessel, and hourly blood samples were obtained for CPK assay to quantitate infarct size. Three days after infarction, [201]thallium scintigraphy was repeated. Neither the size of the infarcts nor the perfusion defects following coronary occlusion were different in the trained and sedentary groups, which strongly suggests that collateral development was not better in the trained dogs.

Left circumflex coronary artery occlusion in sedentary and trained pigs with previously normal coronary arteries produced similar results.[204,205] In the trained animals myocardial flow fell from 0.36 to 0.05 ml/min/g, whereas in control pigs flow decreased from 0.41 to 0.06 ml/min/g. Transmural distribution of flow was similarly affected in the two groups.

Koerner and Terjung[212] trained young rats to run on a treadmill for one hour per day, five days per week. After a training period of 12 to 24 weeks, the animals were anesthetized and the left coronary artery was ligated through a midline sternotomy. Collateral flow to the central ischemic area quantitated with radioactive microspheres was approximately 10% of normal myocardial perfusion in both sedentary and trained animals, and the size of the ischemic portion of the rat left ventricle was similar in the two groups. Thus, the collateral circulation of rats with normal coronary arteries, like that of normal dogs and pigs, appears to be uninfluenced by training.

The lack of effect of exercise on coronary collateral development in animals with normally patent coronary arteries is not surprising. Barnard et al.[213] measured coronary blood flow during maximal exercise in dogs and observed that coronary blood flow increased from 0.91 to 4.24 ml/min/g while the endo/epi flow ratio declined from 1.29 to 1.03. Despite this fourfold increase in flow, vasodilatory reserve was not exhausted since infusion of dipyridamole in the running dogs increased coronary flow further to 6.20 ml/min/g. Hence, maximal exercise expended only 62% of the coronary vascular reserve, making it unlikely that any portion of the myocardium was ischemic. Furthermore, the absence of electrocardiographic evidence of ischemia during maximal exercise also supports the conclusion that the myocardium was adequately perfused. Ball et al.[143] measured coronary flow during various exercise stages in dogs. Although total coronary blood flow increased with each successive increment in speed and incline, the endo/epi ratio actually declined from 1.23 at rest to 1.08 during light and moderate exercise to 0.91 during heavy exercise. Although endocardial flow continued to increase with the more strenuous stages of exercise, it did so at a slower rate than flow to the epicardium. Severe exercise in miniature swine increased myocardial blood flow to 4.04 ml/min/g, while the endo/epi flow ratio remained greater than 1.0.[214] As in dogs, the coronary vascular reserve is not exhausted by exercise in pigs since adenosine infused into running pigs further increased flow by 28%.[215] Thus, there is no evidence that ischemia occurs in exercising animals with normal coronary arteries. Since ischemia is recognized to be the most potent stimulus of coronary collateral development, its absence in these exercising animals markedly reduces the potential for induction of collateral growth. Vasodilatation may be a secondary independent stimulus of collateral transformation, but the studies with chronic pharmacologically induced coronary dilatation suggest it has only a small to moderate effect. Because these training animals have only submaximal coronary vasodilation for approximately one hour each day, it is unlikely that the dilation could be a potent stimulus for collateral development. Thus, exercise programs in animals with normal coronary arteries would not be expected to have any significant effect on the coronary collateral circulation.

In striking contrast to these experimental data and theoretical considerations is the recent report of Knight and Stone.[216] These investigators measured collateral flow with radioactive microspheres during transient balloon occlusion of a coronary artery before and again four weeks after initiation of a daily exercise program. All animals had normal coronary arteries. Although coronary flow to the myocardium was unchanged over the four-week period when measured with all arteries patent, collateral flow during temporary balloon occlusion increased significantly ($p < 0.02$). Thus, endocardial flow increased from 0.62 to 1.02 ml/min/g, while epicardial flow rose from 0.95 to 1.16 ml/min/g. When only myocardial areas in which initial ischemic flows were less than 25% of control flows were considered, four weeks of training increased collateral perfusion of the endocardium from 0.25 to 0.85 ml/min/g ($p < 0.05$). The magnitude of these changes in collateral flow is indeed startling. Knight's dogs were studied in the conscious state and each animal was used as its own control. These differences distinguish this report from the others described above. But until these results are confirmed by other studies, the significance of these data cannot be fully evaluated.

2. *Prior Coronary Occlusion*

Several investigators have studied the consequences of an exercise training program commencing after coronary occlusion. This type of experiment, however, would reveal an effect of exercise on the collateral circulation only if there were a striking stimulation of growth and transformation. Ischemia following coronary occlusion is clearly a potent stimulus of collateral development and is itself able to induce restoration of normal resting flow in the perfusion territory of the obstructed vessel. The effect of additional minor stimuli would, therefore, be obscured. Only a second major stimulus would have a chance of being detected in this setting. Perhaps this accounts for the preponderance of negative results when exercise has been evaluated in an animal model with prior coronary occlusion.

Kaplinsky et al.[217] were perhaps the first to study the effects of exercise in dogs with coronary occlusions. During the first week following ligation of the left anterior descending coronary artery, selected dogs began to run for 30 minutes each day at 4 mph and 10% incline. After five weeks coronary angiography was performed in the trained animals and sedentary controls followed by postmortem coronary injection of a gelatin-barium sulphate mass. All studies showed the same degree of collateralization in the two groups. However, collateral flow was not directly quantitated, and therefore the accuracy of the authors' conclusions may be criticized.

Schaper and his colleagues[144,218,219] have also generally found that exercise does not promote coronary collateral development in dogs with prior coronary occlusions. In one early study[218] ameroid constrictors were implanted around the left circumflex coronary artery of dogs and the animals started on a daily program of running at 9 km/h and 10° incline for 30 minutes.

Training commenced three days after surgery and, therefore, before total occlusion, and continued until six weeks following angiographic documentation of vessel obstruction. There was no difference in peripheral coronary pressure in the distal left circumflex artery between trained and sedentary animals. Measurements of transmural flow with radioactive microspheres during pharmacologic vasodilatation (to simulate the exercise state) revealed relative hypoperfusion of the endocardium. The authors reasoned that the endocardial flow defect might, under selected conditions, result in endocardial ischemia. Since most collaterals in the canine myocardium are located in the subepicardium, it was believed that the physical separation of the endocardial ischemic stimulus and epicardial locus of collaterals might have contributed to the lack of effect of exercise in this canine model. To this end it was felt the pig might be a better animal model. In a second protocol,[219] ameroid constrictors were implanted around both the left circumflex and right coronary arteries of dogs. Daily training at 10 mph and 10% grade for one hour commenced one week after surgery and continued for six weeks. The hearts of sedentary and trained dogs were subsequently isolated, metabolically supported, and perfused with blood at varying perfusion pressures. Maximal coronary vasodilatation was insured by addition of adenosine to the perfusate. Coronary and collateral blood flows were measured with radioactive microspheres. At all pressures except the lowest of 45 mmHg collateral blood flow in the trained dogs was higher than that in the sedentary animals, but the differences were not statistically significant. Finally, Schaper[144] modified the protocol and exercised dogs for one to three months before and then for 100 days after surgical placement of ameroid constrictors. As above, hearts were isolated and blood flow measured at multiple perfusion pressures during adenosine infusion. Maximal collateral conductance averaged 40% of that of normal coronary arteries in both the trained and sedentary groups. These data thus support the inability of training programs to promote collateral growth beyond that resulting from the coronary occlusion itself.

The left circumflex coronary artery was gradually occluded by an implanted ameroid constrictor in dogs studied by Neill and Oxendine,[220] and training was begun six days after surgery and continued for either five or eight weeks. Each day the dogs ran for 30 minutes at 5 mph and 15% incline. Coronary angiography as well as injection of radioactive microspheres and measurements of retrograde flow were used to analyze the collateral circulation. Although retrograde flow appeared to be significantly higher in trained than sedentary dogs after five weeks of the training program, this difference was no longer apparent after eight weeks. Furthermore, there was no difference in either collateral angiographic score or quantitated collateral flow in the sedentary and trained animals.

Heaton et al.[137] also evaluated the effect of training following compromise of the coronary artery circulation. An ameroid was implanted around the left anterior descending coronary artery and the left circumflex cross-sectional area was diminished by 60 to 90%. In contrast to all of the other studies described above, the dogs were evaluated two weeks following surgery before the beginning of the training program and again after six weeks of either cage confinement or daily one-hour runs at 6 mph and 5% grade. Thus, in this protocol each animal was used as its own control. Furthermore, collateral and coronary flows were measured both at rest and during exercise. As early as two weeks following coronary occlusion resting collateral flow and transmural flow distribution in the perfusion territory of the occluded vessel were again normal. Exercise at 3 mph and 5% grade resulted in increases in both collateralized endocardial and epicardial flows, although the increment in endocardial flow was smaller than the increase in epicardial perfusion. In sedentary animals there was no change in flows after six weeks. In trained animals resting flows were not different after the six-week exercise period. During running the increase in epicardial flows was also similar, but the maximal increase in endocardial flow after completion of the exercise program was 39% higher than before training, a change which was significant ($p < 0.05$). Absolute exercise endocardial flows were, however, not different in the sedentary and trained dogs. This observation underscores the importance of using each animal as its own control. Group comparisons tend to obscure the significance of small, significant changes. Thus, exercise appears to have stimulated endocardial collateral growth resulting in an improvement of vascular reserve.

It is likely that the benefit of exercise following coronary occlusion noted by Heaton et al.[137] represents a transient phenomenon whose significance will fade as the interval following the coronary occlusion increases. The superimposed exercise stimulus probably elicits biochemical alterations which in conjunction with the ischemic stimulus of the coronary occlusion accelerate collateral development. Further depletion of the already severely depressed tissue oxygen and metabolite supply resulting from the increased demands of the exercise state most likely results in further interference with organelle function and membrane stabilization, and perhaps leads to increased production of vasoactive metabolites. Because it is known that dogs with chronic coronary occlusions eventually have restoration of epicardial as well as endocardial vascular reserve during exercise in the myocardium beyond the obstruction,[140,142] the reserve in Heaton's sedentary dogs would probably have increased to equal that in the trained group if the interval between coronary occlusion and animal sacrifice had been prolonged to permit continuation of the natural processes of collateral development and transformation. Suzuki's studies[186] with exercising dogs tend to support this impression. After ligation of the left anterior descending coronary artery he assigned dogs to exercise groups beginning one, two, three, or four weeks after surgery. Because all dogs were sacrificed five weeks after the coronary occlusion, these dogs therefore exercised for four, three, two, and one week, respectively. Despite the low-level exercise of daily 20-minute walks at 2.5 km/h, Suzuki observed an effect on the angiographic appearance of intercoronary anastomoses. Those dogs that began exercise early after coronary occlusion had more collaterals than the groups beginning exercise late.

Therefore, the effect of exercise may be more pronounced when begun soon after coronary occlusion. As the natural collateral development process continues, later addition of a second stimulus is less able to aggravate the state of ischemia, and consequently will have less of an effect. Furthermore, any early acceleration of collateral development caused by exercise would probably become less significant as the duration of occlusion increased, giving the collaterals more time to transform.

Scheel et al.[210] implanted ameroid constrictors around the left circumflex coronary artery of beagles and after three months assigned dogs to either sedentary or exercising groups. The latter dogs ran at 3.5 mph and 25% incline for 45 minutes each day for six to eight weeks. This exercise level had previously been shown to stress beagles to 50% of their maximal oxygen consumption. The hearts were isolated and the coronary arteries cannulated and perfused with blood from a reservoir. Adenosine infusion insured total coronary vasodilation. Coronary flows were measured with flowmeters, while collateral function was evaluated by collecting retrograde flow. Exercise significantly lowered the resistance of the left anterior descending–circumflex and right coronary–circumflex collateral pathways ($p < 0.05$). Furthermore, maximal conductance of the occluded vessel's bed in the trained dogs was 52% of that of an unimpaired vessel, higher than the 34% maximal conductance measured in sedentary beagles. These conclusions are at variance with those of Schaper,[144] who also used an isolated heart preparation to measure vascular reserve and found no difference in sedentary and trained dogs with chronic coronary artery occlusions. Scheel used retrograde flows to evaluate collateral function, while Schaper quantitated collateral flow directly with microspheres. This variation in method may account for the different results, but it is obvious that additional investigations are necessary. It should be noted, however, that even Schaper[219] observed a tendency for collateral resistance to fall (0.27 to 0.19 mmHg/[ml/min]/g) in dogs with prior coronary occlusions in whom heavy endurance training had produced mild cardiac hypertrophy (12% increase in weight).

Coronary collateral development in dogs is probably not significantly stimulated by exercise started after coronary occlusion. But some studies are clearly at variance with this conclusion. As suggested by Schaper and his colleagues,[218] it is possible that the dog model used for these studies may be inappropriate because the presumed additional maximal ischemic stimulus of exercise in the subendocardium is physically separated from the greatest locus of collateral vessels in the subepicardium. Accordingly, Schaper[218] did some preliminary experiments in pigs. Three days after ameroid implantation around the left anterior descending coronary artery pigs were started on an exercise program of daily hour runs at 7 km/h. Exercise continued for six weeks following angiographic documentation of vessel occlusion by the ameroid. Trained pigs had angiographic evidence of increased collateral formation when compared to sedentary controls, and the ratio of peripheral coronary pressure distal to the ameroid to aortic pressure was significantly higher in the exercised animals. Sanders et al.[205] have obtained similar data using microspheres to quantitate collateral flow. Pigs with left circumflex occlusions were exercised for five months. Sedentary animals had collateral flows of 10 ± 2 ml/min/100g, whereas average flows of 21 ± 4 ml/min/100g in trained animals were significantly higher ($p < 0.05$). Perhaps exercise following coronary occlusion in the pig, with its more meager, collateral circulation is a better stimulus.

3. Prior Coronary Stenosis

Exercise in dogs with normal or previously occluded coronary arteries has so far generally either had no effect on collateral development or perhaps caused only a transient acceleration. In the first instance exercise cannot induce myocardial ischemia, while in the second the ischemic stimulus is already maximal or nearly so. Therefore, the chances of finding an exercise effect in these two animal models are predictably low. In the ideal model the baseline stimulus for collateral development would be weak except during periods of exercise. An animal with a stenotic coronary artery would appear to satisfy these conditions. Although coronary constriction does stimulate collateral development, the stimulus is inversely proportional to the antegrade flow through the stenosis (Figure 7-8).[39,157] Therefore, careful selection of the degree of stenosis would minimize the stimulus to collateral growth. But because of the stenosis and the resultant compromised vascular reserve,[221] stress such as exercise would produce metabolic demands in excess of the ability of the coronary circulation to satisfy them, thereby producing ischemia. This ischemia might then stimulate collateral growth and development.

The classical study of Eckstein[157] established the ability of a training program to stimulate collateral growth in dogs with stenotic coronary arteries. Using probes with diameters ranging from 0.75 to 1.3 mm, he constricted the left circumflex artery by snugly tying a ligature around both the vessel and the probe and then removing the latter. Dogs were excluded from the study if no ST-T-wave changes were noted during total occlusion of the vessel. Eckstein reasoned that only dogs that developed signs of ischemia had inadequate spontaneous collateral channels that could profit from a stimulus intended to promote their growth. Dogs selected to be trained ran 3.2 to 4.7 mph at a 30° incline for 60 to 80 minutes. After six to eight weeks all sedentary and trained animals underwent a thoracotomy and the left circumflex artery was cannulated distal to the ligature. Two cannulae were inserted. One was directed proximally to permit collection of antegrade flow through the constriction. This flow measurement was treated as an index of the severity of the stenosis. The more severe stenoses limited antegrade flow the most. The second cannula was directed distally to collect retrograde flow, an index of collateral function. All measurements were made at an adjusted aortic pressure of 100 mmHg. In the sedentary animals, a curvilinear relationship between extent of collateral blood flow and degree of constriction was apparent (Figure 7-9). In the trained animals the curve shifted upward. For any stenosis severity, collateral function as assessed by retrograde flow was significantly greater in the trained than in the sedentary dogs. These data clearly demonstrated an effect of exercise on collateral development.

Schaper[219] attempted to improve Eckstein's experimental protocol by using radioactive microspheres to quantitate collateral flow. He constricted the left circumflex coronary artery by slipping Teflon rings with inner diameters of 1.5−2.0 mm around the vessel. In this manner stenoses of varying severity were produced. Peak reactive hyperemia following release of a transient occlusion of the vessel ranged from 24 to 60% of the control value. Dogs were divided into sedentary and training groups. The latter ran on a treadmill at 10 mph and 10% incline for one hour each day. At the end of six to eight weeks the hearts of all animals were isolated and perfused with blood. Maximal coronary vasodilatation was induced by adenosine infusion. A hyperbolic relationship between the degree of stenosis as evaluated by antegrade flow through it and the collateral blood flow to the myocardium distal to the

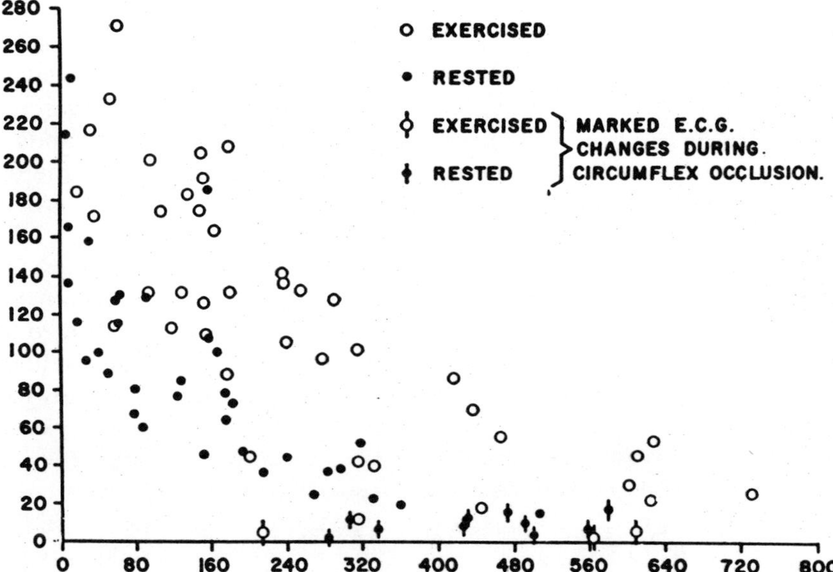

Figure 7-9   Retrograde flow (ml/min/100g) (ordinate) as a function of residual antegrade flow (ml/min/100g) through the proximal coronary artery stenosis (abscissa) in trained (○) and sedentary (●) dogs measured at the time of thoracotomy in the beating, working heart. The overall relationship demonstrating increased retrograde flow in those hearts with the more severe stenoses and therefore the more marked limitation of antegrade flow is similar to that derived by Schaper and Wüsten[39] (see Figure 7-8). In trained dogs the curve is shifted upward. Thus, for any degree of stenosis, collateral flow is higher in the trained dogs. (Reprinted with permission of the American Heart Association from Eckstein.[157])

constriction was evident (Figure 7-8). But unlike Eckstein's results[157] there was no difference between the exercised and the control dogs for comparable stenoses. Perhaps these negative results are related to the scatter of data points in a small group of animals. The tendency for baseline collateral flows to vary greatly in dogs and the wide range of severity of stenoses in Schaper's animals probably contributed to the scatter. In addition, the need to compare flows in two groups of dogs further diminished the chances of finding significant differences.

Cohen et al.[222] successfully overcame all of these technical difficulties. The left circumflex coronary artery of one-year-old male beagles was constricted by tying a ligature around the vessel and an 18- or 19-gauge needle and then removing the latter. The constriction was considered satisfactory if the peak reactive hyperemic response following release of a 15-second left circumflex occlusion was diminished by 50 to 67%. As demonstrated by the cast of a stenosed vessel in Figure 7-10, the diameter of the vessel was decreased by approximately 75–80%, resulting in an average 58 ± 4% decrease in the peak reactive hyperemic response. A balloon occluder and left circumflex flow probe as well as left atrial and aortic catheters were also implanted. Following recovery, all dogs were studied prior to randomization

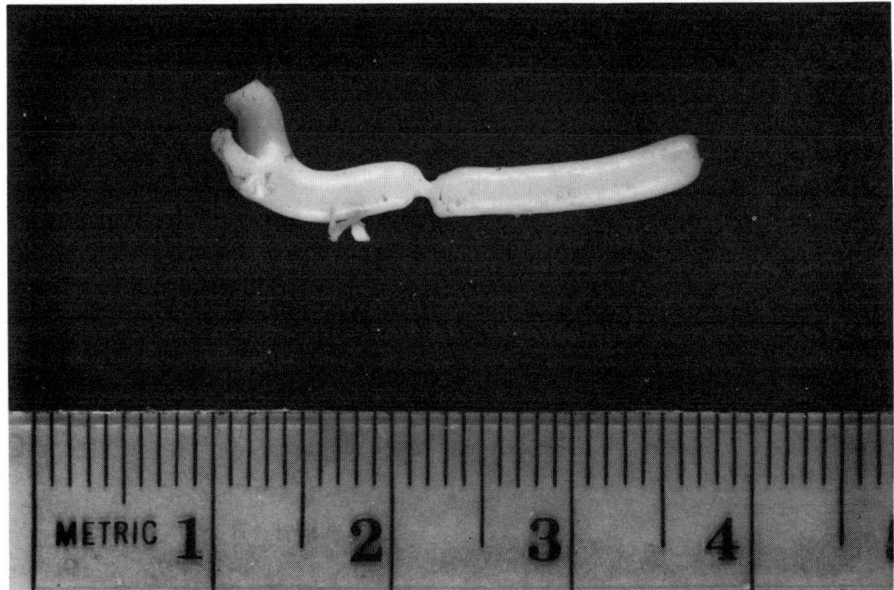

Figure 7-10　　Latex cast of proximal left circumflex artery (LCf) constricted by tying a ligature around the vessel and an interposed 18-gauge needle which was then removed. The diameter of this vessel was reduced by 75% resulting in a 94% decrease in cross-sectional area. This degree of constriction caused a 50–67% diminution of peak reactive hyperemia following release of a 15-sec LCf occlusion. (Reprinted with permission of the American Physiological Society from Cohen et al.[222])

into sedentary and training groups. Hemodynamics were evaluated at rest, and left circumflex collateral blood flow was measured with radioactive microspheres during a one-minute balloon occlusion of the vessel. Following completion of these resting studies all dogs began running on a treadmill. At 6.4 km/h and 12% incline, hemodynamics were again measured before and during left circumflex occlusion. Microspheres with a different radioactive label were injected into the left atrium during the occlusion to again measure collateral flow. After these studies and animal randomization, training was begun. Daily sessions lasted 75 minutes and consisted of sprints at 6.4—11.2 km/h and 6—8% grade as well as endurance runs at 6.4—9.6 km/h and 20% grade. The training period lasted 12 weeks and evidence of a heart rate training effect was evident in all runners. Following the 12-week period, the same resting and exercise hemodynamic and blood flow study done in the first week was repeated. Analysis of the flows in sedentary and trained dogs therefore was not dependent on comparison of group data. Instead, each animal could be used as its own control, and the changes in flow as related to

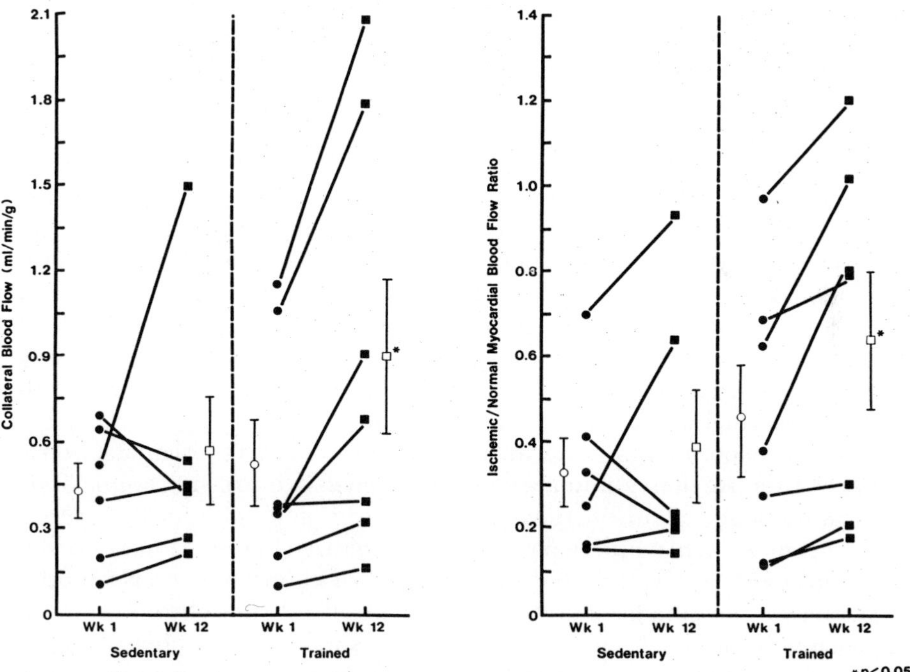

Figure 7-11   Graph demonstrating resting collateral flow (left) and ratio of ischemic or collateral to normal myocardial flow (right) in sedentary dogs confined to a cage for 12 weeks and dogs entered in a training period for the same interval. Whereas there were no consistent changes in sedentary dogs, both absolute collateral flow and the ischemic/normal blood flow ratio were significantly increased in trained animals after 12 weeks. Open symbols represent group means and vertical bars signify ± 1SE. (Reprinted with permission of the American Physiological Society from Cohen et al.[222])

either cage confinement or training could be specifically analyzed without concern that other uncontrolled genetic, biologic, or physiologic variables might be affecting the results.

The collateral flow data in the sedentary and trained beagles as well as the ratios of ischemic to normal myocardial blood flow are presented in Figure 7-11. Resting normal myocardial blood flow in the two groups ranged from 1.2 to 1.6 ml/min/g, while exercise flows increased to approximately $3-4$ ml/min/g. Neither collateral blood flow nor the ischemic/normal myocardial blood flow ratio changed significantly over the 12-week interval in the sedentary dogs at rest (0.42 to 0.58 ml/min/g, 0.33 to 0.39, respectively) or while running (0.68 to 0.95 ml/min/g, 0.22 to 0.27, respectively). Only the inner/outer left ventricular wall blood flow ratio in the ischemic zone measured during exercise increased significantly from 0.52 in week one to 0.67 in week twelve ($p < 0.05$). On the other hand, collateral flow in the trained group was significantly increased after 12 weeks. The 73% increase in resting collateral flow from 0.52 ml/min/g in week one to 0.90 ml/min/g in week twelve ($p < 0.05$) was accompanied by a rise in the ischemic/normal myocardial flow ratio from 0.46 to 0.64 ($p < 0.05$). Even after exclusion of the one trained dog with an exceptionally high collateral flow in week one, the changes in collateral blood flow and the blood flow ratio from week one to week twelve were still significant. Exercise collateral flow doubled over the 12-week training period (1.15 to 2.05 ml/min/g, $p < 0.025$). The inner/outer blood flow ratio did not change from week one to twelve in these animals at rest or during running. The increase in collateral flow in the trained animals, especially in the four dogs with marked rises over the 12-week period, was accompanied by less hemodynamic deterioration when the left circumflex artery was transiently occluded during running. Thus, the collaterals that did develop in these dogs were functionally significant. These observations are consistent with previous studies[135,140] that demonstrated that myocardial dysfunction was reciprocally related to the degree of coronary collateral development and the ischemic/normal myocardial blood flow ratio.

These experiments confirm and extend Eckstein's original observations.[157] Exercise does stimulate collateral growth in exercising animals with critical coronary stenoses. However, the nature and value of the exercise stimulus must be put into perspective. The increase in the resting ischemic/normal blood flow ratio after 12 weeks of a strenuous exercise training program was far smaller than the increase observed after chronic coronary occlusion of shorter duration.[140] In the latter situation the ischemic/normal flow ratio typically increased to 1.0, and this increase was accompanied by dramatic lessening of the degree of left ventricular failure seen in the running dog with coronary occlusion (see Chapter 6). Thus, in the dog, exercise is a weak stimulus of coronary collateral growth, probably because the stimulus is intermittent and the effect on left ventricular function is correspondingly small. Perhaps longer exercise training programs would have more striking effects.

H. Aortic Counterpulsation

Attempts have been made to stimulate collateral development with mechanical devices. Counterpulsation with intraaortic or external inflatable balloons increases diastolic aortic and therefore coronary perfusion pressure. The positive immediate effects of counterpulsation on collateral flow following acute coronary occlusion have already been described. The studies examining the delayed effects of counterpulsation on collateral flow have used only brief one- to two-hour periods of pumping either immediately after acute coronary ligation or during the gradual progressive narrowing occurring after implantation of ameroid constrictors. One would not expect such brief interventions to have any effect on the process of collateral transformation that occurs over a period of weeks to months. Reneman et al.[223] studied the effect of three hours of counterpulsation commenced immediately after abrupt occlusion of the left anterior descending coronary artery in dogs. Peripheral coronary pressure and collateral flow measured with ^{133}Xe intramyocardial depots one hour after discontinuation of the pumping were unchanged from postocclusion levels noted before the start of counterpulsation. Therefore, as expected, short periods of counterpulsation do not have obvious effects on collateral flow beyond the period of counterpulsation. Nonetheless, others have demonstrated that one to two hours of counterpulsation in dogs with occluded or stenotic coronary arteries can diminish mortality and infarct size and improve collateral development.[224−227] However, only coronary angiograms and postmortem coronary injection studies were used for the evaluation, and often the collateral circulation in control dogs that died spontaneously was compared to the collaterals in treated animals sacrificed at significantly longer intervals after the coronary ligation or ameroid implantation. Therefore, the techniques employed were not quantitative, and many of the comparisons may have been biased in favor of the treated animals, which lived longer.

Jacobey et al.[224] embolized plastic microspheres of 297−350 μm diameter down the coronary arteries of dogs, and began two hours of counterpulsation within ten minutes of the embolization. Treated animals had lower mortality rates and smaller infarct sizes. These authors compared postmortem angiograms of control and treated animals that died after similar intervals, and concluded that the collaterals were more abundant in the latter. In additional experiments, they noted that counterpulsation in animals with normal coronary arteries had no effect on the collateral circulation, while pumping six to ten weeks after coronary occlusion had variable effects. Goldfarb et al.[227] noted similar mortality rates in control dogs and animals pumped for two hours after coronary ligation. Coronary angiograms done in the initial three weeks showed no apparent differences between the two groups. The ligated artery was promptly opacified, but runoff was slow. Beyond three weeks, runoff was rapid in all treated animals, while it continued to be slow in nearly 50% of the control dogs. The data of Rosensweig et al.[225,226] reportedly confirmed the efficacy of aortic counterpulsation on collateral development in dogs when performed once during the gradual and progressive narrowing created by implanted ameroid constrictors. However, the conclusions must be regarded as tentative because of the lack of assurance that the angiographic studies in the control and treated groups were performed after similar intervals following the initial surgery.

The effects of counterpulsation on coronary collateral development are still unclear. The studies described above do not truly answer the posed question. As with many of the studies on stimulation of collateral development, further investigations would be necessary to determine the precise role of counterpulsation. But it is obvious that this technique would have limited clinical usefulness, and probably does not deserve as much attention as other potential stimuli such as vasodilators and exercise.

I. Surgical Attempts to Stimulate Intercoronary and Extracardiac Collateral Formation

Today the operation performed for clinical revascularization of ischemic myocardium is the saphenous vein bypass graft. Prior to the introduction of this procedure, however, many attempts, some quite novel, had been made to produce revascularization by stimulating collateral growth and increasing the anastomotic circulation from extracardiac sources. The theory was simple: ischemia would initiate opening of all available intercoronary arterial collaterals; but because intercoronary collaterals might not provide sufficient flow, new anastomoses with extracardiac sources might provide another pathway for blood to supply myocardium with marginal or frankly inadequate perfusion.

1. Inflammatory Pericarditis

Many early efforts focused on production of an inflammatory reaction in the pericardium or epicardium. It was hoped that the inflammatory response would produce neovascularization with anastomotic connections between pericardial and/or mediastinal vessels and the coronary vasculature. Instillation of asbestos,[228] talc,[229,230] carborundum sand,[231] or sodium morrhuate[231] into the pericardial space produced an adhesive pericarditis with highly vascular fibrous adhesions. This inflammatory reaction resulted in decreased mortality when a coronary artery was subsequently ligated,[228,229] smaller infarcts,[228] increased collaterals visualized by postmortem coronary injection of gelatin-barium sulphate mass[228] or aortic injection of a gelatin-ink mixture,[231] and higher retrograde flows from acutely occluded coronary vessels.[230] Following the introduction of talc into the pericardial space in some dogs, sequential proximal ligation of the left anterior descending, left circumflex, and right coronary arteries did not result in death.[229] Epicardial abrasion had the same anatomic[232–234] and functional[232–235] effects.

Berne et al.[236] attempted to quantitate the ability of either asbestos placed on the epicardium or the pericardial fat pad sutured to the heart's surface to induce collateral formation. In dogs with left circumflex stenosis either procedure was performed at the same time as the coronary artery narrowing or six weeks later. Twelve weeks after the intitial surgery peripheral coronary pressure and retrograde flow were measured in all animals. These collateral indices were identical in the dogs with isolated left circumflex stenosis and those with either pericardial fat pad grafts or asbestos-induced pericarditis. Furthermore, postmortem coronary injection of Schlesinger mass failed to differentiate between the various experimental groups. Mac-Lean et al[170] measured collateral flow of empty beating hearts by perfusing the coronary arteries with blood containing 2 vol% D_2O. Acute occlusion of the left anterior descending coronary artery minutes before injection of the tracer decreased myocardial flow distal to the ligature to 7% of normal. This level of flow was no higher in dogs that had had epicardial poudrage four to six months earlier. On the other hand, Leighninger and Beck, advocates of revascularization of ischemic myocardium, had differing results.[230,237–240] Leighninger[230] and Beck and Brofman[239] observed that the Beck I operation combining mechanical or chemical[241] abrasion of the parietal pericardium and surface of the heart, application of an inflammatory agent to the heart's surface, grafting of mediastinal fat to the epicardium, and narrowing of the coronary sinus more than doubled retrograde flow collection from the left circumflex coronary artery of dogs from 3.8 to 8.5 ml/min ($p < 0.001$). This flow increment was associated with a substantial decrease in mortality following occlusion of the left anterior descending coronary artery (26.6% mortality in dogs with and 70% in dogs without this revascularization procedure). Furthermore, this procedure decreased the size of infarcts resulting from coronary ligation by 60 to 70%.[239] The multiple procedures making up the Beck operation also increased retrograde flow when performed separately in experimental animals.[230] In a review of revascularization procedures and their effects, Beck[240] concluded that these manipulations definitely stimulated coronary collateral development. King et al.[242] also quantitated the effect of epicardiectomy on blood flow. At the time of removal of the epicardium, ameroid constrictors were also placed around the left anterior descending and left circumflex arteries. Three weeks later the main left coronary artery was ligated and [86]RbCl injected to measure myocardial flow. Although collateral flow to the jeopardized myocardium of animals with prior epicardiectomy was higher than that in animals without epicardial stripping, the increase was small (6 versus 8 ml/min).

Although the inflammatory response and subsequent vascularization are logical sequelae of the above procedures, it is difficult to imagine that the pericardium and/or mediastinal fat, with their limited sources of arterial inflow, could supply enough blood to the myocardium to affect the ischemic process after occlusion of a coronary artery. In an evaluation of the functional effects of the Beck I operation, Vineberg and Mahanti[243] performed the various parts of this revascularization procedure and simultaneously implanted ameroid constrictors around the left anterior descending and left circumflex coronary arteries. The survival rate in these animals was no better than in dogs with isolated ameroid implantation, and there was minimal evidence of new anastomotic connections with the coronary arterial circulation. The conclusions were equally pessimistic when Vineberg[244] evaluated the functional effects of epicardiectomy.

2. *Coronary Sinus Narrowing and Arterialization*

Beck realized that the neovascularization following scraping of the epicardium and pericardium and instillation of noxious substances in the pericardial space was a slow biological process. He devised a second two-stage Beck operation involving ligation or critical narrowing of the coronary sinus to thicken its walls and increase intrasinus pressure and either direct attachment of an artery (e.g., the subclavian artery) to the ligated or narrowed sinus, or insertion of a bridging venous graft between the coronary sinus and artery. Beck hoped this procedure would result in a more rapid and complete revascularization of the myocardium, and although he and his surgical peers popularized this procedure, Pratt[245] had been the first to suggest that retroperfusion of the capillary bed by introduction of arterial blood into the coronary sinus might have beneficial effects. He forced defibrinated arterial blood into the coronary sinus of freshly extirpated hearts and noted both ventricles continued to contract in a coordinated manner for up to 90 minutes. Roberts et al.[246] created an arteriovenous anastomosis with a glass cannula inserted between the coronary sinus and a systemic artery. Following this arterialization of the coronary sinus the hearts continued to beat from 10 minutes to 26 hours despite multiple coronary artery ligations. Chicago blue dye injected into the coronary sinus of these hearts at a pressure of 100 mmHg produced complete delineation of the myocardium's capillary system.

In addition to arterialization of the heart's venous system in the Beck II operation, the coronary sinus is narrowed or ligated close to its orifice. Although Beck suggested that this be done in order to increase the pressure in the coronary sinus and improve the chances of successful retroperfusion, he, as well as others, had demonstrated that coronary artery ligation following isolated coronary sinus occlusion was associated with a decreased mortality[247−249] and smaller infarct size.[250] Gregg and his co-workers,[247,251] however, demonstrated that chronic coronary sinus occlusion alone did not stimulate collateral development. After acute coronary sinus occlusion they observed that retrograde flow collected distal to the site of coronary ligation was indeed higher than if the coronary sinus were patent, although the contractions of the ischemic muscle were unaffected by this higher "collateral flow."[251] Furthermore, the initially high flows disappeared in chronic experiments. After 30 days of coronary sinus occlusion, retrograde flows had returned to 1.5–5 ml/min, values similar to those observed in control animals with isolated acute coronary artery occlusions.[247]

Beck's initial experience[237,238,252] in dogs following his two-stage procedure demonstrated better survival and smaller infarcts after coronary artery occlusion. Eckstein and colleagues[249,253] also noted an improved survival in dogs with coronary sinus arterialization following coronary artery occlusion. Whereas dogs with surgically created fistulae between the coronary sinus and jugular vein had a 70% mortality within one hour of coronary artery ligation, mortality was reduced to 30% in those animals whose coronary sinuses had previously been constricted. There were no early deaths in those dogs with a subclavian artery–coronary sinus shunt in addition to constriction of the coronary sinus sufficient to raise intrasinus pressures to 50 mmHg.[249,253] In additional animals with staged coronary sinus narrowing and arterialization, survival was maintained despite occlusion of almost all of the coronary arteries.[254,255] One dog's heart continued to beat for 35 minutes after all major coronary arteries were ligated.[254]

Several investigators[256–261] used retrograde flow to determine the effects of combined coronary sinus arterialization and sinus occlusion or constriction on collateral development. All showed an early significant increase in retrograde flow. However, unlike the arterial blood usually collected when a distal coronary artery is permitted to bleed retrogradely, the blood in dogs with the Beck II operation was desaturated, possibly implying that it had passed across a capillary bed. Temporary occlusion of the arterial graft to the coronary sinus promptly increased the collected blood's oxygen saturation and reduced the volume of retrograde flow, although not to the low levels observed in control dogs with coronary ligation in the absence of coronary sinus arterialization. The data of Eckstein and Leighninger[259,261] demonstrate the short-lived direct effect of the arterial graft but persistent effect on the collateral circulation. They performed the Beck II operation in many dogs and studied the effects of the revascularization procedure on retrograde flow following acute coronary occlusion at various time intervals after the initial surgery. Shortly after coronary sinus arterialization, left circumflex retrograde flow was 7.6 ml/min. The flow dropped to 2.8 ml/min when the graft was occluded, and the difference in oxygen content between the blood collected with the graft patent and occluded was 10.9 vol%. Three weeks after arterialization the coronary sinus was ligated and retrograde flow following acute coronary occlusion jumped to 20.8 ml/min. Following graft occlusion retrograde flow was 5.6 ml/min, and the marked difference in blood oxygen content was still apparent. One week later retrograde flow with the graft patent was unchanged, but had increased to 10.0 ml/min when the graft was occluded. One month after the coronary sinus ligation, retrograde flows with the arterial graft patent (30 ml/min) and occluded (28 ml/min) were nearly equal, and the difference in oxygen contents was only 2.1 vol%. By three months the retrograde flow with the graft occluded slightly exceeded that with the graft patent and there no longer was a difference in oxygen contents, which implies that the coronary sinus–arterial graft was no longer functional. At six months retrograde flow with the graft patent was 20.0 ml/min, and 22.0 ml/min with it occluded. Therefore, months after coronary sinus arterialization at a time when the arterial graft was no longer directly affecting collateral blood flow, retrograde coronary flow following acute coronary ligation was still substantially higher than in control animals. The large increases in retrograde flow are presumably related to progressive dilatation of the collateral channels initiated during the period of retroperfusion when the arterial graft was· still patent. It is interesting to note that the high retrograde flows persisted for at least three months following ligation of the arterial graft in dogs whose coronary sinus had been arterialized for three months.[238] Postmortem barium sulphate-gelatin injection studies of the coronary arteries in dogs with chronic aorta–coronary sinus anastomoses revealed many more intercoronary anastomoses than visualized in control animals.[261] In spite of these results supporting collateral growth and development following two-stage coronary sinus arterialization and ligation, Leighninger and Eckstein[262] also demonstrated that retrograde flow was increased to sham-operated dogs. Therefore, some of the reported changes may have been related to the inflammatory effects of pericardiotomy and exposure and drying of the epicardium.

3. Attachment of Vascular Pedicles, Other Tissues, and Foreign Substances to Epicardium

The Beck II operation attempted to supply an alternative source of arterial blood to the heart. Although the operation may have stimulated the development of intercoronary collaterals perhaps because of production of intramyocardial pressure gradients, the graft supplying the arterial blood gradually became functionless. Many other tissues were sutured to abraded epicardium in hopes that anastomoses with the coronary artery circulation would develop through the adhesions, establishing permanent connections with an extracardiac source of arterial blood. Thus, pedicles of pectoral muscle (cardiomyopexy),[263] jejunum (cardiojejunopexy),[264,265] lung (cardiopneumonopexy),[266–275] omentum (cardioomentopexy),[234,276–278] spleen (splenocardiopexy),[279] and deepithelialized skin and subcutaneous tissue[280,281] with preserved vascular attachments were sutured to, or wrapped around, the left ventricle. In these animals the coronary arteries were usually normal. Most of these initial observations documented vastly improved survival rates and smaller infarcts following abrupt coronary ligation in animals several months after the pedicle operation, and a variety of injection and casting techniques demonstrated numerous vascular connections between the grafted tissues and coronary arterial system. After cardiopneumonopexy, Evans blue dye injections into the distal thoracic aorta and determination of relative concentrations in femoral artery and coronary sinus blood suggested that 4 to 19% of coronary blood flow was derived from the graft,[272] while average retrograde flow following cardiomyopexy was triple that in control animals.[263] In Knock's dogs[278] with cardioomentopexy and prior coronary artery occlusions, disruption of the adhesions between myocardium and omentum produced rapid demise of all experimental animals. He also measured extracardiac blood flow to the hearts of control and revascularized animals. Extracardiac flow was never greater than 1.0 ml/min in normal dogs, whereas from 4.6 to 7.7 ml/min was evident in dogs with earlier cardioomentopexy. It was felt that these latter flows were probably underestimations since it was not possible to make the measurements without dividing some of the myocardial-omental adhesions. However, these initial optimistic reports were not always confirmed by others.[243,274,282]

Vineberg and his associates[244,283−286] were intrigued by the ability of the omentum to establish vascular connections with adjacent tissues. They excised pieces of omentum and either wrapped the entire ventricular surface with a free graft or inserted strips into tunnels made in the left ventricular myocardium. In dogs in which ameroid constrictors were simultaneously implanted around the left anterior and left circumflex arteries, vascular connections with the coronary arteries were evident in as few as 8 to 20 days, and mortality and infarction rates were significantly reduced. In Pifarré's dogs with prior epicardiectomy and free omental grafts sutured to the myocardium, multiple small anastomoses between the omental and coronary vessels were identified, although mortality following left circumflex ligation was only slightly reduced.[34] Criollos[287] quantitated the effect of cardioomentopexy on myocardial blood flow by collecting right heart effluent in dogs on right heart bypass. By occluding the aortic root, tissue blood flow was limited to that delivered by extracoronary collaterals. The flow was 8 ml/min. Vineberg[285] also sutured strips of omentum to the subclavian artery and buried the other ends in the left ventricular myocardium. In addition, ameroid constrictors were implanted. After three months, injection of Schlesinger mass into the subclavian artery produced complete opacification of the coronary arterial tree. Thus, the vessels of the omental grafts acted as bridges between the source subclavian artery and recipient coronary artery and established new vascular connections at both ends.

Vineberg[284,288] also sutured pieces of Ivalon sponge to the epicardium. In-vivo cineangiography as well as postmortem injections of Schlesinger mass into the subclavian artery demonstrated flow of the radiopaque substance down the chest wall vessels into the sponge and the myocardial vascular spaces. Multiple mediastinal vessels could be seen to penetrate the sponge. This revascularization procedure prolonged survival and eliminated infarction following occlusions of the left anterior and left circumflex coronary arteries by ameroid constrictors. Curiously, many of the vessels growing into the sponge did not anastomose with myocardial arterioles. Rather, the sponge vessels acted as bridges between vessels in the pericardium and mediastinum and myocardial sinusoids, which then opened directly into the left ventricular lumen.

4. Internal Mammary Artery Ligation

As described in Chapter 5, anastomoses between the internal mammary and coronary artery systems were easily demonstrated with injections of dyes or radioactive substances into the internal mammary artery at the level of its pericardiophrenic branch. In an attempt to increase this potential extracardiac source of blood, ligation of the internal mammary artery distal to the origin of the pericardiophrenic branch was proposed. It was hoped that this ligation would force more blood down the extracardiac pathways to the heart. In fact, Glover,[289,290] Taber,[291] and Botham[292] measured increases in pressure exceeding 10 mmHg in the internal mammary artery proximal to the site of ligation. Blair's studies[293,294] in dogs six months following bilateral internal mammary artery ligation demonstrated that the extracardiac contribution to coronary blood flow averaged 5.5–9.6 ml/min. This contribution decreased to less than 1 ml/min if the internal mammary arteries were clamped. Acute occlusion of these vessels in normal dogs produced no changes in coronary flow.

Claims that dogs with bilateral internal mammary artery ligations were protected following acute occlusion of coronary arteries upheld the functional benefit of this procedure and further supported the assertion that collateral blood flow was increased.[289,290] When Griffin[295] injected potassium chloride solution into the internal mammary artery of normal dogs, he observed no untoward effects. On the other hand, injection of this solution into the proximal left internal mammary artery weeks to months after its distal ligation resulted in rapid onset of ventricular fibrillation in four of eight experimental animals, again supporting the existence of important anastomoses with myocardial vessels following the surgery.

Despite these data, numerous investigators were unable to document any benefits of internal mammary artery ligation. Thus, reports of no increase in pressure in the proximal segment of the ligated artery,[296–298] lack of significant rises in flow in the severed pericardiophrenic artery following internal mammary artery ligation,[273,296,298,299] and little influence of this procedure on either peripheral coronary pressure or retrograde flow[297,298,300] cast significant doubts on the mechanisms or value of the surgery. Finally, neither Sabiston[273,299] nor Vansant[298] was able to document that internal mammary artery ligation had any salutary effect on survival following acute coronary artery ligation. Because of the uncertainty generated by these latter reports, internal mammary artery ligation was quickly abandoned as a myocardial revascularization procedure.

5. Internal Mammary and Other Systemic Artery Implantation

Evidence that new extracoronary collateral vessels could develop and form connections with the coronary circulation following epicardial abrasion or attachment of a variety of tissues to the epicardium stimulated Vineberg to experiment with the internal mammary artery as an extracardiac source of arterial blood. Mautz and Beck[277] had sutured an intercostal pedicle graft containing both internal mammary arteries to the surface of the left ventricle as early as 1937. They constricted the left anterior descending and left circumflex coronary arteries and in several months saw evidence of large anastomoses. While others experimented with modifications of this pedicle graft,[301] Vineberg[302] first suggested placing the internal mammary artery into a myocardial tunnel. In this and subsequent investigations he and his co-workers[243,284,302−307] adequately demonstrated that arterioles formed to connect this artery to the coronary arterial system. In approximately 50% of animals with normal coronary arteries and 85% of those with ameroid-induced coronary constrictions these anastomoses could be demonstrated by injection of Schlesinger mass into the internal mammary artery, and often the mass passed retrogradely up the patent coronary arteries to leak into the root of the aorta. In the injection studies of Bellman and Frank,[308] from one to four or five large anastomotic connections between the implanted artery and the coronary circulation and a variable number of smaller ones were typically identified. These anastomoses were felt to have developed from the vasa vasorum of the internal mammary artery. Bigelow and colleagues[309] examined these new communications and noted that the channels were lined with endothelium, but were devoid of muscle or elastic tissue.

Animals with implanted vessels were protected from the sequelae of acute coronary ligation,[284,305−307] while abrupt occlusion of the internal mammary artery in those protected animals with prior coronary ligation caused large infarcts.[284,306,307] Further evidence of the functional significance of the implanted artery and its vascular connections is apparent from the experiments in which seven of ten dogs with internal mammary artery implantation (and coronary sinus constriction) survived more than six months after implantation of ameroid constrictors around both the left anterior descending and left circumflex vessels.[243] In contrast, none of the control animals without revascularization survived. Sewell[310−313] modified the Vineberg procedure by implanting the internal mammary artery and vein and surrounding muscle and connective tissue into the myocardial tunnel, and had comparable results. But it was felt necessary to obtain other objective data to support the functional importance of these implanted arteries.

Leighninger[230] measured retrograde coronary flow from the left anterior descending and left circumflex arteries in dogs with internal mammary artery implantation, and found no change in this collateral index when the graft was occluded. Furthermore, he observed that the absolute level of retrograde flow was no greater than that measured in control dogs, and therefore felt that intramyocardial implantation of arteries had no effect on myocardial perfusion. Fuquay[314] measured antegrade flows in the implanted internal mammary artery of two dogs with a bubble-type flowmeter, and concluded that the flow was less than 1 ml/min. Using an electromagnetic flowmeter in dogs two to five months after internal mammary artery implantation, Yokoyama[315] measured negligible flows in implanted vessels that had remained patent. Abel[316] and Barner[317] noted similar results. These low flows would not be expected to affect the myocardium importantly. In fact, Barner,[317] using a right heart bypass preparation, derived ventricular function curves in normal dogs and animals with prior implants and chronically occluded left anterior descending arteries. Whereas acute occlusion of the coronary artery shifted the function curve downward and to the right, there was no change when the implanted artery was obstructed, which suggests that the myocardium had little dependence on whatever blood flow passed through the vessel.

Others have documented substantially higher flows and greater functional significance of the implanted arteries. Vineberg et al.[307] measured the flow in implanted internal mammary arteries in dogs in which a coronary artery had been chronically occluded. When the perfusion pressure was equal to that in the carotid arteries, flow ranged from 3 to 21 ml/min. That this flow was not merely the result of arteriovenous shunting was demonstrated in one animal whose heart stopped after exsanguination. Perfusion of the implanted internal mammary artery with oxygenated blood led to resumption of beating, and the 40% oxygen saturation of the blood draining from the coronary sinus was evidence that the blood had traversed a capillary bed. Others who measured internal mammary artery flow either directly by collecting right heart effluent in dogs on right heart bypass,[287] with an electromagnetic flowmeter,[318,319] or with [85]Kr washout[320] have noted average flows ranging from 14 to 63 ml/min. Tschopp's indirect measurements[321] with ^{86}Rb also supported increased "nutritive capillary flow" in dogs with arterial implants. Provan et al.[318] measured internal mammary artery flows at various time intervals after implantation of the internal mammary artery. Immediately after surgery flow averaged 5.6 ml/min and was unchanged for the first six weeks. Thereafter, a linear increase in flow to a maximum of 28 ml/min was observed 30 weeks after implantation. Obviously, flow could not be expected to increase until sufficient connections between the internal mammary and coronary arterial systems had been established. Using electromagnetic flowprobes on the implanted internal mammary artery and normal left circumflex artery in dogs with occluded left anterior descending vessels, Mittmann[322] measured average resting flow through the implant of 9.0 ml/min, while flow to the rest of the left ventricle was 43 ml/min. During running exercise, flow to both the implant and left circumflex doubled. It appears, thus, that arterial implants can form anastomotic connections with the coronary circulation and deliver significant quantities of blood to the myocardium.

Although the implanted arteries are capable of delivering blood to the heart, their functional value cannot be inferred because much of the blood could flow into the venous system, bypassing the capillaries where exchanges with the myocardial cells occur. Vineberg[284,306] wrapped the proximal left anterior descending coronary artery of dogs with cellophane. The resulting inflammatory reaction and fibrosis caused narrowing of the vessel. Those dogs that also had internal mammary artery implantation ran much longer on a treadmill and had fewer difficulties than animals without myocardial revascularization. Perhaps more direct proof of the myocardial effect of blood flowing down an implanted artery is found in Smith's study.[323] Blood delivered to the myocardium through a simulated implanted internal mammary artery transported substrates that were actively used in the metabolism of the heart.

Finally, Reis and colleagues[324] showed that the implanted arteries had a definite effect on ventricular function. Dogs were instrumented with left circumflex ameroid constrictors and snares around the left anterior descending coronary artery. One year later the snares were pulled to occlude the encircled artery. Ten of twelve dogs with bilateral internal mammary artery implantation survived arterial occlusion, whereas five of seven without revascularization succumbed from 2 minutes to 24 hours after occlusion. The implants protected the heart from ventricular arrhythmias and electrocardiographic changes of myocardial ischemia. Force-velocity and length-tension ventricular function curves were derived in nine dogs with implants one week after occlusion of the left anterior descending artery. In six of the nine, ventricular function was significantly impaired after the implants were occluded, and was restored when flow resumed in the implanted arteries. Peak isometric left ventricular pressure also decreased strikingly when the implants were occluded. Of the three dogs without apparent effect of the implanted arteries, the left circumflex was not occluded in one and the left anterior descending had not been adequately snared in another. Thus, in these experimental animals, salutary functional effects of implanted arteries were obvious.

Other investigators have implanted femoral arteries into the left ventricular myocardium.[325,326] Although coronary occlusion in these animals increased the patency rate of the grafts, the flows were unaffected.[326] Femoral artery flows measured by electromagnetic flowmeter immediately before implantation of the arterial graft into the left ventricular myocardium averaged 84 ml/min.[326] After implantation, flows ranged from 6 to 17 ml/min. Eight to 62 weeks later flow through the graft had increased to 11−28 ml/min. Kemp et al.[325] measured flow by injecting ^{85}Kr into the graft and following isotope washout from the myocardium. Tissue flow 12 months following surgery was 90 ml/min/100g. These measurements suggest that the graft, with its connections to the coronary arterial system, may provide appreciable quantities of arterial blood to the myocardium.

Subclavian,[274,313] carotid,[273,274,327] and splenic[328] arteries have also been used as myocardial implants. It was felt that the larger size of these vessels might increase the patency rate. Although protection against the sequelae of acute coronary occlusion may have been demonstrated, flow measurements through the mature grafts have produced conflicting data.

6. Direct Perfusion of the Myocardial Wall

Impressed with the importance of the endomural circulation in lower vertebrates (see Chapters 1 and 5), some investigators attempted to perfuse the myocardium directly from the left ventricular cavity. Either the two limbs of a U-shaped segment of carotid artery with multiple perforations pulled through the left ventricular wall from the inside[329] or a T-tube with the horizontal branches embedded in the subendocardium and the vertical branch extending into the cavity[330] has been employed. Injections into the arterial graft or T-tube demonstrated many communicating vessels coursing into the myocardium. Lower mortality following ligation of the left anterior descending artery and smaller infarct size have also been documented.[329] Sen et al.[331] perforated the entire thickness of the left ventricle with a 1.2-mm-diameter cannula. An average of 20 punctures/cm^2 in the left anterior descending perfusion territory appeared to protect the heart also. Those dogs with left ventricular acupuncture had lower mortality and smaller infarcts after coronary occlusion than control dogs. In dogs sacrificed at eight weeks the tracts in the left ventricular wall persisted as spaces between muscle fibers without endothelial lining.

Thus, multiple approaches to the development of extracoronary collaterals have demonstrated that new anastomoses can form in the myocardium. Of course, the operative nature of the techniques makes them unsuitable for most clinical situations, and when myocardial revascularization is required, the more direct saphenous vein bypass graft is now preferred. Many of the vascular connections between the coronary and extracardiac arterial beds forming after one of the revascularization procedures described above may be too small to have functional value, but merely their demonstration is important. Although collateral transformation of preexisting channels, as described in Chapter 5, is well accepted, one must wonder whether under some conditions formation of new intercoronary collaterals also might be possible.

Coronary collaterals respond to vasoactive metabolites and pharmacologic agents and can be stimulated to develop. Further investigations are necessary before the precise biochemical and/or biophysical stimuli of collateral development are identified. Once the process that controls collateral growth is better understood, it may be possible to select agents that can accelerate and even initiate collateral transformation. It is clear that the level of myocardial oxygen consumption and probably other less well defined factors influence the process of myocardial necrosis independent of the amount of collateral flow.[332,333] However, goals of limiting the amount of myocardial necrosis following coronary occlusion and minimizing other sequelae may in large measure depend on our future ability to control the coronary collateral circulation.

References

1. Cohen MV: Quantitation of collateral and ischemic flows with microspheres and diffusible indicator. *Am. J. Physiol.* 234:H487–H495, 1978.

2. Patterson RE, and Kirk ES: Apparent improvement in canine collateral myocardial blood flow during vasodilation depends on criteria used to identify ischemic myocardium. *Circ. Res.* 47:108−116, 1980.

3. Eckstein RW, Roberts JT, Gregg DE, and Wearn JT: Observations on the role of the Thebesian veins and luminal vessels in the right ventricle. *Am. J. Physiol.* 132:648−653, 1941.

4. Fischl SJ, Sonnenblick EM, and Kirk ES: Collateral blood flow in the border zone following acute coronary occlusion. (abstr) *Am. J. Cardiol.* 35:136, 1975.

5. Hirzel HO, Nelson GR, Sonnenblick EH, and Kirk ES: Redistribution of collateral blood flow from necrotic to surviving myocardium following coronary occlusion in the dog. *Circ. Res.* 39:214−222, 1976.

6. Kirk ES, and Hirzel HO: Critical role of coronary collateral blood flow in the pathophysiology of myocardial infarction. In *Coronary Heart Disease: 3rd International Symposium Frankfurt* (eds M Kaltenbach, P Lichtlen, R Balcon, and W-D Bussmann). Georg Thieme, Stuttgart, 1978, pp 11−20.

7. Factor SM, Sonnenblick EH, and Kirk ES: The histologic border zone of acute myocardial infarction—Islands or peninsulas? *Am. J. Pathol.* 92:111−124, 1978.

8. Gross GJ, Buck JD, Warltier DC, and Hardman HF: Separation of overlap and collateral perfusion of ischemic canine myocardium: Important considerations in the analysis of vasodilator-induced coronary steal. *J. Cardiovasc. Pharmacol.* 4:254−263, 1982.

9. Brazzamano S, Mays AE, Rembert JC, and Greenfield JC Jr: Increase in collateral blood flow following repeated coronary artery occlusion and nitroglycerin administration. *Circ. Res.* 54:204−207, 1984.

10. Zuberbuhler RC, and Bohr DF: Responses of coronary smooth muscle to catecholamines. *Circ. Res.* 16:431−440, 1965.

11. Fam WM, and McGregor M: Effect of nitroglycerin and dipyridamole on regional coronary resistance. *Circ. Res.* 22:649−659, 1968.

12. Winbury MM, Howe BB, and Hefner MA: Effect of nitrates and other coronary dilators on large and small coronary vessels: An hypothesis for the mechanism of action of nitrates. *J. Pharmacol. Exp. Ther.* 168:70−95, 1969.

13. Norton JM, and Detar R: Adenosine and isolated coronary vascular smooth muscle. (abstr) *Physiologist* 13:273, 1970.

14. Schnaar RL, and Sparks HV: Response of large and small coronary arteries to nitroglycerin, NaNO$_2$, and adenosine. *Am. J. Physiol.* 223:223−228, 1972.

15. Cohen MV, and Kirk ES: Differential response of large and small coronary arteries to nitroglycerin and angiotensin: Autoregulation and tachyphylaxis. *Circ. Res.* 33:445−453, 1973.

16. Imai S: Effects of nifedipine on heart and coronary circulation. In *1st International Nifedipine "Adalat" Symposium: New Therapy of Ischemic Heart Disease* (eds K Hashimoto, E Kimura, and T Kobayashi). University of Tokyo Press, Tokyo, 1975, pp 23−30.

17. Takeda K, Nakagawa Y, Katano Y, and Imai S: Effects of coronary vasodilators on large and small coronary arteries of dogs. *Jpn. Heart J.* 18:92−101, 1977.

18. Kamitani T, Nakano K, Mori J, et al: Local specificity in responses of canine coronary vessels to oxygen deficiency and antianginal drugs. *Arch. Int. Pharmacodyn. Ther.* 225:257−274, 1977.

19. Harder DR, Belardinelli L, Sperelakis N, et al: Differential effects of adenosine and nitroglycerin on the action potentials of large and small coronary arteries. *Circ. Res.* 44:176−182, 1979.

20. Vatner SF, Pagani M, Manders WT, and Pasipoularides AD: Alpha adrenergic vasoconstriction and nitroglycerin vasodilation of large coronary arteries in the conscious dog. *J. Clin. Invest.* 65:5−14, 1980.

21. Forman R, and Kirk ES: Comparative effects of vasodilator drugs on large and small coronary resistance vessels in the dog. *Cardiovasc. Res.* 14:601−606, 1980.

22. Tomoike H, Ootsubo H, Sakai K, et al: Continuous measurement of coronary artery diamter in situ. *Am. J. Physiol.* 240:H73−H79, 1981.
23. Noguchi K, Tomoike H, Ootsubo H, et al: Difference in site and time course of coronary dilating effects of trapidil, nitroglycerin and dipyridamole in anesthetized dogs. *J. Pharmacol. Exp. Ther.* 219:809−814, 1981.
24. Macho P, Hintze TH, and Vatner SF: Regulation of large coronary arteries by increases in myocardial metabolic demands in conscious dogs. *Circ. Res.* 49:594−599, 1981.
25. Macho P, and Vatner SF: Effects of nitroglycerin and nitroprusside on large and small coronary vessels in conscious dogs. *Circulation* 64:1101−1107, 1981.
26. Vatner SF, and Hintze TH: Effects of a calcium-channel antagonist on large and small coronary arteries in conscious dogs. *Circulation* 66:579−588, 1982.
27. Hintze TH, and Vatner SF: Dipyridamole dilates large coronary arteries in conscious dogs. *Circulation* 68:1321−1327, 1983.
28. Cohen MV: Coronary steal in awake dogs: A real phenomenon. *Cardiovasc. Res.* 16:339−349, 1982.
29. Wichmann J, Löser R, Diemer HP, and Lochner W: Pharmacological alterations of coronary collateral circulation: Implication to the steal-phenomenon. *Pflügers Arch. Ges. Physiol.* 373:219−224, 1978.
30. Wichmann J, Lochner W, Löser R, and Diemer HP: The pressure-resistance relationships of regional resistances within the coronary circulation and the steal phenomenon. *Basic Res. Cardiol.* 73:607−617, 1978.
31. Parratt JR, Ledingham IM, and McArdle CS: Effect of a coronary vasodilator drug (carbochromen) on blood flow and oxygen extraction in acute myocardial infarction. *Cardiovasc. Res.* 7:401−407, 1973.
32. Flameng W, Schaper W, and Lewi P: Multiple experimental coronary occlusion without infarction: Effects of heart rate and vasodilation. *Am. Heart J.* 85:767−776, 1973.
33. Flameng W, Wüsten B, and Schaper W: On the distribution of myocardial flow. Part II: Effects of arterial stenosis and vasodilation. *Basic Res. Cardiol.* 69:435−446, 1974.
34. Meyer U, Schiffer W, Schulz FW, and Raff WK: The problem of coronary steal phenomenon under the influence of coronary dilators. (abstr) *Naunyn-Schmiedebergs Arch. Pharmacol. Suppl.* 285:R55, 1974.
35. Lochner W, Raff WK, and Meyer U: Comparison of the effect of antianginal drugs with reference to the extravascular component of coronary resistance and the "steal phenomenon." In *Coronary Angiography and Angina Pectoris* (ed PR Lichtlen). Georg Thieme, Stuttgart, 1976, pp 316−324.
36. Cohen MV, Sonnenblick EH, and Kirk ES: Coronary steal: Its role in detrimental effect of isoproterenol after acute coronary occlusion in dogs. *Am. J. Cardiol.* 38:880−888, 1976.
37. Lacroix P, Linee P, and Le Polles JB: Effects of some coronary vasodilator drugs on collateral hemodynamics after chronic myocardial ischemia in the anesthetized dog: Appropriate or inappropriate redistribution? *J. Pharmacol. Exp. Ther.* 204:645−654, 1978.
38. Lochner W, Wichmann J, and Löser R: Physiologic and pharmacologic qualities of coronary collaterals and the steal phenomenon. In *Coronary Heart Disease: 3rd International Symposium Frankfurt* (eds M Kaltenbach, P Lichtlen, R Balcon, and W-D Bussmann). Georg Thieme, Stuttgart, 1978, pp 21−27.
39. Schaper W, and Wüsten B: Collateral circulation. In *The Pathophysiology of Myocardial Perfusion* (ed W Schaper). North-Holland Biomedical Press, Amsterdam, 1979, pp 415−470.
40. Warltier DC, Gross GJ, and Brooks HL: Coronary steal-induced increase in myocardial infarct size after pharmacologic coronary vasodilation. *Am. J. Cardiol.* 46:83−90, 1980.

41. Gross GJ, and Warltier DC: Coronary steal in four models of single or multiple vessel obstruction in dogs. *Am. J. Cardiol.* 48:84−92, 1981.
42. Cohen MV, Downey JM, Sonnenblick EH, and Kirk ES: The effects of nitroglycerin on coronary collaterals and myocardial contractility. *J. Clin. Invest.* 52:2836−2847, 1973.
43. Johansson B, Linder E, and Seeman T: Effects of heart rate and arterial blood pressure on coronary collateral blood flow in dogs. *Acta Physiol. Scand.* 68 (Suppl. 272):33−46, 1966.
44. Gundel WD, Brown BG, and Gott VL: Coronary collateral flow studies during variable aortic root pressure waveforms. *J. Appl. Physiol.* 29:579−586, 1970.
45. Brown BG, Gundel WD, Gott VL, and Covell JW: Hemodynamic determinants of retrograde arterial coronary flow following acute coronary occlusion. (abstr) *Circulation* 46 (Suppl II):II-100, 1972.
46. Brown BG, Gundel WD, Gott VL, and Covell JW: Coronary collateral flow following acute coronary occlusion: A diastolic phenomenon. *Cardiovasc. Res.* 8:621−631, 1974.
47. Chiariello M, Ribeiro LGT, Davis MA, and Maroko PR: "Reverse coronary steal" induced by coronary vasoconstriction following coronary artery occlusion in dogs. *Circulation* 56:809−815, 1977.
48. Gensini GG, Buonanno C, Palacio A, et al: Cinefluorographic control of super selective coronary occlusion in experimental animals. *J. Soc. Motion Picture and Television Engineers* 75:649−651, 1966.
49. Kattus AA, and Gregg DE: Some determinants of coronary collateral blood flow in the open-chest dog. *Circ. Res.* 7:628−642, 1959.
50. Fam WM, and McGregor M: Effect of coronary vasodilator drugs on retrograde flow in areas of chronic myocardial ischemia. *Circ. Res.* 15:355−365, 1964.
51. Pasyk S, Bloor CM, Khouri EM, and Gregg DE: Systemic and coronary effects of coronary artery occlusion in the unanesthetized dog. *Am. J. Physiol.* 220:646−654, 1971.
52. Gregg DE: Coronary vasodilator effects of nitroglycerin during coronary insufficiency. In *The Study of the Systemic, Coronary and Myocardial Effects of Nitrates* (ed GG Gensini). Charles C Thomas, Springfield, Il, 1972, pp 292−296.
53. Nagao T, Murata S, and Sato M: Effects of diltiazem (CRD-401) on developed coronary collaterals in the dog. *Jpn. J. Pharmacol.* 25:281−288, 1975.
54. Pasyk S, Bloor CM, and Gregg DE: Myocardial Xe[133] clearance and its response to vasodilators before, during and after coronary artery occlusion. (abstr) *Fed. Proc.* 27:632, 1968.
55. Grayson J, and Scott C: The action of nitroglycerine and dipyridamole in normal and ischaemic dog heart. *Br. J. Pharmacol.* 53:11−19, 1975.
56. Bache RJ, Ball RM, Cobb FR, et al: Effects of nitroglycerin on transmural myocardial blood flow in the unanesthetized dog. *J. Clin. Invest.* 55:1219−1228, 1975.
57. Schaper W: Effect of drugs on collateral circulation. In *The Pathophysiology of Myocardial Perfusion* (ed W Schaper). North-Holland Biomedical Press, Amsterdam, 1979, pp 471−488.
58. Fukuyama T, and Roberts R: The effect of intravenous nitroglycerin on coronary blood flow and infarct size during myocardial infarction in conscious dogs. *Clin. Cardiol.* 3:317−323, 1980.
59. Fukuyama T, Schechtman KB, and Roberts R: The effects of intravenous nitroglycerin on hemodynamics, coronary blood flow and morphologically and exzymatically estimated infarct size in conscious dogs. *Circulation* 62:1227−1238, 1980.
60. Komer RR, Edalji A, and Hood WB Jr: Effects of nitroglycerin on echocardiographic measurements of left ventricular wall thickness and regional myocardial performance during acute coronary ischemia. *Circulation* 59:926−937, 1979.
61. Jolly SR, and Gross GJ: Improvement in ischemic myocardial blood flow following a new calcium antagonist. *Am. J. Physiol.* 239:H163−H171, 1980.

62. Leighninger DS, Rueger R, and Beck CS: Effect of glyceryl trinitrate (nitroglycerin) on arterial blood supply to ischemic myocardium. *Am. J. Cardiol.* 3:638–646, 1959.

63. Diemer HP, Wichmann J, and Lochner W: Coronary collateral flow: Effect of drugs and perfusion pressure. *Basic Res. Cardiol.* 72:332–343, 1977.

64. Weisse AB, Senft A, Khan MI, and Regan TJ: Effect of nitrate infusions on the systemic and coronary circulations following acute experimental myocardial infarction in the intact dog. *Am. J. Cardiol.* 30:362–370, 1972.

65. Bache RJ: Effect of nitroglycerin and arterial hypertension on myocardial blood flow following acute coronary artery occlusion in the dog. *Circulation* 57:557–562, 1978.

66. Jugdutt BI, Becker LC, Hutchins GM, et al: Effect of intravenous nitroglycerin on collateral blood flow and infarct size in the conscious dog. *Circulation* 63:17–28, 1981.

67. Forman R, Eng C, and Kirk ES: Comparative effect of verapamil and nitroglycerin on collateral blood flow. *Circulation* 67:1200–1204, 1983.

68. Becker LC, Fortuin NJ, and Pitt B: Effect of ischemia and antianginal drugs on the distribution of radioactive microspheres in the canine left ventricle. *Circ. Res.* 28:263–269, 1971.

69. Kjekshus JK: Mechanism for flow distribution in normal and ischemic myocardium during increased ventricular preload in the dog. *Circ. Res.* 33:489–499, 1973.

70. Capurro NL, Kent KM, Smith HJ, et al: Acute coronary occlusion: Prolonged increase in collateral flow following brief administration of nitroglycerin and methoxamine. *Am. J. Cardiol.* 39:679–683, 1977.

71. Gorman MW, and Sparks HV Jr: Nitroglycerin causes vasodilatation within ischaemic myocardium. *Cardiovasc. Res.* 14:515–521, 1980.

72. Cohen MV, Sonnenblick EH, and Kirk ES: Comparative effects of nitroglycerin and isosorbide dinitrate on coronary collateral vessels and ischemic myocardium in dogs. *Am. J. Cardiol.* 37:244–249, 1976.

73. Capurro N, Kent KM, and Epstein SE: Effects of intracoronary and intravenous nitroglycerin on coronary collateral function. *J. Pharmacol. Exp. Ther.* 199:262–268, 1976.

74. Capurro NL, Kent KM, and Epstein SE: Comparison of nitroglycerin-, nitroprusside-, and phentolamine-induced changes in coronary collateral function in dogs. *J. Clin. Invest.* 60:295–301, 1977.

75. Forman R, Kirk ES, Downey JM, and Sonnenblick EH: Nitroglycerin and heterogeneity of myocardial blood flow: Reduced subendocardial blood flow and ventricular contractile force. *J. Clin. Invest.* 52:905–911, 1973.

76. Khouri EM, and Iza AR: The effect of glyceryl trinitrate on coronary collateral flow—A preliminary report. In *Current Topics in Coronary Research: Advances in Experimental Medicine and Biology*, Vol. 39 (eds CM Bloor and RA Olsson). Plenum Press, New York, 1973, pp 191–196.

77. Degenring FH, Curnish RR, Rubio R, and Berne RM: Effect of dipyridamole on myocardial adenosine metabolism and coronary flow in hypoxia and reactive hyperemia in the isolated perfused guinea pig heart. *J. Mol. Cell. Cardiol.* 8:877–888, 1976.

78. Fleckenstein A: On the basic pharmacological mechanism of nifedipine and its relation to therapeutic efficacy. In *3rd International Adalat Symposium: New Therapy of Ischemic Heart Disease* (eds AD Jatene and PR Lichtlen). Excerpta Medica, Amsterdam, 1976, pp 1–13.

79. Gallagher KP, Folts JD, Shebuski RJ, et al: Subepicardial vasodilator reserve in the presence of critical coronary stenosis in dogs. *Am. J. Cardiol.* 46:67–73, 1980.

80. Schaper W, Flameng W, Wüsten B, and Palmowski J: The distribution of coronary and of coronary collateral flow in normal hearts and after chronic coronary

occlusion. In *Current Topics in Coronary Research: Advances in Experimental Medicine and Biology*, Vol. 39 (eds CM Bloor and RA Olsson). Plenum Press, New York, 1973, pp 151−160.

81. Ledingham IM, Marshall RJ, and Parratt JR: Drug-induced changes in blood flow in normal and ischaemic regions of the canine myocardium. (abstr) *Br. J. Pharmacol.* 47:626P−627P, 1973.

82. Davenport N, Goldstein RE, Bolli R, and Epstein SE: Blood flow to infarct and surviving myocardium: Implications regarding the action of verapamil on the acutely ischemic dog heart. *J. Am. Coll. Cardiol.* 3:956−965, 1984.

83. Grayson J, Irvine M, and Parratt JR: Effects of carbochromen and dipyridamole on blood flow and heat production in the normal and ischaemic canine myocardium. *Cardiovasc. Res.* 5:41−47, 1971.

84. Rees JR, and Redding VJ: Effects of dipyridamole on anastomotic blood flow in experimental myocardial infarction. *Cardiovasc. Res.* 1:179−183, 1967.

85. Seeman T: Pharmacological, rheological and surgical attempts to improve myocardial blood flow during coronary occlusion in dogs. *Acta Chir. Scand. Suppl.* 400:1−27, 1969.

86. Henry PD, Shuchleib R, Borda LJ, et al: Effects of nifedipine on myocardial perfusion and ischemic injury in dogs. *Circ. Res.* 43:372−380, 1978.

87. Henry PD, Shuchleib R, Clark RE, and Perez JE: Effect of nifidipine on myocardial ischemia: Analysis of collateral flow, pulsatile heat and regional muscle shortening. *Am. J. Cardiol.* 44:817−824, 1979.

88. Clark RE, Christlieb IY, Henry PD, et al: Nifedipine: A myocardial protective agent. *Am. J. Cardiol.* 44:825−831, 1979.

89. Selwyn AP, Welman E, Fox K, et al: The effects of nifedipine on acute experimental myocardial ischemia and infarction in dogs. *Circ. Res.* 44:16−23, 1979.

90. Nakamura M, Kikuchi Y, Senda Y, et al: Myocardial blood flow following experimental coronary occlusion: Effects of diltiazem. *Chest* 78 (Suppl.):205−209, 1980.

91. Weisse AB, and Regan TJ: A comparison of four potential agents for reducing necrosis after prolonged coronary occlusion. *J. Clin. Pharmacol.* 18:161−173, 1978.

92. Millard RW: Changes in cardiac mechanics and coronary blood flow of regionally ischemic porcine myocardium induced by diltiazem. *Chest* 78 (Suppl.):193−199, 1980.

93. Weintraub WS, Hattori S, Akizuki S, et al: Influence of nifedipine on collateral blood flow during acute ischemia in the dog. *J. Am. Coll. Cardiol.* 3:334−340, 1984.

94. Bache RJ, and Dymek DJ: Effect of diltiazem on myocardial blood flow. *Circulation* 65 (Suppl. I):I-19−I-26, 1982.

95. Bache RJ, Dai X-Z, and Schwartz JS: Effect of nifedipine on myocardial blood flow during exercise in dogs with chronic coronary artery occlusion. *J. Am. Coll. Cardiol.* 3:143−149, 1984.

96. Ribeiro LGT, Reduto LA, Brandon TA, et al: Effects of prostacyclin on hemodynamics, regional myocardial blood flow, infarct size and mortality in experimental myocardial infarction. (abstr) *Clin. Res.* 27:199A, 1979.

97. Jugdutt BI, Hutchins GM, Bulkley BH, and Becker LC: Infarct size reduction by prostacyclin after coronary occlusion in conscious dogs. (abstr) *Clin. Res.* 27:177A, 1979.

98. Jentzer JH, Sonnenblick EH, and Kirk ES: Specificity of prostacyclin as a coronary artery vasodilator. (abstr) *Clin. Res.* 27:177A, 1979.

99. Sapozhkov AV: The effect of vasodilating agents on the collateral coronary circulation and oxygen tension in the myocardium. *Farmakol. Toksikol.* 31:687−690, 1968.

100. Zyvoloski MG, Brooks HL, Gross GJ, and Warltier DC: Myocardial perfusion distal to an acute or chronic coronary artery occlusion: Effects of diltiazem and nifedipine. *J. Pharmacol. Exp. Ther.* 222:494−500, 1982.

101. Gross GR, Warltier DC, and Hardman HF: Comparative effects of two slow channel calcium entry blockers, FR 34235 and nifedipine, on true coronary collateral blood flow. *J. Cardiovasc. Pharmacol.* 6:61−67, 1984.

102. Gopal MA, Neill WA, and Oxendine JM: Effects of nitroprusside on myocardial blood flow in acute regional coronary ischaemia in conscious dogs with and without left ventricular distension. *Cardiovasc. Res.* 17:267−273, 1983.

103. Blumenthal DS, Hutchins GM, Jugdutt BI, and Becker LC: Salvage of ischemic myocardium by dipyridamole in the conscious dog. *Circulation* 64:915−923, 1981.

104. Golenhofen K, Mandrek K, Schaper W, et al: Mechanical activity of isolated canine coronary arteries after coronary occlusion. *Basic Res. Cardiol.* 76:480−484, 1981.

105. Kadatz R: Sauerstoffdruck und Durchblutung im gesunden und koronarinsuffizienten Myokard des Hundes und ihre Beeinflussung durch koronarerweiternde Pharmaka. *Arch. Kreislaufforsch.* 58:263−293, 1969.

106. Franklin D, Millard RW, and Nagao T: Responses of coronary collateral flow and dependent myocardial mechanical function to the calcium antagonist, diltiazem. *Chest* 78 (Suppl.):200−204, 1980.

107. Scholtholt J, Birringer H, Fiedler VB, and Schölkens B: Effects of prostacyclin (PGI$_2$) and adenosine (ASN) on total and regional blood flow of isolated, collateralized dog hearts. *Basic Res. Cardiol.* 76:313−327, 1981.

108. Anrep GV, and Haüsler H: The coronary circulation. I. The effect of changes of the blood-pressure and of the output of the heart. *J. Physiol.* 65:357−373, 1928.

109. Lefemine AA, Low HBC, Cohen ML, et al: Assisted circulation. III. The effect of synchronized arterial counterpulsation on myocardial oxygen consumption and coronary flow. *Am. Heart J.* 64:789−795, 1962.

110. Hirsch LJ, Lluch S, and Katz LN: Counterpulsation effects of coronary blood flow and cardiac oxygen utilization. *Circ. Res.* 19:1031−1040, 1966.

111. Sugg WL, Martin LF, Webb WR, and Ecker RR: Influence of counterpulsation on aortic right and left coronary blood flow following ligation of the left circumflex coronary artery. *J. Thorac. Cardiovasc. Surg.* 59:345−351, 1970.

112. Powell WJ Jr, Daggett WM, Magro AE, et al: Effects of intra-aortic balloon counterpulsation on cardiac performance, oxygen consumption, and coronary blood flow in dogs. *Circ. Res.* 26:753−764, 1970.

113. Feola M, Haiderer O, and Kennedy JH: Intra-aortic balloon pumping (IABP) at different levels of experimental acute left ventricular failure. *Chest* 59:68−76, 1971.

114. Shaw J, Taylor DR, and Pitt B: Effects of intraaortic balloon counterpulsation on regional coronary blood flow in experimental myocardial infarction. *Am. J. Cardiol.* 34:552−556, 1974.

115. Weber KT, and Janicki JS: Coronary collateral flow and intra-aortic balloon counterpulsation. *Trans. Am. Soc. Artif. Int. Organs* 19:395−401, 1973.

116. Watson JT, Willerson JT, Fixler DE, et al: Changes in collateral coronary blood flow (CCBF) distal to a coronary occlusion during intra-aortic balloon pumping (IABP). *Trans. Am. Soc. Artif. Int. Organs* 19:402−407, 1973.

117. Gill CC, Wechsler AS, Newman GE, and Oldham HN Jr: Augmentation and redistribution of myocardial blood flow during acute ischemia by intraaortic balloon pumping. *Ann. Thorac. Surg.* 16:445−453, 1973.

118. Watson JT, Willerson JT, Fixler DE, and Sugg WL: Temporal changes in collateral coronary blood flow in ischemic myocardium during intra-aortic balloon pumping. *Circulation* 50 (Suppl. II): II-249−II-254, 1974.

119. Bleifeld W, Franken G, Meyer J, and Bussmann W-D: The response of mechanical performance, coronary blood flow and myocardial oxygen consumption of the normal and failing dog heart to intraaortic balloon pulsation. *Basic. Res. Cardiol.* 69:379−401, 1974.

120. Saini VK, Hood WB Jr, Hechtman HB, and Berger RL: Nutrient myocardial blood flow in experimental myocardial ischemia: Effects of intraaortic balloon counterpulsation and coronary reperfusion. *Circulation* 52:1086−1090, 1975.

121. Willerson JT, Watson JT, and Platt MR: Effect of hypertonic mannitol and intraaortic counterpulsation on regional myocardial blood flow and ventricular performance in dogs during myocardial ischemia. *Am. J. Cardiol.* 37:514−519, 1976.

122. Watson JT, Fixler DE, Platt MR, et al: The influence of combined intra-aortic balloon counterpulsation and hyperosmotic mannitol on regional myocardial blood flow in ischemic myocardium in the dog. *Circ. Res.* 38:506−513, 1976.

123. Goldfarb D, Conti CR, Brown BG, and Gott VL: Treatment of severe cardiogenic shock by diastolic augmentation after ligation and division of the left circumflex coronary artery in dogs. *J. Thorac. Cardiovasc. Surg.* 51:783−796, 1966.

124. Brown BG, Goldfarb D, Topaz SR, and Gott VL: Diastolic augmentation by intra-aortic balloon: Circulatory hemodynamics and treatment of severe, acute left ventricular failure in dogs. *J. Thorac. Cardiovasc. Surg.* 53:789−804, 1967.

125. Gewirtz H, Ohley W, Williams DO, et al: Effect of intraaortic balloon counterpulsation on regional myocardial blood flow and oxygen consumption in the presence of coronary artery stenosis: Observations in an awake animal model. *Am. J. Cardiol.* 50:829−837, 1982.

126. Raff WK, Kosche F, and Lochner W: Herzfrequenz und extravasale Komponente des Coronarwiderstandes. *Pflügers Arch. Ges. Physiol.* 323:241−249, 1971.

127. Raff WK, Kosche F, and Lochner W: Extravasale Komponente des Coronarwiderstandes und Coronardurchblutung bei steigendem enddiastolischen Druck. *Pflügers Arch. Ges. Physiol.* 327:225−233, 1971.

128. Raff WK, Kosche F, and Lochner W: Die extravasale Komponente des Coronarwiderstandes bei Steigerung der linksventrikulären Druckanstiegsgeschwindigkeit durch Isoproterenol. *Pflügers Arch. Ges. Physiol.* 325:323−333, 1971.

129. Raff WK, Kosche F, and Lochner W: Extravascular coronary resistance and its relation to microcirculation: Influence of heart rate, end-diastolic pressure and maximal rate of rise of intraventricular pressure. *Am. J. Cardiol.* 29:598−603, 1972.

130. Lewis FB, Coffman JD, and Gregg DE: Effect of heart rate and intracoronary isoproterenol, levarterenol, and epinephrine on coronary flow and resistance. *Circ. Res.* 9:89−95, 1961.

131. Pitt B, and Gregg DE: Coronary hemodynamic effects of increasing ventricular rate in the unanesthetized dog. *Circ. Res.* 22:753−761, 1968.

132. Schaper W: Residual perfusion of acutely ischemic heart muscle. In *The Pathophysiology of Myocardial Perfusion* (ed W Schaper). North-Holland Biomedical Press, Amsterdam, 1979, pp 345−378.

133. Russell RE, Chagrasulis RW, and Downey JM: Inhibitory effect of cardiac contraction on coronary collateral blood flow. *Am. J. Physiol.* 233:H541−H546, 1977.

134. Archie JP Jr: Intramyocardial pressure: Effect of preload on transmural distribution of systolic coronary blood flow. *Am. J. Cardiol.* 35:904−911, 1975.

135. Cohen MV, and Yipintsoi T: Myocardial performance and collateral flow after transient coronary occlusion in exercising dogs. *Am. J. Physiol.* 237:H520−H527, 1979.

136. Hill RC, Kleinman LH, Tiller WH Jr, et al: Myocardial blood flow and function during gradual coronary occlusion in awake dog. *Am. J. Physiol.* 244:H60−H67, 1983.

137. Heaton WH, Marr KC, Capurro NL, et al: Beneficial effect of physical training on blood flow to myocardium perfused by chronic collaterals in the exercising dog. *Circulation* 57:575−581, 1978.

138. Hess DS, and Bache RJ: Regional myocardial blood flow during graded treadmill exercise following circumflex coronary artery occlusion in the dog. *Circ. Res.* 47:59−68, 1980.

139. Bache RJ: Effects of exercise on blood flow to collateral-dependent myocardium in the dog. (abstr) *Circulation* 64 (Suppl. IV):IV-117, 1981.

140. Cohen MV, and Yipintsoi T: Restoration of cardiac function and myocardial flow by collateral development in dogs. *Am. J. Physiol.* 240:H811—H819, 1981.

141. Fedor JM, Rembert JC, McIntosh DM,and Greenfield JC Jr: Effects of excercise- and pacing-induced tachycardia on coronary collateral flow in the awake dog. *Circ. Res.* 46:214—220, 1980.

142. Lambert PR, Hess DS, and Bache RJ: Effects of exercise on perfusion of collateral-dependent myocardium in dogs with chronic coronary artery occlusion. *J. Clin. Invest.* 59:1—7, 1977.

143. Ball RM, Bache RJ, Cobb FR, and Greenfield JC Jr: Regional myocardial blood flow during graded treadmill exercise in the dog. *J. Clin. Invest.* 55:43—49, 1975.

144. Schaper W: Influence of physical exercise on coronary collateral blood flow in chronic experimental two-vessel occlusion. *Circulation* 65:905—912, 1982.

145. Capurro NL, Marr KC, Aamodt R, et al: Aspirin-induced increase in collateral flow after acute coronary occlusion in dogs. *Circulation* 59:744—747, 1979.

146. Willerson JT, Powell WJ Jr, Guiney TE, et al: Improvement in myocardial function and coronary blood flow in ischemic myocardium after mannitol. *J. Clin. Invest.* 51:2989—2998, 1972.

147. Willerson JT, Watson JT, Hutton I, et al: The influence of hypertonic mannitol on regional myocardial blood flow during acute and chronic myocardial ischemia in anesthetized and awake intact dogs. *J. Clin. Invest.* 55:892—902, 1975.

148. Hirzel HO, and Kirk ES: The effect of mannitol following permanent coronary occlusion. *Circulation* 56:1006—1015, 1977.

149. Schaper W: Tangential wall stress as a molding force in the development of collateral vessels in the canine heart. *Experientia* 23:595—596, 1967.

150. Schaper W: Der Einfluss physikalischer Faktoren auf das Radialwachstum von Kollateralgefässen im Koronarkreislauf. *Verh. Dtsch. Ges. Kreislaufforsch.* 32: 282—286, 1966.

151. Schaper W: *The Collateral Circulation of the Heart.* North-Holland Publishing Co., Amsterdam, 1971.

152. Scheel KW, Eisenstein BL, and Ingram LA: Coronary, collateral, and perfusion territory responses to aortic banding. *Am. J. Physiol.* 246:H768—H775, 1984.

153. Cuttino JT Jr, Bartrum RJ Jr, Hollenberg NK, and Abrams HL: Collateral vessel formation: Isolation of a transferable factor promoting a vascular response. *Basic Res. Cardiol.* 70:568—573, 1975.

154. Schaper W, DeBrabander M, and Lewi P: DNA synthesis and mitoses in coronary collateral vessels of the dog. *Circ. Res.* 28:671—679, 1971.

155. Ilich N, Hollenberg NK, Williams DH, and Abrams HL: Time course of increased collateral arterial and venous endothelial cell turnover after renal artery stenosis in the rat. *Circ. Res.* 45:579—582, 1979.

156. Zoll PM, and Norman LR: The effects of vasomotor drugs and of anemia upon interarterial coronary anastomoses. *Circulation* 6:832—842, 1952.

157. Eckstein RW: Effect of exercise and coronary artery narrowing on coronary collateral circulation. *Circ. Res.* 5:230—235, 1957.

158. Sewell WH: Physiologic and technical requirements for experimental strong stimulation of coronary collateral arteries. (abstr) *Circulation* 24:1036—1037, 1961.

159. Elliot EC, Jones EL, Bloor CM, et al: Day-to-day changes in coronary hemodynamics secondary to constriction of circumflex branch of left coronary artery in conscious dogs. *Circ. Res.* 22:237—250, 1968.

160. Elliot EC, Bloor CM, Jones EL, et al: Effect of controlled coronary occlusion on collateral circulation in conscious dogs. *Am. J. Physiol.* 220:857—861, 1971.

161. Elliot EC: Hemodynamic evidence of the development of coronary collateral circulation in conscious dogs. In *Current Topics in Coronary Research: Advances in Experimental Medicine and Biology,* Vol. 39 (eds CM Bloor and RA Olsson). Plenum Press, New York, 1973, pp 173—190.

162. Elliot EC, Khouri EM, Snow JA, and Gregg DE: Direct measurement of coronary collateral blood flow in conscious dogs by an electromagnetic flowmeter. *Circ. Res.* 34:374–383, 1974.

163. Gregg DE: The natural history of coronary collateral development. *Circ. Res.* 35:335–344, 1974.

164. Millard RW: Induction of functional coronary collaterals in the swine heart. *Basic Res. Cardiol.* 76:468–473, 1981.

165. Schaper W, Nienaber C, and Gottwik M: The importance of the collateral circulation for myocardial survival. *Acta Med. Scand. Suppl.* 651:29–34, 1981.

166. Schwarz F, Wagner HO, Sesto M, et al: Native collaterals in the development of collateral circulation after chronic coronary stenosis in mongrel dogs. *Circulation* 66:303–308, 1982.

167. Pasyk S, Schaper W, Schaper J, et al: DNA synthesis in coronary collaterals after coronary artery occlusion in conscious dog. *Am. J. Physiol.* 242:H1031–H1037, 1982.

168. Day SB, Gott VL, Lillehei CW, and Wangensteen OH: Development of interarterial intercoronary anastomoses by arteriovenous fistula between pulmonary artery and left atrium. *Proc. Soc. Exp. Biol. Med.* 98:561–563, 1958.

169. Day SB, and Lillehei CW: Experimental basis for a new operation for coronary artery disease: A left atrial-pulmonary artery shunt to encourage the development of interarterial intercoronary anastomoses. *Surgery* 45:487–495, 1959.

170. MacLean LD, Hedenstrom PH, and Rayner RR: Tissue blood flow to the heart: Influence of coronary occlusion and surgical measures. *Circ. Res.* 10:45–50, 1962.

171. Bishop SP, and Bloor CM: Regional myocardial blood flow following coronary occlusion in unanesthetized normal and hypoxemic dogs. (abstr) *Am. J. Cardiol.* 33:127, 1974.

172. Eckstein RW: Development of interarterial coronary anastomoses by chronic anemia. Disappearance following correction of anemia. *Circ. Res.* 3:306–310, 1955.

173. Scheel KW, Brody DA, Ingram LA, and Keller F: Effects of chronic anemia on the coronary and coronary collateral vasculature in dogs. *Circ. Res.* 38:553–559, 1976.

174. Tornling G, Unge G, Skoog L, et al: Proliferative activity of myocardial capillary wall cells in dipyridamole-treated rats. *Cardiovasc. Res.* 12:692–695, 1978.

175. Tornling G, Unge G, Adolfsson J, et al: Proliferative activity of capillary wall cells in skeletal muscle of rats during long-term treatment with dipyridamole. *Arzneimittelforsch.* 30:622–623, 1980.

176. Tornling G, Adolfsson J, Unge G, and Ljungqvist A: Capillary neoformation in skeletal muscle of dipyridamole-treated rats. *Arzneimittelforsch.* 30:791–792, 1980.

177. Vineberg AM, Chari RS, Pifarré R, and Mercier C: The effect of Persantin on intercoronary collateral circulation and survival during gradual experimental coronary occlusion: A preliminary report. *Can. Med. Assoc. J.* 87:336–345, 1962.

178. Laustela E, and Tala P: The effect of dipyridamole on acute left coronary artery occlusion following coronary constriction. *Arzneimittelforsch.* 17:1125–1128, 1967.

179. Asada S, Chiba T, Osawa K, et al: Experimental studies of the effect of long term oral administration of Persantin. *Jpn. Circ. J.* 26:849–855, 1962.

180. Wernitsch W, Richter G, Halmagyi M, and Zeitler E: Die Bedeutung der Entwicklung interkoronarer Kollateralen für das Myokard. *Thoraxchirurgie* 15:637–641, 1967.

181. Halmagyi M, Hempel KJ, Ockenga T, et al: Ergebnisse der oralen Langzeitbehandlung von Schweinen mit 2,6-Bis-(diäthanolamino)-4,8-dipiperidino-pyrimado [5,4-d]pyrimidin vor und nach Coronarocclusion. *Arzneimittelforsch.* 17:272–283, 1967.

182. Fam WM, Ragheb S, and Hoeschen RJ: Augmentation of intercoronary anastomosis by long-term administration of a vasodilator drug, dipyridamole (Persantin). *Can. Med. Assoc. J.* 90:970−973, 1964.

183. Meesmann W, and Bachmann GW: Die Dosisabhängigkeit der Entwicklung von Koronarkollateralen bei Anwendung von Koronardilatantien. *Dtsch. Med. Wochenschr.* 91:1260−1261, 1966.

184. Meesmann W, and Bachmann GW: Pharmakodynamisch induzierte Entwicklung von Koronar-Kollateralen in Abhängigkeit von der Dosis. *Arzneimittelforsch.* 16:501−509, 1966.

185. Schmidt HD, and Schmier J: Erhöhte Toleranz gegen Coronarverschluss durch ein pharmakologisch vermehrtes Gefässnetz. *Arzneimittelforsch.* 16:1058−1064, 1966.

186. Suzuki N: Studies on the prognosis and rehabilitation of the myocardial infarction from the viewpoint of the collateral circulation. *Jpn. Circ. J.* 31:1588−1593, 1967.

187. Rees JR, and Redding VJ: Increase in myocardial collateral capacity following drug-induced coronary vasodilatation: A preliminary report. *Am. Heart J.* 78:224−228, 1969.

188. Schmier J, Kaden F, and Schmidt HD: Augmentation of coronary collaterals and protection against the consequences of coronary ligation following the administration of dipyridamole. *Bruxelles Méd.* 50:617−622, 1970.

189. Lumb G, Singletary HP, and Hardy LB: Collateral circulation following experimental gradual narrowing of the coronary arteries. *Angiology* 13:463−465, 1962.

190. Meester WD, and Van Harn GL: The effect of pentaerythritol tetranitrate pretreatment on experimental coronary occlusion. *Am. Heart. J.* 88:330−337, 1974.

191. Hedges RN Jr, Schmidtke W, and Leslie RE: A possible application of vasodilators in acute coronary occlusion. *Angiology* 12:249−253, 1961.

192. Schaper WKA, Xhonneux R, and Jageneau AHM: Stimulation of the coronary collateral circulation by lidoflazine (R 7904). *Naunyn-Schmiedebergs Arch. Exp. Path.* 252:1−8, 1965.

193. Verheyen A, Xhonneux R, Borgers M, and Reneman RS: Cell proliferation in developing coronary collaterals and the influence of lidoflazine on this process. *J. Mol. Cell. Cardiol.* 8:53−60, 1976.

194. Van Ackern K, Braasch W, Brückner UB, et al: Koronare Kollateralentwicklung nach oraler Langzeitbehandlung mit Nifedipine-erhöhte Überlebensquote nach experimentellem Koronarverschluss. *Arzneimittelforsch.* 24:1577−1581, 1974.

195. Schmier J, van Ackern K, and Brückner U: Investigations on tachyphylaxis and collateral formation after nifedipine whilst taking into consideration the direction of flow and the mortality-rate due to infarction. In *1st International Nifedipine "Adalat" Symposium: New Therapy of Ischemic Heart Disease* (eds K Hashimoto, E Kimura, and T Kobayashi). University of Tokyo Press, Tokyo, 1975, pp 45−52.

196. Schmier J, van Ackern K, Brückner UB, et al: Investigations on the development of collaterals, coronary flow, tachyphylaxis and steal phenomenon in dogs after application of Adalat. In *2nd International Adalat Symposium: New Therapy of Ischemic Heart Disease* (eds W Lochner, W Braasch, and G Kroneberg). Springer-Verlag, Berlin, 1975, pp 92−100.

197. Schmier J, Brückner UB, Mittmann U, and Wirth RH: Intercoronary collaterals and intramyocardial blood distribution in dogs following nifedipine administration compared with controls. In *3rd International Adalat Symposium: New Therapy of Ischemic Heart Disease* (eds AD Jatene and PR Lichtlen). Excerpta Medica, Amsterdam, 1976, pp 42−49.

198. Kanazawa T: The effect of nitrophenyl-dimethyl-dihydropyridine-derivative [BAY a 1040] on intercoronary collateral circulation. In *1st International Nifedipine "Adalat" Symposium: New Therapy of Ischemic Heart Disease* (eds K Hashimoto,

E Kimura, and T Kobayashi). University of Tokyo Press, Tokyo, 1975, pp 53−62.

199. Starey F: Zur Frage der Kollateralenbildung am Koronargefässsystem des Hundes: Der experimentelle Nachweis der Kollateralenbildung am Hundeherzen durch Prenylaminlaktat. *Arzneimittelforsch.* 22:1317−1320, 1972.

200. Mokotoff R, and Katz LN: The effect of theophyllin with ethylenediamine (aminophylline) and of papaverine hydrochloride on experimental myocardial infarction in the dog. *Am. Heart J.* 30:215−230, 1945.

201. Eckstein RW: The ineffectiveness of cortisone on functional coronary interarterial anastomoses. *Circ. Res.* 2:466−470, 1954.

202. Schaper J, Borgers M, Xhonneux R, and Schaper W: Cortisone influences developing collaterals. 1. A morphologic study. *Virch. Arch. (Path. Anat.)* 361:263−282, 1973.

203. Borgers M, Schaper J, Xhonneux R, and Schaper W: Hydrocortisone influences developing collaterals. 2. A cytochemical study. *Virch. Arch. (Path. Anat.)* 361:283−297, 1973.

204. Sanders M, White FC, Peterson TM, and Bloor CM: Effects of endurance exercise on coronary collateral blood flow in miniature swine. *Am. J. Physiol.* 234:H614−H619, 1978.

205. Sanders M, White F, Peterson T, et al: Coronary collateral development with exercise and coronary occlusion in pigs. (abstr) *Med. Sci. Sports* 11:87, 1979.

206. Burt JJ, and Jackson R: The effects of physical exercise on the coronary collateral circulation of dogs. *J. Sports Med. Phys. Fitness* 4:203−206, 1965.

207. Amann L, Meesmann W, Schulz FW, et al: Untersuchungen Über die Kollateralenentwicklung am gesunden Herzen nach körperlichem Training. *Verh. Dtsch. Ges. Kreislaufforsch.* 37:151−154, 1971.

208. Amann L, Meesmann W, Schley G, et al: Der Einfluss gesteigerten Laufbandtrainings auf die Entwicklung von Koronarkollateralen und die Mortalität nach akuter Koronarligatur bei Hunden. (abstr) *Pflügers Arch. Ges. Physiol.* 332:R80, 1972.

209. Cohen MV, Yipintsoi T, Malhotra A, et al: Effect of exercise on collateral development in dogs with normal coronary arteries. *J. Appl. Physiol.* 45:797−805, 1978.

210. Scheel KW, Ingram LA, and Wilson JL: Effects of exercise on the coronary and collateral vasculature of beagles with and without coronary occlusion. *Circ. Res.* 48:523−530, 1981.

211. Cohen MV, Steingart R, and Rao PS: Lack of effect of prior exercise training on infarct size and exercise-induced ischemia after coronary occlusion. (abstr) *Circulation* 70 (Suppl. II):II-178, 1984.

212. Koerner JE, and Terjung RL: Effect of physical training on coronary collateral circulation of the rat. *J. Appl. Physiol.* 52:376−387, 1982.

213. Barnard RJ, Duncan HW, Livesay JJ, and Buckberg GD: Coronary vasodilator reserve and flow distribution during near-maximal exercise in dogs. *J. Appl. Physiol.* 43:988−992, 1977.

214. Sanders M, White FC, and Bloor CM: Myocardial blood flow distribution in miniature pigs during exercise. *Basic Res. Cardiol.* 72:326−331, 1977.

215. Sanders M, White FC, Peterson TM, and Bloor CM: Characteristics of coronary flow and transmural distribution in miniature pigs. *Am. J. Physiol.* 235:H601−H609, 1978.

216. Knight DR, and Stone HL: Alteration of ischemic cardiac function in normal heart by daily exercise. *J. Appl. Physiol.* 55:52−60, 1983.

217. Kaplinsky E, Hood WB Jr, McCarthy B, et al: Effects of physical training in dogs with coronary artery ligation. *Circulation* 37:556−565, 1968.

218. Schaper W, Flameng W, Snoeckx L, and Jageneau A: Der Einfluss körperlichen Trainings auf den Kollateralkreislauf des Herzens. *Verh. Dtsch. Ges. Kreislaufforsch.* 37:112−121, 1971.

219. Schaper W: Influence of physical exercise on myocardial perfusion. In *The Pathophysiology of Myocardial Perfusion* (ed W Schaper). North-Holland Biomedical Press, Amsterdam, 1979, pp 519−533.

220. Neill WA, and Oxendine JM: Exercise can promote coronary collateral development without improving perfusion of ischemic myocardium. *Circulation* 60: 1513−1519, 1979.

221. Gould KL, Lipscomb K, and Hamilton GW: Physiologic basis for assessing critical coronary stenosis: Instantaneous flow response and regional distribution during coronary hyperemia as measures of coronary flow reserve. *Am. J. Cardiol.* 33:87−94, 1974.

222. Cohen MV, Yipintsoi T, and Scheuer J: Coronary collateral stimulation by exercise in dogs with stenotic coronary arteries. *J. Appl. Physiol.* 52:664−671, 1982.

223. Reneman RS, Jageneau AHM, Schaper WKA, et al: Influence of counterpulsation on collateral circulation after acute occlusion of the left anterior descending coronary artery in dogs. *Cardiovasc. Res.* 6:45−53, 1972.

224. Jacobey JA, Taylor WJ, Smith GT, et al: A new therapeutic approach to acute coronary occlusion. II. Opening dormant coronary collateral channels by counterpulsation. *Am. J. Cardiol.* 11:218−227, 1963.

225. Rosensweig J, Borromeo C, Chatterjee S, et al: Treatment of coronary insufficiency by counterpulsation: An experimental study. *Ann. Thorac. Surg.* 2:706−713, 1966.

226. Rosensweig J, and Chatterjee S: Mechanical augmentation of coronary circulation in the ischemic heart: Angiographic and hemodynamic correlation with prolonged survival. *J. Thorac. Cardiovasc. Surg.* 6:839−847, 1967.

227. Goldfarb D, Friesinger GC, Conti CR, et al: Preservation of myocardial viability by diastolic augmentation after ligation of the coronary artery in dogs. *Surgery* 63:320−327, 1968.

228. Schildt P, Stanton E, and Beck CS: Communications between the coronary arteries produced by the application of inflammatory agents to the surface of the heart. *Ann. Surg.* 118:34−45, 1943.

229. Thompson SA, and Raisbeck MJ: Cardio-pericardiopexy; The surgical treatment of coronary arterial disease by the establishment of adhesive pericarditis. *Ann. Intern Med.* 16:495−520, 1942.

230. Leighninger DS: A laboratory and clinical evaluation of operations for coronary artery disease. *J. Thorac. Surg.* 30:397−410, 1955.

231. Heinbecker P, and Barton WA: Operation for development of collateral circulation to the heart. *J. Thorac. Surg.* 9:431−438, 1940.

232. Beck CS, Tichy VL, and Moritz AR: Production of a collateral circulation to the heart. *Proc. Soc. Exp. Biol. Med.* 32:759−761, 1935.

233. Beck CS, and Tichy VL: The production of a collateral circulation to the heart. I. An experimental study. *Am. Heart J.* 10:849−873, 1935.

234. Pifarré R, and Hufnagel CA: Epicardiectomy and omental graft in acute myocardial infarction. *Am. J. Surg.* 115:589−593, 1968.

235. Stanton EJ, Schildt P, and Beck CS: The effect of abrasion of the surface of the heart upon intercoronary communications. *Am. Heart J.* 22:529−538, 1941.

236. Berne RM, Jones RD, and Cross FS: Evaluation of procedures designed to enhance coronary collateral blood flow. *Circ. Res.* 10:142−147, 1962.

237. Beck CS, and Leighninger DS: Operations for coronary artery disease. *JAMA* 156:1226−1233, 1954.

238. Beck CS, and Leighninger DS: Operations for coronary artery disease. *Ann. Surg.* 141:24−37, 1955.

239. Beck CS, and Brofman BL: The surgical management of coronary artery disease: Background, rationale, clinical experiences. *Ann. Intern. Med.* 45:975−988, 1956.

240. Beck CS: Symposium on coronary artery disease: Blood supply to ischaemic

myocardium distal to the occlusion of a coronary artery. *Dis. Chest* 31:243–252, 1957.

241. Leighninger DS, Einsel IH, Rueger RG, and Beck CS: Intercoronary arterial channels produced by chemical agents. *Am. J. Cardiol.* 6:949–951, 1960.

242. King RD, Steiner SH, and Heimburger IL: Effect of epicardiectomy on myocardial blood flow. *J. Thorac. Cardiovasc. Surg.* 51:660–666, 1966.

243. Vineberg A, and Mahanti BC: Evaluation of experimental myocardial revascularization operations by ameroid coronary artery constriction. *Surgery* 47:748–764, 1960.

244. Vineberg AM, Kato Y, and Pirozynski WJ: Experimental revascularization of the entire heart: Evaluation of epicardiectomy, omental graft, and/or implantation of the internal mammary artery in preventing myocardial necrosis and death of the animal. *Am. Heart J.* 72:79–93, 1966.

245. Pratt FH: The nutrition of the heart through the vessels of Thebesius and the coronary veins. *Am. J. Physiol.* 1:86–103, 1898.

246. Roberts JT, Browne RS, and Roberts G: Nourishment of the myocardium by way of the coronary veins. (abstr) *Fed. Proc.* 2:90, 1943.

247. Thornton JJ, and Gregg DE: Effect of chronic cardiac venous occlusion on coronary arterial and cardiac venous hemodynamics. *Am. J. Physiol.* 128:179–184, 1939.

248. Beck CS, and Mako AE: Venous stasis in the coronary circulation: An experimental study. *Am. Heart J.* 21:767–779, 1941.

249. Smith G, Demming J, Eleff M, and Eckstein RW: Further studies on the effect of arteriovenous fistulas and elevations of sinus pressure on mortality rates following acute coronary occlusions. *Circulation* 6:262–266, 1952.

250. Gross L, Blum L, and Silverman G: Experimental attempts to increase the blood supply to the dog's heart by means of coronary sinus occlusion. *J. Exp. Med.* 65:91–108, 1937.

251. Gregg DE, and Dewald D: The immediate effects of the occlusion of the coronary veins on collateral blood flow in the coronary arteries. *Am. J. Physiol.* 124:435–443, 1938.

252. Beck CS: Revascularization of the heart. *Ann. Surg.* 128:854–861, 1948.

253. Eckstein RW, Smith G, Eleff M, and Demming J: The effect of arterialization of the coronary sinus in dogs on mortality following acute coronary occlusion. *Circulation* 6:16–20, 1952.

254. Beck CS, Hahn RS, Leighninger DS, and McAllister FF: Operation for coronary artery disease. *JAMA* 147:1726–1731, 1951.

255. Hahn RS, and Beck CS: Revascularization of the heart: A study of mortality and infarcts following multiple coronary artery ligation. *Circulation* 5:801–809, 1952.

256. Bailey CP, Geckeler GD, Truex RC, et al: Arterialization of the coronary sinus. *JAMA* 151:441–449, 1953.

257. Eckstein RW, Hornberger JC, and Sano T: Acute effects of elevation of coronary sinus pressure. *Circulation* 7:422–436, 1953.

258. Hahn RS, Kim M, and Beck CS: Revascularization of the heart. Observations on the circulation following arterialization of the coronary sinus. *Am. Heart J.* 44:772–780, 1953.

259. Bailey CP, Truex RC, Angulo AW, et al: The anatomic (histologic) basis and efficient clinical surgical technique for the restoration of the coronary circulation. *J. Thorac. Surg.* 25:143–168, 1953.

260. Bakst AA, Costas-Durieux J, Goldberg H, and Bailey CP: Protection of the heart by arterialization of the coronary sinus. II. Coronary flow in dogs with aortico-coronary sinus anastomosis. *J. Thorac. Surg.* 27:442–454, 1954.

261. Eckstein RW, and Leighninger DS: Chronic effects of aorta-coronary sinus anastomosis of Beck in dogs. *Circ. Res.* 2:60–72, 1954.

262. Leighninger DS, and Eckstein RW: Further observations on aorta to coronary sinus anastomosis of Beck in dogs. *Proc. Soc. Exp. Biol. Med.* 87:564−567, 1954.

263. Bakst AA, Boley SJ, Morse W, and Loewe L: Experimental surgical treatment of occlusive coronary artery disease. I. Use of pedicled pectoral muscle grafts. *Angiology* 8:308−315, 1957.

264. Key JA, Kergin FG, Martineau Y, and Leckey RG: A method of supplementing the coronary circulation by a jejunal pedicle graft. *J. Thorac. Surg.* 28:320−329, 1954.

265. Baronofsky ID, Hannon DW, and Turback CE: Cardiojejunopexy for coronary artery disease: An experimental study. *Surgery* 39:3−6, 1956.

266. Carter BN: Discussion of revascularization of the heart. *Ann. Surg.* 128:861−862, 1948.

267. Carter BN, Gall EA, and Wadsworth CL: An experimental study of collateral coronary circulation produced by cardiopneumonopexy. *Surgery* 25:489−509, 1949.

268. Bloomer WE, Stern H, and Liebow AA: Application of induced pulmonary arterial collateral circulation as collateral supply to the heart. *Proc. Soc. Exp. Biol. Med.* 86:202−203, 1954.

269. Smith FR: Coronary artery collateral circulation developed by heart-lung graft. *Anat. Rec.* 113:95−100, 1954.

270. Harken DE, Black H, Dickson JF III, and Wilson HE III: De-epicardialization: A simple, effective surgical treatment for angina pectoris. *Circulation* 12:955−962, 1955.

271. Kline JL, Stern H, Bloomer WE, and Liebow AA: The application of an induced bronchial collateral circulation to the coronary arteries by cardiopneumonopexy. I. Anatomical observations. *Am. J. Pathol.* 32:663−693, 1956.

272. Vidone RA, Kline JL, Pitel M, and Liebow AA: The application of an induced bronchical collateral circulation to the coronary arteries by cardiopneumon-opexy. II. Hemodynamics and the measurement of collateral flow to the myocar-dium. *Am. J. Pathol.* 32:897−925, 1956.

273. Sabiston DC Jr, and Blalock A: Physiologic and anatomic determinants of coro-nary blood flow and their relationship to myocardial revascularization. *Surgery* 44:406−423, 1958.

274. Bowles LT, Tepper R, Coryllos E, et al: An experimental evaluation of operations for revascularization of the heart. *J. Thorac. Cardiovasc. Surg.* 40:375−382, 1960.

275. Mobin-Uddin K, Viamonte M Jr, Martinez LO, et al: Experimental prevention of myocardial infarction by bronchial collateral circulation. *JAMA* 208:301−306, 1969.

276. O'Shaughnessy L: An experimental method of providing a collateral circulation to the heart. *Br. J. Surg.* 23:665−670, 1936.

277. Mautz FR, and Beck CS: The augmentation of collateral coronary circulation by operation. *J. Thorac. Surg.* 7:113−129, 1937.

278. Knock FE: Cardioomentopexy and implantation of multiple omental loops for revascularization of the heart. *Surg. Forum* 9:230−232, 1958.

279. Tanabe S: An experimental study of the development of vascular branches from the splenic pedicle attached to the myocardial lesion. *Nippon Kyobu Geka Gakkai Zasshi* 25:960−970, 1977.

280. Neumann CG, Moran RE, von Wedel J, et al: Reduction of coronary artery blood flow preparatory to revascularization of the heart via pedicled flap of skin. *Plast. Reconstr. Surg.* 13:85−94, 1954.

281. Von Wedel J, Lord JW Jr, Neumann CG, and Hinton JW: Revascularization of the heart by pedicled skin flap: An experimental study investigating the functions of extracoronary anastomoses. *Surgery* 37:32−53, 1955.

282. Burchell HB: Adjustments in coronary circulation after experimental coronary occlusion: With particular reference to vascularization of pericardial adhesions. *Arch. Intern. Med.* 65:240−262, 1940.

283. Vineberg A, Pifarré R, and Mercier C: An operation designed to promote the growth of new coronary arteries, using a detached omental graft: A preliminary report. *Can. Med. Assoc. J.* 86:1116–1118, 1962.

284. Vineberg A: Experimental background of myocardial revascularization by internal mammary artery implantation and supplementary technics, with its clinical application in 125 patients: A review and critical appraisal. *Ann. Surg.* 159:185–207, 1964.

285. Vineberg A, and Syed AK: Arterial vascular pathways from subclavian arteries to coronary arterioles created by free omental myocardial implants: A preliminary report. *Can. Med. Assoc. J.* 97:399–401, 1967.

286. Vineberg A: Revascularization of the right and left coronary arterial systems: Internal mammary artery implantation, epicardiectomy and free omental graft operation. *Am. J. Cardiol.* 19:344–353, 1967.

287. Criollos RL, AlShamma AM, and Roe BB: Direct measurement of extracoronary blood flow after revascularization procedures. *Ann. Thorac. Surg.* 4:151–158, 1967.

288. Vineberg A, and Deliyannis TD: The sponge operation for myocardial revascularization: An experimental study. *Can. Med. Assoc. J.* 78:610–612, 1958.

289. Glover RP, Davila JC, Kyle RH, et al: Ligation of the internal mammary arteries as a means of increasing blood supply to the myocardium. *J. Thorac. Surg.* 34:661–678, 1957.

290. Glover RP, Kitchell JR, Kyle RH, et al: Experiences with myocardial revascularization by division of the internal mammary arteries. *Dis.Chest* 33:637–657, 1958.

291. Taber RE, and Marchioro T: Observations on the hemodynamic effects of experimental internal mammary artery ligation. *Arch. Surg.* 76:781–785, 1958.

292. Botham RJ, Rowe GG, and Gale JW: Experimental evaluation of systemic and coronary arterial pressure response associated with ligation of the internal mammary and subclavian arteries. *Am. Heart J.* 58:719–725, 1959.

293. Blair CR, Roth RF, and Zintel HA: Evaluation of internal mammary artery ligation for relief of angina pectoris. *Surg. Forum* 8:345–348, 1957.

294. Blair CR, Roth RF, and Zintel HA: Measurement of coronary artery blood-flow following experimental ligation of the internal mammary artery. *Ann. Surg.* 152:325–329, 1960.

295. Griffin JC Jr, Hardy JD, and Turner MD: Does internal mammary ligation increase arterial flow to the myocardium? *Surg. Forum* 8:325–327, 1957.

296. Zagnoni C, and Ziliotto P: Considerazioni e raffronti sopra l'intervento di legatura delle arterie mammarie interne (Operazione di Davide Fieschi) (studio critico sperimentale). *Acta Chir. Ital.* 14:511–538, 1958.

297. Hurley RE, and Eckstein RW: Effect of bilateral internal mammary artery ligation on coronary circulation in dogs. *Circ. Res.* 7:571–573, 1959.

298. Vansant JH, and Muller WH Jr: Experimental evaluation of internal mammary artery ligation as a method of myocardial revascularization. *Surgery* 45:840–847, 1959.

299. Sabiston DC Jr, and Blalock A: Experimental ligation of the internal mammary artery and its effect on coronary occlusion. *Surgery* 43:906–912, 1958.

300. Glover RP, Kitchell JR, Davila JC, and Barkley HT Jr: Clinical and experimental study of bilateral internal mammary artery ligation (Bimal) for the relief of angina pectoris. (abstr) *Circulation* 20:701–702, 1959.

301. Sewell WH, and Davalos PA: Factors influencing collateral arterial formation from pedicles on the surface of the hearts of dogs. *Angiology* 13:231–240, 1962.

302. Vineberg AM: Development of an anastomosis between the coronary vessels and a transplanted internal mammary artery. *Can. Med. Assoc. J.* 55:117–119, 1946.

303. Vineberg AM, and Jewett BL: Development of an anastomosis between the coronary vessels and a transplanted internal mammary artery. *Can. Med. Assoc. J.* 56:609–614, 1947.

304. Vineberg AM: Development of anastomosis between the coronary vessels and a transplanted internal mammary artery. *J. Thorac. Surg.* 18:839−848, 1949.

305. Vineberg AM, and Niloff PH: The value of surgical treatment of coronary artery occlusion by implantation of the internal mammary artery into the ventricular myocardium: An experimental study. *Surg. Gynecol. Obstet.* 91:551−561, 1950.

306. Vineberg A, and Miller D: Functional evaluation of an internal mammary coronary artery anastomosis. *Am. Heart J.* 45:873−888, 1953.

307. Vineberg A, Munro DD, Cohen H, and Buller W: Four years' clinical experience with internal mammary artery implantation in the treatment of human coronary artery insufficiency including additional experimental studies. *J. Thorac. Surg.* 29:1−32, 1955.

308. Bellman S, and Frank HA: Vascular channels established by implantation of a systemic artery into the myocardium. *Ann. Surg.* 147:425−442, 1958.

309. Bigelow WG, Basian H, and Trusler GA: Internal mammary artery implantation for coronary heart disease: A clinical follow-up study one to eight years after operation. *J. Thorac. Cardiovasc. Surg.* 45:67−78, 1963.

310. Sewell WH: Physiological background, coronary arteriography, and the pedicle operation for coronary arterial insufficiency. *J. Natl. Med. Assoc.* 55:299−305, 1963.

311. Sewell WH: Application to coronary arteries of the basic principles governing the development of collateral arterial channels. *Circulation* 27:705−707, 1963.

312. Sewell WH: A basic physiological approach to myocardial revascularization. *Conn. Med.* 27:76−78, 1963.

313. Sewell WH: Coronary cinearteriography and pedicle operation in diagnosis and treatment of coronary insufficiency. *Surgery* 55:99−104, 1964.

314. Fuquay MC, Carey LS, Dahl EV, and Grindlay JH: Myocardial revascularization: A comparison of internal mammary and subclavian artery implantation in the laboratory. *Surgery* 43:226−235, 1958.

315. Yokoyama M, and Sakakibara S: Blood flow measurements in internal mammary artery implanted into the myocardium. *Ann. Thorac. Surg.* 13:155−162, 1972.

316. Abel RM, Reis RL, Yarbrough JW, et al: Determinants of flow through internal mammary artery implants. *Ann. Surg.* 175:607−613, 1972.

317. Barner HB, Kaiser GC, Mudd JG, et al: Internal mammary artery implantation: Effects upon coronary flow and ventricular function. *J. Thorac. Cardiovasc. Surg.* 56:43−50, 1968.

318. Provan JL, Hammond GL, and Austen WG: Flowmeter studies of internal mammary artery function after implantation into the left ventricular myocardium. *J. Thorac. Cardiovasc. Surg.* 52:820−828, 1966.

319. Malette WG, Schneider B, and Tait IB: "Demand" and internal mammary artery implantation. *Circulation* 35 (Suppl. I):I-152−I-154, 1967.

320. Kakvan M, Carriere S, Levy R, and Gagnon E: Evaluation of collateral myocardial blood flow following long term implantation of the internal mammary artery in the dog. *RI Med. J.* 54:458−461, 480, 1971.

321. Tschopp HM, Rakušan K, Gudbjarnason S, and Bing RJ: Physiologic studies on revascularization of the dog heart. *J. Thorac. Cardiovasc. Surg.* 55:466−478, 1968.

322. Mittmann U, Allenberg JR, Heger W, and Schmier J: Entwicklung und Kapazität von anschlusskollateralen bei regionaler Mangeldurchblutung des Myokards. *Thoraxchirurgie* 22:317−320, 1974.

323. Smith PE, Mobin-Uddin K, Lombardo C, and Jude J: Metabolic studies of blood infused into the myocardium. *J. Thorac. Cardiovasc. Surg.* 53:566−571, 1967.

324. Reis RL, Enright LP, Staroscik RN, and Hannah H III: The effects of internal mammary artery implantation on cardiac function and survival following acute coronary artery occlusion. *Ann. Surg.* 171:9−16, 1970.

325. Kemp HG, Zaroff LI, Heinle RA, et al: Myocardial revascularization: Free arterial grafts in nonischemic dogs. (abstr) *Circulation* 36 (Suppl. II): II-159, 1967.

326. Baird RJ, Cohoon WJ, Spratt EH, and Williams WG: Myocardial revascularization with femoral artery and vein autografts. *Can. J. Surg.* 10:474−482, 1967.
327. Sabiston DC Jr, Fauteux JP, and Blalock A: An experimental study of the fate of arterial implants in the left ventricular myocardium: With a comparison of similar implants in other organs. *Ann. Surg.* 145:927−938, 1957.
328. Bloomer WE, Vidone RA, and Liebow AA: Implantation of the splenic artery into the myocardium as a source of collateral circulation. *Yale J. Biol. Med.* 36:295−305, 1964.
329. Goldman A, Greenstone SM, Preuss FS, et al: Experimental methods for producing a collateral circulation to the heart directly from the left ventricle. *J. Thorac. Surg.* 31:364−374, 1956.
330. Massimo C, and Boffi L: Myocardial revascularization by a new method of carrying blood directly from the left ventricular cavity into the coronary circulation. *J. Thorac. Surg.* 34:257−264, 1957.
331. Sen PK, Udwadia TE, Kinare SG, and Parulkar GB: Transmyocardial acupuncture: A new approach to myocardial revascularization. *J. Thorac. Cardiovasc. Surg.* 50:181−189, 1965.
332. Müller KD, Klein H, and Schaper W: Changes in myocardial oxygen consumption 45 minutes after experimental coronary occlusion do not alter infarct size. *Cardiovasc. Res.* 14:710−718, 1980.
333. Fujiwara H, Ashraf M, Sato S, and Millard RW: Transmural cellular damage and blood flow distribution in early ischemia in pig hearts. *Circ. Res.* 51:683−693, 1982.

The Biological Role of Coronary Collaterals

Both animal studies and clinical evaluations in man have demonstrated that coronary collaterals are present in all normal hearts and, when stimulated by myocardial ischemia and/or hypoxia, undergo a striking histologic transformation that converts thin-walled conduits into muscular arterioles. Although the precise biophysical and/or biochemical mediators of this transformation are unknown, ischemic myocardium does produce an extractable substance which initiates neovascularization in suitable biological assay systems. Whereas nontransformed collaterals are essentially devoid of smooth muscle and therefore are unable to respond to metabolic or pharmacologic stimuli, well-formed collaterals can autoregulate and dilate following administration of nitrates and other selected vasodilators. The reactivity of transformed collaterals is closer to that of epicardial conductance vessels than intramyocardial resistance arterioles. Coronary collateral vessels cannot completely normalize coronary reserve in myocardial regions deprived of their natural antegrade coronary artery flow but they do have the capacity to restore normal resting flow and even normal flow during physiologic stresses such as exercise. Although coronary collaterals may develop or become evident only when coronary arterial stenoses become critically narrowed, anastomotic channels clearly are not merely markers of the severity of the underlying disease. Collaterals have numerous salutary functional effects, including limitation of infarct size, preservation of regional myocardial and global left ventricular function, enhancement of cardiac performance during exercise and other stresses, and improvement of survival. Because of these acknowledged beneficial effects, attempts have been undertaken to stimulate collateral growth before and after outward manifestations of ischemic heart disease become apparent. No satisfactory stimulus has yet been identified but exercise and chronic administration of some vasodilator agents hold promise. Future efforts should be directed at discovery of suitable methods which can be used to manipulate the coronary collateral circulation successfully. Successful stimulation of collateral development would help to preserve cardiac integrity and attenuate the deleterious sequelae of coronary obstructive disease.